CLINICAL CORRELATION
with Diagnostic Implications in
DERMATOLOGY

CLINICAL CORRELATION with Diagnostic Implications in DERMATOLOGY

Editor-in-Chief

Biju Vasudevan MD (DVL) FRGUHS
Associate Professor
Department of Dermatology
Base Hospital
Barrackpore, West Bengal, India

Assistant Editors

Shekhar Neema MD (DVL)
Assistant Professor
Department of Dermatology
Command Hospital
Kolkata, West Bengal, India

Ankan Gupta MD (DVL)
Assistant Professor
Department of Dermatology
Christian Medical College and Hospital
Vellore, Tamil Nadu, India

Editorial Advisory Committee

Rajesh Verma MD (DVL)
Consultant
Department of Dermatology
Skin Centre, Base Hospital
Lucknow, Uttar Pradesh, India

Manas Chatterjee MD (DVL)
Senior Advisor, Professor and Head
Department of Dermatology
INHS Asvini
Mumbai, Maharashtra, India

Foreword

Rajan S Grewal

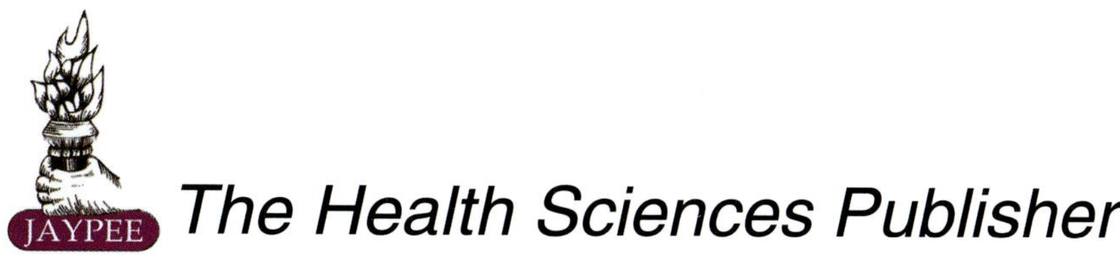

New Delhi | London | Panama

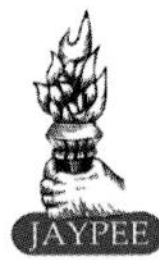

Jaypee Brothers Medical Publishers (P) Ltd

Headquarters

Jaypee Brothers Medical Publishers (P) Ltd
4838/24, Ansari Road, Daryaganj
New Delhi 110 002, India
Phone: +91-11-43574357
Fax: +91-11-43574314
Email: jaypee@jaypeebrothers.com

Overseas Offices

J.P. Medical Ltd
83 Victoria Street, London
SW1H 0HW (UK)
Phone: +44 20 3170 8910
Fax: +44 (0)20 3008 6180
Email: info@jpmedpub.com

Jaypee Brothers Medical Publishers (P) Ltd
17/1-B Babar Road, Block-B, Shaymali
Mohammadpur, Dhaka-1207
Bangladesh
Mobile: +08801912003485
Email: jaypeedhaka@gmail.com

Jaypee-Highlights Medical Publishers Inc
City of Knowledge, Bld. 235, 2nd Floor, Clayton
Panama City, Panama
Phone: +1 507-301-0496
Fax: +1 507-301-0499
Email: cservice@jphmedical.com

Jaypee Brothers Medical Publishers (P) Ltd
Bhotahity, Kathmandu
Nepal
Phone: +977-9741283608
Email: kathmandu@jaypeebrothers.com

Website: www.jaypeebrothers.com
Website: www.jaypeedigital.com

Inquiries for bulk sales may be solicited at: jaypee@jaypeebrothers.com

Clinical Correlation with Diagnostic Implications in Dermatology

First Edition: **2017**

ISBN: 978-93-86322-66-1

Printed at Sanat Printers

Dedicated to

My family, teachers and patients

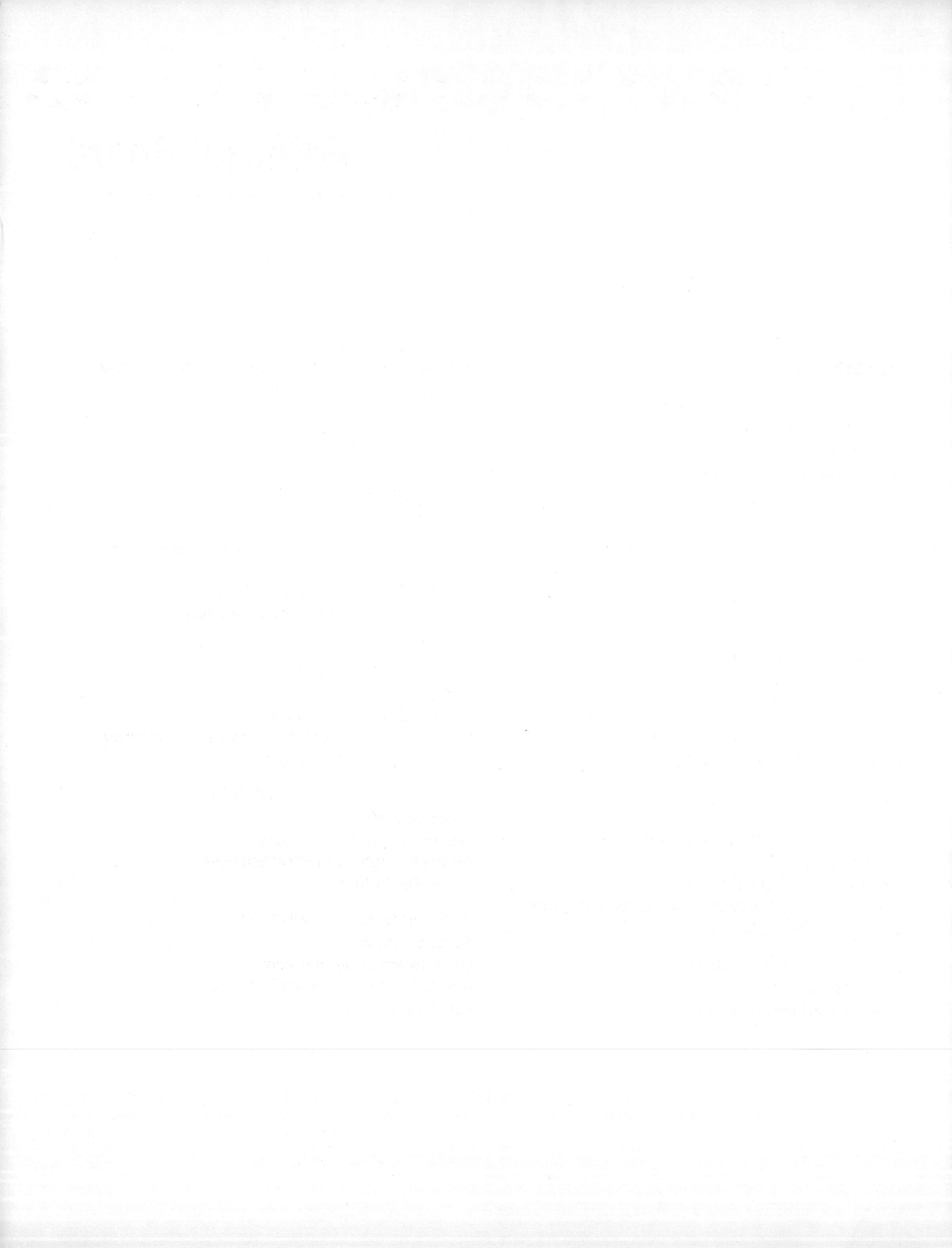

Editorial Board

Contributors

Aarti Sarda MD (DVL)
Senior Resident
KPC Medical College
Kolkata, West Bengal, India

Abhishek De MD (DVL)
Associate Professor
Calcutta National Medical College
Kolkata, West Bengal, India

Aditi Bhagat MD (DVL)
Consultant
Currae Hospital
Thane, Maharashtra, India

Ajay Chopra MD (DVL)
Head
Department of Dermatology
Base Hospital, Delhi Cantt
Delhi, India

Akhilesh Shukla MD (DVL)
Consultant Dermatologist
Skin and Hair Clinic
New Delhi, India

Akshi Bansal MD (DVL)
Resident
Department of Dermatology
Bangalore Medical College
and Research Institute
Bengaluru, Karnataka, India

Amina Asfiya MD (DVL)
Senior Resident
Department of Dermatology
Yenepoya Medical College
Mangaluru, Karnataka, India

Amit Bahuguna MD (DVL)
Cl Spl (Dermatology and Venereology)
155 Base Hospital
Tezpur, Assam, India

Anagha S MD (DVL)
Fellow (Dermatosurgery)
Department of Dermatosurgery
Bangalore Medical College and Research Institute
Bengaluru, Karnataka, India

Ananta Khurana MD (DVL) DNB MNAMAS
Assistant Professor
RML Hospital and PGIMER
New Delhi, India

Anju George MD (DVL) DNB FRGUHS
Consultant Dermatologist
RMV Hospital
Bengaluru, Karnataka, India

Ankan Gupta MD (DVL)
Assistant Professor
Christian Medical College and Hospital
Vellore, Tamil Nadu, India

Ankur Talwar MD (DVL)
Assistant Professor
Department of Dermatology
Hind Institute of Medical Sciences
Consultant Dermatologist
Talwar Skin Institute
Lucknow, Uttar Pradesh, India

Anupam Das MD (DVL)
Senior Resident
Department of Dermatology
KPC Medical College and Hospital
Kolkata, West Bengal, India

Anuradha Babu DNB
Consultant Dermatologist
Aster Medcity Hospital
Kochi, Kerala, India

Archana S MD (DVL)
Associate Consultant Dermatologist
Bengaluru, Karnataka, India

Asad Ansari DDVL
Senior Resident
Calcutta National Medical College
Kolkata, West Bengal, India

Aseem Sharma MD (DVL) MBA
Senior Registrar
Lokmanya Tilak Municipal Medical College and Hospital
Mumbai, Maharashtra, India

Ashwani Kumar MD (Internal Medicine)
Base Hospital, Delhi Cantt
Delhi, India

Bhumika S MD FRUGHS
Consultant Dermatologist
Cuti-Sculpt Clinic
Bengaluru, Karnataka, India

Bhushan Madke MD (DVL)
Associate Professor
Jawaharlal Nehru Medical College
Wardha, Maharashtra, India

Biju Vasudevan MD (DVL) FRGUHS
Associate Professor
Base Hospital
Barrackpore, West Bengal, India

Boby Krishna DNB MNAMS DermSurg Fellow
Consultant Dermatologist and Cosmetologist
NIMS Medicity
Thiruvananthapuram, Kerala, India

Brijesh C MD (DVL)
Consultant Dermatologist
Sanjivani Hospital
Kochi, Kerala, India

Debdeep Mitra MD (DVL) DNB
Graded Specialist Dermatology
Base Hospital, Delhi Cantt
Delhi, India

Deepak Vasisht MD (DVL)
Assistant Professor
Command Hospital
Pune, Maharashtra, India

Deepashree Daulatabad MD (DVL) DNB
Senior Resident
Department of Dermatology and STD
University College of Medical Sciences and GTB Hospital
Delhi, India

Disha Dabbas MD (DVL)
Cl Spl, Military Hospital
Meerut, Uttar Pradesh, India

Divya Gorur K MD (DVL) FRGUHS
Senior Resident
Department of Dermatology
Bangalore Medical College and Research Institute
Bengaluru, Karnataka, India

Eswari L MD (DVL) FRGUHS
Assistant Professor
Bangalore Medical College and Research Institute
Bengaluru, Karnataka, India

GK Singh MD (DVL)
Cl Spl (Dermatology)
Military Hospital
Ahmedabad, Gujarat, India

Gopikrishanan Anjaneyan MD (DVL) DNB
Assistant Professor
Department of Dermatology
Amrita Institute of Medical Sciences
Kochi, Kerala, India

Govind Mittal MD (DVL) FRGUHS
Consultant Dermatologist and Dermatosurgeon
Bengaluru, Karnataka, India

Harish Shetty MD (DVL)
Senior Consultant Dermatologist
Kaya Skin Clinic
Hyderabad, Telangana, India

Harish Prasad MD (DVL) FRGUHS
Consultant Dermatologist
Apollo, HCG Cancer Hospital and VITAL Clinic
Bengaluru, Karnataka, India

Indrashis Podder MD (DVL)
Consultant Dermatologist
Kolkata, West Bengal, India

Ishad Aggarwal MD (DVL)
Consultant Dermatologist
Purnam Medicare
Kaya Skin Clinic and Pristine
Kolkata, West Bengal, India

Kanhaiya Patidar MBBS
Resident (Dermatology)
Armed Forces Medical College
Pune, Maharashtra, India

Kingshuk Chatterjee DNB MNAMS MRCPS (Glasgow)
Assistant Professor
Department of Dermatology
Calcutta School of Tropical Medicine
Kolkata, West Bengal, India

Kirti S Jangid MD (DVL)
Consultant Dermatologist
Mumbai, Maharashtra, India

Krishna Talukdar MD (DVL)
Associate Professor and In-Charge Head
Jorhat Medical College and Hospital
Jorhat, Assam, India

Lakshmi DV MD (DVL) FRGUHS
Senior Resident
Department of Dermatology
Bangalore Medical College and Research Institute
Bengaluru, Karnataka, India

Lekshmipriya B MD (DVL)
Graded Specialist (Derm and Ven)
151 Base Hospital
Guwahati, Assam, India

Maheshwari NS DVD FRGUHS (Pediatric Dermatology)
Consultant Dermatologist
Bengaluru, Karnataka, India

Malcolm Pinto MD (DVL)
Assistant Professor
Department of Dermatology
Yenepoya Medical College
Mangaluru, Karnataka, India

Mary Thomas DNB
Consultant Dermatologist
Poornima Hospital
Bengaluru, Karnataka, India

Meenaz Khoja DDV
Consultant Dermatologist
GMF Ruby Hall Clinic and MMF Joshi Hospital
Pune, Maharashtra, India

Nagendra Beniwal DNB
Assistant Professor
Military Hospital
Kirkee, Pune, Maharashtra, India

Nagesh TS MD (DVL) DNB
Associate Professor
Sapthagiri Institute of Medical Sciences
and Research Center
Bengaluru, Karnataka, India

Navya Handa MD (DVL)
Associate Consultant
Max Hospital
New Delhi, India

Neetu Bhari MD (DVL)
Department of Dermatology, Venereology and Leprology
All India Institute of Medical Sciences
New Delhi, India

Nidhi Sharma MD (DVL)
Senior Resident
Calcutta National Medical College
Kolkata, West Bengal, India

Niharika Lal MD (DVL)
Assistant Professor
Department of Dermatology
ESI-PGIMSR and ESIC Medical College
Kolkata, West Bengal India

Nikita Lodha DNB
Consultant Dermatologist
Clear Skin Clinic
Mumbai, Maharashtra, India

Nirmal Krishna B MD (DVL)
Assistant Professor
Department of Dermatology
Christian Medical College
Vellore, Tamil Nadu, India

Pallavi Ailawadi MD (DVL) DNB
Senior Resident
Maulana Azad Medical College
and Lok Nayak Hospital
New Delhi, India

Parul Thakur MD (DVL) DNB
Associate Dermatologist
Alok Clinic
Panvel, Maharashtra, India

Piyush Kumar MD (DVL)
Associate Professor
Katihar Medical College
Katihar, Bihar, India

Preema Sinha MD (DVL)
Assistant Professor
Department of Dermatology
Armed Forces Medical College
Pune, Maharashtra, India

Priyadarshini Kharge DDVL FRGUHS
Consultant Pediatric Dermatologist
Department of Dermatology
Bangalore Medical College and Research Institute
Bengaluru, Karnataka, India

Priyanka Borde Bisht DNB (DV)
Consultant Dermatologist
Skin City Clinic
Pune, Maharashtra, India

Rahul Arora MD (DVL)
Senior Resident
University College of Medical Sciences
New Delhi, India

Rajan S Grewal VSM
Commandant—Command Hospital (Southern Command)
Professor
Department of Dermatology
Armed Forces Medical College and
Command Hospital (Southern Command)
Pune, Maharashtra, India

Rajesh Kumar Mandal MD (DVL)
Assistant Professor
Department of Dermatology
North Bengal Medical College
Darjeeling, West Bengal, India

Rajeshwari Dabbas MD (DVL)
Assistant Professor
Air Force Command Hospital
Bengaluru, Karnataka, India

Resham Vasani MD (DVL) DNB
Consultant Dermatologist
Anand Polyclinic
Mumbai, Maharashtra, India

Ruby Venugopal MD (DVL)
Dermatologist
Command Hospital (Western Command)
Chandigarh, India

Sacchidanand S MD (DVL) DHA FRCP
Director
Department of Medical Education
Government of Karnataka
Karnataka, India

Sahana M Srinivas DNB DVD FRGUHS (Pediatric Dermatology)
Consultant Pediatric Dermatologist
Indira Gandhi Institute of Child Health
Bangaluru, Karnataka, India

Saloni Katoch MD (DVL)
Consultant Dermatologist
Columbia Asia Hospital
Bengaluru, Karnataka, India

Samipa S Mukherjee DDV DDVL FRGUHS
Consultant Pediatric Dermatologist and
Dermatotrichologist
Cutis Academy of Cutaneous Sciences
Bengaluru, Karnataka, India

Samujjala Deb MD (DVL) FRGUHS
St. John's Medical College and Hospital
Bengaluru, Karnataka, India

Sanjay Singh MD (DVL)
Department of Dermatology, Venereology and Leprology
All India Institute of Medical Sciences
New Delhi, India

Sankeerth V MD FRGUHS
Consultant Dermatologist and Cosmetologist
Apollo Spectre Hospitals
Bengaluru, Karnataka, India

Savitha AS MD (DVL)
Assistant Professor
Department of Dermatology
Sapthagiri Institute of Medical Sciences
Bengaluru, Karnataka, India

Shekhar Neema MD (DVL)
Assistant Professor
Command Hospital
Kolkata, West Bengal, India

Sherina Laskar MD DNB MSc
Resident Physician
Department of Dermatology
Gauhati Medical College
Guwahati, Assam, India

Shilpa Garg DNB (DV)
Consultant Dermatologist
Sir Ganga Ram Hospital
New Delhi, India

Shilpa K MD (DVL) FRGUHS
Assistant Professor
Department of Dermatology
Bangalore Medical College and Research Institute
Bengaluru, Karnataka, India

Shreyaswini Pujary DNB
Consultant Dermatologist
Kaya Skin Clinic
Mumbai, Maharashtra, India

Shruthi C MD (DVL)
Department of Dermatosurgery
Bangalore Medical College and Research Institute
Bengaluru, Karnataka, India

Siddharth Sonthalia MD (DVL) DNB
Director and Consultant
Skinnocence – The Skin Clinic
Gurugram, Haryana, India

Soumya Jagadeesan MD (DVL)
Assistant Professor
Department of Dermatology
Amrita Institute of Medical Sciences
Kochi, Kerala, India

Sriharsha Talabhukta MD (DVL)
Assistant Professor
Gayatri Vidya Parishad Healthcare and Medical Technology
Visakhapatnam, Andhra Pradesh, India

Sujala S Aradhya MD FRGUHS
Consultant Dermatologist and Dermatosurgeon
Sujala Polyclinic and Laboratory
Bengaluru, Karnataka, India

Sukesh Mathapathi MD (DVL) DNB
Consultant Dermatotrichologist and Hair Transplant Surgeon
Bengaluru, Karnataka, India

Sumit Gupta MD (DVL)
Consultant (Dermatology)
New Delhi, India

Suneil Gandhi MD (DVL) DNB
Consultant Dermatologist
Reviva Skin Clinic
Surat, Gujarat, India

Surajit Gorai MD (DVL)
Consultant (Dermatology)
Bardhaman, West Bengal, India

Tanmay Padhi MD (DVL)
Assistant Professor
Veer Surendra Sai Institute of Medical Sciences and Research
Sambalpur, Odisha, India

Tanumay Raychaudhury MD (DVL)
Consultant
Tata Medical Centre
Kolkata, West Bengal, India

Tarang Goyal MD (DVL)
Professor and Head
Department of Dermatology, Venereology and Leprosy
Muzaffarnagar Medical College
Muzaffarnagar, Uttar Pradesh, India

Vinitha Varghese MD (DVL)
Associate Professor
Department of Dermatology
Amrita Institute of Medical Sciences
Kochi, Kerala, India

Vishal Sharma MD (DVL) DNB
Cl Spl
Command Hospital (Northern Command)
Udhampur, Jammu & Kashmir, India

Foreword

The fascinating panoramic canvas of dermatology portrayed through its myriad clinical presentations puts the oft-quoted adage 'A picture is worth a thousand words'; in the shade.

In the era of exponential advancements in technology driven, skill-based dermatology, with its alluring commercial bottom line, this unique book is a refreshingly informative achievement. It fortifies the foundations of conventional dermatology; which one speculates, is not the flavor of the season amongst the young achievers, who seem enamoured by the reward-oriented conveyor belt of procedure-based interventions.

This book elucidates clinical approaches to a multitude of dermatological disorders with their dilemmas and diagnostic implications. We are sanguine that it will be a boon for clinicians, and the entire medical fraternity, including postgraduates, academicians, practitioners; and even MBBS students. The contemporary chapters with their educative scientific contents will be a value addition in our comprehension of pragmatic approaches to patients who present with various dermatologic, genitourinary and leprology conditions. It shall also help the readers to navigate through the common differential diagnosis, and customize the investigations, to arrive at the accurate diagnosis, in the best interests of our patients, who ought to be the ultimate beneficiaries.

This book with its unique format, provides cohesive clinicodiagnostic insights to enhance our perspective as a quantum force multiplier. It encompasses recent advances in the clinical, investigational, diagnostic and therapeutic arenas, thereby adding substantially to the knowledge quotient. The format also ensures simplicity of learning in a reader-friendly manner.

We are confident that this book will be of immense value in the field of dermatology. Its uncomplicated and informative contents should make it a 'must have' for students, faculty, practitioners and healthcare professionals.

Rajan S Grewal VSM MD
Commandant—Command Hospital (Southern Command)
Professor
Department of Dermatology
Armed Forces Medical College
and Command Hospital (Southern Command)
Pune, Maharashtra, India

Preface

The idea of *Clinical Correlation with Diagnostic Implications in Dermatology* was born due to the felt need for a book which would help everyone dealing with dermatological manifestations to decide their approach to these conditions. Similar titles do exist in other specialties, but there was a vacuum when it came to books with an approach to dermatological manifestations.

This is a dream project meant primarily for postgraduates in dermatology to help them in their approach to various dermatological conditions and also help them in preparing for their cases In practical examinations. It is however equally beneficial for practising dermatologists, undergraduates and other specialists to define their approach when they come across any dermatological manifestation.

Every topic has been chosen keeping the relevance to the above matter and the approach, both clinical and investigational is complemented by relevant images. Common dermatological disorders, interesting and exam-oriented topics are presented with an algorithmic kind of approach. Multiple questions and answers in a logical fashion leading to a clinical diagnosis and relevant investigations to confirm the diagnosis, form the pattern for all chapters.

The contributors have been chosen from all over the country with utmost care and they are all young academicians who are designing such approaches regularly and who are likely to be the real guiding forces in dermatology in the near future. Section editors of different sections have reviewed the chapters and have made their contributions to both the text and images.

The book aims to be a benchmark for approach towards dermatological disorders. The logically flowing question-and-answer format following a clinical case presentation lends a unique approach towards managing the various conditions. All members who have contributed to the book have been duly acknowledged. The book has 25 sections with 129 chapters. We hope the sincere efforts of the entire editorial team will live up to the expectations of all concerned.

Biju Vasudevan

Acknowledgments

All faculty members, residents and staff of Department of Dermatology, Armed Forces Medical College, Pune, Maharashtra, and Bangalore Medical College, Bengaluru, Karnataka, India.

Contents

Section 17: Infections-1 (Bacterial, Mycobacterial and Fungal)

Lakshmi DV

Section 18: Infections-2 (Viral and Parasitic)

Ruby Venugopal

Section 19: Mucosal Disorders

Anupam Das

Section 20: Nutritional Disorders

Priyadarshini Kharge

Section 21: Autoimmune Connective Tissue Disorders

Nirmal Krishna B

Section 22: Connective Tissue Disorders

Navya Handa

SECTION 1

Drug Reactions

Savitha AS

CHAPTER 1

Toxic Epidermal Necrolysis

Asad Ansari, Shekhar Neema

Case study Toxic Epidermal Necrolysis

Presenting Complaints

Doctor, I suddenly started developing red, painful lesions over my trunk which gradually spread to my limbs and face. It was accompanied by blister formation on some parts of the body. I also developed fever and oral ulcers simultaneously.

Setting

Dermatology outpatient department.

History of Present Illness

A 35-year-old male patient was brought to dermatology outpatient department with complaints of the sudden development of red, flat and painful lesions over his trunk for the past 1 day. The lesions gradually spread to involve the face, neck and upper limbs. Few of the lesions became fluid filled. The patient also developed high-grade fever, reddening of eyes and painful oral ulcers simultaneously. He complains of pain and difficulty in swallowing food.

The patient was started on tablet phenytoin (dilantin sodium) 20 days back for epilepsy.

General Physical Examination

Patient appears toxic, but well oriented to time, place and person.

- Temperature: 40°C
- Pulse: 110 beats/min (bpm)
- Respiration: shallow and regular
- Blood pressure (BP): 110/80 mm Hg
- Pallor: Present.

Systemic Examination

No abnormality detected.

Dermatologic Examination

Dusky-red macular eruptions occur all over the trunk, face and upper limbs. Epidermal detachment with flaccid bullae is seen at some sites. Few tense bullae are seen over the palms. Some atypical target lesions are also seen. Tangential pressure on involved erythematous skin caused the separation of the epidermis (pseudo-Nikolsky sign) (Figs 1 and 2). Oral mucosa involved with ulceration and hemorrhagic crusts on lips. Redness of conjunctiva is seen.

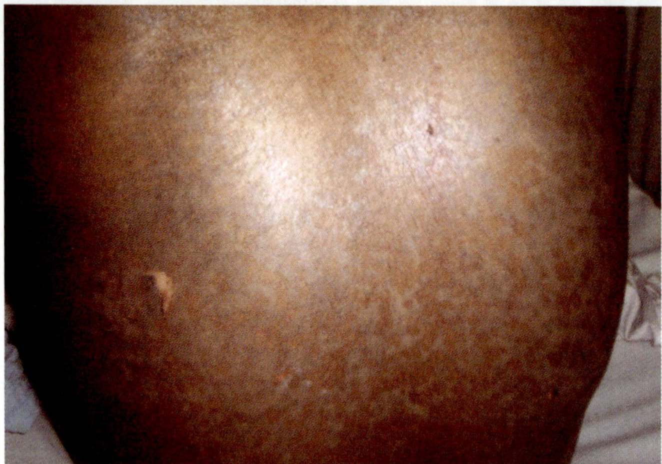

Fig. 1: Back of the patient showing multiple purpuric macules with impending bulla formation and pseudo-Nikolsky sign positive

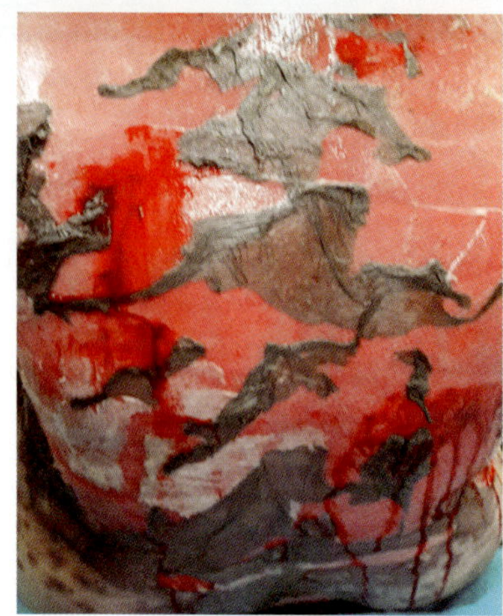

Fig. 2: Progression of condition showing extensive involvement

Q1. What is the most likely diagnosis?

a. Toxic epidermal necrolysis (TEN)
b. Pemphigus vulgaris
c. Staphylococcal scalded skin syndrome
d. Paraneoplastic pemphigus

Ans: **a.** Toxic epidermal necrolysis (Lyell's syndrome). Presence of erythematous macular eruptions over trunk and upper limbs, targetoid lesions, bullae, painful oral mucosal ulceration, pseudo-Nikolsky sign and history of ingestion of phenytoin 20 days prior to appearance of lesions suggests diagnosis of TEN.

Q2. What are the risk factors and causative factors of TEN?

Ans: The risk factors and causative factors of TEN are described in Table 1.

Q3. Which are the common drugs implicated in TEN?

Ans: More than 100 drugs have been implicated to leading to Stevens-Johnson syndrome (SJS)/TEN. The most common include:

Table 1: Risk factors and causative factors of TEN

Risk factors	*Causative factors*
• Women (M:F = 0.6:1) • Increasing age (risk increases after the 4th decade) • Immunosuppression, e.g. human immunodeficiency virus (HIV) infection • Lymphoma • Collagen vascular disorders • Slow acetylators	• Drugs • Infections: Mycoplasma pneumonia, viral illness • Immunization • Following bone marrow transplantation

- Allopurinol
- Aromatic anticonvulsants: Phenytoin, carbamazepine, phenobarbital, lamotrigine
- Antibiotics:
  - Sulfonamides including sulfasalazine, sulfamethoxazole
  - Aminopenicillins
  - Cephalosporins
  - Quinolones
  - Macrolides
  - Tetracyclines
- Nonsteroidal anti-inflammatory drugs (NSAIDs): Diclofenac, oxicams
- Antifungals
- Nevirapine.

Q4. What is the pathogenesis of TEN?

Ans: The medications cause widespread apoptosis of keratinocytes leading to TEN. Apoptosis can be due to:

- Induction of upregulation of Fas-ligand by keratinocytes: Death receptor-mediated apoptotic pathway.
- Drug interaction and activation of CD8+ cytotoxic cells releasing perforin and granzyme-B that destroy keratinocytes.
- Activation of CD8+ T-cells and natural killer (NK)-cells to secrete granulysin, which causes keratinocyte death.

Q5. What are the histopathological findings in TEN?

Ans: Early lesions: Apoptotic keratinocytes in the basal and suprabasal layers of epidermis. Late lesions: Subcorneal blister with confluent necrosis of the upper lying epidermis and a sparse perivascular lymphocytic infiltrate, satellite cell necrosis (close contact between necrotic keratinocytes and mononuclear cells). CD8+ lymphocytes and macrophages are seen in epidermis while the papillary dermis primarily contains CD4+ lymphocytes.

Q6. What are the differential diagnoses?

Ans: Differential diagnoses include:

- Stevens-Johnson syndrome
- Erythema multiforme major
- Acute generalized exanthematous pustulosis
- Staphylococcal scalded skin syndrome
- Acute syndrome of apoptotic pan-epidermolysis (ASAP)
- Bullous fixed drug eruption (FDE).

Q7. How do we differentiate between SJS and TEN?

Ans: Stevens-Johnson syndrome and TEN both have almost similar presentation. The main difference is the extent of body surface area (BSA) involvement (Table 2). Systemic symptoms are seen more prominently in TEN than in SJS. Mortality rate varies from 1% to 5% in SJS to more than 30% in TEN.

Q8. How do we determine the prognosis of TEN?

Ans: The prognosis of TEN is determined by SCORTEN (SCORe of Toxic Epidermal Necrosis). It is based on seven independent risk factors which are assessed on the 1st day of hospitalization. 1 point is assigned to each risk factor. Greater the score, higher is the risk of mortality (Tables 3 and 4).

Table 2: Body surface area (BSA) involvement

Clinical entity	*% of BSA detachment*
SJS	<10%
SJS-TEN overlap	10–30%
TEN	>30%

Abbreviations: SJS, Stevens-Johnson syndrome; TEN, toxic epidermal necrolysis.

Table 3: Prognostic factors of TEN

Prognostic factors	*Points*
Age > 40 years	1
Heart rate > 120 beats/min	1
Epidermal detachment > 10%	1
Cancer or hematological malignancy	1
Serum urea > 10 mmol/L	1
Serum bicarbonate < 20 mmol/L	1
Serum glucose > 14 mmol/L	1

Q9. What are the complications of TEN?

Ans: Complications of TEN include:

- Fluid and electrolyte imbalances, renal insufficiency
- Adult respiratory distress syndrome
- Multiorgan failure and death (due to sepsis: *Staphylococcus aureus* and *Pseudomonas aeruginosa*)
- Insulin resistance
- Long-term sequelae: Scarring of skin and mucous membranes, symblepharon, conjunctival synechiae, entropion, phimosis, vaginal synechiae, nail dystrophy and hair loss.

Q10. How do you manage a case of TEN?

Ans: All patients of TEN should be immediately transferred to intensive care unit (ICU) or burns unit. Supportive treatment is very important in reducing mortality.

- Prompt withdrawal of the causative/suspected drug. A checklist of any medication ingested within last 2 months is enlisted with corresponding date of initiation, dosage and indication for the same.
- Maintain hemodynamic equilibrium with prompt fluid and electrolyte replacement. Fluid requirements are two-thirds of that of a patient with second-degree burns with similar BSA involvement.
- Maintain a temperature of 28–30°C
- Strict aseptic precautions and topical antibiotics to prevent secondary infection
- Early caloric replacement through nasogastric tube
- Skin, blood, sputum and urine samples should be cultured periodically
- Good nursing care with biological dressings of the denuded areas. Avoid any debridement
- Ophthalmological consultation with good eye-care to prevent sequelae
- Oral care to prevent infections
- An "Allergy card" to be issued to patient at the time of discharge enlisted with offending drug

Table 4: SCORTEN: Independent risk factors

SCORTEN	*Probability of death (%)*
1	3.2
2	12.1
3	35.8
4	58.3
5 or more	90

and drugs of similar biochemical structure, cross-reacting drugs and counsel the patient.

Specific treatments include:

- Cyclosporine in doses of 3–5 mg/kg/day and taper after 7 days.
- Intravenous immunoglobulin (IVIg) in doses of 2 g/kg given over 3–4 days
- Systemic steroids: Controversial role. If required to use, use in high doses for short duration only
- Cyclophosphamide (100–300 mg/day)
- Plasmapheresis
- N-acetyl cysteine (2 g every 6th hourly)
- Tumor necrosis factor-alpha (TNF-α) antagonists, e.g. infliximab, etanercept.

Q11. What is the role of prophylactic systemic antibiotics in management of TEN?

Ans: Prophylactic antibiotics are initiated only in cases of clinical infection/culture proven sepsis or when there is neutropenia or an increase in bacterial counts of a single strain on the swabs. They need to be given in a higher dose than usual because of large amount of protein loss in TEN. Otherwise it is avoided due to possibility of cross-reactivity with the drug that initiated the TEN and also due to risk of infection with resistant organisms. Sterile handling and maintenance of asepsis is more important.

Q12. Why role of corticosteroids is controversial in TEN?

Ans: Systemic corticosteroids prolong wound healing, increase the risk of infection, mask early signs of sepsis, and may precipitate gastrointestinal bleeding, thus increasing mortality. Once a large area of dermis is uncovered, i.e. more than 20% of BSA, the advantages of the treatment would be far outweighed by its drawbacks. Hence, it is advisable to start within the first 72 hours of onset in a patient with a still limited skin surface involvement to prevent widespread diffusion, and continued for 3–5 days followed by rapid tapering.

CHAPTER 2

Drug Hypersensitivity Syndrome

Anupam Das, Biju Vasudevan

Case study Drug Hypersensitivity Syndrome

Presenting Complaints

Doctor, I have developed these scaly red rashes all over the body, over the last 4 days. I also have noticed that my urine is yellow in color. I was taking a medication for chronic headache since the last 4 weeks.

Setting

Intensive care unit (ICU).

History of Present Illness

A 38-year-old man presented with fever and red scaly lesions distributed all over the body, present for the preceding 4 days. To start with, there were a few lesions over the face and neck, but gradually they progressed to involve the entire body. The patient is anorectic and drowsy. The color of urine is deep yellow. He suffers from chronic headache, possibly due to migraine; for which he was prescribed carbamazepine, 4 weeks prior to the onset of the lesions, by a local doctor.

General Physical Examination

Patient looks ill, oriented to time, place and person.

- Temperature: 102°F
- Pulse: 124 beats/min
- Blood pressure (BP): 110/70 mm Hg
- Respiratory rate: 32 breath/min
- Anemia and icterus present (Fig. 1). Facial edema present.

Systemic Examination

Hepatomegaly present.

Dermatological Examination

- Morbilliform rash with exfoliation: Distributed throughout the body
- Characteristic facial edema and plenty of pustules distributed on the face.

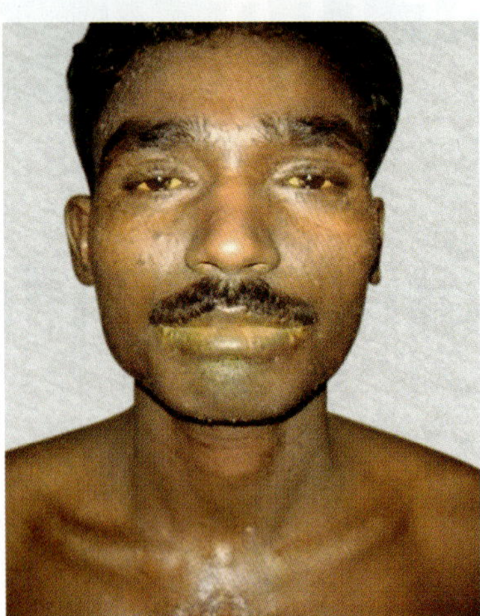

Fig. 1: Drug hypersensitivity syndrome (DHS) showing icterus and morbilliform rash on face

Q1. What is the most likely diagnosis?

a. Erythema multiforme
b. Acute generalized exanthematous pustulosis
c. Drug reaction with eosinophilia and systemic symptoms (DRESS)
d. Stevens-Johnson syndrome (SJS)-Toxic epidermal necrolysis (TEN)

Ans: c. DRESS. The typical history, onset of lesion 4 weeks after taking carbamazepine, sparing of mucosae, facial edema, icterus, liver enlargement and ill look of the patient clinches the diagnosis.

Q2. What are the diagnostic features of DRESS?

Ans: Diagnostic features of DRESS include:

- Rash developing more than 3 weeks after the introduction of medicine
- Symptoms persist more than 2 weeks after discontinuation of drug
- Fever more than 38°C
- Multiorgan involvement
- Eosinophilia (>1,500 absolute eosinophils)
- Lymphocyte activation (lymphocytosis, atypical lymphocytosis, lymphadenopathy)
- Frequent reactivation of herpes viruses human herpes virus 6 (HHV-6), human herpes virus 7 (HHV-7). Epstein-Barr virus (EBV), cytomegalovirus (CMV).

Q3. What are the drugs implicated in the causation of DRESS?

Ans: The most common drugs implicated in the causes of DRESS:

- Anticonvulsants (phenobarbitone, phenytoin, lamotrigine, carbamazepine)
- Long-acting sulfonamides
- Allopurinol
- Nevirapine
- Abacavir
- Dapsone
- Minocycline
- Vancomycin.

Q4. What are the cutaneous lesions associated with DRESS?

Ans: The cutaneous lesions associated with DRESS:

- Morbilliform rash
- Exfoliative erythroderma
- Facial edema
- Superficial pustules typically on the face
- Purpuric macules similar to SJS/TEN.

Q5. What are the types of internal organ involvement in DRESS?

Ans: Types of internal organ involvement:

- Organ dysfunction associated with acute episode: Colitis, encephalitis, aseptic meningitis, hepatitis, interstitial nephritis, interstitial pneumonitis, respiratory distress syndrome, sialadenitis, myocarditis, orchitis, myositis, parotitis
- Late sequelae with an autoimmune basis: Syndrome of inappropriate secretion of antidiuretic hormone (SIADH), thyroiditis, Graves' disease, diabetes mellitus, systemic lupus erythematosus (SLE).

Q6. What are the key points in the pathogenesis of DRESS?

Ans:

- Defective detoxification of reactive oxidative metabolites by the liver
- Genetic predisposition [human leukocyte antigen (HLA) predilection]
- Coinfection with HHV 6 plays important role
- Release of interleukin-5 from drug-specific T cells, leading to eosinophilic activation and initiation of inflammatory cascade.

Q7. What are the laboratory findings which provide additional support to the diagnosis?

Ans: Laboratory findings:

- Hemogram: Neutrophilia, eosinophilia, hemolytic anemia, atypical lymphocytosis, thrombocytopenia

- Liver function test: Elevated transaminases, alkaline phosphatases, prothrombin time and bilirubin
- Renal function test: Elevated urea and creatinine
- Chest X ray: Features of respiratory distress syndrome
- Histopathology: Parakeratosis, intracorneal pustule, spongiosis, mixed perivascular infiltrate.

Q8. Which drug causing DRESS is most commonly associated with renal dysfunction?

a. Phenytoin
b. Dapsone
c. Allopurinol
d. Amoxicillin

Ans: c. Allopurinol.

Q9. Which drugs are associated with lung involvement?

Ans: Drugs associated with lung involvement:

- Minocycline
- Abacavir.

Q10. What are the treatment options available for DRESS?

Ans:

- Withdrawal of all suspected medications
- Supportive management (maintenance of ambient temperature, fluid electrolyte balance and an aseptic environment)
- Systemic steroids: Oral prednisolone 40–60 mg/day for a minimum duration of 8–12 weeks or even longer
- N-acetyl cysteine (1.0–1.5 mg/kg) if hepatitis is present
- Immunosuppressives like azathioprine, cyclosporine
- Intravenous immunoglobulins.

Q11. What are the HLA associations with drug hypersensitivity syndrome (DHS)?

Ans: The human leukocyte antigen (HLA) associations with DHS:

- Allopurinol: HLA-B-5801
- Carbamazepine: HLA-B-1502.

Q12. What is the most common anticonvulsant causing DRESS?

a. Carbamazepine
b. Valproic acid
c. Phenytoin
d. Phenobarbitone

Ans: a. Carbamazepine

Q13. What are the diagnostic features of dapsone hypersensitivity syndrome?

Ans: The diagnostic features of dapsone hypersensitivity syndrome include:

- The morbilliform rash typically begins 4 weeks after starting the drug
- The rash heals with a typical desquamation
- Eosinophilia is absent
- Liver involvement in the form of both hepatocellular and obstructive jaundice
- Hypoalbuminemia is typical.

CHAPTER 3

Acute Generalized Exanthematous Pustulosis

Soumya Jagadeesan

Case study Acute Generalized Exanthematous Pustulosis

Presenting Complaints

Doctor, I have developed a red rash with tiny yellow bumps on my body since 2 days. It started on my back and is now spreading all over and I have high fever too.

History of Present Illness

A 25-year-old male presented to the emergency with acute onset of high-grade fever and a generalized rash of 24 hours duration. The symptoms started with high-grade fever and simultaneously, the patient noticed a reddish rash, initially on the back, which later spread to involve the proximal limbs and rest of the trunk. There were multiple tiny yellowish bumps seen along with the rash (Figs 1 and 2). Patient gave history of intake of Cefuroxime tablets for urinary tract infection, 2 days prior to the onset of symptoms. No history of involvement of eye or oral cavity present.

General Physical Examination

Well built and nourished. No pallor/icterus.

- Temperature: 100°F
- Pulse: 90 beats/min
- Blood pressure (BP): 110/70 mm Hg
- Systems: Within normal limits.

Dermatological Examination

Widespread edematous erythema on the face, trunk and limbs (upper limbs more than lower limbs, more on the proximal aspects) covered with numerous discrete, non-follicular pustules (<5 mm in diameter) which are seen to be coalescing on the palms. No vesicles/bullae/erosions seen. No mucosal erosions seen. No scalp scaling. No significant nail changes.

Laboratory tests revealed significant leukocytosis with neutrophilia and mild eosinophilia. Bacterial and fungal cultures of the pustular lesions were negative.

Q1. What is the most likely diagnosis?

a. Pustular psoriasis
b. Acute generalized exanthematous pustulosis (AGEP)
c. Stevens-Johnson syndrome
d. Subcorneal pustular dermatosis

Ans: b. Acute generalized exanthematous pustulosis. Also known as toxic pustuloderma, it is a type of severe cutaneous adverse drug reaction (SCAR). The presence of preceding drug intake, presence of fever with exanthematous rash and sterile non-follicular pustules are in favor of the diagnosis.

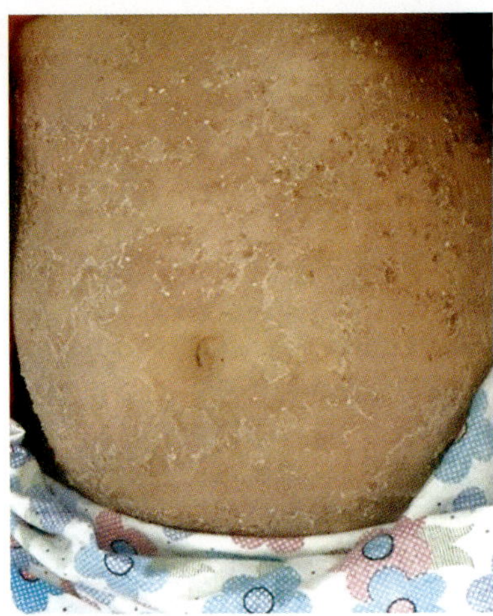

Fig. 1: Trunk showing scaly erythematous rash and pustules

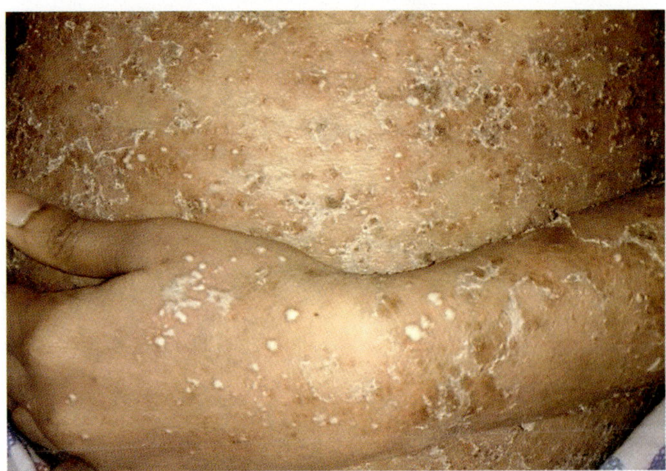

Fig. 2: Close up of same patient as in Figure 1 showing the pustules

Q2. How do you diagnose AGEP?

Ans: Acute generalized exanthematous pustulosis is diagnosed based on clinical grounds and the history of drug intake.Histological examination may be done to rule out other causes of pustular eruptions. Gram stain and pus culture may be done to rule out infectious causes.

Diagnostic criteria for AGEP was established by an International Committee of Experts: the European Study of Severe Cutaneous Adverse Reactions (EuroSCAR), as for drug reaction with eosinophilia and systemic symptoms (DRESS). The scoring system takes into account the clinical pattern (presentation, evolution), biological data and histological findings. The scale is used retrospectively by consensus groups to classify cases as definitive, probable, possible or excluded.

Q3. What are the clinical features of AGEP?

Ans: Acute generalized exanthematous pustulosis eruption generally begins on the face or intertriginous areas and rapidly extends to the trunk and limbs with a diffuse or patchy distribution. The characteristic feature is the rapid development of hundreds of non-follicular, sterile, pinhead-sized pustules on a background of edematous erythema with flexural accentuation. The eruption usually occurs a few hours to a few days after the administration of the offending drug. A localized variant also has been described. The pustular rash is occasionally accompanied by facial edema and nonspecific lesions such as purpura, atypical target lesions, blisters, or vesicles. Severe cases of AGEP may present with atypical target lesions and coalescent pustules, resulting in superficial erosions and a clinical picture similar to SJS-TEN.

Q4. Which of the following diseases mimic AGEP the most?

a. Subcorneal pustular dermatosis
b. Pustular psoriasis
c. Drug hypersensitivity syndrome
d. Miliaria pustulosa.

Ans: b. Pustular psoriasis is one of the most important differential diagnoses (DDs) of AGEP. Other important DDs include pustular variant of DRESS, subcorneal pustular dermatosis, pustular vasculitis and SJS/TEN.

Q5. How will you differentiate AGEP from pustular psoriasis?

Ans: The difference between AGEP and pustular psoriasis has been described in Table 1.

Q6. What are the etiopathogenic factors involved in AGEP?

Ans: Drugs are implicated in approximately 90% of the cases of AGEP. There are also a few reports of AGEP being associated with viral, bacterial or parasitic infections, spider bites and herbal medication. However, in some cases, the cause remains undetermined.

The immunopathogenesis of AGEP is not fully known. AGEP appears to be a drug-specific, CD4- and CD8-T-lymphocyte mediated immune reaction that results in CXCL8 production directly by T cells and indirectly by keratinocytes. CXCL8 is a potent neutrophil-attracting chemokine. AGEP and its

Table 1: Difference between AGEP and pustular psoriasis

Parameters	*AGEP*	*Pustular psoriasis*
Age	Mostly adults, can occur in any age	Mostly adults
History of drug intake	Almost always present	Usually not present
History of psoriasis	Possible	Usually present
Clinical characteristics	Rapid development of dozens to hundreds of non-follicular, sterile, pinhead-sized pustules on a background of edematous erythema with flexural accentuation	Discrete scaly plaques or generalized scaling with pustules may be seen. Lakes of pus may be seen. More prolonged course
Fever	High, acute	Prolonged
Arthritis	Rare	Frequent
Histology	Spongiform subcorneal and/or intraepidermal pustules, edema of papillary dermis, vasculitis, exocytosis of eosinophils, single-cell necrosis of keratinocytes. Psoriasiform acanthosis not seen	Subcorneal and/or intraepidermal pustules, papillomatosis, acanthosis, psoriasiform epidermal hyperplasia is a distinguishing feature

Abbreviation: AGEP, acute generalized exanthematous pustulosis.

systemic involvement might reflect the effects of circulating interleukin-17 (IL-17) and IL-22. These inflammatory cytokines are secreted by CD4+, Th-17 and Th-22 T lymphocytes.

Recessively inherited mutations in the *IL36RN* gene encoding the IL-36 receptor antagonist (IL-36Ra) have been found in generalized pustular psoriasis. Mutations in *IL36RN* have also been found in a very small subset of patients with AGEP. This finding suggests that generalized pustular psoriasis and AGEP may share a common pathogenetic pathway, making it difficult in some cases to distinguish between the two entities.

Q7. What are the drugs most commonly responsible for AGEP?

Ans: Antibiotics: Mostly macrolides (azithromycin, erythromycin, spiramycin) and betalactam group of drugs (amoxicillin, cefaclor, cefuroxime, cephalexin and penicillin) are likely to cause AGEP. Interestingly, sulfonamides are less likely to cause AGEP. The other drugs implicated are quinolones, (hydroxy) chloroquine, terbinafine, itraconazole, diltiazem, nifedipine, carbamazepine, metronidazole, mercury, acetaminophen, allopurinol, diclofenac, etc.

Q8. What are the laboratory tests recommended in AGEP?

Ans: Leukocytosis with marked neutrophilia (>7,000/μL) and sometimes eosinophilia may be seen. Other acute inflammatory markers may be elevated. Gram stain and pus culture may be done which will be negative.

Patch testing with one or multiple suspected drugs may be useful in identifying the cause of AGEP. Patch testing is generally performed 4–6 weeks after the disease resolution. A positive test can confirm a suspected drug as the cause of AGEP. However, a negative result does not exclude that a certain drug is the causative agent.

Q9. What are the histopathological features of AGEP?

Ans: Two histological patterns may be seen: (1) spongiform intraepidermal pustules, papillary edema and a mixed upper dermal perivascular inflammatory infiltrate; or (2) a leukocytoclastic vasculitis with neutrophil collections both below and within the epidermis, suggesting passive neutrophil elimination via the overlying epidermis. The presence of eosinophils in the inflammatory infiltrate is a helpful pointer to a drug cause. Psoriatic changes like acanthosis and papillomatosis are usually absent.

Q10. What are the complications of AGEP?

Ans: Cutaneous manifestations of AGEP are often associated with high fever, asthenia, elevated neutrophil count and a nonspecific inflammatory syndrome. Acute skin failure and the accompanying complications can also occur in the very severe cases. Systemic involvement is generally rare in AGEP. However, a recent study had demonstrated hepatitis, cholestasis, renal, pulmonary and bone marrow involvement in patients with AGEP. More studies are needed to determine the extent of systemic involvement in AGEP.

Q11. Discuss the management of AGEP.

Ans: Acute generalized exanthematous pustulosis is generally a self-limiting disease. Management strategies include:

- Immediate withdrawal of the offending drug. In patients taking multiple drugs, the drugs suspected to be the cause of AGEP should be discontinued and patients should be counseled to avoid re-exposure to the same drug.
- Supportive care: Patients with severe forms of the disease are hospitalized and care should be given to maintain thermoregulation, fluid-electrolyte balance, nutritional support, avoidance of infections and other supportive measures. In the pustular phase, moist dressings and antiseptic solutions may be used for relief of pruritus and prevention of bacterial superinfection. In the desquamation phase, emollients may be helpful in restoring the skin barrier function.
- Symptomatic treatment of pruritus and skin inflammation: Medium potency topical corticosteroids are preferred along with oral antihistamines. In severe cases, some authors consider systemic corticosteroids/other immunomodulators.

CHAPTER 4

Fixed Drug Eruption

Sumit Gupta

Case study Fixed Drug Eruption

Presenting Complaints

Doctor, I have a large dark round painful spot on my genitalia since yesterday.

Setting

Dermatology outpatient department.

History of Present Illness

Patient was suffering from diarrhea from 2 days and had taken an antibiotic after 24 hours. He suddenly developed a circular raised lesion on the glans penis associated with burning sensation and itching. The lesion appeared on an already hyperpigmented region on glans penis.

He gives history of appearance of similar lesion at the exact same location in the past which he associates with bouts of diarrhea. On further prodding, he gives history of intake of one tablet norfloxacin-tinidazole fixed-dose combination every time he suffers from diarrhea. His diarrhea resolves effectively with just one dose, but the lesion on his penis troubles him for at least a week.

Patient is an unmarried male with no history of any sexual encounter. There is no history of any trauma to the penis.

General Examination and Systemic Examination

No abnormality detected.

Dermatological Examination

Single, well-circumscribed violaceous plaque 2 cm × 2.5 cm on the dorsal aspect of glans penis (Fig. 1). No lymphadenopathy could be detected.
Oral cavity examination: Normal.
Ocular examination: Conjunctiva appears normal.

Q1. What is the most likely diagnosis?

a. Fixed drug eruption (FDE)
b. Erythema multiforme
c. Herpes simplex
d. Behçet syndrome

Ans: a. Fixed drug eruption. Appearance of such a lesion at a fixed location (glans penis), which heals with hyperpigmentation and history of recurrence after intake of the same medicine, points towards the diagnosis of FDE.

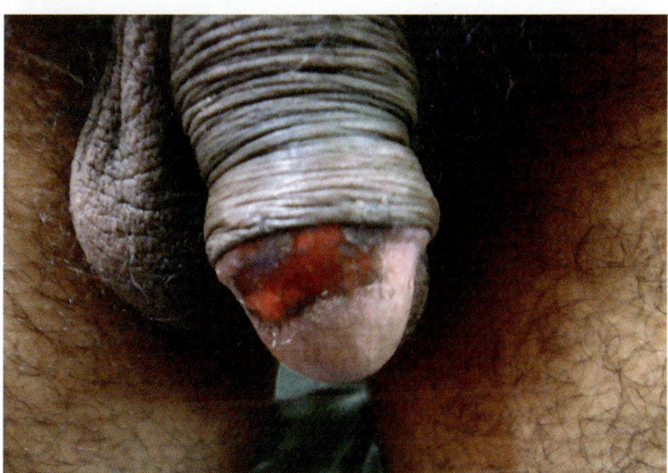

Fig. 1: Solitary dusky plaque on the dorsum of glans

Q2. Which of the following is NOT true about clinical features of FDE?

a. Generalized bullous FDE is an uncommon maximal variant, which is difficult to differentiate from toxic epidermal necrolysis (TEN).
b. Lips, hands, genitalia and occasionally oral mucosa are favored sites.
c. The lesions may flare within few hours of drug intake.
d. Systemic symptoms, like fever and malaise, are seen commonly.

Ans: d. Systemic symptoms, like fever and malaise, are commonly seen.

Q3. What are the clinical manifestations of FDE?

Ans: The typical/classical clinical presentation of FDE is distinct. In the acute phase, FDEs present as solitary, well-demarcated, edematous, violaceous, hyperpigmented, circular, or oval plaques. Bullae and subsequent erosions occur occasionally. The hyperpigmentation persists long after the acute eruption resolves, and many patients present with no active inflammation. Multiple satellite lesions can appear in adjacent skin and sometimes become confluent. Although FDE may present on almost any part of the body; lips, palms, soles, genitalia (especially male genitalia) and oral mucosa are favored sites. After intake of the offending drug, FDE appears within minutes up to several hours (~30 min to 8 hours). Lesions are often associated with burning and itching in the lesions. General symptoms such as fever, nausea, dysuria, abdominal cramps and diarrhea are rare.

Q4. What are the different morphological variants of FDE?

Ans: The different clinical appearances of FDE are:
- Pigmenting FDEs
- Nonpigmenting FDEs
- Bullous FDEs
- Multifocal FDEs
- Erythema multiforme, like FDEs
- Linear FDEs
- Generalized bullous/TEN, like FDEs
- Wandering FDEs

Q5. Which of the following is NOT true about causative agents of FDE?

a. Some drugs cause FDE predominantly at specific sites.
b. Multisensitivity is more common than monosensitivity.
c. Pseudoephedrine has shown to cause nonpigmenting FDE.
d. Tetracyclines cause FDE on genitalia more than any other site.

Ans: b. Multisensitivity is more common than monosensitivity. Monosensitivity refers to occurrence of FDE by one causative drug only. When several drugs induce FDE in the same patient it is known as multisensitivity. The most common reason for multisensitivity is cross-sensitivity between chemically-related drugs such as tetracyclines. Less frequently, multisensitivity can occur due to polysensitivity, where two or more chemically unrelated drugs either induce the identical FDE lesion or each drug causes flare-ups in separate lesions. Some cases of FDE can be induced by a drug combination, but not by the individual constituents. It has also been claimed that recurrences of FDE can be induced in nonspecific fashion by mast cell degranulators such as strawberries or other foods, acetylsalicylic acid, bacterial toxins or physical stimuli such as friction. These mast cell degranulators lead to a rapid local release of preformed cytokines such as tumor necrosis factor (TNF) from mast cells and serve as the stimulus for reactivating memory T cells in old FDE lesions.

Q6. Which are the common drugs causing FDE?

Ans: In general, antibiotics [tetracyclines, quinolones amoxicillin, rifampin, trimethoprim-sulfamethoxazole (TS)], imidazole group of antiprotozoal agents, analgesics (paracetamol, piroxicam, mefenamic acid), muscle relaxants (chlormezanone), anti-epileptics (carbamazepine) and sedatives are the most frequent culprit drugs. In addition TS and tetracyclines in India have been reported as the most frequent causes of FDE.

Q7. What is the pathogenesis of FDE?

Ans: According to the new subclassification of delayed type IV immune reactions, FDE is a type IVc reaction in which CD8+ cytotoxic T cells play the predominant role. It has been shown that autoaggressive $\alpha\beta$+CD8+ memory T cells that persist in the epidermis of the FDE sites play a central role in flare-ups. It has been hypothesized that drugs stimulate keratinocytes in the involved site to a TNF-dependent and rapid expression of intercellular adhesion molecule-1 (ICAM-1). Thus, CD8+ T cells persisting in old FDE sites can be immediately stimulated by ICAM-1. These CD8+ T cells are capable, after stimulation by ICAM-1 to promptly release target amounts of the cytokine interferon-gamma (IFN-γ), which results in the inflammatory flare-up reaction at the site. It is further presumed that elevated expression of FAS in lesional keratinocytes and the increased cytotoxicity of CD8+ T cells induce apoptosis of lesional keratinocytes, predominantly in the basal layer, by means of FAS-FAS ligand interaction. On the other hand, transient intraepidermal migration of CD4+ T cells into active FDE lesions occurs. These regulatory CD4+ T cells are capable of releasing large amounts of interleukin-10 (IL-10), inducing resolution of the flare-up reaction.

Individual reports of the occurrence of FDE in relatives of the first-degree point to the genetic basis of the disease. Tetracyclines, acetylsalicylic acid, TS and ibuprofen were the causative drugs in these reports. Statistically significant correlations have been reported between TS-induced FDE and HLA-A30 (human leukocyte antigen) or the haplotype HLA-A30 B13 Cw6.

Q8. What are the histopathological features of FDE?

Ans: In its classical form, the histopathology of FDE reveals a reaction pattern with lichenoid or erythema multiforme-like changes. The acute phase is characterized by dyskeratosis, hydropic degeneration of the basal cells, dermal edema and a perivascular lymphocytic infiltrate of the upper dermis. Residual pigmentation in the healing phase is accompanied by hyperpigmentation of the basal layer and pigment-laden macrophages in the upper dermis.

Atypical histopathological reaction patterns such as leukocytoclastic vasculitis, neutrophilic reaction and a predominantly dermal reaction without pigment incontinence in what is termed nonpigmented FDE have been reported. In addition, cases with positive immunofluorescence have been described.

Q9. Which of the following statements is NOT true about provocation tests in FDE?

a. The appropriate time of performing the re-challenge is 1 week after the original eruption.
b. Testing is done with a subtherapeutic initial dose, which is gradually increased up to standard dose until a positive result is obtained.
c. Topical provocation tests give positive test reactions usually only at lesional skin.
d. The Kramer algorithm from 1979 with Food and Drug Administration (FDA) modifications has the best diagnostic certainty for drug reactions.

Ans: a. The appropriate time of performing the re-challenge is 1 week after the original eruption.

Q10. What are the provocation tests for FDE?

Ans: In most settings, FDEs are diagnosed on clinical grounds. However, to ascertain the causative drug with confidence, some tests are sometimes essential, especially in cases of multiple drug intake. To establish cause and effect relationship, Kramer algorithm from 1979 with FDA modifications has the best diagnostic certainty for most drug reactions. The algorithm consists of following steps: Challenge, Dechallenge, Rechallenge and Exclusion in addition to the following criteria: Biological Plausibility, Class Effect and Dose Relationship. Rechallenge is the paramount active step necessary to establish causation. It is performed by either systemic or topical provocation.

Systemic provocation is the gold standard in diagnosing FDE. Testing with a subtherapeutic initial dose, e.g. with one-eighths of a tablet, that is increased every 12–24 hours up to a whole tablet, is a suitable method. A positive test result is a flare-up reaction on a FDE lesion within 10–30 min up to 10–18 hours. The optimal time point for systemic provocation is not defined, but it is generally advised to wait at least 4 weeks after resolution of signs and symptoms to avoid false-negative results due to a refractory period.

Topical provocation testing is an alternative diagnostic method, especially for children and in cases of generalized bullous FDE; it is a safe diagnostic first step. The various kinds of skin tests, such as open, patch, photopatch, prick, scratch and intradermal tests, have been tried for the diagnosis of drug eruptions. Among these, the patch test has been the most commonly used method in FDEs.

Q11. How do you manage FDE?

Ans: Treatment:

- Discontinuation of the administered drugs is the first step
- Use of systemic antihistamines with topical corticosteroids is usually necessary to treat the lesions; however, extensive lesions and those surmounted with bullae often require treatment with systemic corticosteroids.
- If lesions are eroded or blister roofs are removed, oral antibacterials may be necessary to prevent secondary infection.
- Protection from recurrence is the most important goal. Effort must be made to ascertain the offending drug. Patients should be advised to avoid not only the offending drug, but sometimes also the drugs that are chemically related to it.

SECTION 2

Bullous Disorders

Soumya Jagadeesan

CHAPTER 5

Pemphigus Vulgaris

Vishal Sharma, Biju Vasudevan

Case study Pemphigus Vulgaris

Presenting Complaints

Doctor, I have been suffering from ulcers in the mouth since last 8 months and have now developed blisters on my body.

Setting

Dermatology outpatient department.

History of Present Illness

A 35-year-old male presented with complaints of oral ulceration of 8 months duration and blisters on the body of 2 months duration. He also complains of difficulty in swallowing solid food associated with pain and bleeding from the gums. There is no history of photosensitivity, drug intake, joint pains or itching.

General Physical Examination and Systemic Examination

No abnormality detected.

Dermatological Examination

- Multiple flaccid bullae present over the chest, abdomen and legs (Fig. 1)
- Nikolsky's sign positive
- Multiple erosions in the oral cavity and gingiva along with crusting of lips (Fig. 2).

Q1. What is the most likely diagnosis?

a. Pemphigus vulgaris (PV)

b. Toxic epidermal necrolysis

c. Pemphigus foliaceus

d. Bullous pemphigoid

Ans: a. Pemphigus vulgaris; presence of oral ulcers with flaccid bulla over the body with Nikolsky's sign positivity is a hallmark of PV.

Q2. How will you distinguish the condition from pemphigus foliaceus, bullous pemphigoid and toxic epidermal necrolysis (TEN)?

Ans: Pemphigus foliaceus does not produce oral lesions and pemphigoid has large intact tense blisters associated with pruritus and oral lesions are rare. In case of TEN, the history is short and there will be history of drug intake with causal relationship and other mucosal surfaces will also be involved.

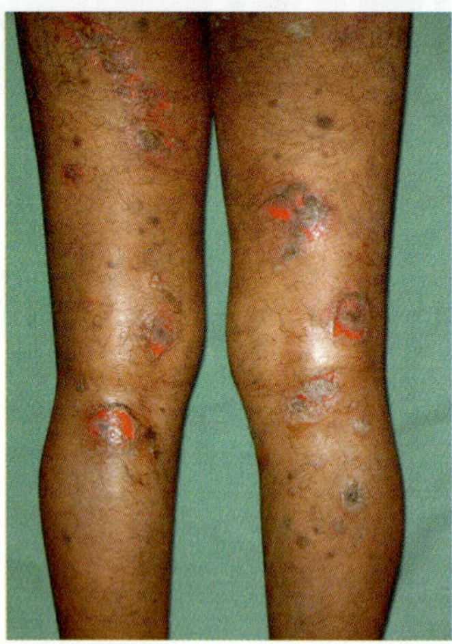

Fig. 1: Multiple flaccid bullae and erosions on lower limbs

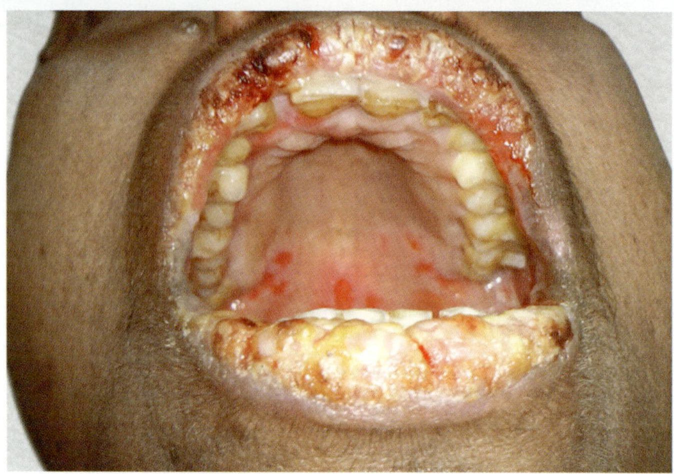

Fig. 2: Multiple oral erosions and crusting of lips

Q3. How will you confirm the diagnosis?

Ans: Diagnosis is made on clinical grounds. Tzanck smear, skin biopsy and direct immunofluorescence are the tests done to confirm the diagnosis.

Q4. What is Tzanck smear and what are the findings in PV?

Ans: Tzanck smear is a very simple and rapid technique. In case of blistering disorders, the intact roof of a blister is opened along one side, folded back and the floor is gently scraped. The material thus obtained is smeared onto a microscopic slide, allowed to air dry, and stained with Giemsa stain. It reveals multiple acantholytic cells (Tzanck cells). A typical Tzanck cell is a large round keratinocyte with a hypertrophic nucleus, hazy or absent nucleoli, and abundant basophilic cytoplasm. The basophilic staining is deeper peripherally on the cell membrane ("mourning edged" cells) due to the tendency of the cytoplasm to get condensed at the periphery, resulting in a perinuclear halo.

Q5. What are the findings of skin biopsy?

Ans: The characteristic-histologic finding is suprabasilar separation or blister formation with acantholysis. The basal cells remain attached to the basement membrane but lose their contact with neighboring cells and as a result, they appear as a "row of tomb stones".

Q6. What are the antibodies involved in PV?

Ans: The autoimmune target of pemphigus is desmoglein, a cadherin type of cell-to-cell adhesion molecule found in the desmosomes. There are three isotypes of desmoglein (Dsg): Dsg1, Dsg2 and Dsg3. Dsg1 and Dsg3 are usually restricted to the stratified squamous epithelia, where blister formation occurs in pemphigus. Patients with pemphigus have anti-Dsg1 and/or anti-Dsg3 immunoglobulin G (IgG) autoantibodies. IgG1 and IgG4 are the most common subclasses of antibodies in patients with active disease, but IgG4 is more pathogenic and indicates the activity of the disease. In PV, both anti-Dsg1 and Dsg3 are present.

Q7. What is the use of direct and indirect immunofluorescence findings in PV?

Ans: Direct immunofluorescence (DIF) is a one-step procedure used to detect and localize immunoreactants deposited in vivo in the patient's skin or mucosa. The immunoreactants include antibodies, complement components and fibrinogen. Indirect immunofluorescence (IIF) is a two-step procedure used to identify circulating autoantibodies to cutaneous or mucosal structures in a patient's serum. These antibodies are most commonly of IgG or IgA classes. The hallmark of pemphigus is the finding of IgG autoantibodies against cell surface keratinocytes. The diagnosis of pemphigus is questioned if DIF is negative. However there is imperfect correlation between DIF and disease activity in patients.

Q8. Which test is used for assessment of disease activity?

Ans: Besides clinical improvement, enzyme-linked immunosorbent assay (ELISA) for anti-Dsg1 and anti-Dsg3 antibodies are more specific and sensitive markers of disease activity.

Q9. What is the role of diet in PV?

Ans: The possible etiologic role of dietary factors in the development and exacerbation of pemphigus has recently been documented. Among the enormous variety of chemical compounds that are present in the diet; thiols, isothiocyanates, phenols and tannins seem to be responsible for induction of pemphigus in genetically predisposed subjects. It is advisable for pemphigus patients to reduce the consumption of foods and drinks with a high content of the above chemical compounds.

Q10. What are the drugs causing PV?

Ans: Drugs containing sulfhydryl groups, like penicillamine and captopril, are the drugs causing PV.

Q11. What are the diseases associated with PV?

Ans: Autoimmune disorders like myasthenia gravis and thymoma. Malignancies like Castleman's disease can also be associated with PV.

Q12. What is paraneoplastic pemphigus (PNP)?

Ans: Paraneoplastic pemphigus was first described by Anhalt et al. in 1990. PNP affects organ systems other than the integument and thus, the term "paraneoplastic autoimmune multiorgan syndrome (PAMS)" has been suggested as a more appropriate name for the syndrome. It may be considered as an example of a rare paraneoplastic phenomenon that occurs as an autoimmune disorder, initiated by a lymphoreticular neoplasm. PNP is associated mostly with non-Hodgkin's lymphoma, chronic lymphocytic leukemia and Castleman's disease.

Paraneoplastic pemphigus can be identified by the following features:

- Painful, recalcitrant stomatitis and a polymorphous cutaneous eruption that may be bullous/lichenoid/resembling erythema multiforme or a drug eruption or graft versus host disease
- Histologic findings showing lichenoid change/acantholysis/interface change
- Direct immunofluorescence studies showing fishnet pattern of IgG and complement (C3) deposition similar to PV along with a linear/granular pattern of complement deposition along the basement membrane
- Serum autoantibodies that bind simple, columnar and transitional epithelia
- Serum autoantibodies against Dsg1 and Dsg3, as well as members of the plakin family of epithelial proteins.

Along with the treatment or resection of the underlying neoplasm, the disease has to be treated as an autoimmune disorder, though the disease, especially the stomatitis may be refractory to the usual modalities of treatment. Rituximab may be useful in recalcitrant cases.

Q13. What are the treatment modalities of PV?

Ans: Systemic steroids along with adjuvant immunosuppressive agents like cyclophosphamide, cyclosporine, mycophenolate mofetil and azathioprine are mainstays. Steroids are administered orally at 1–2 mg/kg or in form of pulse therapy with either methylprednisolone or dexamethasone. Treatment regimens can start with both steroids and immunosuppressive agents together and gradually steroids can be tapered off. Other therapies include gold, plasmapheresis, intravenous immunoglobulin (IVIg) and extracorporeal photochemotherapy.

Q14. Enumerate the management of PV during acute phase?

Ans: The management of PV during active phase of the disease necessitates intensive care, preferably in intensive care unit (ICU) till the acute skin failure is under control, besides definitive treatment for the underlying disease. The supportive management involves skin care, barrier nursing, maintenance of fluid and electrolytes, ambient temperature with proper nutritional support.

Q15. What is dexamethasone cyclophosphamide pulse (DCP) therapy?

Ans: This regime was first used in the treatment of PV by Pasricha et al., modified from the use in rheumatoid arthritis. The entire treatment is divided into four phases as per the protocol:

1. Phase I: Patients receive monthly doses of 100 mg of dexamethasone dissolved in 500 mL of 5% dextrose by slow IV infusion over 2 hour on 3 consecutive days along with 500 mg of cyclophosphamide in the infusion on day 2. In between, the patients receive 50 mg of oral cyclophosphamide daily and this is continued in monthly cycles till patient achieves remission.
2. Phase II: Patients are in remission but monthly DCP therapy and daily oral cyclophosphamide are continued for 9 months.
3. Phase III: Only oral cyclophosphamide 50 mg was given to patients for an additional 9 months.
4. Phase IV: All treatments were withdrawn and patients are followed up for relapse, if any.

Q16. What is gold therapy in PV?

Ans: Oral or IV gold preparations along with steroids were used earlier. Parenteral sodium thiomalate or aurothioglucose 25 mg/week, later increased to 50 mg/week has been used alone or with steroids. Side effects includes bone marrow toxicity, renal toxicity and cutaneous allergic reactions.

Q17. What is the role of rituximab in PV?

Ans: Rituximab is a chimeric monoclonal antibody directed against CD20 and acts by causing death of CD20 positive cells (cells of β cell lineage, which produce the autoantibodies) by complement-dependent cytotoxicity and antibody-dependent cellular cytotoxicity.

Q18. What are the indications of rituximab therapy?

Ans: Rituximab is indicated in PV patients who fail to respond adequately to conventional treatment modality, or in whom systemic corticosteroids and/or other immunosuppressants are contraindicated or cause severe adverse effects requiring its discontinuation. It is also indicated in patients who relapse following treatment with conventional drugs.

Q19. What are the treatment protocols with rituximab therapy?

Ans: The various treatment protocols followed include:

- Lymphoma protocol: Most commonly followed protocol. Rituximab is administered at a dose of 375 mg/m^2 body surface area weekly for 4 weeks.
- Rheumatoid arthritis protocol: Two doses of rituximab 1 g is administered at an interval of 15 days. It is increasingly used by dermatologists and advantages over the lymphoma protocol include less cost and fewer infusions.
- Combination therapy: Rituximab has been used in combination with IVIg, immunoadsorption and dexamethasone pulse therapy
- Long-term rituximab treatment with regular infusions every 4 weeks or 12 weeks following an induction cycle of infusions every week.

Q20. What is the mortality rate in PV?

Ans: Until the introduction of system corticosteroids, PV was an almost invariably fatal disease with a mortality rate of up to 90%. After the advent of corticosteroids in the 1950s, the mortality rate decreased dramatically. Mortality rates continued to decline, more slowly in the 1970s to an average of 60% and have remained essentially unchanged during the past 2 decades between 5% and 15%, with the concurrent use of immunosuppressive agents.

CHAPTER 6

Pemphigus Foliaceus

Deepashree Daulatabad

Case study Pemphigus Foliaceus

Presenting Complaints

Doctor, I am developing a lot of itchy and scaly rashes and a few blisters over my scalp, face, chest and upper back since the past 2 months.

Setting

Dermatology out-patient department.

History of Present Illness

A 35-year-old gentleman presented with complaints of multiple itchy, crusted, red raised lesions over the scalp, face, chest and the upper back since 2 months. The patient had also noticed occasional fluid filled lesions over the same sites which ruptured within a day, leaving behind erosions. The patient continues to develop two-three such lesions daily, with extension of the preexisting lesions. There is no history of any oral or genital lesions. There is no history of any new drug intake prior to the onset of the lesions. The patient also denied any systemic complaints.

General Physical Examination and Systemic Examination

No abnormality detected.

Dermatological Examination

- Multiple crusted papules and plaques present over an erythematous base, in a predominantly seborrhoeic distribution involving the scalp, face, chest and the upper back (Figs 1 and 2).
- Occasional intact flaccid vesicles and bullae containing clear fluid and demonstrating a positive bulla spread sign. Perilesional Nikolsky sign positive but direct Nikolsky negative.
- Oral and genital mucosa: Within normal limits, with no evidence of erosions or ulceration

Q1. What is the most likely diagnosis?

a. Pemphigus vulgaris
b. Pemphigus foliaceus
c. Bullous pemphigoid
d. IgA pemphigus

Ans: b. Pemphigus foliaceus.

Presence of predominantly crusted papules and plaques with occasional flaccid bullae in a seborrhocic distribution with sparing of the mucosa, in a middle-aged individual, is highly suggestive of pemphigus foliaceus. Positive bulla spread sign and Nikolsky test also favor the diagnosis of an intraepidermal blistering disorder.

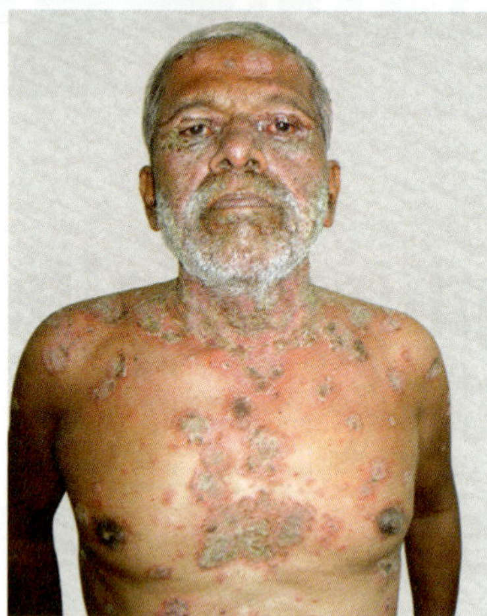

Fig. 1: Extensive scaly crusted plaques on scalp, face and upper chest

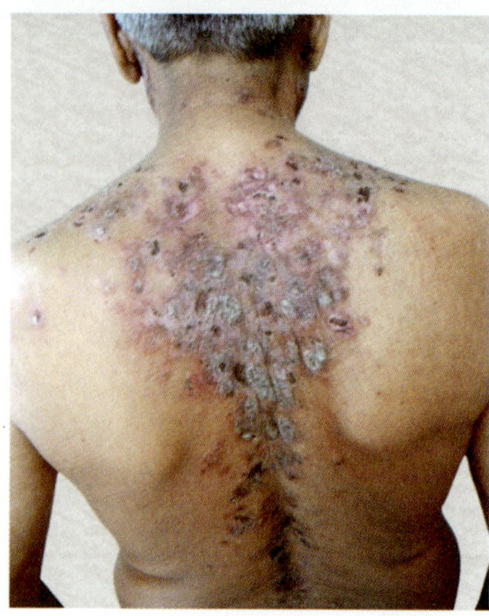

Fig. 2: Similar lesions on upper back

Q2. Which bed-side test can help you reach a diagnosis?

Ans: Demonstration of acantholytic cells in a Tzanck smear can reliably help in making the diagnosis of an intraepidermal blistering disorder which includes both pemphigus foliaceus and pemphigus vulgaris. Both these conditions will demonstrate acantholytic cells, but the latter shows rounder cells with a higher nucleocytoplasmic ratio whereas the former has flatter acantholytic cells with a smaller nucleocytoplasmic ratio in the background of lymphocytes, neutrophils and occasional eosinophils.

Q3. In pemphigus foliaceus, what is the target antigen and its molecular weight?

a. Desmoglein 1, 160 kDa
b. Desmoglein 1, 130 kDa
c. Desmoglein 3, 160 kDa
d. Desmoglein 3, 130 kDa

Ans: a. Desmoglein 1, 160 kDa.

Pemphigus foliaceus is an autoimmune blistering disorder. Sera of the patients contain circulating pathogenic antibodies against the extracellular aminoterminal domain of desmoglein-1, a 160-kDa desmosomal cadherin. The location of this antigen explains the clinical manifestation of the disease. Desmoglein-1 is expressed more strongly in skin from the upper torso than from the lower torso or scalp and it is weakly expressed in mucosae, thus accounting for the predominant involvement of upper torso with lack of mucosal involvement in pemphigus foliaceus.

Q4. How will you confirm the suspected diagnosis?

Ans: Skin biopsy from a fresh intact vesicle for hemotoxylin and eosin staining will demonstrate the presence of a cleft or split in the superficial epidermis either in the granular layer or just beneath the stratum corneum. The cleft contains acantholytic keratinocytes, some neutrophils and fibrin. The dermis shows a mixed inflammatory infiltrate of eosinophils and neutrophils. The older lesions of pemphigus foliaceus demonstrates acanthosis, hyperkeratosis and focal parakeratosis along with the presence of dyskeratotic cells in the granular layer, the latter (dyskeratotic cells) are lacking in pemphigus vulgaris.

Direct immunofluorescence from perilesional skin demonstrates immunoglobulin G (IgG) and C3 deposition in a fishnet pattern among the keratinocytes, which is higher in intensity at the superficial part of the epidermis.

Indirect immunofluorescence is positive in 85% cases.

Enzyme-linked immunosorbent assay demonstrates antibodies against desmoglein -1. Immunoblotting may demonstrate the target antigen. Electron microscopy demonstrates loss of desmosomes, detachment of keratin tonofilaments and dyskeratosis.

Q5. What are the various intraepidermal immunobullous disorders and how do you classify them?

Ans: The various intraepidermal immunobullous disorders are classified as under:

- Pemphigus vulgaris:
  - Variant: Pemphigus vegetans

- Pemphigus foliaceus:
  - Variant: Pemphigus herpetiformis
  - Variant: Pemphigus erythematosus
  - Variant: Endemic pemphigus
- Induced pemphigus
- Intercellular IgA dermatosis
- Paraneoplastic pemphigus.

Q6. What are the main clinical variants of pemphigus foliaceus and how do you recognize them?

Ans: There exist two main clinical variants of pemphigus foliaceus—pemphigus herpetiformis and pemphigus erythematosus.

- *Pemphigus herpetiformis*: A rare and atypical variant that clinically resembles dermatitis herpetiformis (grouped pruritic papules and vesicles on an erythematous base) but on immunofluorescence, resembles pemphigus foliaceus (intercellular staining for IgG). Histopathology reveals subcorneal pustules, eosinophilic spongiosis or features of dermatitis herpetiformis with no acantholysis. Circulating IgG autoantibodies against either desmoglein-1 or desmoglein-3 or neither antigen may be found. The disease is usually benign and eventually evolves into the classical form of pemphigus foliaceus or rarely into pemphigus vulgaris.
- *Pemphigus erythematosus (Senear–Usher syndrome)*: This is another rare form of pemphigus foliaceus that clinically as well as immunologically resembles a combination of lupus erythematosus and pemphigus foliaceus. In addition to the features of pemphigus foliaceus, patients also develop erythematous scaly lesions over the nose and malar areas, resembling the butterfly rash of cutaneous lupus erythematosus. Photo-exacerbation is often noted and strict photo protection is advisable. On direct immunofluorescence again, both intercellular IgG and C3 in the epidermis as well as a granular IgG and C3 at the basement membrane zone is observed. Circulating antibodies against desmoglein-1 and antinuclear antibodies can be detected, but the disease rarely progresses to systemic lupus erythematosus. Association with myasthenia gravis or thymoma has been observed.

Q7. What do you understand by fogo selvagem?

Ans: Fogo selvagem (meaning *wild fire* in Portuguese) is another name for endemic pemphigus foliaceus or Brazilian pemphigus foliaceus that is endemic to certain parts of South America. It mainly affects children and young adults and shows temporal and familial clustering in the endemic zones, suggestive of some infectious etiology. Clinically, patients develop flaccid bullae that rupture to leave behind superficial erosions. Classically, the patients have a burnt appearance and complain of burning sensation, particularly on sun exposure and hence the name, fogo selvagem. Histologically and immunopathologically, it resembles the classical pemphigus foliaceus.

Q8. How will you manage this patient?

Ans: Pemphigus foliaceus is usually a benign disease of long duration.

Supportive therapy: Local skin care of the lesions is of utmost importance. Daily bathing or cleaning of the lesions as well as scalp hygiene are essential. A bland emollient dressing can prevent friction and further development of new lesions secondary to trauma. Topical steroid preparation or a combination of steroid-antibiotic (in case of infected lesions) can help in early healing of the lesions.

In case of extensive skin involvement, strict input-output charting along with close monitoring of the pulse rate, BP, temperature and electrolytes is a must. Adequate hydration should be ensured via oral or intravenous route as the patient is prone to develop dehydration secondary to excessive fluid loss. In the presence of secondary infection, presumptive broad spectrum oral or intravenous antibiotics may have to be initiated. Further antibiotics should be guided by the blood and pus culture sensitivity reports.

An initial hematological and biochemical work up in the form of a complete hemogram, liver and renal function tests, fasting blood glucose and lipid profile is a must. Since this is an autoimmune blistering disorder, the specific therapy deals with immunosuppression. Any other cause of immunosuppression like HIV, diabetes or drug-induced immunosuppression should be evaluated. Evaluation for an occult focus of infection like tuberculosis, urinary tract infection, secondary infection of the lesions, etc. should be evaluated and treated.

Specific therapy: The disease specific therapeutic options include daily oral steroids, steroid pulse therapy along with adjuvants like cyclophosphamide, azathioprine, cyclosporine, mycophenolate mofetil, methotrexate, nicotinamide with tetracyclines and dapsone. In severe or recalcitrant cases, intravenous immunoglobulins can be used. Rituximab has also shown promising results.

Q9. What are the potential complications of this disease?

Ans: When localized, the disease is not life-threatening, but an extensive skin involvement can lead to skin failure. The potential complications are as enumerated:

- Acute skin failure
- Dehydration due to excessive fluid loss from skin
- Secondary skin infections
- Hypothermia
- Hypoproteinemia
- Electrolyte imbalance
- Acute renal failure, mostly prerenal in origin, secondary to excessive fluid loss
- Sepsis
- Multiorgan failure secondary to sepsis
- High output cardiac failure secondary to skin failure.

Q10. What is the prognosis of this disease?

Ans: Pemphigus foliaceus has a chronic but benign disease course.

CHAPTER 7

Subepidermal Blistering Disorders

Mary Thomas

Case study Subepidermal Blistering Disorders

Presenting Complaints

Doctor, I have multiple large blisters on my body along with itching for the past 2 weeks.

Setting

Dermatology inpatient department.

History of Presenting Complaints

A 60-year-old man presented with multiple blisters on his trunk and limbs for the past 2 weeks. The blisters started as reddish itchy lesions and later became fluid filled. These blisters would not burst spontaneously and when they were scratched and ruptured, they formed raw areas. These lesions later healed with dark pigmentation. There was no history of involvement of the oral cavity, genitalia, face or scalp. There was no history of previous medications, photosensitivity, gluten intolerance and no significant family history.

General Physical Examination and Systemic Examination

No abnormality detected.

Dermatological Examination

- Multiple tense vesicles and bullae present on the trunk and limbs (Figs 1 and 2).
- Few urticarial plaques interspersed.
- Few erosions with crusting, healing with hyperpigmentation.
- Mucosal surfaces, face and scalp are spared.

Q1. What is the most likely diagnosis?

a. Bullous pemphigoid
b. Pemphigus vulgaris
c. Dermatitis herpetiformis
d. Cicatricial pemphigoid

Ans: a. Bullous pemphigoid.

Q2. What is the clinical differential diagnosis of subepidermal bullous disorders?

Ans: Clinical differential diagnosis has been described in Table 1.

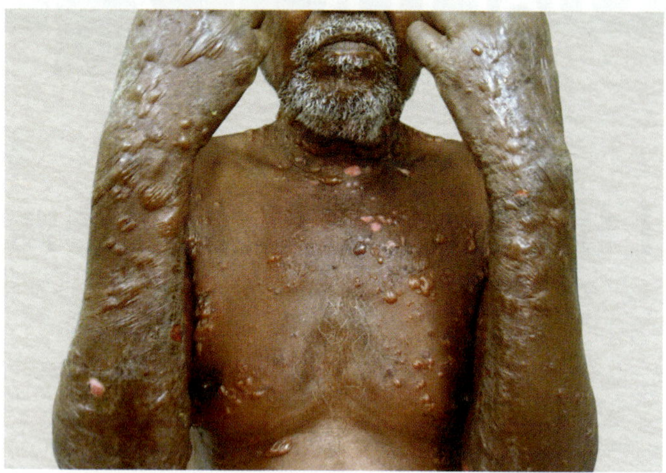

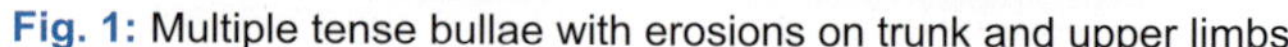

Fig. 1: Multiple tense bullae with erosions on trunk and upper limbs

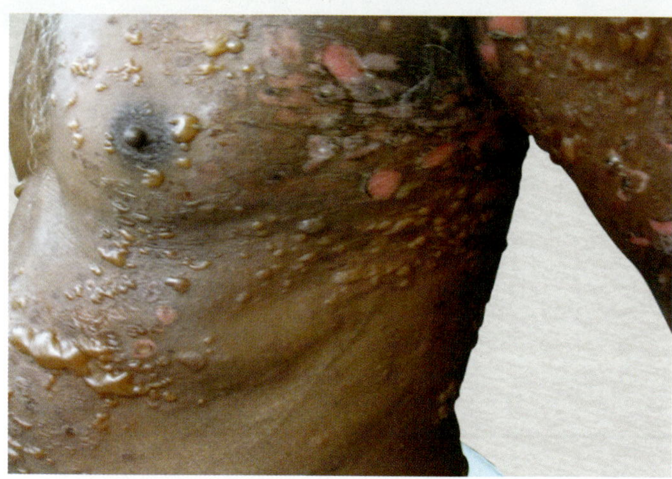

Fig. 2: Similar lesions on left side of trunk

Table 1: Clinical differential diagnosis of subepidermal bullous disorders

	Diagnosis	*Age*	*Cutaneous involvement*	*Mucosal/systemic*	*Course*
1.	Bullous pemphigoid (BP)	60 years	Multiple fluid filled vesicles which rupture with crusting and erosions Heals with hyperpigmentation. Lower limbs > upper limbs > trunk	Rare	Benign
2.	Epidermolysis bullosa acquisita (EBA)	Elderly	Multiple tense bullae, milia and scars. Trauma prone sites	Spared	Chronic course with exacerbations and remissions
3.	Epidermolysis bullosa (EB)	Childhood	Multiple bullae which rupture to form erosions, primarily on trauma prone sites. Heal with scarring. Features vary with type. Trauma prone sites, bony prominences	May be involved	Chronic progressive
4.	Porphyria cutanea tarda	Sporadic: Adulthood Genetic: Childhood	Multiple bullae on the sun exposed areas, especially the face, ears and backs of the hands. Onycholysis, hypertrichosis. Aggravated by alcohol and estrogens	Spared. Rarely hepatic	Chronic relapsing and remitting
5.	Dermatitis herpetiformis (DH)	Between second and fourth decade	Multiple tense bullae of varying sizes. New blisters form around healing old blisters forming "a cluster of jewels." Intensely pruritic chronic grouped papules and vesicles distributed symmetrically on extensor surfaces, buttocks, hairline and nuchal region	Rare. Gluten sensitive enteropathy	Remitting and relapsing
6.	Chronic bullous disease of childhood (CBDC)	Occurs before 5 years of age	Lower trunk, genital area, and thighs May also affect the scalp	Perioral and mucosal involvement present	Vancomycin, lithium, diclofenac intake. Course is chronic and spontaneous remission usually occurs after an average of 3–4 years
7.	Linear immunoglobulin A (IgA) disease	Two peaks: teens and sixth decade	DH type: Extensor surfaces BP type: Flexural. Erythema multiforme type: Annular or grouped papules, vesicles and bullae	Oral cavity and eyes are the most commonly affected	Drugs, lymphoproliferative disorders, infections, ulcerative colitis, systemic lupus erythematosus (SLE). Chronic relapsing course

Contd...

Contd...

	Diagnosis	Age	Cutaneous involvement	Mucosal/systemic	Course
8.	Bullous lupus erythematosus	Adults	Tense bullae arising from erythematous or normal appearing skin. Some lesions are hemorrhagic. Sun exposed areas	Involved. SLE features	Depends on systemic involvement
9.	Pemphigoid gestationis	Women in child-bearing age group. Second trimester to immediate post-partum period	Extremely pruritic, polymorphic eruption–urticarial plaques, bullae, pruritic papules. Abdomen (involves umbilicus), unlike pruritic papules and plaques of pregnancy	Spared	May recur in subsequent pregnancies
10.	Mucous membrane pemphigoid (MMP)	Adults	Tense bullae similar to BP Predominantly mucosal involvement	Prominent mucosal involvement with extensive scarring. Solid organ malignancy	Chronic progressive

Q3. What are the bedside clinical tests that can be performed to differentiate pemphigus from pemphigoid?

Ans: The following bedside clinical tests can be performed to differentiate BP from pemphigus:

Nikolsky's sign: Slight rubbing of the skin results in the formation of an intraepidermal cleft manifesting as a blister. This sign is positive in pemphigus but absent in BP. This sign has also been used to monitor disease activity.

Bulla spread sign: The '"bulla spread sign"' refers to the extension of a blister to adjacent unblistered skin when pressure is put on the top of the bulla. While a regular rounded border is observed in BP and other subepidermal blistering disorders, irregular angulated border is seen in pemphigus vulgaris.

Q4. What bedside laboratory test would you do to support your diagnosis?

Ans: *Tzanck smear*: Bullous pemphigoid shows scarcity of epithelial cells and an abundance of leukocytes, particularly eosinophils with leukocyte adherence on Tzanck smear.

Q5. How do you confirm the diagnosis?

Ans: *Skin biopsy*: A skin biopsy taken from a recent blister from a nonfrictional site is ideal. More than one site should be biopsied in cases of polymorphous eruption. For immunofluorescence, a specimen taken from a perilesional site should be sent in Michael's solution. The histological findings along with differential diagnosis are listed in Table 2.

Q6. What is the pathogenesis of bullous pemphigoid?

Ans: Immunoglobulin G autoantibodies against bullous pemphigoid antigen (BPAg) 1 and 2 located in the basement membrane lead to clefting at the level of the lamina lucida.

Table 2: Histological findings to confirm the diagnosis

	Diagnosis	Histopathology	DIF	IIF
1.	Bullous pemphigoid	Subepidermal blister with prominent eosinophil infiltration	Linear band of C3 and IgG at the basement membrane zone. Salt split skin revealed IgG on the blister roof	Circulating IgG to BMZ in 70–80% of the patients Serum levels of autoantibodies against BPAg 2 correlate with disease activity
2.	EBA	Subepidermal blister with mixed infiltrate	Linear band of IgG and C3 at BMZ. Salt split skin: Antibodies bind to the floor of the blister	IgG and C3 against type VII collagen
4.	Porphyria cutanea tarda	Subepidermal bulla with festooning of dermal papillae. Cell poor infiltrate	Vessels show homogenous and intense fluorescence as well as in the dermal-epidermal junction	Often negative for circulating antibodies

Contd...

Contd...

	Diagnosis	Histopathology	DIF	IIF
5.	DH	Subepidermal blister at the level of the lamina lucid with neutrophilic abscesses in the dermal papillae Dermal infiltrate of neutrophils	Granular IgA1 deposits in the dermal papillae	Often negative for circulating IgA antibodies
6.	CBDC/Linear IgA disease	Subepidermal bullae with a collection of neutrophils along the basement membrane	Linear pattern of IgG and C3 along the basement membrane Salt split skin is positive on the epidermal side in 60–70% of the cases.	Circulating IgA antibodies are rare (7–30% of the cases) and IIF should be performed to dismiss other dermatoses such as BP
7.	Bullous LE	Subepidermal cleft with a neutrophilic infiltrate in the upper dermis. Perivascular lymphocytic infiltrate Thickened BMZ Vacuolar interface dermatitis	Perilesional skin shows granular BMZ granular IgG and C3 deposit along BMZ Salt split skin: Deposits on floor of blister	Subdivided into type 1 and 2 depending on the presence or absence respectively of type VII collagen
8.	Pemphigoid gestationis	Basal cell vacuolization Subepidermal cleft Papillary dermal edema with eosinophilic infiltrate	Linear C3 deposits in the BMZ in 100% of the cases. Linear IgG deposits in the BMZ are found in 30–40% of the cases Salt split skin: Fluorescence on the epidermal side	Circulating antibodies of the IgG1 subclass in 10–20%. HG factor positive
9.	MMP	Subepidermal bulla with thickened collagen in the dermis indicating scarring	Linear IgG and C3 deposits in the BMZ IgA in the BMZ occurs in 20% of the cases Salt split skin: Positivity in the epidermal and dermal side	Rarely positive

Abbreviations: DIF, direct immunofluorescence; IIF, indirect immunofluorescence; BMZ, basement membrane zone; BPAg, bullous pemphigoid antigen; LE, lupus erythematosus

Bullous pemphigoid antigen 1:
- 230 kDa
- Intracellular portion of hemidesmosome.

Bullous pemphigoid antigen 2:
- 180 kDa, type XVII collagen
- Transmembranous protein with a collagenous extracellular domain.

Q7. What are the precipitating factors of BP?

Ans: The following have been found to precipitate BP:
- Mostly sporadic
- Ultraviolet light
- Radiation therapy
- Percutaneous endoscopic gastrostomy
- Burns
- Scars
- Adhesive dressing.

Q8. Name some diseases that occur in association with BP.

Ans: The following disease may occur in association with BP:
- Diabetes mellitus
- Pernicious anemia
- Lichen planus
- Psoriasis
- Multiple sclerosis
- Nephropathy
- Eosinophilia
- Elevated IgE
- Various malignancies.

Q9. What are the drugs associated with bullous pemphigoid?

Ans: The following drugs have been implicated in BP:
- Furosemide
- Ibuprofen
- Nonsteroidal anti-inflammatory drugs
- Captopril
- Penicillamine
- Antibiotics.

Q10. What best describes the histopathology of bullous pemphigoid?

a. Subepidermal cleft with neutrophils
b. Subepidermal cleft with eosinophils
c. Intraepidermal cleft with eosinophils

d. Suprabasal cleft with lymphocytes

Ans: b. Subepidermal cleft with eosinophils.

Q11. What are the newer investigations for BP?

Ans: Newer investigations to diagnose BP include:
- Immunoelectron microscopy
- Immunoblotting
- Immunoprecipitation
- Enzyme-linked immunosorbent assay
- Immunohistochemistry.

Q12. What are the variants of BP?

Ans: Some of the important variants of BP are:
- Childhood BP
- Urticarial BP
- Vesicular BP
- Vegetative BP
- Pemphigoid nodularis
- Localized BP
- Erythrodermic BP
- Acral BP
- Drug induced BP
- 105 kDa Ag anti P 105 pemphigoid.

Q13. What are the treatment options for this patient?

Ans: The treatment options for this patient are as follows:
- *First-line treatment*: Immunosuppressive agents to control disease
  - Systemic prednisone: Daily oral/pulsed rarely
  - Cyclophosphamide
  - Azathioprine
  - Mycophenolate mofetil
  - Methotrexate
  - Cyclosporine A
- *Others*: anti-inflammatory agents
  - Dapsone
  - Tetracyclines and nicotinamide
  - Intravenous immunoglobulins
  - High potency topical steroids
- *Newer drugs*:
  - Rituximab
  - Intravenous immunoglobulin
  - Plasma exchange.

Q14. What is the prognosis of BP?

Ans: Self-limiting disease with a chronic relapsing and remitting course.

SECTION 3

Nevi and Vascular Malformations/Tumors

Deepashree Daulatabad

CHAPTER 8

Verrucous Epidermal Nevus

Bhushan Madke

Case study **Verrucous Epidermal Nevus**

Presenting Complaints

Doctor, please have a look at this skin abnormality which is present on my nose. As far as I remember this skin problem is present since birth. I noticed that this abnormality has become more prominent and rough to feel in past few years. Please help me.

Setting

Dermatology outpatient department.

History of Presenting Illness

An 18-year-old boy, presented with the chief complaint of a single rough linear raised lesion on his nose present since birth. It has progressively increased in size to the present condition. He gives no history of any systemic illness.

General Examination and Systemic Examination

No abnormality detected.

Dermatological Examination

A single verrucous linear line of coalescing papules measuring 4 × 0.5 centimeter is present on the nose (Fig. 1). There is no oozing, scaling or crusting.

Q1. What is your diagnosis?

a. Nevus sebaceous
b. Warts
c. Linear verrucous epidermal nevus
d. Linear hypertrophic lichen planus

Ans. c. Linear verrucous epidermal nevus. It is feature of cutaneous mosaicism.

Q2. What is cutaneous mosaicism?

Ans: The term mosaicism refers to the occurrence of two or more genotypically different cell populations derived from a single zygote within an individual. It happens due to postzygotic mutation. Cutaneous mosaicisms are the clinical expression of these disorders.

Q3. What is the pattern followed by mosaic disorders?

Ans: Cutaneous diseases that reflect mosaicism are distributed along certain patterns and forms. The prototype for patterns of cutaneous mosaicism is the Blaschko's line system, originally described in 1901 by Alfred Blaschko.

Q4. What are Blaschko's lines?

Ans: These are invisible lines within human skin that indicate keratinocyte migration pathway during

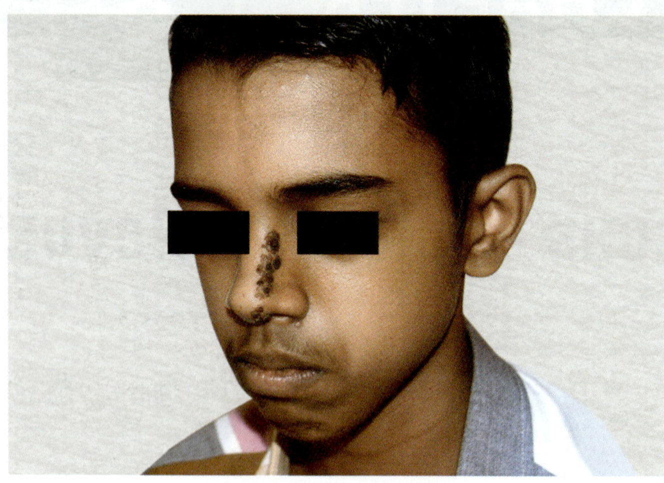

Fig. 1: Linear verrucous coalescing papules on nose

embryonic life. They are not visible in normal condition but become apparent in certain cutaneous disorders.

Q5. What are the patterns described by Alfred Blaschko for mosaic disorders?

Ans: Patterns of Blaschko's lines:

Type 1a: Blaschko lines, narrow bands
Type 1b: Blaschko lines, broad bands
Type 2: The "Checkerboard" pattern
Type 3: The Phylloid pattern
Type 4: Patchy pattern without midline separation
Type 5: Lateralization pattern.

Q6. Describe verrucous epidermal nevus.

Ans: Verrucous epidermal nevi (VEN) are characterized by brownish or skin-colored papules and/or plaques, with a verrucous or velvety surface, following the Blaschko lines. It originates from keratinocytes.

Q7. What are the forms in which epidermal verrucous nevus can present?

Ans: Forms of epidermal verrucous nevus:

- Localized
- Systematized
- Nevus unius lateralis
- Ichthyosis hystrix
- ILVEN (Inflammatory Linear Verrucous Epidermal Nevus).

Q8. What is the histopathology of VEN?

Ans: Hyperkeratosis, acanthosis, papillomatosis are seen in most of the patients with VEN. Depending upon different types, picture may vary like in ichthyosis hystrix: epidermal hyperkeratosis is the prominent finding. In ILVEN: psoriasiform hyperplasia with chronic inflammatory infiltrate and alternate bands of ortho and parakeratosis are seen.

Q9. What is Epidermal nevus syndromes?

Ans: Epidermal nevus syndromes (ENSs) are a group of rare complex disorders characterized by the presence of skin lesions known as epidermal nevi associated with additional extracutaneous abnormalities, most often affecting the brain, eye and skeletal systems. Solomon defines epidermal nevus syndrome as a sporadic neurocutaneous linkage of congenital ectodermal defects in the skin, brain, eyes, and/or skeleton.

- Angora hair nevus syndrome—characterized by lanugo-like depigmented hypertrichosis developing along the Blaschko's lines.
- Becker nevus syndrome—characterized by the presence of a Becker nevus in association with hypoplasia of the ipsilateral breast or other skin-related, muscular, or skeletal defects usually of the same side of the body.
- CHILD syndrome—congenital hemidysplasia with ichthyosiform nevus and limb defects
- Garcia-Hafner-Happle syndrome—characterized by characterized by epidermal nevus in association with acanthosis nigricans, and neurological abnormalities like seizures, intellectual impairment, cortical atrophy, and underdevelopment of corpus callosum.
- Nevus comedonicus syndrome—presents as confluent clusters of dilated follicular orifices that are plugged with keratin. This gives the appearance of aggregated open comedones present in a Blaschkoid pattern.
- Phacomatosis pigmentokeratotica—characterized by multiple organoid nevi with sebaceous differentiation, a speckled lentiginous nevus, and skeletal and neurologic abnormalities. It may or may not be associated with extracutaneous manifestations.
- Proteus syndrome—a hamartomatous disorder associated overgrowth of skin, connective tissue, fat, bones and other tissues.

- Schimmelpenning syndrome—characterized by sebaceous nevus with cerebral anomalies, coloboma and lipodermoid of the conjunctiva.
- Type 2 segmental Cowden disease—characterized by the association of nonorganoid epidermal nevus with Cowden disease.

Q10. What are the treatment options for verrucous epidermal nevus?

Ans: Treatment options for verrucous epidermal nevus are:

- Surgical excision
- Carbon dioxide laser
- Radiofrequency ablation
- Electrocautery.

Q11. What is the prognosis?

Ans: Prognosis:

- Usually appears after birth and enlarges in size up to puberty.
- Epidermal nevi in flexural areas may be macerated, infected and cause significant discomfort.
- May be seen as a part of epidermal nevus syndrome.
- Rarely it may turn into basal cell carcinoma or squamous cell carcinoma.

CHAPTER 9

Nevus Sebaceous

Kingshuk Chatterjee

Case study Nevus Sebaceous

Presenting Complaints

Doctor, my daughter has developed an orange-colored elevation over the scalp since last 4 years. There is no pain or itching. She is also not growing hair in that region.

Setting

Dermatology outpatient department.

History of Present Illness

An 8-year-old girl presented with complaints of progressive thickening of skin over the occipital area of scalp with orange discoloration, for last 4 years. It was not associated with any itching or pain. Her mother revealed that she did not have hair in that area. There was no history of similar illness in the family. There was no history of birth trauma or trauma during assisted delivery.

General Physical Examination and Systemic Examination

No abnormality detected.

Dermatological Examination

- A circumscribed 5 × 3 cm yellowish-orange plaque over the occipital area of scalp (Fig. 1).
- Verrucous surface.
- Alopecia over the plaque.

Q1. What is the diagnosis?

a. Linear verrucous epidermal nevus
b. Nevus sebaceous
c. Basal cell carcinoma
d. Plane Warts

Ans: b. Nevus sebaceous.

Q2. How do you make a diagnosis of nevus sebaceous?

Ans: The diagnosis is primarily based on clinical grounds alone. The most common presentation is a circumscribed, round/oval/linear, smooth/verrucous, yellowish-orange plaque over the scalp, face or neck leading to alopecia. Mehregan and Pinkus have described three stages for these lesions. The early infantile stage is characterized by papillomatous hyperplasia and immature hair follicles. In the second stage of pubertal expansion, hormonally driven development of sebaceous glands and maturation of apocrine glands are seen. The final stage is characterized by development of benign and malignant neoplasms in adult life.

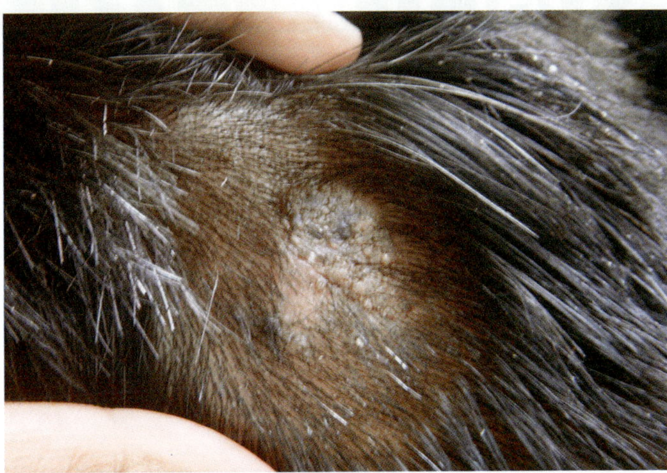

Fig. 1: Orange yellow plaque on scalp with some hyperpigmentation interspersed

Q3. Which neoplasms are likely to develop in a case of nevus sebaceous?

Ans: Neoplasms are likely to develop have been listed in Table 1.

Q4. All of the following can be considered as differentials for nevus sebaceous except?

a. Aplasia cutis
b. Pseudopelade of Brocq
c. Early juvenile xanthogranuloma
d. Solitary mastocytoma

Ans: b. Pseudopelade of Brocq. This is a progressive cicatricial alopecia, developing as an idiopathic entity or secondary to a number of dermatoses, e.g. lichen planus.

All the other three should be considered as close differentials for nevus sebaceous. In early infancy, aplasia cutis may pose a similar picture but has a smooth, papyraceous surface with complete loss of hair. Distinctive domed and papulonodular lesions, progressing rapidly, are characteristic features for xanthogranuloma. Formation of wheal on stroking (Darier's Sign) will be positive in case of mastocytoma along with histological presence of mast cells.

Table 1: Types of neoplasms

Benign	*Malignant*
Syringocystadenoma papilliferum	Basal cell carcinoma
Trichoblastoma	Squamous cell carcinoma
Trichilemmoma	Keratoacanthoma
Apocrine cystadenoma	Sebaceous carcinoma
Nodular hidradenoma	Apocrine carcinoma
Syringoma	Adnexal carcinoma
Infundibuloma	Porocarcinoma

Q5. What are the syndromes in association with nevus sebaceous?

Ans: Schimmelpenning-Feuerstein-Mims syndrome, also known as linear sebaceous nevus syndrome. This is characterized by nevus sebaceous, usually on the face along with variable ipsilateral anomalies of the central nervous system, ocular anomalies and skeletal defects. SCALP syndrome is composed of nevus sebaceous, central nervous system malformations, aplasia cutis congenita, limbal dermoid and pigmented nevus.

Q6. What is the origin of nevus sebaceous?

Ans: This is an organoid hamartoma, composed of epidermal, follicular, sebaceous and apocrine elements. It is postulated to originate from genomic mosaicism of stem cells that expand along the distribution of the lines of Blaschko. Such mosaicism has recently been incriminated to maternal transmission of human papillomavirus DNA to fetal ectodermal stem cells.

Q7. What is the next best step in the management of this girl?

a. Intralesional corticosteroid injection
b. Radiofrequency ablation
c. Full thickness dermal and epidermal excision
d. Masterly inactivity

Ans: c. Full thickness dermal and epidermal excision. Presence of asymptomatic verrucous plaque with alopecia is suggestive toward the diagnosis of nevus sebaceous of Jadassohn, at the second stage of development. The first stage is characterized by papillomatous epithelial hyperplasia with underdeveloped hairs. The last stage is characterized by development of benign and malignant epithelial neoplasms. Though the risk of malignancy is not high enough to warrant prophylactic excision in each and every case, a full thickness excision results in better cosmesis and reduces the risk of recurrences.

Q8. What are the alternative treatment modalities for nevus sebaceous?

Ans: The alternative treatment modalities are:

- Photodynamic therapy
- CO_2 laser resurfacing
- Dermabrasion.

CHAPTER 10

Vascular Malformation

Sahana M Srinivas

Case study 1 Capillary Hemangioma (Infantile Hemangioma)

Presenting Complaints

Doctor my child is having red skin lesions on the face noticed after 2 weeks of birth and is increasing in size gradually from past 6 months.

Setting

Outpatient department.

History of Presenting Illness

An 8-month-old male child presented with complaints of asymptomatic red skin lesions on left forehead, left eyelid and left cheek from 2 weeks of age. Mother gives history that the skin lesions are increasing in size from past 6 months. She also complains that her child is not able to open her left eye completely. Child is otherwise normal with no similar lesions elsewhere on the body. There is no history of eye abnormalities or suggestive of any neurological involvement.

General Physical Examination and Systemic Examination

No abnormality detected.

Dermatological Examination

- Well-defined bright red dome-shaped papules coalescing to form large plaque with lobulated surface measuring 10 cm × 6 cm present on the left forehead extending to left upper eyelid, left lower eyelid and left cheek.
- Noncompressible on palpation, partially blanching on pressure.
- Oral mucosa, ocular mucosa, palms, soles and scalp—within normal limits.

Q1. Based on the history and clinical examination, what is the most likely diagnosis?

a. Infantile hemangioma (segmental type)
b. Port-wine stain
c. Epidermal verrucous nevus
d. Congenital hemangioma

Ans: a. Infantile hemangioma. Diagnosis is made on clinical grounds. The characteristic natural history of hemangioma (that is lesions noticeable after birth with slowly proliferating phase for the next 6 months) along with the morphology and site suggests a diagnosis of infantile hemangioma.

Q2. Enumerate the clinical features of infantile hemangioma?

Ans: Clinical features are:

- Infantile hemangioma or capillary hemangioma is the most common benign soft tissue tumor of childhood.
- Have distinctive life cycle, characterized by proliferative phase for 9–12 months, and occasionally till 18–24 months in early infancy, followed by an involutional phase leading to complete spontaneous regression in most children, leaving residual fibrous tissue.
- They can occur on any part of the body as solitary or multiple lesions, but most commonly involve the head and neck regions. Facial hemangiomas develop along the four facial segments.

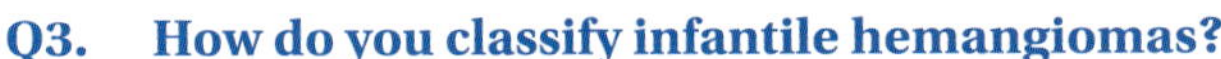

Q3. How do you classify infantile hemangiomas?

Ans: Infantile hemangiomas can be classified as:

- Hemangiomas may occur as superficial, deep or mixed type.
- Superficial hemangiomas present as bright red, dome shaped to lobulated papules, plaques, nodules (Fig. 1). They are rubbery in consistency, noncompressible on palpation and partially blanch with pressure.
- Deep hemangiomas present as subcutaneous partially compressible nodules and tumors often with an overlying blue hue, prominent venous network or telangiectasias (Fig. 2).
- Combined hemangiomas have both superficial bright red component and deeper blue nodular component (Fig. 3).

Based on the anatomical site, it can be classified into localized (77%), segmental (18%) (Fig. 4) and multifocal type (5%).

Q4. What is the estimated rate of complete involution in infantile hemangiomas?

a. 30% by 3 years
b. 50% by 5 years
c. 70% by 7 years
d. >90% by 9–10 years
e. All of the above are correct

Ans: e. All of the above. Infantile hemangioma will not involute with normal skin, but with residual changes like telangiectasias, atrophy, scarring or fibrofatty tissue.

Q5. Enumerate the risk factors associated with hemangioma situated on functionally threatening sites?

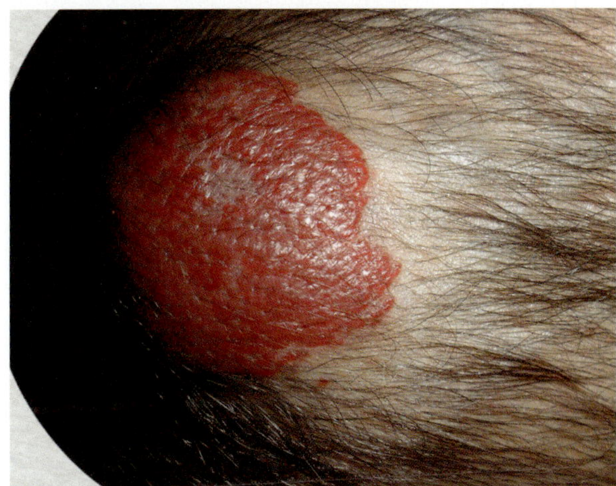

Fig. 1: Superficial type of hemangioma on the scalp

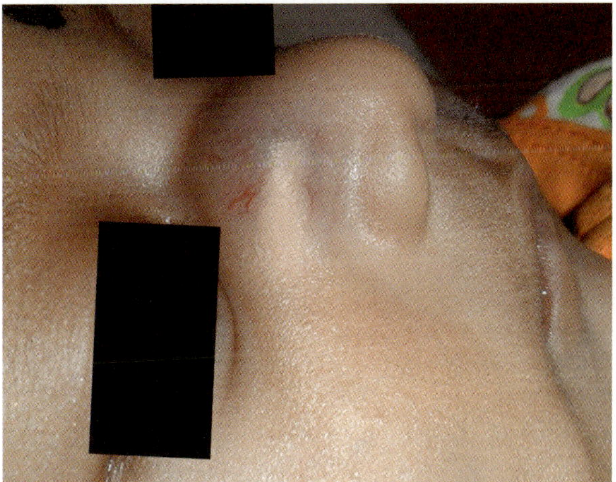

Fig. 2: Deep hemangioma with telangiectasias on the right ala of nose

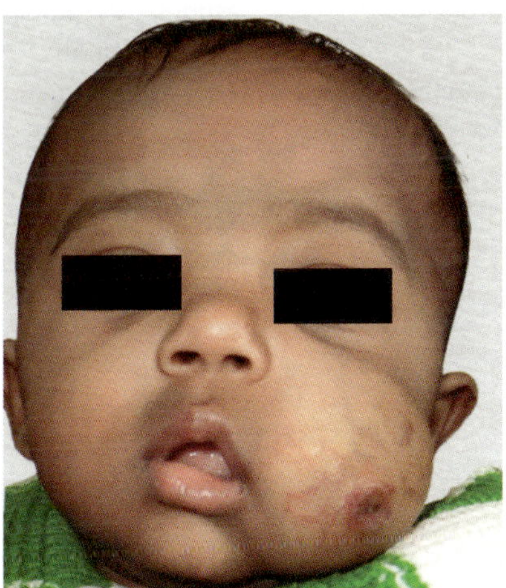

Fig. 3: Combined hemangioma on the right cheek with superficial and deep component

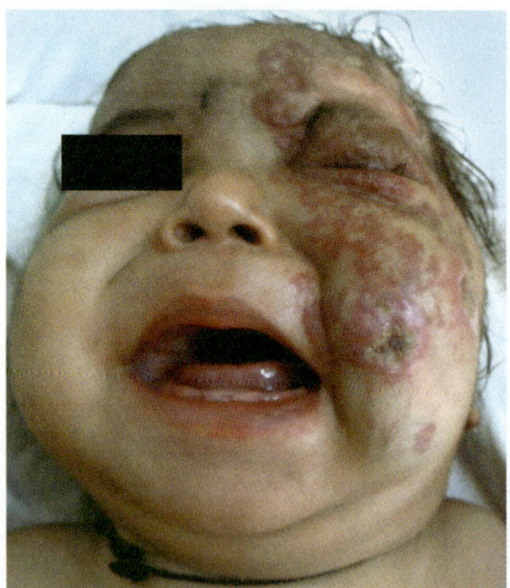

Fig. 4: Segmental hemangioma

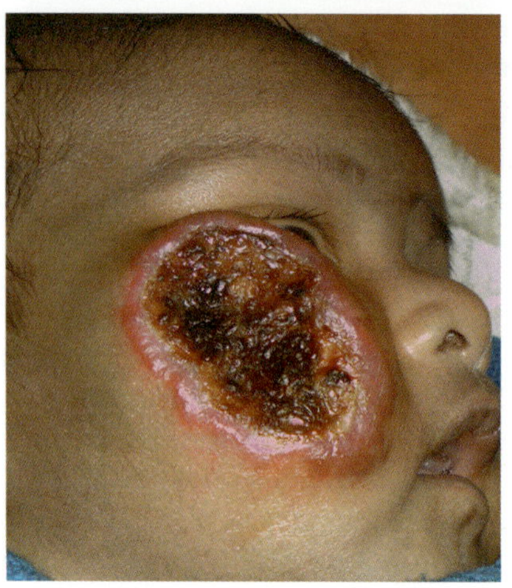

Fig. 5: Ulcerated hemangioma

Ans: The risk factors associated with hemangiomas located on different anatomical sites are listed in Table 1.

Q6. What are complications associated with infantile hemangiomas?

Ans: Complications depend on the type and location of hemangiomas. Common complications associated with infantile hemangioma are:

Table 1: Location and morphology of infantile hemangioma and associated risks

Anatomic location/ Morphology	*Associated risk*
Large segmental facial	PHACES* syndrome
Nasal tip, ear, large facial (especially with prominent dermal component)	Permanent scarring and disfigurement
Periorbital and retrobulbar	Ocular axis occlusion, astigmatism, amblyopia, tear-duct occlusion
Segmental mandibular (beard area) and central neck	Airway hemangioma
Perioral, lips	Ulceration, disfigurement
Lumbosacral hemangiomas	Tethered spinal cord, genital and vesicorenal anomalies (imperforate anus, abnormal genitalia, skin tags, bony sacral anomalies)
Perianal, axilla, neck	Ulceration, bleeding, infection, scarring
Multiple hemangiomas	Hepatic involvement with risk of congestive heart failure and hypothyroidism

*PHACES syndrome: P, posterior fossa and other brain malformations; H, hemangioma; A, arterial anomalies typically of the aortic branches (aortic branch vessels); C, cardiac defects and coarctation of the aorta; E, eye anomalies; S, sternal defects and supraumbilical raphe.

- Ulcerations (Fig. 5)
- Bleeding
- Infections
- High output cardiac failure
- Ocular complications
- Airway obstructions } Site dependent complications
- Interference with feeding } Site dependent complications
- Obstruction of external auditory meatus.

Q7. What are the systems involved in infantile hemangiomas?

Ans: In 10–25% of the cases, multiple lesions are present, and may indicate systemic involvement. Evaluation for hepatic involvement is recommended in infants with 5 or more lesions. Visceral hemangiomatosis may occur without cutaneous lesions as well. Visceral hemangiomas may rarely involve lungs, gastrointestinal tract (GIT), central nervous system (CNS), intestine, brain, eyes, spleen, oral mucosa and renal systems.

Q8. What are the syndromes associated with infantile hemangiomas?

a. PHACES syndrome
b. LUMBAR syndrome
c. PELVIS syndrome
d. SACRAL syndrome
e. All of the above

Ans: d. All of the above.

Q9. When should you consider hemangiomas for complete evaluation and investigations?

Ans:
- Many of the hemangiomas that are single and are not life-threatening do not require any evaluation. They resolve spontaneously without any treatment.

- Hemangiomas that should be considered for complete evaluation and aggressive therapy are those that are life-threatening or function-threatening, like hemangiomas present on periocular region, nasal tip, ear (extensive), lips, genitalia or perineum, large facial hemangiomas, hemangiomas present on beard area, lumbosacral, multiple and segmental hemangiomas.

Q10. What are the investigations to be done while evaluating an infantile hemangioma?

Ans: Infantile hemangiomas generally require no investigations, as the diagnosis is clinically evident. In certain cases (as outlined above), the following are required:

- Doppler ultrasound to differentiate deep hemangiomas with vascular malformation.
- Magnetic resonance imaging, computed tomography scan and radiography imaging.
- Ophthalmological evaluation if eyelid involvement is present.
- Complete blood count, liver function test, coagulation studies, stool examination, echocardiography, ECG, abdominal and CNS imaging.
- Direct laryngoscopy for airway involvement.

Q11. What are the other differential diagnoses to be considered for infantile hemangioma?

Ans: Other differential diagnoses to be considered are:

- Congenital hemangiomas (rapidly involuting and noninvoluting congenital hemangioma)
- Capillary malformation (Port-wine stain)
- Kaposiform hemangioendothelioma
- Tufted angiomas
- Pyogenic granuloma
- Infantile myofibromatosis
- Venous and lymphatic malformations.

Q12. How do you differentiate rapidly involuting and noninvoluting congenital hemangiomas?

Ans: Differences between rapidly involuting congenital hemangioma (RICH) and noninvoluting congenital hemangiomas (NICH) are listed in Table 2.

Q13. What are the goals of management of infantile hemangioma?

Ans: Goals of management of infantile hemangioma are:

- Prevention or reversal of life-threatening or function-threatening complications.
- Prevention of permanent disfigurement, diminution of psychosocial stress for the patient and family.
- Avoidance of aggressive or detrimental interventions in lesions that may have excellent prognosis without treatment.
- Prevention or treatment of ulceration to lower scarring, infection and pain.

Q14. What is the first line of therapy in hemangiomas which are life-threatening and function threatening?

Ans: First line of therapy includes:

- Propranolol, a beta blocker, is the first-line therapy for hemangiomas requiring treatment.
- It is given at the dosage of 2–3 mg/kg body weight 8 hourly until clinically evident results are achieved, and then maintained on 0.5–1 mg/kg body weight. Studies have shown long-term usage of around 9–12 months would prevent recurrences.
- Contraindicated in children with bradycardia, bronchial asthma, heart failure, hypotension, hypoglycemia, CNS vascular anomalies.

Table 2: Differences between RICH and NICH

Infantile hemangioma	*RICH*	*NICH*
Absent, precursor or present at birth	Fully developed at birth	Fully developed at birth
Rapid postnatal proliferation	Intrauterine proliferation	Proportionate growth
Slow spontaneous involution	Rapid involution after the first year	Do not involute spontaneously
More common in girls	Equal prevalence or slightly more common in girls	Slightly more common in boys
Lobular endothelial proliferation during proliferative phase; fibrofatty tissue during involution	Capillary lobules within fibrotic stroma containing thin-walled vessels, hemosiderin	Lobules of small, thin-walled vessels with large central vessel; dilated, dysplastic veins between lobules; "hobnailed" endothelial cells lining intralobular vessels
GLUT1-positive, Lewis Y antigen-positive	GLUT1-negative, Lewis Y antigen-negative	GLUT1-negative

Abbreviations: GLUT1, glucose transporter 1

- Pre-evaluation of blood pressure, ECG, echocardiography, chest X-ray and blood sugars is necessary.
- Adverse reactions include hypoglycemia, hypotension, bradycardia, sleep disruption, acrocyanosis and diarrhea.

Q15. What are the other treatment modalities for infantile hemangiomas?

a. Active nonintervention
b. Supportive therapy
c. Topical—corticosteroids, intralesional steroid, timolol, imiquimod
d. Systemic treatment—oral propranolol, corticosteroids, interferon-alpha, vincristine, cyclophosphamide and bleomycin
e. Surgical modalities—excision, laser therapy, sclerotherapy, embolization and radiotherapy
f. All of the above

Ans: f. All of the above.

Active nonintervention:

- Education of parents about the natural course of infantile hemangioma
- Regular follow up to assess the course of the lesion
- To address emotional and psychological issues raised due to cosmetic disfigurement.

Supportive therapy:

- Bland emollients
- Saline soaks and topical antibiotics for ulcerated lesions
- Oral antibiotics for secondary infection.

The different treatment modalities are listed in Table 3.

Table 3: Different treatment modalities

Therapeutic options	*Indications*
Topical corticosteroids	Superficial hemangioma or precursor lesions in attempt to prevent/alter proliferative phase
Intralesional corticosteroids	Accessible sites such as the lip, cheek, nasal tip glabellar and periocular areas
Imiquimod 5% cream	Superficial hemangioma in "cosmetically sensitive" areas
Timolol 0.5% lotion	Single, superficial hemangiomas with no deep component <4–5 cm
Systemic corticosteroids (1–4 mg/kg/day)	Life or function-threatening hemangiomas—airway, hepatic, periorbital, hemangiomas with persistent ulceration or at sites where significant disfigurement is likely
Vincristine (1–1.5 mg/m^2/week)	Life or function-threatening hemangiomas resistant to treatment with systemic steroids
Interferon-α2a, b (3 μm/m^2/day or QOD)	Life or function-threatening infantile hemangioma in older children (particularly in infants >1 year of age when risk of neurotoxicity is lower)
Surgical excision/debulking	Function-threatening infantile hemangioma (periorbital), hemangioma where scarring/anetoderma are expected (large, pedunculated or painfully ulcerated hemangioma)
Pulsed dye laser (595 nm)	Ulcerated hemangiomas, superficial hemangiomas
Bare-fiber (Nd:YAG)	Deep hemangioma in life- or function-threatening areas

Abbreviation: Nd:YAG, neodymium-doped yttrium-aluminum garnet

Case study 2 Port-wine Stain

Presenting Complaints

Doctor my child is having red skin lesions on the face since birth, the lesions are nonprogressive in nature.

Setting

Dermatology outpatient department.

History of Presenting Illness

A 5-year-old female child presented with complaints of asymptomatic red skin lesions on left forehead, left upper eyelid, left cheek and left side of upper lip from birth. Mother gives history that the skin lesions are not increasing in size and have been persistent as it is from birth. There is history of seizures in the child for which the child is on anticonvulsants from past 4 years. Child is otherwise normal with no similar lesions elsewhere on the body. There is no history suggestive of eye or hearing abnormalities.

General Physical Examination

Child is conscious and alert. Child has normal development with height and weight at the 50th percentile with normal progress on her growth curve. General physical examination and vitals are normal. There is no facial asymmetry.

Systemic Examination

No abnormality detected.

Dermatological Examination

- Well-defined dark red macule measuring 12 cm × 8 cm present on the left forehead extending to left upper eyelid, left lower eyelid, left cheek and left upper lip not crossing the midline.
- Smooth on palpation and does not blanch on pressure.
- Oral mucosa, ocular mucosa, palms, soles and scalp—within normal limits.

Q1. Based on the history and clinical examination, what is the most likely diagnosis?

a. Port-wine stain (PWS)
b. Infantile hemangioma
c. Nevus Anemicus
d. Salmon patch

Ans: a. Port-wine stain. Presence of nonprogressive, non-blanchable macule with unilateral distribution on the face suggests the possibility of PWS. Association of PWS with seizures may point toward Sturge-Weber syndrome (SWS).

Q2. How do you diagnose PWS?

Ans: Diagnosis of PWS:

- Diagnosis is made on clinical grounds. PWS, also called as nevus flammeus, presents as well to ill-defined pink to bright red macules at birth seen most commonly on the face, but can occur anywhere on the body including mucosae (Fig. 6). They tend to darken with age and may develop small nodules leading to a cobble stoned appearance.

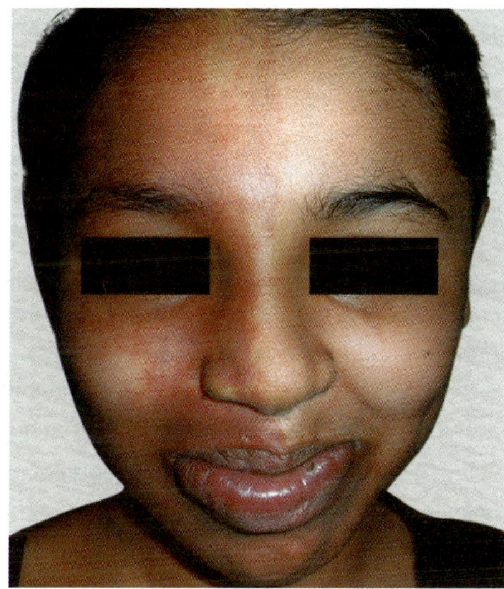

Fig. 6: Facial port-wine stain with slight hypertrophy of lower lip

- Port-wine stains are mostly unilateral in distribution. Facial PWS may be associated with ocular and neurological abnormalities.

Q3. How do you confirm your diagnosis?

Ans: Though PWS is a clinical diagnosis, skin biopsy can be done to rule out other disorders. Skin biopsy shows proliferation and ectasia of thin and thick walled vessels with lumina of varying diameter in the upper dermis.

Q4. What are the other vascular abnormalities associated with PWS?

Ans: Various vascular abnormalities associated with PWS are hemangiomas, arteriovenous fistulae, nevus anemicus, pyogenic granuloma and tufted angiomas.

Q5. What are other associated features to look for in facial PWS?

a. Ocular abnormalities
b. Grand mal epilepsy
c. Subnormal intelligence
d. Contralateral hemiparesis
e. All of the above

Ans: e. All of the above.

Facial PWS in the distribution of trigeminal nerve can be associated with SWS. Ocular abnormalities are present in 40% of these patients and include ipsilateral glaucoma, buphthalmos, congestion, strabismus and loss of vision. Glaucoma is seen in two-thirds of cases in infancy. Grand mal type convulsions usually occur within first year of life. There may be other associated features like behavioral problems, subnormal intelligence, contralateral hemiparesis, EEG abnormalities and intracranial calcification on CT scan.

Q6. What are the changes that occur in PWS?

Ans: Port-wine stain darkens with age, and secondary proliferative lesions like vascular blebs (pyogenic granuloma-like lesions) may develop on PWS. Rarely basal cell carcinoma has been reported to occur in PWS. Soft tissue swelling and bony overgrowth may develop under a PWS.

Q7. What are the other syndromes associated with PWS?

Ans: Syndromes associated with PWS are listed in Table 4.

Q8. How do you differentiate PWS from infantile hemangiomas?

Ans: Early PWS may resemble infantile hemangioma. Congenital onset, static nature without rapid proliferation differentiates PWS from hemangioma.

Q9. What are the treatment modalities for PWS?

a. Laser therapy
b. Surgery
c. Radiation therapy
d. Cryotherapy

Ans: a. Laser therapy. Flashlamp-pumped tunable pulsed dye laser is the treatment of choice for PWS. It is done in several sessions 6–8 weeks apart. It is associated with mild scarring and pigmentary changes.

Table 4: Syndromes associated with PWS

Syndromes	*Clinical features*
Klippel-Trenaunay syndrome (KTS)	PWS, venous and lymphatic malformation, bony and soft tissue hypertrophy
Parkes-Weber syndrome	PWS, venous varicosities, limb hypertrophy, arteriovenous fistulae
Phakomatosis pigmentovascularis	PWS, extensive nevus flammeus, pigmentary nevus, aberrant Mongolian spots, nevus anemicus, Beckers nevus, renal agenesis, features of SWS and KTS
Proteus syndrome	Overgrowth of multiple tissues, asymmetry, exostosis, disfigurement of skull, macrocephaly, partial gigantism of hands or feet, hemangioma, PWS, lipomas, lymphangioma, verrucous epidermal nevi
Cobb syndrome	Spinal cord angioma overlaid by segmental PWS or cavernous hemangioma
Bannayan-Riley-Ruvalcaba syndrome	Macrocephaly, mixed vascular malformation, subcutaneous and visceral lipomas, skeletal defects
Beckwith-Wiedemann syndrome	Facial PWS, macroglossia, omphalocele, visceral hyperplasia, hemihypertrophy
Von Hippel-Lindau disease	PWS, bilateral retinal angiomatosis, cerebellar or medullary hemangioma
Rubenstein-Taybi syndrome	Mental retardation, broad thumbs and great toes, high palate, crowded teeth, PWS
Wyburn-Mason syndrome	Ipsilateral PWS, unilateral retinal arteriovenous malformation, ipsilateral aneurismal arteriovenous malformation
Coat's disease	Ipsilateral PWS, retinal telangiectasias

CHAPTER 11

Angiokeratoma

Navya Handa

Case study Angiokeratoma

Presenting Complaints

Patient has developed multiple bleeding small dark lesions on my scrotum since the last 1 year.

Setting

Dermatology outpatient department

History of Present Illness

A 28-year-old man, presented to the dermatology outpatient department with complaints of small, dark lesions on his scrotum since 1 year, which were insidious in onset and have gradually increased in number and size with associated mild itching. Patient notices blood on his undergarments that he attributes to scratching these lesions. These lesions are otherwise asymptomatic and he has no medical problems.

General Physical Examination and Systemic Examination

No abnormality detected.

Dermatological Examination

- Multiple red to violaceous discrete papules of size 2–4 mm over the scrotum which do not blanch on pressure (Fig. 1)
- Surrounding skin is excoriated.

Q1. What is the most likely diagnosis?

a. Angiokeratoma of Fordyce
b. Angiokeratoma corporis diffusum
c. Kaposi sarcoma
d. Pyogenic granuloma.

Ans: a. Angiokeratoma of scrotum (Fordyce).

Diagnosis of angiokeratoma corporis diffusum should be considered in any patient presenting with scrotal angiokeratomas. Kaposi sarcoma can mimic angiokeratoma clinically but lesions are typically larger and more nodular. HIV testing should be done in these cases.

Q2. What are angiokeratomas?

Ans: Angiokeratomas are characterized by dilation of superficial vessels with hyperkeratosis of the overlying epidermis. There is evidence that local venous hypertension plays a part in its development.

Q3. Which are the different types of local angiokeratomas?

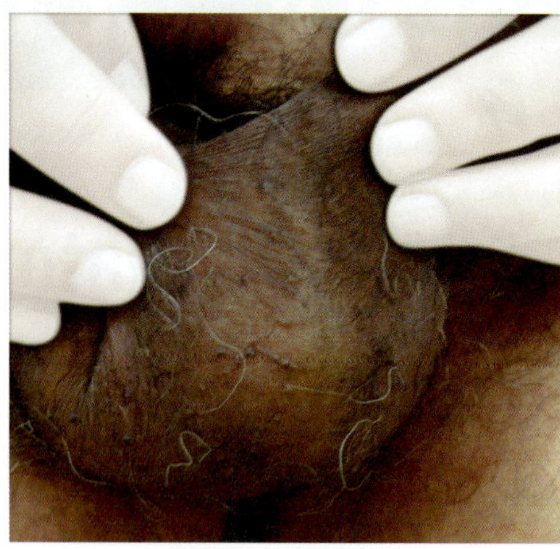

Fig. 1: Red and dark papules on scrotum

Ans: Types of local angiokeratoma are as follows:

- *Angiokeratoma circumscriptum:* It is a vascular malformation of ectatic vessels in the papillary dermis. It presents as a blue-black color hyperkeratotic vascular plaque, usually present from birth. It is often found on the extremities and bleeds on trauma. It progressively becomes verrucous and does not remit with age.

  Differential diagnoses:
  - *Verrucous hemangioma*: Histologically, it involves the dermis and subcutaneous fat whereas angiokeratoma involves only papillary dermis.
  - Localized lymphatic malformations (microcystic) which are not hyperkeratotic
  - *Acral pseudolymphomatous angiokeratoma of children (APACHE)*: It has pseudolymphomatous histology rather than a true angiokeratoma.
- *Angiokeratoma of Mibelli*: Autosomal dominant inheritance with variable penetrance. Most often affects females younger than 20 years. Site; most often found on dorsa of hands and feet, and less commonly observed over elbows, knees, shoulders and ear lobes. Multiple, 3–5 mm, dark red papules with verrucous surface. Associated with recurrent chilblains and acrocyanosis. It can also present as asymptomatic ulceration of fingertips.
- *Angiokeratoma of scrotum (Fordyce)*: The most common of the angiokeratomas, angiokeratoma of the scrotum, also called as Angiokeratoma of Fordyce is more common in males with peak incidence after the third decade. They are typically asymptomatic, 2–5 mm, blue-to-red papules with a scaly surface located on the scrotum which may bleed spontaneously or after trauma.
- *Solitary papular angiokeratoma*: This presents in the age group of 10–40 years over the lower extremities and is usually acquired as a response to trauma. Clinically patient presents with 2–10 mm, blue-black papules or plaques. Differential diagnoses include viral wart, melanocytic naevi and malignant melanoma.
- *Angiokeratoma of vulva*: Lesions analogous to those of angiokeratoma of Fordyce develop over the vulva. Usually occur in older women, in younger women history of use of oral contraceptive pills should be asked for.

Q4. Which are the generalized angiokeratomas?

Ans: Angiokeratoma corporis diffusum is the characteristic generalized angiokeratoma. It is the dermatological hallmark of several rare inherited lysosomal disorders like Fabry's disease, fucosidosis, galactosialidosis, GM1 gangliosidosis, etc. out of which it is most commonly associated with Fabry's disease. Fabry's disease is an X-linked recessively-inherited disorder caused by the deficiency of the enzyme alpha-galactosidase. These patients present with verrucous, deep red to blue-black papules between the umbilicus and the knees, with a predilection for the scrotum, penis, lower back, thighs, hips and buttocks. Patients may also present with fever and painful hands and feet. Ocular, renal, cardiac and central nervous system are also involved. Differential diagnoses include other types of angiokeratoma, purpura, angioma serpenginosum, erythromelalgia, rheumatoid arthritis and rheumatic fever.

Q5. What are the histological findings of angiokeratoma?

Ans: It is characterized by dilated vascular channels in the papillary dermis with the overlying epidermis showing compact hyperkeratosis, acanthosis and papillomatosis. The elongated rete ridges tend to enclose the dilated vascular channels.

Q6. How will you confirm the diagnosis?

Ans: Localized angiokeratomas are diagnosed clinically which can be differentiated and hence confirmed from other simulating conditions histologically.

Lysosomal storage disorders can be diagnosed by distinct deficient enzyme analysis and electron microscopy. Fabry's disease can be differentiated by electron microscopic examination by the characteristic lamellar (zebra like) inclusions within endothelial cells and other cell types. Urine examination of these patients shows maltese crosses of lipid globules on polarizing microscopy.

Q7. How will you treat a patient of angiokeratoma?

Ans: The lesions can be treated, if desired.

- Local excision—in cases where number of lesions are few.
- Cryotherapy—may heal with residual hypopigmentation and scarring
- Electrocautery.
- Laser-Erbium or CO_2 laser to remove the hyperkeratotic acanthotic epidermis, followed by PDL which targets hemoglobin.
- Deficient enzyme replacement and genetic counseling in case of angiokeratoma corporis diffusum
- Symptomatic treatment is required in cases where systemic involvement is seen.

CHAPTER 12

Melanocytic Nevus

GK Singh

Case study Melanocytic Nevus

Presenting Complaints

Doctor, I have a black spot on my upper lip since birth. Is there a need to remove it?

Setting

Dermatology outpatient department

History of Presenting Complaint

A 19-year-old boy presents with a solitary, blackish skin lesion on the upper lip since birth. It has grown in size proportionately with age. It is not associated with pain or itching. He wants to get it removed if it is likely to create any problems later.

General and Systemic Examination

No abnormalities detected.

Dermatological Examination

Solitary, brownish-to-blackish nodule with coarse hair on the surface, present over philtrum area over the upper lip, measuring 1 cm × 1.5 cm (Fig. 1). No bleeding/oozing/crusting over lesion.

Q1. What is your diagnosis?

a. Melanocytic nevus
b. Melanoma
c. Basal cell carcinoma
d. Blue nevus

Ans: a. Melanocytic nevus

Q2. What is a melanocytic nevus?

Ans: Melanocytic nevi are normal, benign proliferations of melanocytes. Although the risk of a nevus evolving into a melanoma is extremely small, melanocytic nevi are both risk factors for melanoma and precursors of melanoma. Prevalence of melanocytic nevi varies with ethnicity and races; however, they are generally considered to be present in between 1% and 2% of newborns and adults.

Q3. What is the differential diagnosis of a melanocytic nevus?

Ans: Freckles, lentigines, melanoma, basal cell carcinoma, blue nevus.

Q4. How do you classify melanocytic nevus?

Ans: Melanocytic nevus can be classified as Congenital and Acquired.

Congenital nevi are deeply pigmented and present at birth. These increase in proportion to the increase

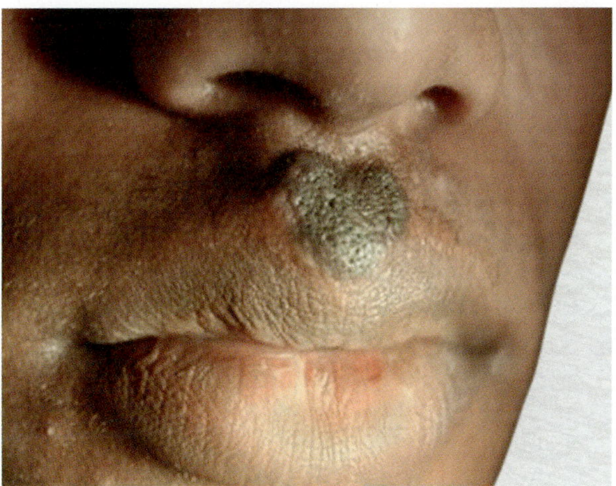

Fig. 1: Congenital melanocytic nevus

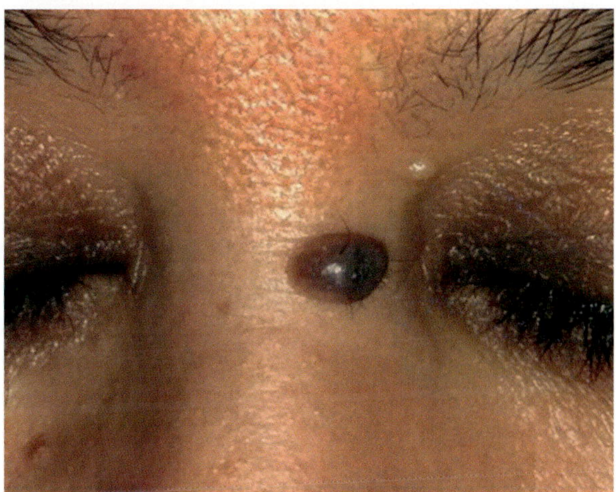

Fig. 2: Acquired compound melanocytic nevus

in the size of the infant and may become more pigmented and hairy. A significant proportion of these nevi fade within first 1–2 years. Most of the congenital nevi are dermal or compound melanocytic nevi with nevus cells typically extending more deeply into the dermis (within appendages and even into striated muscle and fat) than those of acquired nevi.

Acquired nevi develop later in life and arise as a benign cluster of melanocytic nevus cells arising as a result of proliferation of melanocytes at the dermal-epidermal junction. Further types depend on the extent of migration of these cells from the dermoepidermal junction to the dermis (types discussed later) (Fig. 2).

Histopathologically types of melanocytic nevus are theque, junctional nevus, compound nevus and intradermal nevus.

Theque: A group of melanocytes (generally four or more) in contact with the basal layer of the epidermis but budding downward into the dermis.

Junctional nevus: A pigmented melanocytic nevus in which there is presence of theques of melanocytes at the dermal-epidermal junction. A few nevus cells are usually observed scattered in the underlying dermis.

Compound nevus: A pigmented melanocytic nevus in which the histological features include both junctional activity and the presence of nevus cells in the dermis. Such nevi usually contain melanin may be clinically hyperpigmented.

Intradermal nevus: A melanocytic nevus in which there is little or no abnormality of melanocytes in the epidermis. There is presence of packets of nevus cells in the dermis. Melanin pigmentation is often absent and such nevi may be clinically nonpigmented.

Q5. Is there any classification of congenital melanocytic nevus? How they are different from each other?

Ans: As per American National Institutes of Health (NIH) consensus definition, these nevi are categorized according to size. Small congenital nevi are defined as under 1.5 cm in diameter, large as having a diameter between 1.5 cm and 20 cm and giant nevi as having a diameter of 20 cm or more. The differentiating features are illustrated below in Table 1.

Table 1: Differentiating features of congenital melanocytic nevus

Subtype	*Pathology*	*Significance*	*Treatment*
Small (<1.5 cm) may appear in the first 2 years of life	Deeper nevus cells exhibiting a tendency to extend deeply in relation to skin appendages	Very small risk of melanoma	None, other than self-examination. Consider excision in sites where review is difficult such as the scalp
Large (1.5 to 20 cm)	Deeper nevus cells exhibiting a tendency to extend deeply in relation to skin appendages	Increased risk of melanoma	Excise if technically feasible with good cosmetic result
Giant (>20 cm)	Deeper nevus cells exhibiting a tendency to extend deeply in relation to skin appendages. May be associated with benign but atypical proliferations such as hamartomas	Increased risk of melanoma especially if over the trunk and associated with many satellite nevi. Lifetime risk likely to be less than 14%.	Removal of risk not possible because such lesions cannot be fully excised. Surgical decisions should be deferred to assess spontaneous improvement in the first few years of life

Q6. Will you recommend any investigation in the diagnosis of this case?

Ans: The above case does not require any investigation for diagnosis. However, once excised lesion should be sent for histopathological examination to rule out any remote possibility of malignant changes.

Q7. Is there any role of imaging study in diagnosing congenital melanocytic nevus?

Ans: No. An MRI scan should only be considered in babies with nevi over the cranium or spine to exclude significant leptomeningeal melanocytosis. Symptomatic neurocutaneous melanosis is rare, so the value of scanning seems questionable in the absence of neurological signs. Regular neurological examination, however, is more important.

Q8. When should you suspect that such a lesion could be a malignancy?

Ans: When there is a history of sudden change in the size or shape of the lesion or change in the surface or bleeding from the lesions.

Q9. How are you going to treat this case?

Ans: He requires simple excision and suturing for cosmetic reason.

Q10. Is there any role of Lasers in the treatment of congenital melanocytic lesions?

Ans: These can be treated with following lasers but results are not satisfactory as compared to surgical excision and there is higher chance of recurrence. High-energy pulsed carbon dioxide laser, Erbium:YAG laser, normal-mode ruby laser, Q-switched ruby laser, Q-switched alexandrite laser can be tried.

Q11. What are the treatment options available for large or giant congenital lesion?

Ans: Serial excision, use of tissue expanders, flap surgeries or tissue grafts are the options for surgical treatment of larger nevus. These also depend upon size and site of lesions.

Q12. Do you think there is requirement of genetic counseling for the parents of children of congenital nevus for next pregnancy?

Ans: Congenital nevi are essentially considered to be developmental abnormalities of the skin, with a very low risk of recurrence in subsequent pregnancies. So, there is no need of genetic counseling. However, reassurance is always required.

Q13. Is there any lifetime risk of developing malignancy in congenital melanocytic nevus?

Ans: There have been several attempts to estimate the lifetime risk; most of the studies give values between 4.6% and 14%. Overall, it is giant nevus which has more chances to develop malignancy than small congenital nevus.

Q14. What are the nevi thought to be variants of congenital melanocytic nevi but which appear in childhood? What are the salient differences between them?

Ans: Nevus spilus and agminate Spitz nevus are thought to be variants of congenital melanocytic nevus which appear in childhood. The salient differences are given in Table 2.

Q15. Which are the Lasers that can be used to treat acquired melanocytic nevi?

Ans: The spectrum of lasers used ranges from the green lasers (pulsed dye, Q-switched, and neodymium:yttrium aluminum garnet [Nd:YAG-532] to the far-infrared lasers [CO_{2-} 10,600 nm] and erbium [Er:YAG- 2940 nm). Junctional nevi respond to Q-switched/normal mode pigment lasers, whereas for the compound and dermal nevi, pulsed ablative laser (CO_2/Er:YAG) are better options.

Q16. What is the basic difference between acquired melanocytic nevus and dermal melanocytic lesions?

Ans: Acquired melanocytic nevus is benign tumor of melanocyte develops from epidermal melanocytes

Table 2: Salient differences between nevus spilus and agminate Spitz nevus

Types	*Clinical pathological relation*	*Significance*	*Treatment*
Speckled nevus (nevus spilus)	Commonly nevi arising in a macular lentigo with subtle increase in melanocyte number	Uncommon cases of melanoma described arising in such nevi	Education about self-examination.
Agminate Spitz nevus	Spitzoid proliferations arising in a macular area of pigmentation. Usually appear in childhood where a group of Spitz nevi develop on skin with background hyperpigmentation like speckled nevus	Similar to a speckled nevus but with spitzoid elements	Review at intervals and excise changing elements within

Table 3: Halo and Mayerson's nevi

Subtypes	*Clinicopathological relation*	*Significance*	*Treatment*
Halo nevus	Dense lymphocytic infiltrate in the early phase and subsequent removal of nevus cells. Clinically presents as central hyperpigmented macules with surrounding depigmented macule in circular shape giving halo like appearance	None. Thought to result from immunologically-mediated host responses to a nevus	None in the absence of atypical features clinically. Can be excised if cosmetically desired
Meyerson's nevus	Benign nevus with overlying spongiosis of the epidermis. Clinically presents as nevus with surrounding halo of eczema	None	The eczematous component should be treated and the nevus reexamined

that have completed their migration from the neural crest to the dermal–epidermal junction in fetal life, proliferated and then senesced (i.e. ceased proliferation), come to resemble cells of neural or fibroblast lineage. By contrast, the dermal melanocytic lesions are believed to arise from dermal melanocytes that have become arrested in the dermis during fetal life and tissue modeling and have not reached their normal site in the basal layer of the epidermis; e.g. Mongolian spot, nevus of Ito and nevus of Ota.

Q17. Is there any relation to underlying disease and number of melanocytic nevus?

Ans: Patients with atopic dermatitis may have significantly lower nevus counts than age-matched controls. Children with Turner's syndrome, leukemia-treated patients and recipients of renal transplants have increased numbers of nevi on the body.

Q18. What is an atypical (dysplastic) nevus? What is the clinical significance of this lesion? How it is to be treated?

Ans: Unlike typical acquired melanocytic nevus, an atypical (dysplastic) nevus, the melanocyte proliferation continues so that the nevus continues to grow in size beyond the "usual" size, and the junctional proliferative component may show some features reminiscent of an early melanoma, resulting in some irregularity of shape and color clinically. However, eventually they mature as compound or dermal nevus and behave benign. Long-term significance of these lesions is being markers of risk of melanoma and precursor lesions for melanoma.

Solitary lesion should be removed in its entirety with a 2 mm clinical margin and subjected to pathological examination to exclude *in situ* melanoma. Such nevi should never be punch biopsied or an incisional biopsy taken from them.

Q19. What are halo and Meyerson's nevi?

Ans: Halo and Meyerson's nevi have been described in Table 3.

Q20. What is blue nevi?

Ans: A blue or blue-black melanocytic nevus is relatively common nevus comprising of aberrant collections of pigment-producing but benign melanocytes, in the dermis rather than at the dermoepidermal junction. Because of the presence of deep pigmentation within a refracting colloidal medium (Tyndall effect), the brownish-black pigment present contributes a bluish cast to such lesions, thereby explaining the name. Blue nevi are benign usually symmetric lesions, typically occur on the distal extremities or scalp, but they can occur at any site.

SECTION 4

Pediatric Dermatology

Sahana M Srinivas

CHAPTER 13

Pustular Lesions in Neonates

Divya Gorur K, Amina Asafiya

Case study Pustular Lesions in Neonates

Presenting Complaints

Doctor, my baby has pus-filled lesions on the face since birth.

History of Presenting Illness

A one-week-old baby presented with tiny pus-filled lesions on face since birth. The lesions started on the chin and gradually progressed to involve neck and forehead. The lesions gradually increased in size too and then ruptured to leave behind brownish discolored areas. No history of fever, feeding difficulty, topical application, atopy or phototherapy was present. The infant was otherwise well.

Birth History

Baby was born of nonconsanguineous marriage, full term normal vaginal delivery. There is no history of any maternal illness during pregnancy. BCG and OPV were given next day of delivery.

General Physical Examination and Systemic Examination

No abnormality detected

Dermatological Examination

- Multiple superficial papules and pustules present on chin, neck and forehead. Few hyperpigmented macules present over the chin.
- Palms and Soles—Normal
- Mucosae, hair and nails—Normal

Q1. What is your most likely diagnosis?

a. Bullous impetigo
b. Erythema toxicum neonatorum
c. Transient neonatal pustular melanosis
d. Miliaria pustulosa

Ans: c *Transient neonatal pustular melanosis (TNPM)*: An idiopathic pustular eruption that heals with brown pigmented macules. TNPM is more common in neonates of dark skin color. The lesions are almost invariably present at birth with 1–3 mm, flaccid, superficial, fragile pustules with no surrounding erythema. Usually distributed over chin, neck, forehead, back, and buttocks, even palms and soles may be involved.

Table 1: Differentiation of pustular eruptions in neonates

Condition	*Onset*	*Clinical features*	*Investigation*
ETN	Onset 1–4 years of life. Persists up to 10 days	Erythematous macules, papules, pustules located on trunk, back, upper arm and face (Fig. 1). Described as flea bitten appearance	Wright's stain from lesions demonstrate eosinophils
Miliaria pustulosa	Can present any time in neonatal period. Lesions resolve in 2–3 weeks. Predisposed by warm, humid temperature	Pustules admixed with lesions of miliaria rubra, over flexures, back, forehead and neck (Fig. 2)	Wright's stain shows squamous cells
Neonatal acne	Onset in first few weeks of life; may persist up to 3 months	Tiny papulopustules over nose, forehead and cheeks	Typical clinical appearance. Investigations are not needed
Infantile acropustulosis	Can rarely present at birth. Commonly at 3 months of life, with each crop of lesions lasting upto 2 weeks	Recurrent crops of itchy, 1–4 mm vesicopustules on the palms and soles, dorsa of the feet, hands and fingers, ankles, wrists and forearms. Scattered lesions may also be seen on face, scalp and trunk	Wright's stain shows neutrophils with few eosinophils
Eosinophilic pustulosis	Onset is first 6 months of life. Recurrence may be present	Starts as pustules on erythematous base on scalp and progress to involve any site except mucosa	Wright's stain demonstrates eosinophils

Q2. What are the different clinical phases in TNPM?

Ans: Three phases:

1. First phase—Superficial vesiculopustules: 2–10 mm at birth, around nipple and pressure sites.
2. Second phase—Fine collarette of scales around resolving pustules.
3. Third phase—Postinflammatory hyperpigmented brown macules persisting up to 3 months.

Q3. What will the Gram stain from the pustules show?

Ans: Gram stain will show plenty of neutrophils. Bacterial culture is negative.

Q4. Describe the histopathology of transient neonatal pustular melanosis?

Ans: Pustular lesions show intra- or subcorneal collections of neutrophils with a few eosinophils.

The pigmented macules demonstrate basal and supra-basal increase in pigmentation, without any pigmentary incontinence.

Q5. How will you manage the case?

Ans: TNPM needs no treatment and it resolves spontaneously.

Q6. What are the noninfective neonatal dermatoses presenting as pustular eruptions?

Ans:
- Erythema toxicum neonatorum (ETN)
- Transient pustular melanosis
- Miliaria pustulosa
- Infantile acropustulosis
- Eosinophilic pustulosis
- Acne neonatorum
- Benign neonatal cephalic pustulosis
- Pustular psoriasis
- Pustular eruption of transient myeloproliferative disorder.

Q7. How will you differentiate these conditions?

Ans: Differentiation of pustular eruptions in neonates has been described in Table 1.

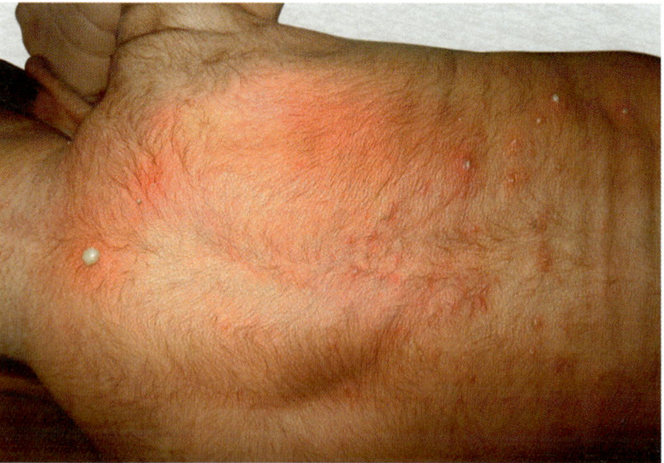

Fig. 1: Erythema toxicum: Multiple pustules on erythematous base and few erythematous macules on back

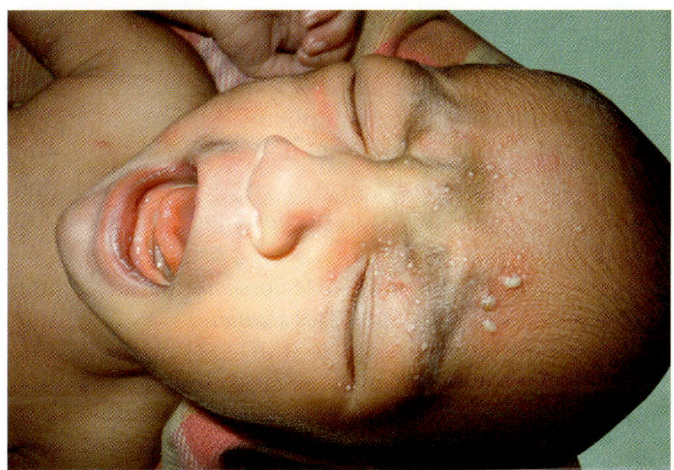

Fig. 2: Miliaria pustulosa: Multiple erythematous papules and pustules on forehead

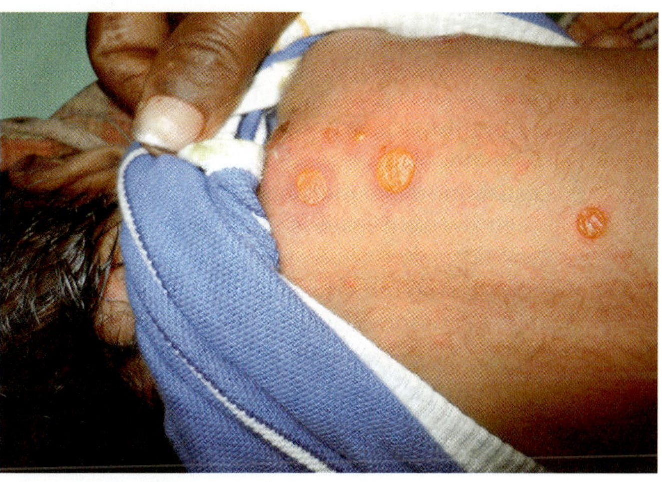

Fig. 3: Bullous impetigo: Multiple pustules on the back

Q8. What are the neonatal pustular dermatoses of infective etiology?

Ans:
- *Bacterial:*
  - Bullous impetigo (*Staphylococcus aureus*) (Fig. 3)
  - Folliculitis (*Staphylococcus aureus*, Streptococcus, gram-negative bacteria)
  - Ecthyma (*Staphylococcus aureus*)
  - Ecthyma gangrenosum (*Pseudomonas aeruginosa*)
  - Congenital syphilis (*Treponema pallidum*)
- *Viral:*
  - Neonatal herpes simplex (herpes simplex virus)
  - Congenital herpes (intrauterine infection by herpes simplex virus)
  - Neonatal varicella (varicella zoster virus)
  - Cytomegalic inclusion disease (Cytomegalovirus)
  - Congenital Epstein-Barr virus syndrome (Epstein-Barr virus)
- *Fungal:*
  - Congenital candidiasis (*Candida albicans, Candida glabrata)*
  - Neonatal candidiasis (*Candida albicans, Candida parapsilosis)*
  - Pityrosporum folliculitis (Malassezia sp.)
- *Parasites:*
  - Scabies (*Sarcoptes scabiei*)

Q9. How will you differentiate the infectious conditions?

Ans: Differentiation of the infectious conditions causing neonatal pustular dermatoses has been described in Table 2.

Table 2: Differentiation of the infectious conditions of neonatal pustular dermatoses

Class	*Cause*	*Distinguishing features*
Bacterial	Group A/B Streptococcus, *Listeria monocytogenes, Pseudomonas aeruginosa, Staphylococcus aureus*, Other gram-negative organisms	Other signs of sepsis usually present. Elevated band count, positive blood culture; Gram stain of intralesional contents shows polymorphic neutrophils
Fungal	Candida	Presents within 24 hours after birth if congenital, after one week if acquired during delivery. Thrush is common. Potassium hydroxide preparation of intralesional contents shows pseudohyphae and spores
Spirochetal	Syphilis	Rare. Lesions on palms and soles. Suspect if results of maternal rapid plasma reagin or venereal disease research laboratory test positive or unknown
Viral	Cytomegalovirus, Herpes simplex, Varicella zoster	Crops of vesicles and pustules appear on erythematous base. For herpes simplex and varicella zoster, Tzanck test of intralesional contents shows multinucleated giant cells

Q10. A neonate presenting with pustules; how will you proceed to manage the case?

Ans:
- Maternal diseases such as vulvovaginal candidiasis, genital herpes, syphilis and scabies should be ruled out.
- Distribution and morphology of lesions, the time when the skin lesions appeared and how they evolved.
- Signs of systemic disease in newborns as fever or hepatosplenomegaly should be enquired.
- *Gram stain*: Gram-positive bacteria such as Staphylococcus and Streptococcus, Gram negative; also to identify the cellular composition of the inflammatory infiltrate.
- *KOH mount*: In case of fungal elements, for the detection of dermatophytosis, infections caused by Malassezia or Candida spp.
- *Tzanck smear*: Presence of multinucleated cells and inclusion bodies suggestive of herpes infection.
- Direct examination of lesion scraping can identify mites such as *Sarcoptes scabiei.*
- In doubtful cases—Syphilis serology, culture of pustules contents or skin biopsy.

CHAPTER 14

Neonatal Erythroderma

Lakshmi DV

Case study Neonatal Erythroderma

Presenting Complaints

Doctor, my baby has developed redness and scaling all over the body since 2 days.

Setting

Dermatology outpatient department

History of Present Illness

Informant: Mother—A 2-week-old male baby, first born of a nonconsanguineous marriage, was brought by the mother with generalized scaling and redness since 2 days. The rash was noticed over the face initially, and then eventually spread to involve the trunk and abdomen. No history of atopy in the family. Maternal history and prenatal history was uneventful. The baby has scaling over the scalp since birth.

General Physical Examination

Child is irritable. Weight: 3.5 kg
BMI—18 kg/m^2, Pulse—100 bpm

Systemic Examination

No abnormality detected

Dermatological Examination

Generalized erythema and scaling present with cradle cap over the vertex (Figs 1 and 2) and scalp hair appears normal. Waxy scaling is present in the retroauricular area and nasolabial fold. Scaling and erythema present over the eyelids, forehead with relative sparing of perinasal and perioral area. Scaling is however present in the nasolabial folds. Axilla, cubital fossa, groin, popliteal area, neck folds are also involved. Scaling and erythema are also seen over the genital area and groin folds. Palms and soles, perianal, perineum regions are spared. No areas of local tenderness. Oral and genital mucosa normal. Eyes normal. Nails appear normal.

Q1. What is the most likely diagnosis?

Ans: Neonatal erythroderma

Q2. What is the most probable cause?

a. Infantile seborrheic dermatitis
b. Atopic dermatitis
c. Drug-induced erythroderma
d. Netherton syndrome

Ans: a. Seborrheic dermatitis

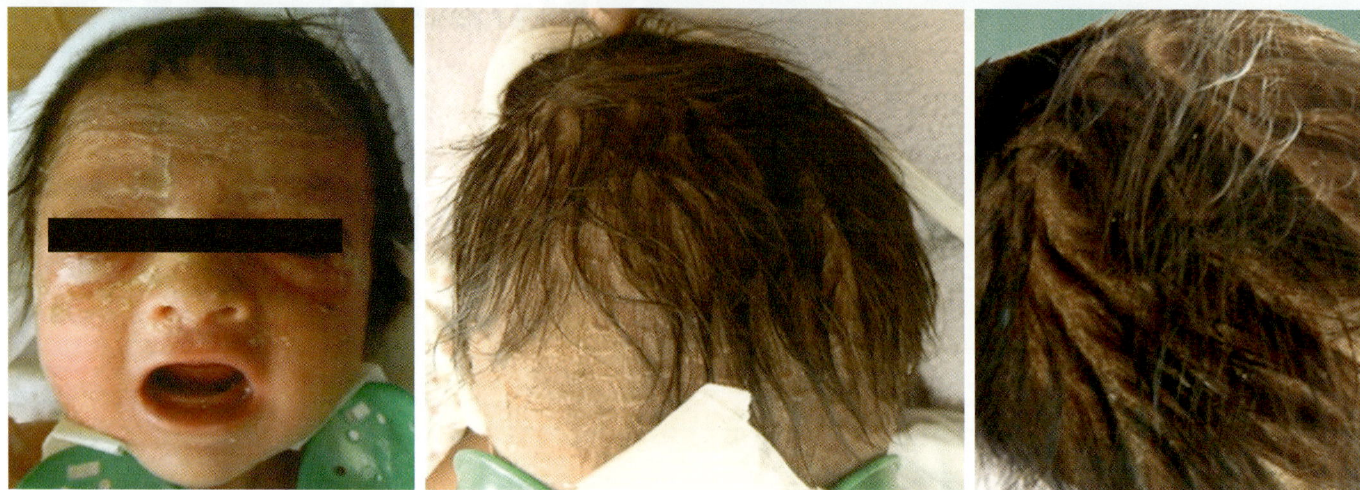

Fig. 1: Erythema and scaling over the forehead, scalp and nasolabial areas

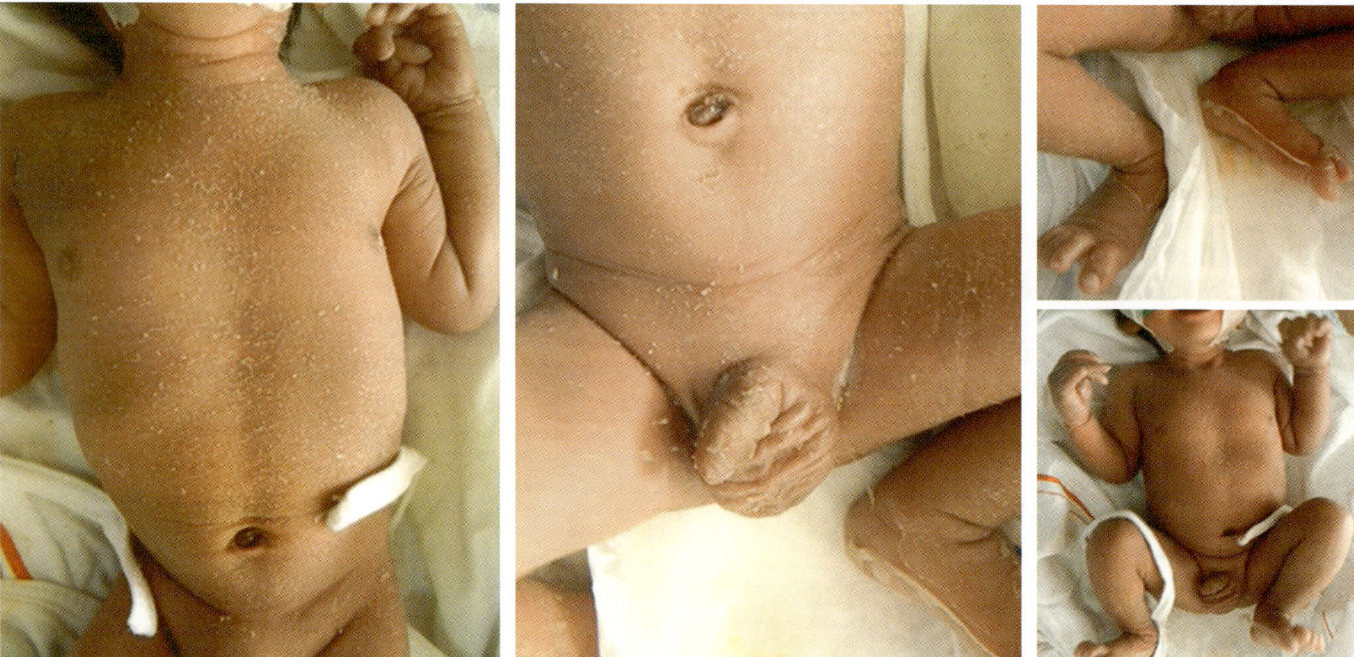

Fig. 2: Generalized erythema and scaling, involvement of genital area

Q3. What are the distinguishing features that favor the diagnosis?

Ans: Distinguishing features:

- Presence of prominent cradle cap since birth
- Greasy nature of scales accentuated in seborrheic areas and flexures
- Diaper area involvement favors seborrheic dermatitis
- No features of sepsis/failure to thrive/alopecia/hepatosplenomegaly clinically and systemic examination are normal
- Absence of atopy in family members.

Q4. What are the primary causes of neonatal erythroderma?

Ans: The primary causes of neonatal erythroderma are described in Table 1.

Table 1: Causes of neonatal erythroderma

Ichthyosis	Nonbullous ichthyosiform erythroderma (NBIE), bullous ichthyosiform erythroderma (BIE), Netherton syndrome, Conradi-Hunermann syndrome, Sjogren-Larsson syndrome, lamellar ichthyosis, trichothiodystrophy
Infections	Staphylococcal-scalded skin syndrome, scarlet fever, neonatal candidiasis, toxic shock syndrome
Infestations	Norwegian scabies
Immunodeficiency/ Immunocompromised state (ICD)	Omenn syndrome, graft vs host disease
Drug induced	Boric acid toxicity, ceftriaxone, vancomycin, antiepileptics, sulfonamides, antitubercular drugs, homeopathic, indigenous
Metabolic/Nutritional disorders	Disorders of biotin deficiency, Essential fatty acid deficiency, Kwashiorkor, acrodermatitis enteropathica, cystic fibrosis, Leiner's disease
Other disorders	Infantile seborrheic disorders, atopic dermatitis, psoriasis, pityriasis rubra pilaris (PRP), diffuse cutaneous mastocytosis

Q5. What are the diagnostic clues in a case of neonatal erythroderma?

Ans:
- Erythroderma + Failure to thrive + Alopecia + (Lymphadenopathy + Hepatosplenomegaly) = Primary immunodeficiency disorders
- Erythroderma + Failure to thrive + Alopecia (bamboo hair) = Netherton syndrome
- Erythroderma + History of Collodion baby= Nonbullous ichthyosiform erythroderma
- Erythroderma + Blistering (superficial) = Bullous ichthyosiform erythroderma
- Erythroderma + Blistering + Diarrhea + Flushing + Hypotension + Pruritus = Mastocytosis
- Erythroderma + Spared areas + Follicular hyperkeratosis + Palmoplantar keratoderma = PRP

Q6. What are the different types of scales which distinguish causes of erythroderma?

Ans: Types of scales:
- *Fine scales*: Atopic dermatitis
- *Bran-like scales*: Seborrheic dermatitis
- *Plate-like scales*: Lamellar ichthyosis
- *Double-edged scales*: Netherton syndrome

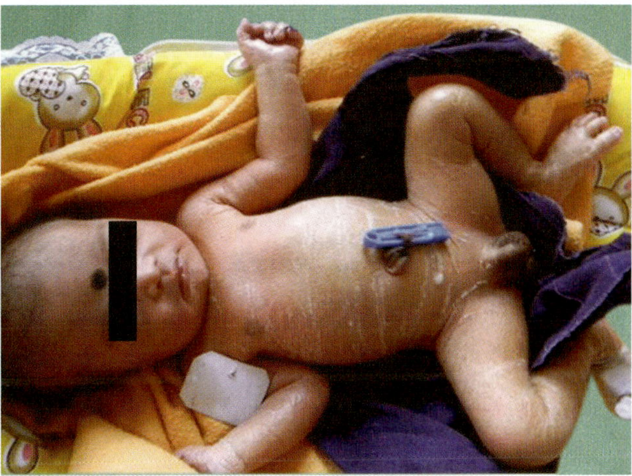

Fig. 3: Physiological desquamation

Q7. What is erythroderma desquamativum?

a. Leiner's disease
b. Omenn syndrome
c. Netherton syndrome
d. Job syndrome

Ans: a. *Leiner's disease*: It is caused by defect of complement protein C5 characterized by seborrheic dermatitis, severe diarrhea and failure to thrive.

Q8. What is physiological desquamation?

Ans: Physiological desquamation of neonatal skin generally takes place 24–36 hours after delivery and may not be complete until the 3rd week of life (Fig. 3). Desquamation at birth is an abnormal phenomenon and is indicative of postmaturity, intrauterine anoxia, or congenital ichthyosis. Unlike erythroderma, no erythema is present and it is a transient phenomenon.

Q9. What is the amount of transepidermal water loss (TEWL) in newborn and its significance in neonatal erythroderma?

Ans: In neonatal erythroderma TEWL is high. Insensible water loss is a measure of skin surface area to body weight ratio, and infants have larger body surface area compared to adults. Thus, more TEWL occurs. In premature infants, due to immaturity of stratum corneum, there is greater TEWL.

Q10. What are the laboratory investigations to be performed in a case of erythroderma?

Ans: Laboratory investigations which need to be performed in a case of erythroderma, have been described in Box 1.

Box 1

Baseline and specific laboratory investigations to be performed

Baseline investigations
- Complete hemogram, liver and renal function tests, serum electrolytes, random blood glucose estimation.
- Gram's stain for bacteria and bacterial culture
- Tzanck test
- Demonstration of *Sarcoptes scabiei*
- Microscopic analysis of hair shaft abnormalities
- Potassium hydroxide (KOH) stain for demonstration of mycelia/spores and fungal culture
- Skin biopsy for microscopic pathology

Specific investigations
- Serum zinc and alkaline phosphatase levels
- Sweat chloride levels
- Lipid profile including essential fatty acid levels
- Evaluation of humoral and cellular immunity; immunoglobulin A (IgA), IgG, IgM, IgE, complement component, T and B lymphocytes
- Biotinidase/holocarboxylase synthetase levels
- Plasma amino acid levels and urine organic acids

Q11. What are the distinguishing factors between atopic dermatitis and seborrheic dermatitis?

Ans: Distinguishing factors between atopic dermatitis and seborrheic dermatitis have been described in Table 2.

Q12. Is there a need to follow-up these infants with neonatal erythroderma secondary to seborrheic dermatitis?

Ans: Yes. Seborrheic dermatitis has good prognosis, but these infants can eventually develop atopic dermatitis. Some authors believe that infantile seborrheic dermatitis is a variant of atopic dermatitis.

Q13. Are breastfed babies more susceptible to develop neonatal erythroderma in biotinidase deficiency than formula-fed babies?

Ans: Yes. Biotin is in lower concentration in human milk. Breast-fed babies with biotinidase deficiency may become symptomatic earlier than formula-fed infants. Biotinidase deficiency presents later (mean age of onset 3 months) with hypotonia, lethargy, and seizures; the skin lesions resemble acrodermatitis enteropathica while in holocarboxylase synthetase deficiency, they are acutely ill with ketoacidosis, dehydration, and coma, and most of them die within the first week if untreated. Hence, with early biotin substitution, all skin and neurological symptoms are completely reversible in biotinidase deficiency.

Q14. Which are the metabolic disorders associated with acrodermatitis like exfoliative erythema?

Table 2: Distinguishing factors between atopic dermatitis and seborrheic dermatitis

Atopic dermatitis	*Seborrheic dermatitis*
• Erythroderma rare in neonatal period • Positive family history of atopy • Dermatitis characterized by vesicles and exudation • Sparing of napkin area and axilla • Itching only after 3 months of age	• Presents in first few months of life • Inflammatory, yellowish scaling on the scalp • Neck, axilla and groins • Erythematous patches are well demarcated and less pruritic • Diarrhea, failure to thrive

Table 3: Role of histopathology in neonatal erythroderma

Histopathological patterns	*Features*	*Underlying disease*
Psoriasiform pattern	Confluent parakeratosis, hyperkeratosis, hypogranulosis, suprapapillary thinning of the epidermis, regular acanthosis often with clubbed rete ridges. No spongiosis	Psoriasis, Netherton syndrome, pityriasis rubra pilaris, cystic fibrosis, acrodermatitis enteropathica
Spongiform pattern	Focal edematous parakeratosis, acanthosis or hyperkeratosis, spongiosis, sometimes spongiotic vesicles, mild or intense lymphocyte exocytosis	Infantile seborrheic disorders, atopic dermatitis, allergic contact dermatitis, DiGeorge syndrome, severe combined immunodeficiency
Ichthyosiform pattern	Compact orthohyperkeratosis, normal or thickened granular layer, follicular ostial plugs, No or few inflammatory cells	Ichthyosis, Neonatal cutaneous T cell lymphoma

Ans: Acrodermatitis like features:
- Maple syrup urine disease
- Deficiency of arginine
- Neonatal citrullinemia
- Deficiency of carbamoyl phosphate synthetase.

Q15. What is the role of histopathology in neonatal erythroderma?

Ans: The diagnostic value in erythroderma is not specific but can be helpful (Table 3).

Q16. What are the complications of neonatal erythroderma?

Ans:
- Septicemia

- Infections
- Hypoalbuminemia
- Hyperpyrexia
- Hypernatremic dehydration
- Renal failure
- Dermatopathic enteropathy
- High output cardiac failure
- Failure to thrive.

Q17. What are the principles in management of neonatal erythroderma?

Ans:
- Correction of hematological, biochemical and metabolic imbalance
- Prevention and treatment of infections
- Ambient humidity and temperature
- Correction of caloric and protein intake
- Maintenance of fluid and electrolyte balance
- Prevention of hyperpyrexia
- Maintenance of skin barrier by topical application of bland emollients, wet dressings, topical steroids (if needed) and use of systemic antibiotics
- Treatment of specific disease.

Q18. How would you manage the above case?

Ans: Bland emollients and topical hydrocortisone over cradle cap with general principles of management of erythroderma (Fig. 4).

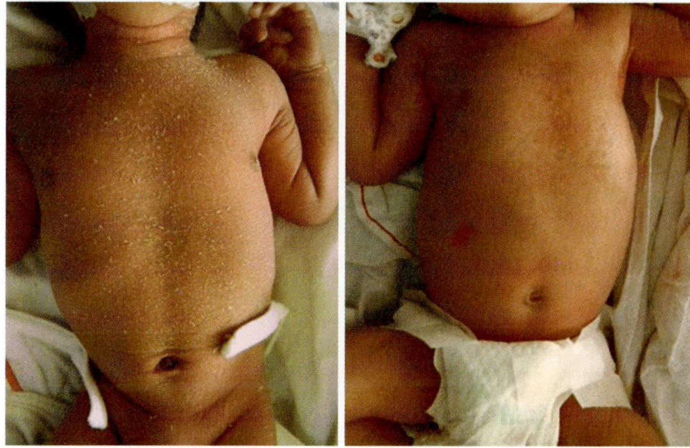

Fig. 4: Pre- and postphotographs showing marked improvement

Q19. What is the role of ambient humidity in neonatal erythroderma?

Ans: Insensible water loss is inversely proportional to body weight and maturity. Radiant warmer, phototherapy increases body temperature and peripheral blood flow and increases TEWL. Temperature in double walled humidified incubators gives ambient humidity that provides a thermal neutral environment and conserves total body water.

Q20. What is the prognosis?

Ans: The prognosis depends on underlying condition. Conditions such as drug-induced erythroderma, infantile seborrheic dermatitis, staphylococcal scalded skin syndrome and nutritional deficiencies respond well to treatment. Psoriatic and ichthyotic erythroderma need systemic drugs (Acitretin). In Immunodeficiency and inherited metabolic conditions prognosis is poor and variable.

CHAPTER 15

Epidermolysis Bullosa

Sahana M Srinivas

Case study Dystrophic Epidermolysis Bullosa

Presenting Complaints

Doctor, my child is getting recurrent blisters all over the body from birth. My child also gets severe pain and itching in the areas of blistering and is not able to do daily activities.

Setting

Dermatology outpatient department

History of Present Illness

A 3-year-old male child presented with multiple blisters all over body from birth. Child was born at term and was born out of consanguineous marriage. Natal and postnatal history was normal. Developmental milestones were normal. Blisters are painful and occur repeatedly on face, extremities and trunk. These blisters rupture within a day to form raw areas which leave behind light-colored areas and scarring. The child has restricted mobility in the hands. The blisters occur after trivial trauma and increased during summer season. There was history of oral lesions and nail involvement. There is no history of feeding problems. There was history of death in the elder sibling at 6 months of age due to similar symptoms. There is no history of photosensitivity, ocular involvement or gastrointestinal involvement in the child. Child is immunized till date.

General Physical Examination

Child is conscious, alert and not in pain. Vitals—normal, pallor—present.
Height and weight of the child was less than 50th percentile.

Systemic Examination

No abnormality detected

Dermatological Examination

- Multiple erosions and bullae present on forehead, upper arms, and forearms, dorsum of hands, lower back, elbow joint, gluteal region, knee joint, lower legs and feet
- Multiple atrophic scarring, milia and postinflammatory hypopigmentation present on face, elbow joint, trunk, knee joint, lower legs, hands and feet
- *Scalp*: Cicatricial alopecia present on parietal region
- *Oral mucosa*: Normal
- Teeth caries present
- *Palms and soles*: Atrophic scarring with milia present on dorsum of hands and feet. Flexion contractures of fingers and toes present (pseudosyndactyly)
- *Nails*: Total dystrophy of finger and toe nails.

Q1. What is the most likely diagnosis?

a. Dystrophic epidermolysis bullosa (DEB)
b. Junctional epidermolysis bullosa (JEB)
c. Porphyria
d. Epidermolysis bullosa acquisita

Ans: a. Dystrophic epidermolysis bullosa. Presence of bullae, erosions, atrophic scarring, milia, flexion contractures of fingers and toes (pseudosyndactyly), total nail dystrophy and cicatricial alopecia suggests the diagnosis of epidermolysis bullosa (EB) dystrophic variant.

Q2. How do you diagnose epidermolysis bullosa?

Ans: Diagnosis of EB is mainly clinical, based on history and clinical examination. There are various types of EB. There are no criteria but the hallmarks of the disease are mechanical fragile skin, easily inducible blisters and erosions from birth or early infancy. Other clinical features suggestive of EB are exuberant granulation tissue, atrophic scarring, milia, nail dystrophy, palmoplantar keratoderma, oral ulcers, dyspigmentation, alopecia, finger contractures, pseudosyndactyly, dental caries, enamel hypoplasia and various other systemic abnormalities.

Q3. What are the various types of epidermolysis bullosa?

Ans: Recent classification of epidermolysis bullosa is given below in Table 1.

Table 1: Classification of epidermolysis bullosa (EB)

Type	*Major types*	*Subtypes*
EB simplex (EBS)	Suprabasal	Acral peeling skin syndrome
		EBS superficialis (EBSS)
		Acantholytic EBS (EBS-acanth)
		Skin fragility syndromes
	Basal	EBS, localized (EBS-loc)
		EBS, generalized severe (EBS-gen sev)
		EBS, generalized intermediate (EBS-gen intermed)
		EBS with mottled pigmentation (EBS-MP)
		EBS, migratory circinate (EBS-migr)
		EBS, autosomal recessive K14 (EBS - AR K14)
		EBS with muscular dystrophy (EBS–MD)
		EBS with pyloric atresia (EBS-PA)
		EBS-Ogna (EBS-og)
		EBS, autosomal recessive-BP230 deficiency
		EBS, autosomal recessive-exophilin 5 deficiency
Junctional EB (JEB)	JEB, generalized	JEB, severe generalized
		JEB, generalized intermediate
		JEB, with pyloric atresia
		JEB, late onset
		JEB, with respiratory and renal involvement
	JEB, localized	JEB, localized (JEB - loc)
		JEB, inversa
		JEB-LOC syndrome (Laryngo-onycho-cutaneous syndrome)
Dystrophic EB (DEB)	Dominant DEB (DDEB)	DDEB, generalized (DDEB-gen)
		DDEB, acral (DDEB-ac)
		DDEB, pretibial (DDEB-pt)
		DDEB, pruriginosa (DDEB-pr)
		DDEB, nails only (DDEB-na)
		DDEB, bullous dermolysis of newborn (DDEB-BDN)
	Recessive DEB (RDEB)	RDEB, generalized severe
		RDEB, generalized intermediate
		RDEB, inversa
		RDEB, localized
		RDEB, pretibial
		RDEB, pruriginosa
		RDEB, centripetalis
		RDEB, bullous dermolysis of newborn
Kindler syndrome		

Q4. How will you confirm the diagnosis?

Ans: Although diagnosis of EB is clinical, laboratory tests are necessary to determine the type of epidermolysis bullosa (simplex, junctional or dystrophic variant). Skin biopsy must be sent for ultrastructural examination to confirm the subtype of EB.

Q5. Which among the following tests is the most feasible for confirming type of EB in our setting?

a. Immunofluorescence antigen mapping
b. Transmission electron microscopy
c. Molecular testing
d. All of the above

Ans: a. Immunofluorescence antigen mapping. Monoclonal antibodies are used in antigen mapping in finding the likely mutated protein, thus determining the subtype of EB. This test is simple and available in India and is less expensive than other tests. A panel of four antibodies, namely collagen IV, keratin 14, laminin 332, collagen VII are used to determine the level of blistering. Antibodies to type XVII collagen, plectin, α6β4 integrin are used to categorize subtype of EB. The other useful tests are:

- *Transmission electron microscopy*: Visualizes the various components of dermoepidermal junction, but this test is very expensive and requires expertise opinion.
- *Molecular testing:* Available at few centers in India; is very expensive and considered to determine the mode of genetic transmission, prenatal diagnosis and few rare types of EB.

Q6. How do you take a skin biopsy in epidermolysis bullosa?

Ans: Biopsy should be taken from unaffected skin. Micro blister can be induced by rubbing the skin with fingertip or pencil eraser. Skin should be stroked 30–40 times to induce the blister. Incision and punch biopsy is avoided. Shave biopsy should be done in EB.

Q7. How can the many types of epidermolysis bullosa be differentiated from each other clinically?

Ans: Types of epidermolysis bullosa have been described in Table 2.

Table 2: Types of epidermolysis bullosa (EB) (Figs 1 to 5)

Type of EB	*Cutaneous features*	*Extracutaneous features*
EBS (Simplex EB)	Onset is at birth or infancy, localized or generalized blisters, heals with postinflammatory hypopigmentation, rarely milia and scarring, dystrophic nails, scalp normal	Systemic involvement rare. Hoarse cry due to laryngeal involvement seen in generalized variant, gastroesophageal reflux, rarely pyloric atresia and duodenal atresia
JEB (Junctional EB)	Onset at birth or infancy, extensive generalized blistering, heals with atrophic scarring, rarely milia, nonscarring alopecia, nail dystrophy, paronychia, bulbous finger tips, microstomia, ankyloglossia	Dysphagia, esophageal strictures, fissures, gastroesophageal reflux, urethral stenosis, corneal blisters, erosions, scarring, exposure keratitis, tracheolaryngeal stenosis, hoarseness, excessive caries, enamel hypoplasia. Malignancy rare, death more in first year of life
DEB (Dystrophic EB)	Onset at birth, blistering generalized, bony prominences, atrophic scarring, milia formation prominent, scarring alopecia, flexion contractures, total nail dystrophy, mitten appearance of hands (90–100%), pseudosyndactyly	Anemia, growth retardation, ankyloglossia, microstomia, atrophic tongue, enamel hypoplasia absent, dysphagia, constipation, anal fissures, urethral stenosis, nephropathy, postinfectious glomerulonephritis, symblepharon, renal failure, multiple squamous cell carcinoma by adult age, death can occur by 3rd to 4th decade

Q8. What are complications associated with epidermolysis bullosa?

Ans: Complications include severe infection, septicemia, malnutrition, growth retardation, anemia, fluid and electrolyte imbalance, respiratory failure, renal failure, heart disease, skin cancer (metastatic squamous cell carcinoma), impairment of quality of life, failure to thrive and death.

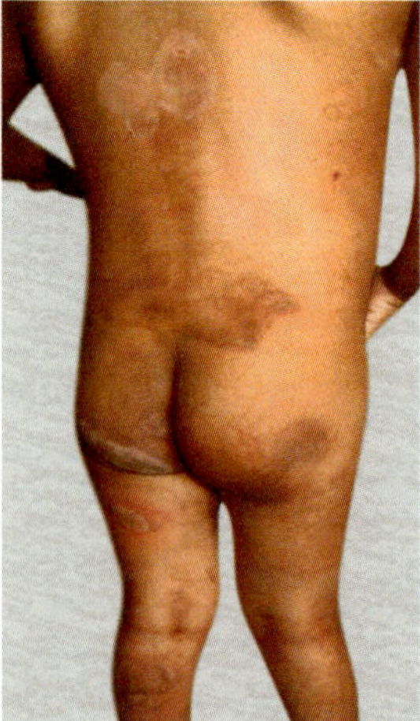

Fig. 1: Epidermolysis bullosa simplex showing bullae on gluteal region and postinflammatory hypopigmentation on back

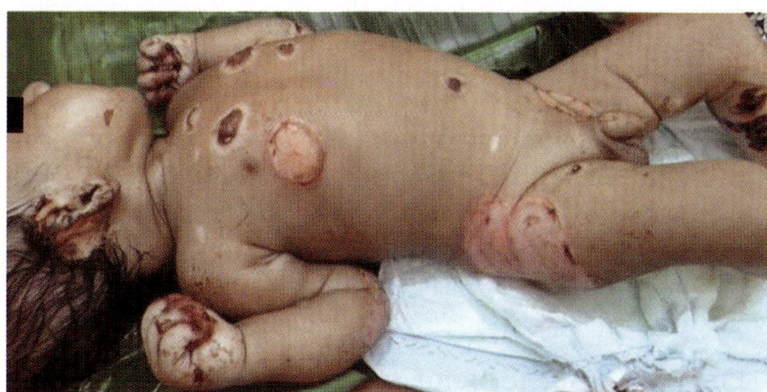

Fig. 2: Epidermolysis bullosa simplex with generalized involvement

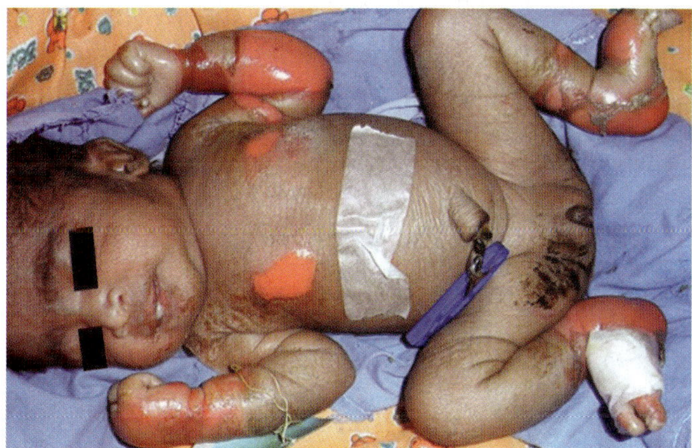

Fig. 3: Severe erosions seen on trunk and extremities in newborn child in junctional epidermolysis bullosa

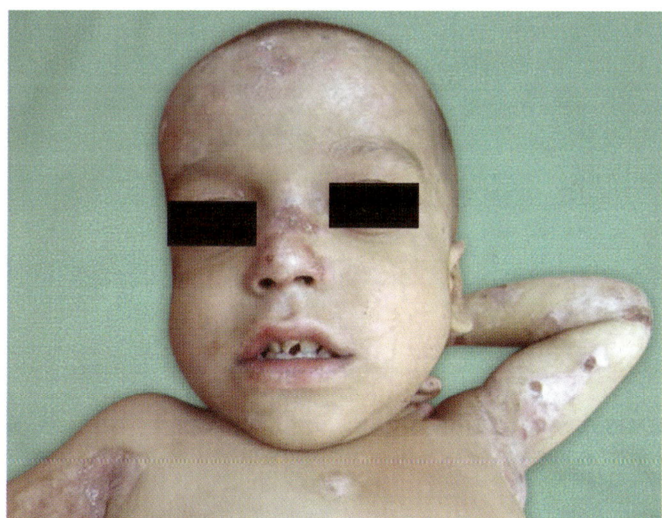

Fig. 4: Dystrophic epidermolysis bullosa showing atrophic scarring, milia on face and upper limbs

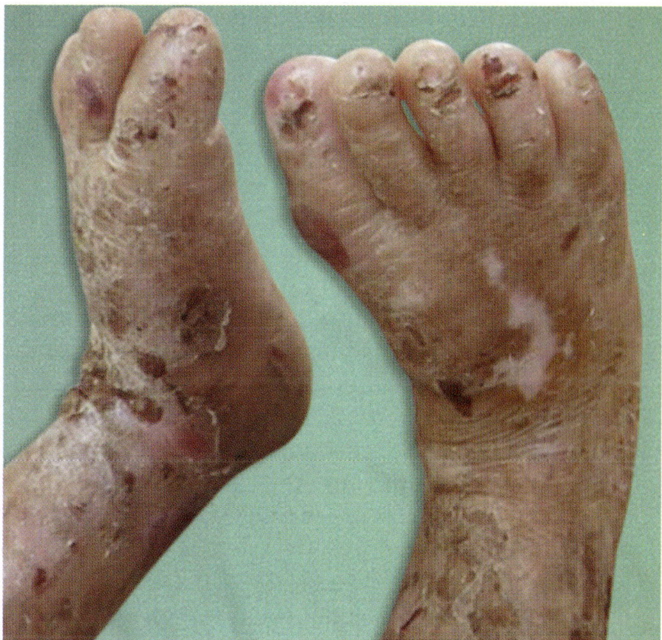

Fig. 5: Scarring, postinflammatory hypopigmentation and total nail dystrophy in dystrophic epidermolysis bullosa

Q9. Which is the best treatment option for epidermolysis bullosa?

a. Supportive therapy and general skin care
b. Wound care
c. Prevention and treatment of infections
d. Management of extracutaneous complications
e. All of the above.

Ans: e. All of the above.

Q10. What are the treatment principles in epidermolysis bullosa?

Ans: Treatment principles:

Supportive therapy and general skin care: Treatment of EB is mainly supportive as there is no curative therapy.

- Counseling all family members about the disorder and the regular follow-up
- Caregivers must be taught to handle the child gently to prevent new blisters. Lift the baby by head and buttocks
- Multiple handlers for the child should be avoided
- Environment should not be too warm. Nursing the child in incubators should be avoided
- Parents should be taught to pop the blisters by using lancet or sterile needle. Needle should pierce from one end of the blister to other end without deroofing, allowing slow drainage

- Daily bathing with mild cleansers
- Diapers with no elastic or soft cotton diapers must be used. Clothing should be loose soft cotton with seams covered
- Hanging skin trimmed. Nails should be cut regularly
- Moisturizers like liquid paraffin to be used all over the body except on raw wounds to prevent itching and for lubrication
- Prevention of trauma in elderly children
- Palms and soles must be kept dry in summer season. Cotton mittens can be used to prevent itching
- Maintenance of good nutrition
- Parents should be empathetic toward their children to boost their confidence (support groups are there for help)

Wound care

- Wound dressing should start from legs, face and scalp
- *There are two types of wound care*: Raw wound and healing wound
- Moisturizers should be applied for dry and healing wound
- Dressing are mainly three layered.
  - *1st layer/primary layer*: Nonsticky, silicone nonadherent woven mesh-like dressing/ Mepitel/Vaseline impregnated gauze/burns mesh/collagen dressings
  - *2nd layer/secondary layer*: Absorptive dressings, foam-based dressings used. Mepilex if available can be used/dressing pad
  - *3rd layer*: To hold the dressing in place. Mepitac or roller gauze can be used.

Prevention and treatment of infections

- Inspection of wounds regularly for purulent exudates
- Regularly swab for culture and sensitivity should be done
- Choice of antibiotic is based on culture sensitivity.

Management of extracutaneous complications: Multidisciplinary approach is necessary to manage complications. Epidermolysis bullosa team consists of trained nurses, dermatologist, pediatrician, gastroenterologist, dentist, ophthalmologist, plastic surgeon, dietician, occupational therapist and geneticist.

Q11. What is the prognosis of epidermolysis bullosa?

Ans: Prognosis depends on the type and subtype of EB

- Most EB children, particularly EBS, DDEB have normal life expectancy
- Herlitz JEB, RDEB, Dowling-Meara type have highest risk of mortality in first year of life.
- Metastatic squamous cell carcinoma is seen in adulthood.

Q12. In a nutshell, what are the steps involved in an approach to a case of epidermolysis bullosa?

Ans: Steps involved in an approach to a case of epidermolysis bullosa have been shown in Flowchart 1.

Flowchart 1: Steps involved in an approach to a case of epidermolysis bullosa

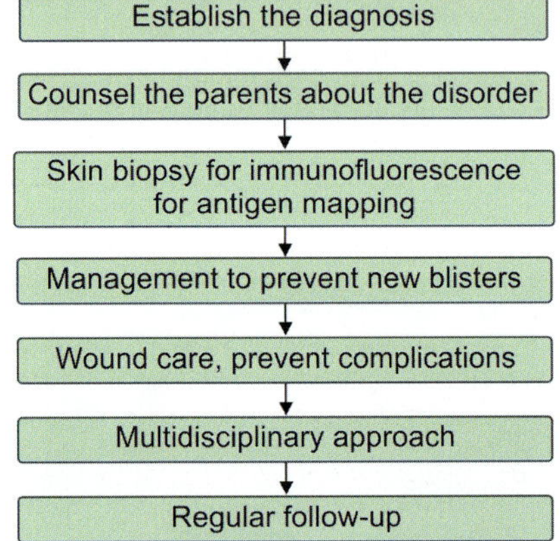

CHAPTER 16

Ichthyosis

Samipa S Mukherjee

Case study Ichthyosis

Presenting Complaints

A 10-year-old child is brought by parents with complaints of dry skin having started a few months after birth not being alleviated by the use of routine over the counter moisturizers.

Setting

Dermatology outpatient department

History of Present Illness

The child was born to non-consanguineous parents, full-term normal delivery, with normal developmental milestones, no history suggestive of a collodion membrane at birth and started developing dry skin over the body since 3 months of age. The accentuation of scaling was prominent over the extensor areas with marked exacerbation during winter season. The child also had a history of recurrent cold and cough, suggestive of an atopic diathesis.

General Physical Examination and Systemic Examination

No abnormality detected.

Dermatological Examination

- Light white to gray scales covering mainly the extensor surfaces of extremities and trunk.
- "Pasted on" large scales present over bilateral shin.
- Flexures spared.
- Follicular keratotic papules present over the lateral aspect of the arms and thighs.
- Hyperlinearity of palms and soles noted.

Q1. What is the most likely diagnosis?

a. Ichthyosis vulgaris
b. X-linked recessive ichthyosis
c. Lamellar ichthyosis
d. Non-bullous congenital ichthyosiform erythroderma.

Ans: a. Ichthyosis vulgaris. The presence of fine light white to gray scales sparing the flexures, hyperlinearity of palms and soles, keratosis pilaris and atopic diathesis suggests a diagnosis of ichthyosis vulgaris (Fig. 1).

Q2. How do you diagnose ichthyosis vulgaris?

Ans: Ichthyosis vulgaris is majorly diagnosed on the presence of clinical features. Confirmation of the diagnosis can be done on histopathology which shows compact orthohyperkeratosis, reduced rete-

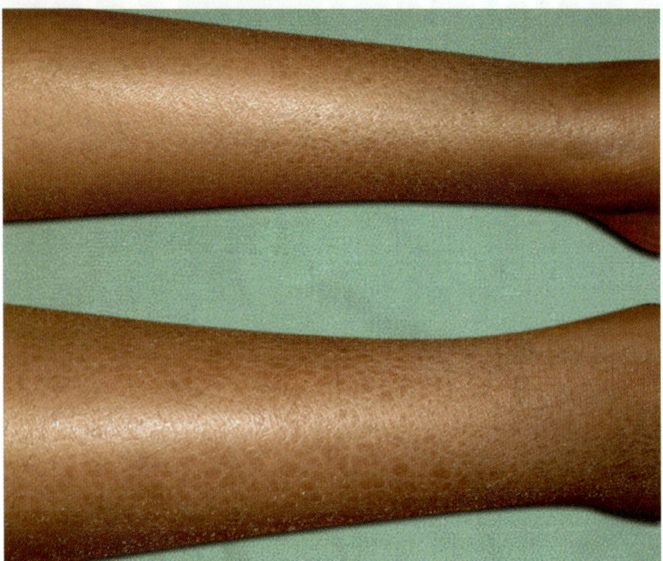

Fig. 1: Fine scales in ichthyosis vulgaris

papillae pattern and hypogranulosis as opposed to hypergranulosis in X-linked recessive ichthyosis.

Q3. Which of the following is the genetic defect in ichthyosis vulgaris?

a. Steroid sulfatase deficiency
b. Filaggrin (FLG gene) deficiency
c. Transglutaminase deficiency
d. Phytanic acid oxidase deficiency.

Ans: b. Filaggrin deficiency. Ichthyosis vulgaris is inherited in a semidominant pattern and is characterized by the loss of function of FLG gene which encodes profilaggrin. Filaggrin is responsible for keratin filament aggregation conferring barrier function to the skin and also hydration of stratum corneum via its break down products. This gene has been implicated in atopic dermatitis.

Q4. What are the differences between the three major congenital ichthyoses?

Ans: The differences between the three major congenital ichthyoses are described in Table 1.

Table 1: Differences between three major congenital ichthyoses

Feature	*Ichthyosis vulgaris*	*X-linked recessive ichthyosis*	*Lamellar ichthyosis*
Pathogenesis	Defective filaggrin	Steroid sulfatase deficiency	Transglutaminase 1 mutation
Onset	After 3 months of life	Within 3 months of life	At birth
Type of scale	Fine light white to gray	Smaller, darker with dirty appearance	Plate-like quadrangular
Associated feature	Hyperlinearity of palms and soles, keratosis pilaris	Cryptorchidism, corneal opacities	Ectropion, nail involvement
Course of disease	Improves with age	Does not improve with age	Remains life long
Histopathology	Hypogranulosis	Hypergranulosis	Hypergranulosis with mitotic figures

Q5. How do you classify ichthyosis?

Ans: Congenital ichthyosis and acquired ichthyosis.

- Congenital ichthyosis is further classified as:
  - Autosomal dominant:
    - Bullous ichthyosiform erythroderma
    - Ichthyosis bullosa of Siemens
    - Ichthyosis vulgaris
  - Autosomal recessive:
    - Lamellar ichthyosis
    - Non-bullous congenital ichthyosiform erythroderma
  - X-linked recessive ichthyosis
- Acquired ichthyosis is further classified as:
  - Malignancy associated
  - Infection associated
  - Metabolic disease associated
  - Endocrine disorder related
  - Connective tissue disorders related
  - Granulomatous disease related
  - Drug-induced.

Q6. What are the types of scales seen in ichthyosis?

Ans: Different types of scales are:

- *Ichthyosiform scale*: Large polygonal scales—ichthyosis vulgaris.
- *Hystrix-like scale*: Porcupine spine-like, muddy brown or gray color scaling over verrucous lesion (generalized or nevoid)—ichthyosis hystrix.
- *Mauserung desquamation*: Circumscribed patchy scaling with focal desquamation or moulting of scale—ichthyosis bullosa of Siemens.
- *Carapace-like scale*: Branny semiadherent scale with turned up edges, pasted on appearance—ichthyosis vulgaris.
- *Coat of armor*: Rigid, taut, yellow brown adherent hyperkeratotic skin—Harlequin ichthyosis.

- *Plate-like scale*: Large polygonal, thick, rigid dark brown firmly adherent arranged in mosaic pattern—lamellar ichthyosis.
- *Double-edged scale*: Ichthyosis linearis circumflexa—Netherton syndrome.
- *Corrugated/ridged scale*: Brown, waxy, ridged scaling after subsidence of erythroderma—bullous ichthyosiform erythroderma.

Q7. What are the clinical features of lamellar ichthyosis?

Ans: Lamellar ichthyosis is characterized by the presence of dark brown, large and plate-like scales forming a mosaic pattern (Fig. 2). The scales are adherent to the center with free edges. Ectropion and eclabium with hypoplasia of the nasal and auricular cartilage can occur. Palmoplantar keratoderma in varying severity, scarring alopecia, loss of eyebrows and eyelashes may be a common finding.

Q8. Which are the ichthyotic disorders which have a collodion membrane at presentation?

Ans: Collodion membrane:

- Autosomal recessive congenital ichthyosis
  - Lamellar ichthyosis
  - Congenital ichthyosiform erythroderma
  - self-healing collodion baby
- Autosomal dominant lamellar ichthyosis
- Sjögren-Larsson syndrome
- Trichothiodystrophy
- Infantile Gaucher disease
- Neutral lipid storage disease
- Hay-Wells syndrome.

Q9. How does a harlequin ichthyosis differ from lamellar ichthyosis?

Ans: Harlequin ichthyosis is an autosomal recessive disease associated with significant morbidity and mortality. It is clinically characterized by premature newborns who are encased in a hard, armor-like covering which is grayish yellow in color with an offensive odour restricting movements. The tautness of skin with severe eclabium, ectropion, microcephaly, hypoplastic nose gives a grotesque appearance. The child succumbs to systemic complications of prematurity, respiratory distress, sepsis, hypothermia and hypernatremic dehydration.

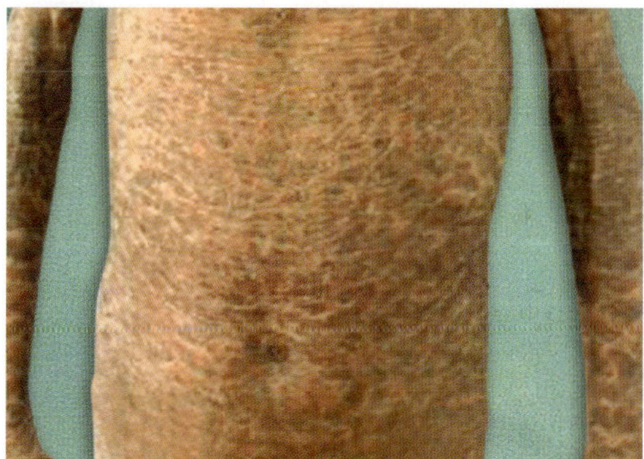

Fig. 2: Large plate-like scales in lamellar ichthyosis

Q10. What are the extracutaneous manifestations of ichthyosis?

Ans: Extracutaneous manifestations:

- Hearing loss due to retention of scales in the external auditory canal
- Dysphonia due to keratinization of the vocal cords
- Hypotrichosis
- Nail dystrophies
- Anhidrosis or hypohidrosis
- Neurological involvement—Sjögren-Larsson syndrome
- Musculoskeletal disorders—chondrodysplasia punctata
- Sensorineural deafness—KID syndrome
- Mental retardation—trichothiodystrophy.

Q11. What are the primary symptoms of ichthyosis and its pathomechanism?

Ans: The primary symptoms of ichthyosis and its pathomechanism are described in Table 2.

Q12. What is the role of wet wrap therapy in ichthyosis?

Ans: Wet wrap therapy is a technique where the patient is smeared with lubricant and other topical medications followed by the patient donning a wet close fitting cotton garment covering the entire body with a second dry layer of garment or wrapping with strips of cotton cloth/Elastocrepe bandages. The

Table 2: Primary symptoms of ichthyosis and its pathomechanism

Pathomechanism	*Symptom*
Abnormal quality or quantity of scales	Dryness and scales
Abnormal thickness of stratum corneum	Fissures and erosions, keratoderma
Skin inflammation	Erythema
Barrier failure	Infections, poikilothermia
Secondary infections	Pruritus
Obstruction of adnexal ducts	Anhidrosis
Stiffness of skin	Ectropion

Table 3: Mechanism of action of common additives in creams and ointments

Mechanism of action	*Ingredient*
Hydration	NaCl, urea and glycerol
Lubrication	Petrolatum and other lipids
Keratolysis	Alpha hydroxyl acids, urea >5%, salicylic acid and propylene glycol
Modulators of differentiation	Retinoids and calcipotriol
Antimicrobials	Mupirocin and fusidic acid

therapy helps in rehydrating the stratum corneum—alleviating dryness, scaling and pruritus.

Q13. What is the mechanism of action of common additives in creams and ointments?

Ans: The mechanism of action of common additives in creams and ointments are given in Table 3.

Q14. What is used in the treatment of mild to moderate ichthyosis?

Ans: Emollients with urea can be used for adults whereas glycerol is recommended for children and plain liquid paraffin for infants. Keratolytics may be used in moderate to severe disease in adults and severe disease in children.

Q15. How do oral retinoids help in ichthyosis?

Ans: Retinoids have keratolytic effects that facilitate shedding of scales from the surface and prevent excessive hyperkeratosis thus leading to a normalized thickness and improved function of the epidermis. Both isotretinoin and aromatic retinoids (acitretin and etritinate) have been found effective in the management of ichthyosis. Since acitretin has a longer half-life of elimination than isotretinoin, it is best avoided in female patients considering pregnancy in the near future where isotretinoin may be the preferred choice.

Q16. Which are the special scenarios in ichthyotic conditions where systemic retinoids may not be beneficial?

Ans: Oral retinoids are contraindicated for use in KID syndrome where the keratitis may be aggravated due to the use of oral retinoids. Also oral retinoids enhance skin fragility. It is therefore recommended to issue special caution while using oral retinoids in cases of epidermolytic hyperkeratosis where the chances of skin fragility may be increased.

Q17. What is the role of retinoic acid metabolism blocking agents?

Ans: An alternative to synthetic retinoid treatment is to manipulate the endogenous level of all trans-retinoic acid by blocking its cellular catabolism in the skin. The compounds used include liarozole (0.1g/day) and rambazole.

Q18. Which are the various syndromes in ichthyosis and what are their genetic defects and inheritance patterns?

Ans: The various syndromes in ichthyosis and their genetic defects and inheritance patterns are given in Table 4.

Table 4: Syndromes, inheritance and genetic defects in ichthyosis

Syndrome	*Inheritance*	*Genetic defect*
Sjögren-Larsson syndrome	Autosomal recessive	Fatty aldehyde dehydrogenase deficiency
Refsum's disease	Autosomal recessive	Phytanoyl-CoA hydroxylase
Conradi-Hünermann-Happle Syndrome	X-linked dominant	Emopamil binding protein
CHILD syndrome	X-linked dominant	NSDHL gene
Netherton syndrome	Autosomal recessive	SPINK5
IFAP syndrome	X-linked recessive ichthyosis	Zinc metalloproteinase

CHAPTER 17

Palmoplantar Keratoderma

Resham Vasani, Shreyaswini Pujary

Case study Palmoplantar Keratoderma

Presenting Complaints

Doctor, my 5-year-old son has thickening of palms and soles since birth. It started as a focal area of thickening at birth and has now extended to involve the entire palms and soles with recent appearance of lesions over the elbow and knees.

Setting

Dermatology outpatient department

History of Present Illness

Informant: Mother (reliable informant): The child was born of a non-consanguineous marriage as a normal full-term delivery and cried immediately after birth. The child had focal areas of thickened skin at birth over the palms and soles, which further extended over a period of 2–3 years to involve the entire palms and soles. There are, areas of thickened skin occurring over the elbows and knees since the past 4 months. There was no other abnormality. There was no history of similar complaints in parents or in the elder sibling aged 8 years.

General Examination and Systemic Examination

No abnormality detected.

Dermatological Examination

There is generalized thickening over the palms and soles (Fig. 1) with transgrediens to the lateral aspects of the feet and dorsa of the hands (Figs 2A and B). There are well-defined erythematous hyperkeratotic plaques over the elbows and knees (Figs 3A and B). The palms and soles appear macerated, have an erythematous base with associated malodor. The dorsa of hands show peeling of skin in large sheets. Nails show evidence of dystrophy with Beau's lines. Rest of the dermatological examination including that of the scalp/oral cavity/teeth/genitals/hair was normal.

Q1. What is the provisional diagnosis?

a. Vorner keratoderma
b. Greither's disease
c. Mal de Meleda syndrome
d. Unna-Thost keratoderma

Ans: c. Mal de Meleda syndrome.

- The patient has lesions since early months of life: it is a case of congenital keratoderma.
- Palmoplantar keratoderma (PPK) is extending onto the dorsal aspect of the hands and feet as

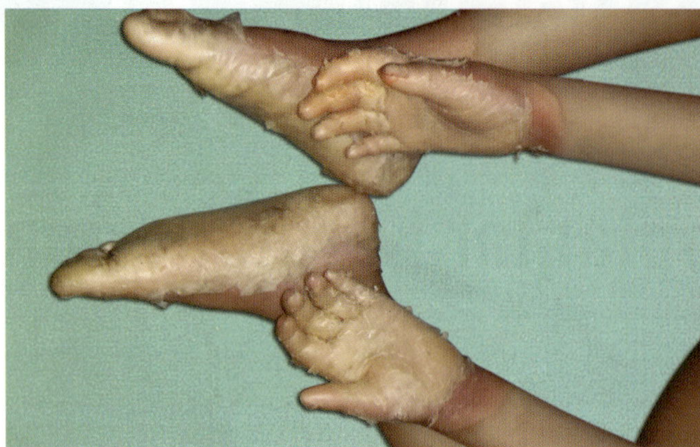

Fig. 1: Generalized thickening of skin over the palms and soles

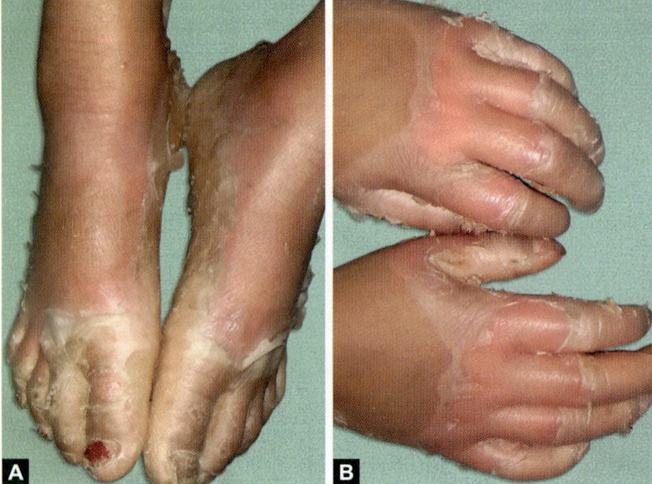

Figs 2A and B: Transgrediens to the lateral aspects of the feet and dorsa of the hands

well as onto the elbows and knees—that suggests it is a transgradient keratoderma.

- Severity of the disease increased with the age—demonstrating progradiens
- No other abnormalities—unlikely as a part of some syndrome.

The differential diagnosis of a patient with diffuse keratoderma without associated features presenting in early childhood are:

- *Vorner's keratoderma*: Epidermolytic non-transgradient keratoderma having early onset, diffuse keratoderma with dorsal sparing, history of blistering and fissuring and histological study demonstrating epidermolytic hyperkeratosis.
- *Unna-Thost keratoderma*: Non-epidermolytic non-transgradient keratoderma with onset in early childhood beginning with thick hyperkeratosis starting over the soles and progressing to involve the palms with dorsal sparing.
- *Greither's disease or acral keratoderma of Sybert*: Progressive keratoderma with onset at the age of 8–10-year-old and improving with age. Lesions are diffuse but transgradient hyperkeratosis with patchy lesions on knees and elbows can present. Erythema at the margins with hyperhidrosis may present. Can also be associated with Raynaud's-like vasomotor disturbance.
- *Mal de Meleda*: Onset soon after birth, as a palmoplantar erythema and progress to characteristic thickened exfoliative hyperkeratosis. Characteristically bilateral PPK that is diffuse and cuff-like (glove and stocking) with sharp margins and a yellow tone. It is transgradient and progradient. Becomes more severe with age. Can

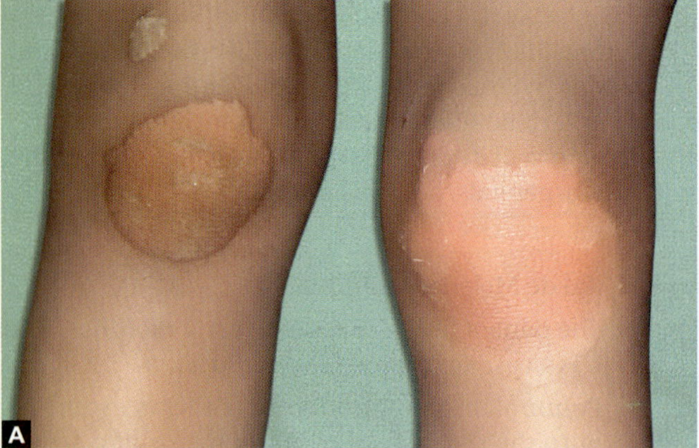

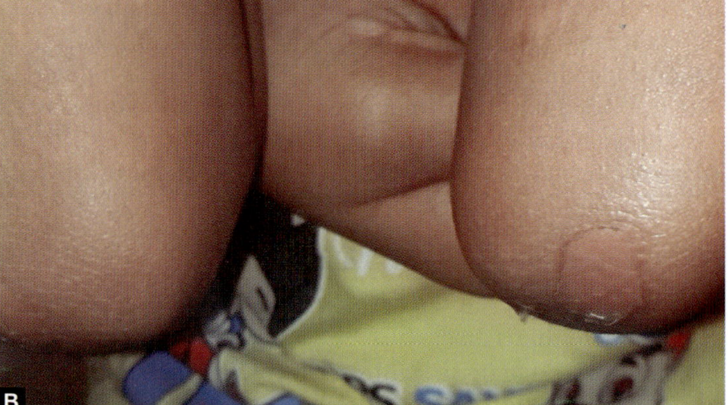

Figs 3A and B: Well-defined erythematous hyperkeratotic plaques over the elbows and knees

be complicated by hyperhidrosis with subsequent microbial infection leading to malodorous and painful lesions. Nagashima is a milder form of Mal de Meleda and is a milder transgradient variant, with few cases reported.

Considering the clinical presentation Mal de Meleda is the best fit and is the clinical diagnosis in this case.

Q2. How do you classify PPK?

Ans:
- Based on history: Inherited and acquired
- Clinical pattern as:
  - Diffuse keratodermas: Whole of the palmar or plantar epidermis is abnormally and uniformly thickened.
  - Focal (or aerate or nummular): Areas of palmoplantar skin undermost pressure are disproportionately thickened. The lesions may be painful.
  - Striate: Overlaps clinically with focal keratoderma, but the lesions are mostly longitudinal, particularly on the fingers, where the lesion overlies flexor tendons.
  - Punctate (papular or disseminated): Consists of multiple scattered discrete round lesions.
- The keratodermas can additionally be classified into three subgroups:
  - Simple keratodermas with PPK as the sole manifestation.
  - Complex keratodermas associated with lesions of non-volar skin, hair, teeth, nails, and/or sweat glands, including the ectodermal dysplasias.
  - Syndromic keratodermas with associated abnormalities of other organs, including deafness, cardiomyopathy and cancer.

Q3. What are the various clinical patterns of keratoderma?

Ans:
- Transgradient keratoderma: Extends beyond palmoplantar skin contiguously. Confluent hyperkeratosis extends around the whole digit.
- Cicatrizing keratodermas are those in which constricting bands appear around digits, usually distal to proximal interphalangeal joints.

Q4. Enumerate diffuse and focal keratodermas.

Ans: The enumeration of diffuse and focal keratodermas are given in Table 1.

Table 1: Diffuse and focal keratodermas

Diffuse keratodermas	*Focal keratodermas*
Epidermolytic keratoderma (Vörner)	Wachters keratoderma
Non-epidermolytic keratoderma (Thost-Unna)	Focal keratoderma with oral leukokeratosis
Loricrin keratoderma (Camisa; variant Vohwinkel)	Pachyonychia congenita type 1 (Jadassohn-Lewandowsky)
Autosomal dominant transgradient keratoderma (Greither; Sybert)	Pachyonychia congenita type 2 (Jackson-Lawler)
Keratoderma with scleroatrophy (Huriez)	Howel-Evans syndrome
Mal de Meleda	Striate keratoderma (Brunauer-Fohs-Siemens syndrome)
Palmoplantar and periorificial keratoderma (Olmsted)	Hidrotic ectodermal dysplasia (Clouston syndrome)

Q5. Which are the keratodermas with extracutaneous features?

Ans:
- *Howel-Evans syndrome*: Keratoderma with oesophageal carcinoma—(focal PPK with oral lesions).
- *Naxos disease*: Striate keratoderma, woolly hair and arrhythmogenic right cardiomyopathy.
- *Carvajal syndrome*: Striate keratoderma, woolly hair and dilated left cardiomyopathy.
- *Vohwinkel syndrome*: Cicatrizing keratoderma with hearing loss; papular lesions becoming confluent, starfish keratosis is the classical feature. Mild sensorineural hearing impairment present.
- *Papillon-Lefèvre syndrome*: Keratoderma with severe periodontitis and other pyogenic infections.
- *Richner-Hanhart syndrome*: Oculocutaneous tyrosinemia, corneal ulcers, painful keratoses and progressive mental impairment.

Q6. Which are the keratodermas associated with carcinoma?

Ans:
- *Howel-Evans syndrome* is a hereditary focal hyperkeratosis of palms and soles associated with esophageal carcinoma.
- *Papillon-Lefèvre syndrome*: Keratoderma with periodontitis. Malignant melanoma has been reported as a complication of this syndrome.
- *Keratoderma with scleroatrophy*: Huriez syndrome is associated with squamous and verrucous carcinomas.
- *Familial punctate keratoderma* is associated with various internal organ malignancies.
- *Filiform PPK* with cancer of the breast, colon and kidney.
- *Acquired PPK* can be paraneoplastic.

Tripe palms is a form of acquired palmar keratoderma with a thickened moss-like or velvety structure characterized by exaggerated dermatoglyphics of the palmar aspect of the hands. It is commonly associated with lung and stomach malignancies.

- *Bazex's acrokeratosis paraneoplastica* is a form of acquired PPK seen in association with neoplasia of upper aerodigestive tract.
- *Arsenical keratoderma* is associated with PPK with internal malignancy commonly affecting the lung and bladder.

Q7. Which are the keratodermas associated with hearing impairment?

Ans: Vohwinkel syndrome, Bart-Pumphrey syndrome, mitochondrial PPK with hearing impairment. Due to the defect in connexin function, hereditary keratoderma is associated with hearing loss.

Q8. What are the causes of acquired PPK?

Ans: The causes of acquired PPK are described in Table 2.

Table 2: Causes of acquired palmoplantar keratoderma (PPK)

Inflammatory skin conditions	Psoriasis, Reiter's disease, dermatitis, lupus erythematosus, lichen planus, lichen nitidus and pityriasis rubra pilaris
Infections	Reiter syndrome, dermatophyte fungal infection, syphilis, late yaws, crusted scabies and extensive viral warts (in immunosuppressed)
Circulatory problems	Lymphedema
Secondary to inherited conditions that may not usually result in keratoderma	Ichthyosis, ectodermal dysplasia, epidermolysis bullosa and erythrokeratoderma
Medications and toxins	Iodine, lithium, glucan, halogenated weed killers, arsenic, digoxin and chemotherapeutic agent used in cancer treatment
Internal illness	Myxedema and internal malignancies
Miscellaneous	Keratoderma climactericum

Q9. What are the complications of keratodermas?

- Pain
- Abnormalities in gait
- Secondary infection
- Long standing cases can develop carcinoma.

Q10. Describe the management of PPK.

Ans: Treatment targets at removal of hyperkeratosis with the following:

- Physical debridement
- Emollients
- Keratolytic agents (salicylic acid 5–20% ointment, benzoic acid)
- Propylene glycol (40–60%) in aqueous cream under occlusion softens the hyperkeratotic material)
- Topical vitamin A analogs
- Topical vitamin D analogs
- Systemic retinoids (isotretinoin and acitretin)
- For the treatment of hyperhidrosis regular potassium permanganate soaks or aluminum chloride hexahydrate lotion is useful

Secondary infection is treated with appropriate antifungal agents and antibiotics.

CHAPTER 18

Staphylococcal Scalded Skin Syndrome

Saloni Katoch

Case study Staphylococcal Scalded Skin Syndrome

Presenting Complaints

Doctor, my 25-day-old baby has been having fever since 5 days and skin rashes since 4 days.

Setting

Neonatal intensive care unit (NICU)

History of Presenting Illness

A 25-day-old, full-term, vaginally delivered, male neonate is referred by the pediatrician for skin rashes of 4 days duration. The neonate was apparently alright 6 days back when the mother noticed that the baby was being very irritable, was crying excessively on being held and was feeding poorly. The fever developed a day later and was followed by the skin rash. The rashes were initially red in color, started over the face and then progressed to become widespread over the body. The rashes evolved over a period of 48 hours forming blisters of varying sizes, most of which have now ruptured to leave behind raw areas.

General Physical Examination

- Neonate is febrile and irritable
- Pulse: 170 beats/min
- BP: 70/50 mm Hg
- Respiratory rate: 50 cycles/min.

Systemic Examination

Within normal limits

Dermatological Examination

- Few flaccid bullae and multiple erythematous erosions present in the periorificial areas, trunk and flexural surfaces (Figs 1 and 2).
- Perioral crusting with radial fissures seen.
- Areas of desquamation present over the trunk (Fig. 3).
- Nikolsky sign: Positive.

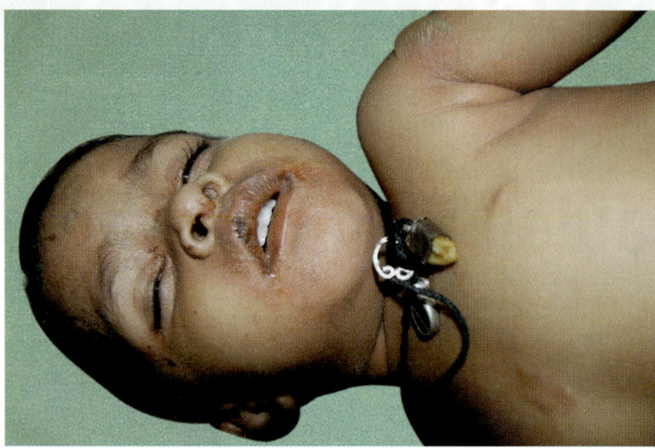

Fig. 1: Multiple erythematous erosions and crusts present in the periorificial areas

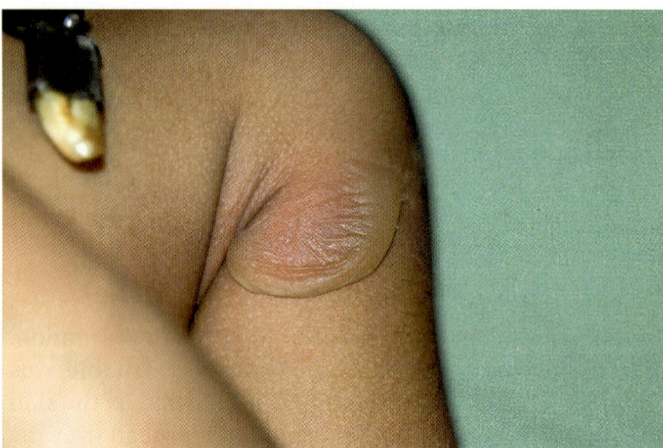

Fig. 2: A flaccid bulla on left forearm

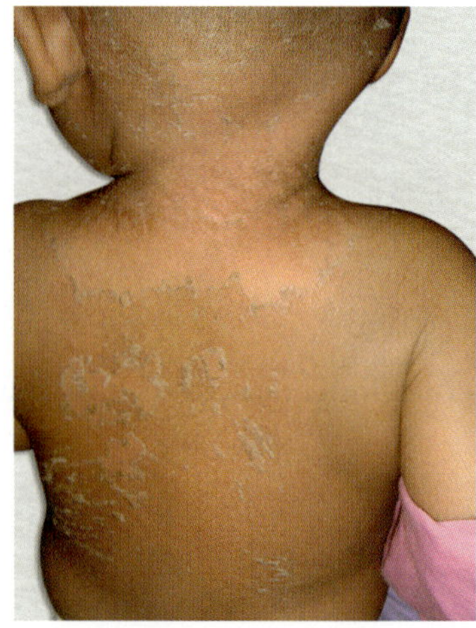

Fig. 3: Areas of desquamation present over the trunk

Q1. What is the most likely diagnosis?

a. Toxic epidermal necrolysis (TEN)
b. Epidermolysis bullosa
c. Staphylococcal scalded skin syndrome (SSSS)
d. Bullous ichthyosiform erythroderma.

Ans: c. Staphylococcal scalded skin syndrome. The characteristic history pointing towards skin tenderness (baby crying excessively on being held), evolution of the rash, perioral crusting with radial fissures and other examination findings, sparing of the mucosal surfaces and a positive Nikolsky sign are in the favor of the diagnosis.

Q2. What is SSSS? Describe its clinical features.

Ans: Staphylococcal scalded skin syndrome, also known as Ritter's disease or pemphigus neonatorum is a toxin mediated exfoliative dermatosis caused by *Staphylococcus aureus* characterized by widespread erythema, blistering and denudation of skin.

- There is an evident or an occult focus of infection with hematogenous dissemination of the epidermolytic toxin (ET).
- It is commonly seen in neonates, infants and children less than 5 years and this incidence is attributed to poor renal excretion of the toxin and inadequate neutralizing antitoxin antibodies.
- Adults may be affected when there is an underlying immunosuppression, renal failure, malignancy or alcohol abuse.
- The clinical features are as follows:
  - The initial event is usually a localized staphylococcal infection (purulent conjunctivitis, otitis media, nasopharyngeal infection or pyogenic skin infection).
  - A few days later, patient develops fever, irritability and skin tenderness.
  - This is followed by widespread erythema progressing to tissue paper like wrinkling of skin and blisters which denude easily to leave behind raw painful areas resembling a generalized scalding burn with a predilection for the periorificial and flexural surfaces (Figs 1 to 3).
  - Perioral crusting with radial fissures and associated edema is typical of SSSS: "Sad man facies".
  - The infants and children do not appear toxic unless they have developed complications.
  - Resolves with superficial desquamation, with healing complete within 7–14 days.

- Prognosis is good in children with early administration of antibiotics, the mortality is low (2%).
- Adult mortality is higher (10%), due to increased likelihood of sepsis.

Q3. What are the key points in etiopathogenesis of SSSS?

Ans: Etiopathogenesis:

- Hematogenous dissemination of ETs (exfoliatin A and B) produced by certain strains (usually phage group II) of *S. aureus* from a focus of localized infection.
- Exfoliatin A and B are serine proteases which behave as desmoglein 1 specific molecular scissors, cleaving the cell adhesion molecule and resulting in superficial epidermal blisters.
- Blisters do not form in the lower epidermis or mucous membrane as desmoglein 3 maintains cell-to-cell adhesion in these areas and compensates for the loss of desmoglein 1: "the desmoglein compensation theory".

Q4. How do you diagnose SSSS?

- The diagnosis is usually clinical. The characteristic clinical pattern of skin tenderness, widespread erythema, scarlatiniform rash evolving into tissue paper like wrinkling of skin and flaccid bullae which rupture easily to leave behind painful erosions with a predilection for the periorificial and flexural areas, followed by superficial desquamation during the phase of resolution suggests a diagnosis of SSSS.
- Nikolsky sign is found to be positive.
- Tzanck smear from a freshly denuded area reveals acantholytic cells without inflammatory cells.
- Histopathology reveals an intraepidermal cleavage with splitting beneath and within the stratum granulosum.

Q5. What investigations should one carry out in this case?

Ans: Investigations:

- *To find out foci of infection*: Swabs are taken from the conjunctiva, nares, nasopharynx, external auditory canal, umbilical stump and skin for Gram staining and culture.
- *Blood cultures*: Positive in less than 5% of pediatric patients as the disease is toxin mediated.
- Swabs and culture of blister fluid do not usually grow staphylococci as the blisters are due to a hematogenously disseminated toxin.
- *Skin biopsy*: Intraepidermal split between the granular and spinous layers.
- *To detect the exfoliative toxins*: Slide latex agglutination and ELISA.
- *WBC count*: May be normal or elevated.
- *Serum electrolytes*: To detect abnormalities due to widespread disruption of barrier function.

Q6. How would you like to proceed with the management?

Ans: Management:

- Staphylococcal scalded skin syndrome in neonates can be life-threatening and may lead to NICU outbreaks, hence, appropriate preventive measures should be initiated.
- *General measures*: Incubators to maintain body temperature and humidity, management of potential fluid and electrolyte abnormalities.
- *Supportive skin care*: Nonadherent dressings to areas with blistering and erosions (petrolatum impregnated gauze), saline compresses and mupirocin ointment to clear impetiginized areas.
- *Parenteral antistaphylococcal antibiotic (cloxacillin and flucloxacillin)*: For eradication of *S. aureus* and are given for a duration of 7–10 days. Alternative drugs are erythromycin, cephalosporins and clindamycin. Injections of gentamicin/amikacin may be added if there is a secondary gram-negative infection. Vancomycin would be the drug of choice in case of methicillin-resistant *S. aureus* infections.

Q7. What are the complications of SSSS?

Ans: Complications:

- Fluid and electrolyte disturbances and hypothermia (acute skin failure)
- Secondary gram-negative infection (*Pseudomonas aeruginosa*)
- Sepsis
- Pneumonia
- Cellulitis
- Osteomyelitis
- Septic arthritis
- Necrotizing fasciitis.

Q8. What precautions are to be taken to prevent NICU outbreaks?

- Isolation of the affected neonate and contacts.
- Strict aseptic measures while handling the baby to prevent cross infection to other neonates.
- Strict infection control measures like handwashing and cohort of at-risk neonates.

- Identification and treatment of symptomatic and asymptomatic carriers of *S. aureus*

Q9. What are the differential diagnosis of SSSS?

- Bullous impetigo
- Toxic epidermal necrolysis
- Epidermolysis bullosa
- Bullous ichthyosiform erythroderma
- Bullous mastocytosis
- Neonatal pemphigus
- Scalding burns.

Q10. How would you differentiate between SSSS and toxic epidermal necrolysis?

Ans: The differentiation between SSSS and toxic epidermal necrolysis are described in Table 1.

Q11. What is Nikolsky sign and where is it found to be positive?

Ans: Nikolsky's sign:

- Nikolsky sign is a clinical sign which indicates intraepidermal cleavage and differentiates intraepidermal from subepidermal blisters.
- It is best elicited by applying lateral pressure with the thumb or finger pad on skin over a bony prominence, the shearing force thus created dislodges the upper layers of the epidermis from the lower ones.
- It is found to be positive in:
  - Pemphigus group of disorders
  - Staphylococcal scalded skin syndrome
  - Ichthyosis bullosa of Siemens ("mauserung phenomenon").

Table 1: Differentiation between SSSS and toxic epidermal necrolysis

Features	*SSSS*	*TEN*
Etiology	Epidermolytic toxin (ET) elaborated by *Staphylococcus aureus*	Drugs, neoplasia, infections, graft versus host disease
Age	Neonates, infants and children	Adults
Mucosal erosions	Absent	Present
Tzanck smear	Acantholytic cells present	Acantholytic cells absent
Histopathology	Superficial subgranular acantholysis Epidermal necrosis absent	Dermal-epidermal separation Full thickness epidermal necrosis
Prognosis	Good, mortality: 2–3%	Poor, mortality: 25–50%

Q12. How would you explain the prognosis to the worried parents?

Ans: Prognosis:

- The disease may look worrisome when denudation of large areas of skin may give the child a scalded appearance, but the prognosis in neonates and children is good with complete recovery.
- In neonates, widespread exfoliation may lead to fluid and electrolyte imbalance and hypothermia and hence, SSSS is considered as a dermatological emergency and should be managed accordingly in the NICU.
- Mortality is low in the pediatric age group (2–3%).

Q13. Which of the following can cause erythroderma in neonates?

a. Infantile seborrheic dermatitis
b. Non-bullous ichthyosiform erythroderma
c. Candidiasis
d. All of the above.

Ans: d. All of the above. Erythroderma is defined as inflammation of skin with erythema and scaling involving more than 90% of the body surface area. It may lead to acute skin failure with impaired thermoregulation, fluid and electrolyte imbalance, protein and calorie loss, failure of barrier function with predisposition to infection and systemic involvement. It is a dermatological emergency and requires a multidisciplinary approach.

Q14. Enumerate causes of erythroderma in neonates.

Ans: Erythroderma in neonates:

- *Infections*: Staphylococcal scalded skin syndrome, toxic shock syndrome and candidiasis.
- *Ichthyosis*: Non-bullous ichthyosiform erythroderma, Conradi-Hunermann syndrome, bullous ichthyosiform erythroderma, Netherton's syndrome.
- *Immunodeficiency*: Omenn's syndrome and graft-versus-host disease.
- *Metabolic disorders*: Disorders of biotin metabolism and essential fatty acid deficiency.
- *Drugs*: Ceftriaxone and vancomycin.
- *Others*: Infantile seborrheic dermatitis, atopic dermatitis, psoriasis, pityriasis rubra pilaris, generalized mastocytosis

CHAPTER 19

Kawasaki's Disease

Priyadarshini Kharge

Case study Kawasaki's Disease

Presenting Complaints

Frantic parents: My child has persistent fever for more than 4 days. He has also developed red eyes, dry lips, red tongue, red rashes, swelling of the hands and legs, extreme tiredness and is very irritable. He is not showing any improvement despite treatment.

Setting

Dermatology outpatient department.

History of Presenting Illness

A 5-year-old boy presented with persisting high to moderate fever of more than 4 days, in spite of oral medications and antibiotics. He also complains of red eyes with no discharge. By the fourth day, he developed dry, cracked lips with a red tongue, generalized red rash and swelling over the limbs. Peeling of skin over the palms and soles was present since 2 days. The child has been irritable and less cooperative. There was no history of any usage of drugs prior to onset, no fluid-filled lesions, generalized peeling of skin, sore throat, joint pains, abdominal pain or blood in urine.

General Physical Examination

- An uncooperative and irritable child, conscious and oriented to person, time and space.
- Temperature: 101°F. Pulse: 120/min.
- Non-pitting edema over the lower limbs predominantly.
- Non-exudative and non-tender cervical lymphadenopathy.

Cutaneous Examination

- Generalized, non-blanchable, non-tender, maculopapular rash over trunk and extremities.
- Oral cavity: Dry, fissured lips. Erythematous (strawberry like) tongue (Fig. 1), genital area: perianal erythema.
- Desquamation over the palms and soles (Fig. 2).

Q1. Based on the above findings, what is the most probable diagnosis?

a. Viral exanthem
b. Kawasaki's disease
c. Measles
d. Staphylococcal scalded skin syndrome

Ans: b. Kawasaki's disease. The classical features of persisting fever for more than 5 days with ocular, oral and skin lesions favor this condition.

Q2. Who gets this disease?

Ans: Children less than 5 years of age are most commonly affected. Incidence in teenagers and adults is very less.

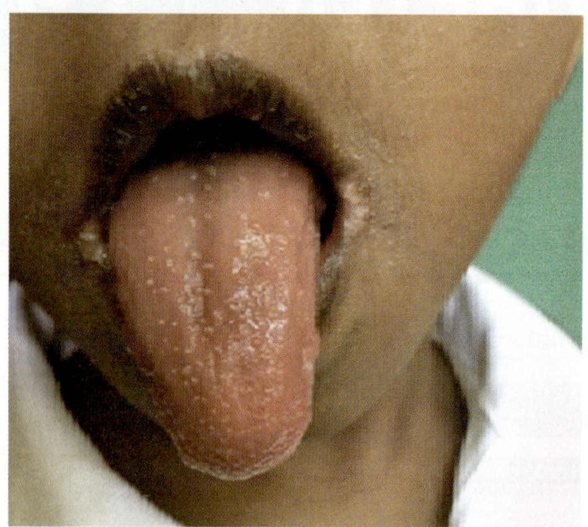

Fig. 1: Strawberry tongue

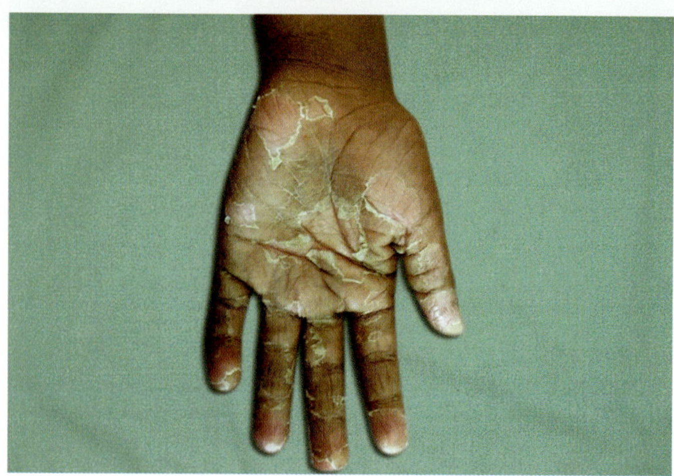

Fig. 2: Desquamation of palms and soles

Q3. How do we diagnose this condition?

Ans: Kawasaki's disease is diagnosed based on the diagnostic criteria formulated by the American Heart Association (AHA) given in Flowchart 1. Fever for 5 days or more with at least 4 of the 5 clinical signs in major criteria is necessary for diagnosis.

Q4. Why is it essential to detect Kawasaki's disease early?

Ans: The disease presents with both typical and atypical features, hence it is important to identify the condition early to prevent systemic and most importantly, cardiac complications. Even without treatment, it is usually self-limiting and resolves spontaneously within 4–8 weeks. But, 20% of untreated children have coronary artery damage and about 2% may die due to a myocardial infarction.

Q5. Is there a causative agent identified?

Ans: There is no specific etiology though multiple viruses and hereditary associations of gene *HLA-BW22J2* and the inositol 1,4,5-triphosphate 3-kinase C (*ITPKC*) gene on band 19q13.2 expressions have been identified. This is specially seen in the Japanese and US populations where this disease is more common.

Q6. What are the rare cutaneous features and complications associated with Kawasaki's disease?

Ans: Rare cutaneous features include pustules, onychomadesis, and erythema multiform like lesions. Other systemic complications include dehydration,

Flowchart 1: Diagnostic criteria of Kawasaki's disease by American Heart Association (AHA)

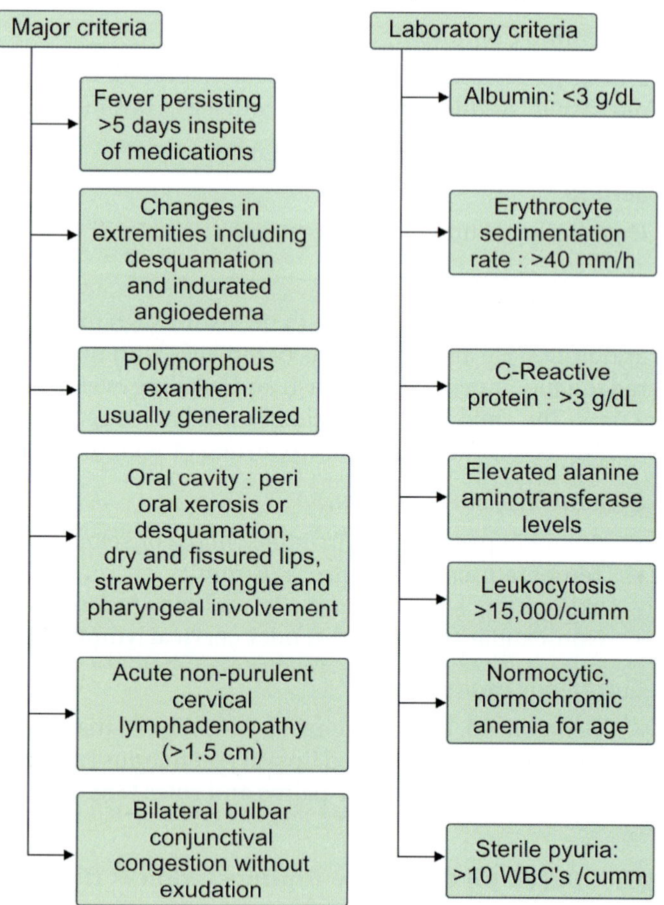

pneumonitis, otitis media, orchitis, urethritis, uveitis and peripheral gangrene.

- *Cardiovascular system*: Dilatation and/or narrowing of the coronary arteries leading to angina, myocardial infarction or sudden death. This is the most important complication that cannot be ignored.
- *Central nervous system*: Stiff neck, aseptic meningitis, unilateral facial palsy and sensori-neural hearing loss.
- *Gastrointestinal features*: Diarrhea, vomiting, abdominal pain, hepatomegaly and jaundice may occur.
- *Musculoskeletal system*: Diffuse arthralgia and arthritis.

Q7. What is the next step of approach in this patient?

a. Symptomatic treatment
b. Wait and watch as it is self-limiting
c. Investigate the child as per AHA guidelines
d. Admission as it can deteriorate if cardiovascular system is involved.

Ans: c. Investigate as per the AHA guidelines. Prompt appropriate treatment is important in case of systemic involvement.

Q8. How do we investigate the children?

Ans: There is no specific diagnostic test for this condition. But, multiple investigations are necessary to evaluate the child. Acute phase reactant levels of erythrocyte sedimentation rate, C-reactive protein and alpha 1 antitrypsin levels are elevated. Three biomarkers that are recently identified include proteins associated with endothelial and myocardial cell injury (filamin C), soluble *LR119* and immune regulators (meprin A) though they are not routinely done in our set up.

A complete blood count to look for thrombocytosis initially and thrombocytopenia in the later stages along with investigations to diagnose leukocytosis, albuminemia, normocytic, normochromic anemia and hypertriglyceridemia should be done.

Serial electrocardiogram and echocardiograms, especially, at diagnosis, at 2 weeks, and at 6–8 weeks after onset, have to be done. Follow-up with the pediatric cardiologist is advised if involvement is noted.

In a suspected incomplete type, an urine investigation is also needed to rule out pyuria.

Q9. What are the treatment options?

Ans: The children have to be admitted once the diagnosis with complications is made. Multidisciplinary team of pediatric dermatologist, pediatrician and pediatric cardiologist is needed. A single large dose of intravenous immunoglobulin (IVIG) of 2 g/kg intravenously over 10–12 hours is given. IVIG is most effective between 5–10 days of illness. If the signs and symptoms fail to resolve or recur within days then, a second dose of IVIG is given.

High-dose aspirin (80–100 mg/kg/day orally in 4 divided doses) is given in the acute phase and continued until day 14 or until the patient has been afebrile for 48–72 hours. Then, low-dose aspirin (3–5 mg/kg/day for 6–8 weeks) as maintenance is given. Reye's syndrome has to be watched for especially if children are susceptible to varicella or viral infections.

If a second dose of IVIG therapy fails, they can be treated with intravenous pulse of methyl prednisolone at a dose of 30 mg/kg for 2–3 hours, once daily for 1–3 days. Alternatively, infliximab 5 mg/kg can be used.

Q10. Will all children need long-term monitoring?

Ans: Reevaluate all children within a week of discharge with a repeat echocardiography. If no evidence of coronary aneurysms, further echo studies are unnecessary. Only children with persistent changes have to be evaluated by the respective consultants. As IVIG affects the efficacy of live vaccines, they should be delayed for at least a year after the last dose is given or repeated after 11 months if given earlier.

CHAPTER 20

Gianotti-Crosti Syndrome (Papular Acrodermatitis of Childhood)

Sahana M Srinivas

Case study Gianotti-Crosti Syndrome (Papular Acrodermatitis of Childhood)

Presenting Complaints

Doctor my child is having itchy skin lesions all over the body from past 1 week. My child also had mild fever and diarrhea 1 week before.

Setting

Dermatology outpatient department

History of Presenting Illness

A 1-year-old male child presented with complaints of itchy skin lesions on the face and extremities of 1 week duration. There was history of mild fever and one episode of diarrhea 1 week before development of rash. Initially the skin lesions started on the face and then appeared on the upper and lower limbs. There were no similar symptoms in the family. No history of drug intake prior to onset of lesions. Child is healthy and immunized till date.

General Physical Examination

Child is alert and conscious. Vitals are normal. Lymphadenopathy—present.

Systemic Examination

No abnormality detected.

Dermatological Examination

- Multiple erythematous to skin colored, discrete and grouped papules present symmetrically on the face, extensor aspect of upper limbs, gluteal region, thighs and lower legs (Figs 1 and 2).
- Koebner's phenomenon present on the lower legs.
- Oral mucosa, palms and soles normal.

Q1. What is the most likely diagnosis?

a. Gianotti-Crosti syndrome
b. Papular urticaria
c. Scabies
d. Atopic dermatitis
e. Lichen planus.

Ans: a. Gianotti-Crosti syndrome (papular acrodermatitis of childhood). Presence of symmetrically distributed monomorphic, erythematous to edematous papules on face and extremities, sparing the trunk suggests the diagnosis of papular acrodermatitis of childhood.

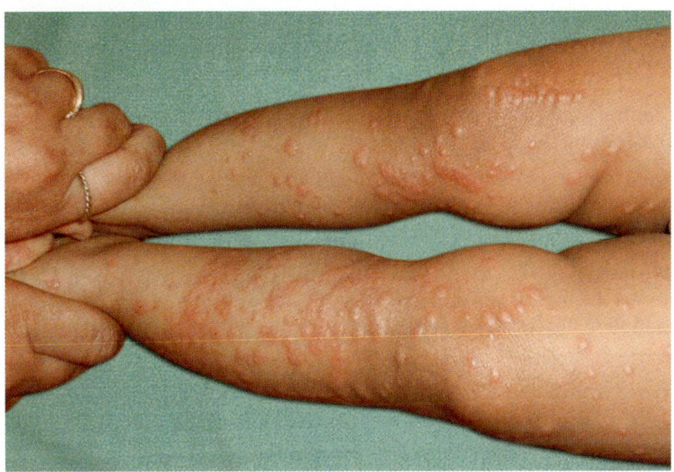

Fig. 1: Multiple erythematous monomorphic papules present bilaterally symmetrically on the extensor aspect of legs

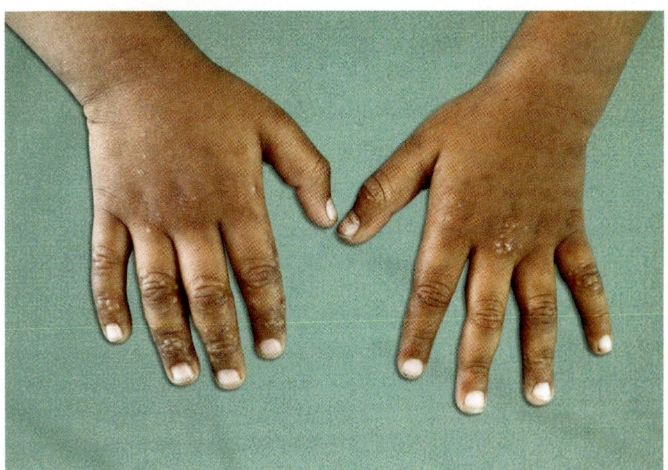

Fig. 2: Similar lesions on the dorsum of hands

Q2. How do you diagnose papular acrodermatitis of childhood?

Ans: Papular acrodermatitis of childhood is diagnosed clinically based on morphology and distribution of lesions. Positive and negative criteria is given here:

Positive Clinical Features

- Monomorphous, flat topped, pink to brown papulovesicles 1–10 mm in diameter on at least three of the following four sites—(1) cheeks, (2) buttocks, (3) extensor surfaces of forearms and (4) extensor surfaces of legs.
- Symmetrical distribution.
- Duration of at least 10 days.

Negative Clinical Features

- Extensive truncal lesions
- Scaly lesions.

Q3. Are there any investigations to confirm the diagnosis?

Ans: Diagnosis is made on clinical grounds. No laboratory investigations are required to confirm the diagnosis. However, leukocytosis and lymphocytosis can be seen. Skin biopsy may be useful to corroborate the diagnosis, but is rarely necessary. If hepatitis B association is considered, serological evaluation is indicated.

Q4. Enumerate the clinical features of papular acrodermatitis of childhood?

Ans: Clinical features:

- Also called as Gianotti-Crosti syndrome, it is a distinctive exanthem of childhood of viral etiology caused by Epstein-Barr virus, hepatitis B, enterovirus, hepatitis A, cytomegalovirus, adenovirus, rotavirus, parvovirus and respiratory syncytial virus.
- It is seen in children between the age group of 1 year and 6 years. Prodrome may be mild with fever, upper respiratory symptoms and lymphadenopathy. Pruritus may be present. Clinically presents with erythematous, edematous, monomorphic papules, papulovesicles distributed symmetrically on face and extremities (Fig. 1). Rarely hemorrhagic or purpuric lesions may occur.
- Trunk is usually (not always) spared.
- Resolution is seen by 8–12 weeks with post-inflammatory hyperpigmentation.

Q5. Is systemic involvement seen in papular acrodermatitis of childhood?

Ans: Systemic involvement is rarely seen. Hepatomegaly and abnormal liver function tests may be present if it associated with hepatitis B.

Q6. Can papular acrodermatitis of childhood occur post-vaccination in children?

Ans: Recently there are reports of papular acrodermatitis of childhood being associated with vaccination. Vaccine reports associated are measles-mumps-rubella, hemophilus, oral polio, Japanese B encephalitis, diphtheria-pertussis-tetanus and hepatitis B vaccines.

Q7. What are the differential diagnoses of papular acrodermatitis of childhood?

Ans: The various differential diagnoses are listed in Table 1.

Table 1: Differential diagnoses of papular acrodermatitis

Disorder	*Characteristic features*
Papular urticaria	Multiple erythematous papules with central punctum present more on the exposed part of the body Not symmetrical and not monomorphic lesions
Scabies	Multiple polymorphic lesions with erythematous papules, excoriated papules, vesicles, bullae distributed on axillae, trunk, periumbilical region, web spaces, extremities and genitalia Intensely pruritic and history of similar complaints in family members
Atopic dermatitis	Pruritus with family history of atopy present Chronic disorder with recurrent lesions on the face, trunk and extremities Eczematous plaques and excoriated papules
Lichen planus	Pruritic, chronic and recurrent Violaceous, polygonal flat topped papules distributed on the volar wrists, forearm, trunk, thighs, ankle region and lower legs Resolves with intensely hyperpigmented macules
Lichenoid drug eruption	History of drug intake prior to onset Generalized lichenoid papules with more of truncal involvement
Unilateral periflexural exanthem	Mild prodrome with fever and upper respiratory infections Unilateral exanthem, starts from one side of the chest near axilla or thigh, later becomes bilateral Morbilliform, scarlatiniform, urticarial, vesicular, reticulated and purpuric Spontaneous resolution in 4–8 weeks
Hand-foot-mouth disease	Elliptical vesicles, vesiculopustules surrounded by erythema on the palms, soles elbow joint, forearm, knee joint, gluteal region, perineum and lower legs Painful small ulcers on buccal mucosa, tongue and palate

Q8. What is the treatment of papular acrodermatitis of childhood?

a. Supportive therapy
b. Topical therapy
c. Antihistamines
d. All of the above.

Ans: d. All of the above.

- *Supportive therapy*: Counseling is the main stay of treatment. Parents should be counseled that it may take 6–8 weeks or more to resolve.
- Topical therapy:
  - Emollients
  - *Topical steroid*: Mild to mid potent steroid can be given for short period to reduce pruritus but it is not going to alter the natural history of the disorder.
- *Antihistamines:* Antihistamines can be given to reduce pruritus.

Q9. What is the prognosis?

Ans: Prognosis is good as it is a self-limiting disorder. Lesions resolve by 2–3 months without any complications.

CHAPTER 21

Viral Exanthem

Sahana M Srinivas

Case study Measles

Presenting Complaints

Doctor, my child is having skin rashes all over the body from 2 days. He is also having fever from past 6 days along with running nose and redness of eyes.

Setting

Dermatology outpatient department

History of Present Illness

A 5-year-old boy, presented to dermatology outpatient department with complaints of asymptomatic skin lesions on face, trunk, and extremities from 2 days. Mother gives a history that her child had fever from past 6 days along with running nose, red eyes, and mild sore throat. Red rashes initially started on the face and then spread to involve the trunk and extremities. There is history of having taken syrup amoxicillin for fever for presumed pharyngitis for 4 days before the onset of rash. There is no history of similar illness in the family members. There was no history of recent travel, exposure to pets, or drug allergy in the past. Child is otherwise healthy and immunized till date.

General Physical Examination

Child is conscious, alert, and not in distress. Child has normal development with height and weight at the 50th percentile with normal progress on his growth curve.
Temperature: 38.2 °C
Pulse: 95 beats/min
Respiratory rate: 26/min
BP: 110/70 mm Hg
No lymphadenopathy.
Conjunctival congestion was present.

Systemic Examination

No abnormality detected.

Dermatological Examination

- Diffuse erythematous maculopapular rash in a confluent pattern present on the face, trunk, upper and lower limbs (Fig. 1).
- *Oral mucosa*: Gray white punctate papules surrounded by erythema present on the buccal mucosa opposite the lower second molar tooth (koplik spots) (Fig. 2).
- Palms, soles, and scalp normal.

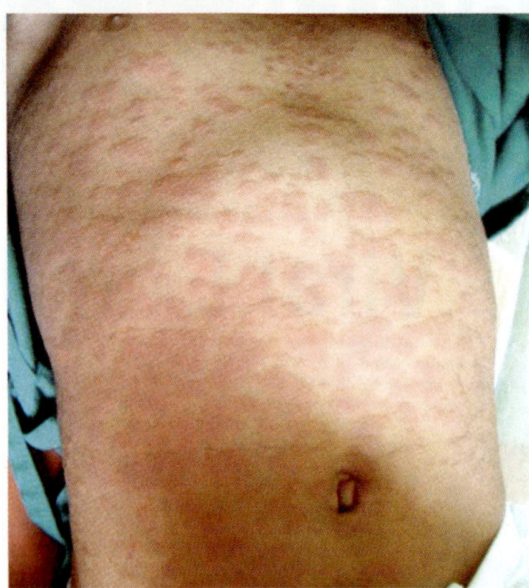

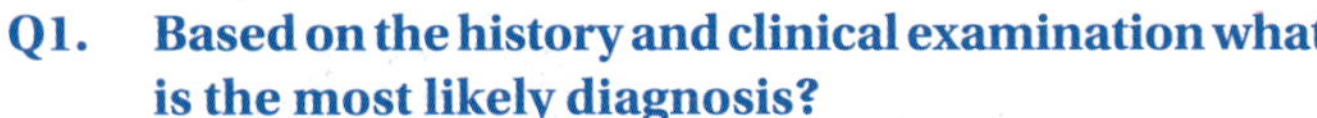

Fig. 1: Diffuse maculopapular rash in a confluent pattern seen in measles

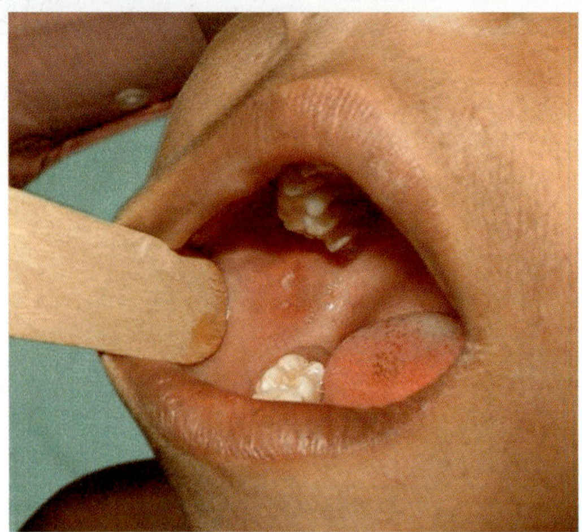

Fig. 2: Koplik spots seen on buccal mucosa in measles

Q1. Based on the history and clinical examination what is the most likely diagnosis?

a. Measles
b. Roseola infantum
c. Rubella
d. Erythema infectiosum
e. Drug reaction
f. Kawasaki disease

Ans: a (Measles)

Diffuse maculopapular rash in a confluent pattern with presence of koplik spots suggests the diagnosis of measles.

Q2. What are the tests done to confirm diagnosis of measles?

a. Measles IgM antibody
b. Virus isolation
c. Lymphopenia
d. Skin biopsy

Ans: Both a and b

Although lymphopenia is seen in viral exanthem, diagnosis of measles can be confirmed by serology testing where there is a fourfold increase in measles IgM antibody titres in acute and convalescent stage. Virus isolation is also confirmatory but is limited to research laboratory only.

Q3. Enumerate the clinical features of measles?

Ans: Clinical features:

- Measles is an acute febrile illness caused by RNA virus of the genus *Morbillivirus* in the Paramyxoviridae family. It spreads by direct contact with infectious droplets through coughing, sneezing, and close personal contact.
- The incubation period is from 10 days to 12 days. Patients are contagious 4 days before the onset of rash and 4 days after the onset of rash. Measles is seen more commonly in preschool children less than 5 years.
- It is characterized by prodromal symptoms of fever, malaise, cough, rhinorrhea, and conjunctival congestion. Clinically they present with characteristic enanthem called koplik spots. Koplik spots are pathognomoic sign of measles. They appear 2 days before and remain until after the onset of rash. They are punctate blue white papules surrounded by erythema on the buccal mucosa adjacent to molars.
- Exanthem appears as diffuse maculopapular confluent rash, initially beginning behind the ears, forehead, and progress toward trunk and extremities. Rash fades by 5–7 days in the same order as their appearance leaving behind branny desquamation.

Q4. What are the complications seen in measles?

Ans: Complications are rarely seen in measles. Hepatosplenomegaly, lymphadenopathy, pneumonia, blindness, encephalitis, otitis media, bronchopneumonia, myocarditis, pericarditis, and transient immunosuppression are some of the complications seen in measles.

Q5. What are the chances of measles occurring in immunized children?

Ans:

- Atypical and modified measles can occur in children immunized with measles vaccine.
- Atypical measles is extremely rare and not seen nowadays as it occurs in those vaccinated with

killed vaccine or in whom live vaccination has failed. There is prodrome of fever, respiratory symptoms, abdominal pain, pleural effusion, and lymphadenopathy along with peripheral petechial, vesicular, or vesiculopustular eruption.

- Modified measles occurs in infants with residual maternal antibodies and in previously vaccinated children. Prodrome and exanthem is very mild and is of shorter duration. Exanthem is limited to extremities, and koplik spots are absent.

Q6. What are the differential diagnoses to be considered in measles?

Ans: The differential diagnoses that should be considered for measles are enumerated in Table 1.

Q7. How do you differentiate viral exanthem from drug reaction?

Ans: Differentiation between viral exanthem and drug reaction is enumerated in Table 2.

Q8. What of the following are correct with respect to management option for measles?

a. There is no specific antiviral therapy for measles
b. Supportive therapy
c. Treatment with vitamin A
d. Immunization of children to prevent spread of measles
e. All of the above

Ans: e. (All of the above)

Supportive therapy

- Counseling
- Topical therapy—emollients or calamine lotion
- Antipyretics
- Antihistamines if pruritus is present
- Lot of fluids.

Treatment with vitamin A: Vitamin A deficiency is associated with severe complications in measles. Vitamin A supplementation is considered if there

Table 1: Differential diagnoses that should be considered for measles

Disorder	*Characteristic features*
Rubella	• Prodrome mild with fever, sore throat, cough, headache • Rash appears within 24 hours of onset of prodromal symptoms, starts on face, neck, and spreads to trunk and extremities • Minute discrete macules as compared to confluent pattern of measles • Painful suboccipital, postauricular, cervical lymphadenopathy
Roseola infantum	• Prodrome of high fever, diarrhea • Abrupt onset of erythematous, macules, and papules • Appears initially on trunk, later spreads to extremities, neck, and face
Erythema infectiosum	• Prodrome mild with fever, pharyngitis, arthritis • Exanthem appears in a characteristic pattern. Initially it appears as facial erythema, more prominent on the cheeks giving the appearance of slapped cheek appearance. After 1-4 days of appearance of facial rash, lacy reticulated erythematous eruption appears on extremities
Infectious mononucleosis	• Fever, pharyngeal inflammation, generalized lymphadenopathy • Exanthem occurs in the form of maculopapular rash, petechial, erythema multiforme, urticarial
Kawasaki disease	• Absence of prodrome of respiratory symptoms, nonexudative conjunctivitis • Rash is polymorphic and predominantly on trunk • Edema over the hands and feet with desquamation • Periungual and perianal desquamation is characteristic
Drug reaction	• History of drug intake • Associated with pruritus • Rashes could be maculopapular, urticaria, vesicles, purpuric macules with central necrosis
Meningococcemia	• Transient maculopapular rash resembles viral exanthem • Fever with petechiae on trunk and extremities, may go for purpura fulminans and multiorgan failure
Dengue fever	• High grade fever, headache, arthralgia, • Transient generalized macular rash develops within 48 hours • Fever subsides within 2–7 days and later reappears after 1–2 days. Generalized maculopapular rash occurs all over the body sparing the palms and soles • Islands of sparing of skin in a background of ocean of erythema are a distinctive pattern seen during resolving phase
Papular-purpuric gloves and socks syndrome	• Progressive erythema, edema on palms and soles, later becomes petechial and purpuric • Sharp demarcation at wrists and ankles. Many involve elbows, knees, buttocks, and dorsum of hands and feet

Table 2: Differentiation between viral exanthem and drug reaction

Viral exanthem	*Drug reaction*
Constitutional symptoms are present	Constitutional symptoms are less
Onset of lesions starts from face, progresses to trunk and extremities, and resolves in same pattern	Abrupt onset of skin lesions
Pruritus absent	Pruritus present
Maculopapular rash	Dusky erythema
Palms and soles may/not be involved	Palms and soles involved
Systemic involvement is less involved	Systemic involvement more common
Investigations—lymphopenia, neutropenia	Eosinophilia present

is a dietary deficiency, and its administration has been associated with 50% reduction in mortality and morbidity associated with measles.

Immunization: Parents should be counseled about the importance of immunization to prevent spread of measles.

Q9. What is the prognosis of measles?

Ans: Prognosis is good with supportive care. Infants, malnourished, and immunodeficient children are at risk for complications. If there is systemic involvement child should be admitted and a pediatrician referral should be taken.

SECTION 5

Disorders of Appendages (Hair and Nail)

Lakshmi DV

CHAPTER 22

Alopecia Areata

Shilpa K

Case study Alopecia Areata

Presenting Complaint

Doctor, my daughter is having a patch of hair loss on her scalp since 1 month.

Setting

Dermatology outpatient department

History of Present Illness

An 8-years-old girl (informant-mother) presented with complaints of patchy hair loss on the scalp since 1 month. It was spontaneous in onset and gradually progressive. Patient had similar lesions about 2 years back for which treatment was taken in the form of ointments following which hair had regrown. There is no history of associated symptoms like itching, pulling of hair by the patient, behavioral abnormalities, or learning difficulties. However mother gave history of recurrent nasal allergies and upper respiratory tract infection in the child since the age of 7 years, and her paternal grandmother was an asthma patient.

General Physical Examination and Systemic Examination

No abnormality detected.

Dermatological Examination

- A single well-defined patch of alopecia in the parietal area on right side of the scalp
- Exclamatory hair present
- Nails showing regular pitting.

Q1. What is the most likely diagnosis?

a. Alopecia areata
b. Tricotillomania
c. Tinea capitis
d. Pseudopelade

Ans: a (Alopecia areata)

Points in favor are:

- A well-defined area of patchy hair loss with no itching, scales, or broken hair shaft
- Similar history in the past with regrowth of hair
- Presence of atopic history in the family and the patient. Typical nail finding with regular pitting.

Q2. How do you diagnose alopecia areata?

Ans:

- Alopecia areata is diagnosed on clinical grounds:
  - Single or multiple patchy areas of baldness with smooth surface
  - Exclamatory hairs at the periphery of the patch
  - Absence of inflammation, itching, scaling, or broken hair
  - Positive hair pull test at the periphery.
- History of atopy or asthma in the patient or family.
- Similar history of patchy hair loss in family or patient with regrowth spontaneously or with treatment.

Q3. How will you confirm the diagnosis?

Ans: It can be confirmed by dermoscopy and biopsy. Autoimmune panel may be performed if required.

Dermoscopy findings include yellow dots, black dots, broken hairs, short vellus hair, and tapering hairs.

The histopathologic features of alopecia areata (AA) depend on the stage of the disease. In the acute stage, terminal hairs are surrounded by bulbar lymphocytes giving an appearance of "swarm of bees". In the subacute stage, decreased anagen while increased catagen and telogen hairs are characteristically found. In the chronic stage, decreased terminal and increased miniaturized hairs are found, with variable inflammation. During recovery, increasing numbers of terminal anagen hairs from regrowth of miniaturized hairs and a lack of inflammation are noted.

Q4. Which factors are involved in the pathogenesis of alopecia areata?

Ans: The pathogenesis of AA is multifactorial. They are:

- Genetic factors—HLA-DR and HLA-DQB1*03
- Atopy
- Other potential offenders proposed in the causation of AA are psychologic stress, anemia, parasitic infestations, hypothyroidism, hyperthyroidism, and diabetes
- Autoimmunity and vitamin D may also be involved.

Q5. What are the various clinical patterns of alopecia areata?

Ans: Ikeda et al. have classified AA into four types based on the course of the disease and associated conditions as shown in the Table 1.

Table 1: Types of alopecia areata

Type	*Presentation*	*Course*
Atopic type	It begins early in life	Mostly (30-75%) progresses to alopecia totalis
Autoimmune type	It is seen in middle-aged groups associated with autoimmune diseases, diabetes mellitus (diabetes is an autoimmune disease by itself)	Progresses to alopecia totalis in 10–50%
Prehypertensive type	It is seen in young adults whose parents were hypertensive	Progresses fastly to alopecia totalis in 40% of cases
Common type	It affects adults aged 20-40 years	Alopecia totalis develops in 5–15%

Based on the number, extent, and body parts; AA can be

- Alopecia areata monolocularis (solitary patch; Fig. 1)
- Alopecia areata multilocularis (multiple patches; Fig. 2)
- *Alopecia totalis*: Involvement of scalp and body hair such as eyebrows, eyelashes, beard, underarm hair, and pubic hair
- *Alopecia universalis*: Involvement of entire body.
- *Ophiasis pattern*: Alopecia areata extending along the posterior occipital and temporal scalp margins (Fig. 3)
- *Sisaipho pattern*: The opposite of ophiasis type, where hairs are lost centrally and spared at the margins of the scalp
- *Alopecia areata incognita (diffuse alopecia areata)*: The typical patchy distribution of hair loss in classical AA is absent, but abrupt and intense hair loss is characteristic
- Linear AA
- Reticulate type
- *Acute diffuse and total alopecia*: A new subtype of AA with a favorable prognosis
- Areas involved other than scalp—beard, axilla, pubic area, extremities, eyebrow (Fig. 4).

Q6. What are the nail changes seen in alopecia areata?

Ans: Nail changes are seen in 29% of adults and 50% of children with AA.

- Regular pits giving scotch plaid appearance
- Geometric punctate leukonychia

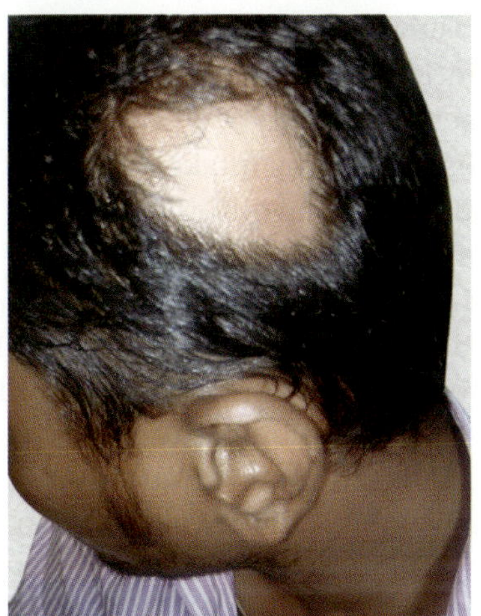

Fig. 1: Alopecia areata—solitary patch

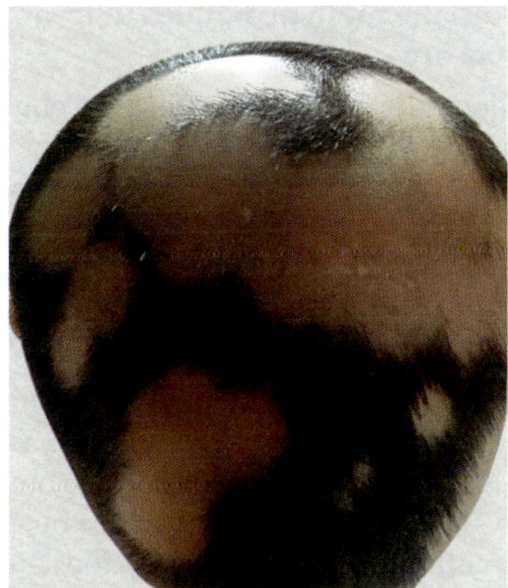

Fig. 2: Alopecia areata—multiple patches

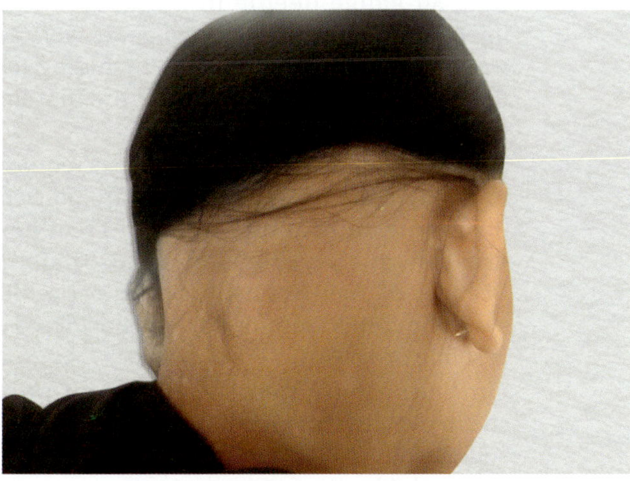

Fig. 3: Alopecia areata—ophiasis pattern

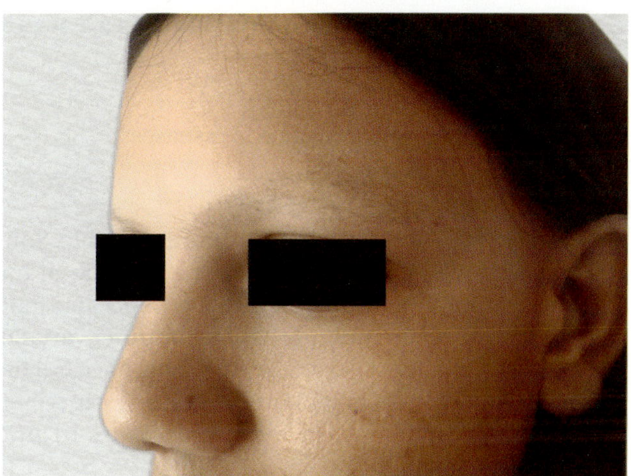

Fig. 4: Alopecia areata of the eyebrow

- Trachyonychia (sandpaper nails)
- Red-spotted lunula
- Periungual erythema
- Beau's lines
- Onychomadesis.

Q7. What are the associations of alopecia areata?

Ans: Associations

- Thyroid disease (8–28%)
- Atopic dermatitis
- Vitiligo
- Diabetes mellitus type 1
- Polyglandular autoimmune syndrome type I
- Collagen-vascular diseases
- Down syndrome
- Psychiatric disorders—anxiety, personality disorders, depression, and paranoid disorders
- Stressful life events in the 6 months before onset.

Q8. How do you grade the severity of the disease?

Ans: Severity assessment

- *Mild*: Three or less patches of alopecia with a widest diameter of 3 cm or less or the disease limited to the eyelashes and eyebrows.
- *Moderate*: Existence of more than three patches of alopecia or a patch greater than 3 cm at the widest diameter without alopecia totalis or alopecia universalis.
- *Severe*: Alopecia totalis or alopecia universalis.
- *Ophiasis*: Severe form in which loss of hair occurs in the shape of a wave at the circumference of the head.

Q9. The poor prognostic factors in alopecia areata are:

a. Early age of onset
b. Family history
c. Concomitant autoimmune diseases
d. All of the above

Ans: d (All of the above)

The natural course of AA is very unpredictable. Some patients may experience only one episode of hair loss during their lifetimes, while others experience recurrences with multiple patches. Further variation occurs during recovery. Some patients have full hair regrowth, yet others remain the same or experience further hair loss. However, indicators of poor prognosis include:

- Extensive loss (especially alopecia totalis and universalis)
- Ophiasis variant
- Nail changes
- Early age of onset
- Duration of more than 1 year
- Family history
- Concomitant autoimmune diseases (e.g., atopy, Hashimoto thyroiditis).

Q10. What are the other conditions that have to be considered as differential diagnosis of alopecia areata and what are the distinguishing features?

Ans: Differential diagnosis incudes:

Scarring alopecia:

- Loss of follicular ostia, atrophy, signs of inflammation. Biopsy may confirm.

Nonscarring conditions include:

- Trichotillomania
  - Incomplete nature of the hair loss.
  - The broken hairs are firmly anchored in the scalp. A wire brush feel as compared to the smooth hair loss of alopecia areata.
  - History of impulsive pulling of hair present.
  - Biopsy may confirm.
- Tinea capitis
  - Scalp may be inflamed in tinea capitis and there is often scaling. Presence of cervical lymphadenopathy.
  - Easy breaking of hair shaft present.
  - Itching may be severe.
  - Demonstration of fungi by KOH is confirmatory.
- Telogen effluvium
  - History of precipitating factor present
  - Diffuse hair loss
  - Positive hair pull test
  - Horizontal and vertical biopsy to confirm.
- Anagen effluvium
  - History of drug intake
  - Sudden onset, diffuse hair loss
- Secondary syphilis
  - Moth eaten alopecia
  - Positive serological test for syphilis
  - Biopsy shows plasma cell infiltrate with endarteritis obliterans
- Loose anagen hair syndrome
  - A disorder of abnormal anagen hair anchorage. It is commonly found in children and has an autosomal dominant inheritance.
  - Light microscopy of the hair bulb shows crumpled sock appearance.

Q11. What are the main principles in treating a case of alopecia areata?

Ans: Management of patients with AA is a challenging task as a number of risk factors have been implicated in its etiology. No definitive cure has been established, and treatment has focused mainly on containing disease activity. Spontaneous remission may occur.

Treatment options include:

- Glucocorticoids
  - *Topical steroids*: Fluocinolone acetonide cream, fluocinolone scalp gel, betamethasone valerate lotion, and clobetasol propionate ointment—very good option in children because of their painless application and wide safety margin.
  - *Intralesional steroids*: Triamcinolone acetonide (10 mg/mL) is administered using a 0.5-inch long 30-gauge needle in multiple 0.1 mL injections approximately 1 cm apart every 4-6 weeks, for circumscribed AA involving less than 50% of the scalp. They are the first line treatment in most cases.
  - *Systemic corticosteroids*: The dosages required to maintain hair regrowth in AA are between 0.5 mg/kg and 1.5 mg/kg daily. Treatment duration can range from 1 month to 6 months. Because of their extensive side effect profile systemic corticosteroids are not considered as first line drugs.
  - *Oral mini-pulse steroids*: Oral mini-pulse therapy with corticosteroids has been successfully used for the treatment of AA with minimal side effects. Given on two consecutive days a week: Tab prednisolone 40–80 mg/day.

- Minoxidil
  - Minoxidil 5% has shown considerable results in the management of AA.
- Anthralin
  - 0.5–1% anthralin cream to be applied everyday for 20–30 min for 2 weeks, gradually increasing exposure duration until low-grade erythema and pruritus develops. Then, same duration to be continued for 3–6 months, suitable agent for children under 10 years of age.
- Calcineurin inhibitors phototherapy
  - Oral PUVA (psoralen plus ultraviolet A), topical PUVA, and PUVA sol can be given in case of alopecia totalis and universalis.
- Contact sensitizers
  - For AA involving more than 50% of scalp contact sensitizers like diphenylcyclopropenone and squaric acid dibutyl ester can be used.
- Miscellaneous
  - Topical retinoids like tazarotene, capsaicin, prostaglandin analogs, PRP (platelet-rich plasma), excimer laser, oral simvastatin.

CHAPTER 23

Androgenetic Alopecia

Sukesh Mathapathi

Case study Androgenetic Alopecia

Presenting Complaints

Doctor, my scalp is going bald and my hairs are getting thinner day by day since 6–8 years.

Setting

Dermatology outpatient department

History of Present Illness

A 30-year-old male presented with complaints of thinning and loss of hair since 6–8 years, leading to balding of scalp in a patterned manner (Fig. 1). Family history of similar balding in father is present.

General Physical and Systemic Examination

No abnormality detected.

Dermatological Examination

- Thinning of hair and loss of hair is noted mainly over bitemporal and vertex areas. Occipital area is relatively spared—corresponds to grade IV of Hamilton Norwood classification.
- Trichoscopy shows hair diameter diversity is more than 20% (anisotrichosis), predominance of follicles with single hair, vellus hairs are more than terminal hairs on the above areas.

Q1. What is the most likely diagnosis?

a. Androgenetic alopecia

b. Telogen effluvium

c. Diffuse alopecia areata

d. Senile alopecia

Ans: a [Androgenetic alopecia (AGA)]

Progressive thinning of hair with balding of bitemporal and vertex areas corresponding to Grade IV Hamilton Norwood classification in a 30-year-old male; trichoscopy showing hair diameter diversity more than 20% suggests the diagnosis of AGA.

Q2. How do you diagnose androgenetic alopecia?

Ans: Androgenetic alopecia is diagnosed mainly on clinical grounds and trichoscopy. Biopsy is confirmatory in atypical cases (not much used compared to use in male pattern hair loss).

Q3. What are the commonly used clinical grading classifications in male and female androgenetic alopecia?

Ans: Most commonly followed classification:

Male—Norwood (Hamilton Norwood)

Female—Ludwig/Sinclair.

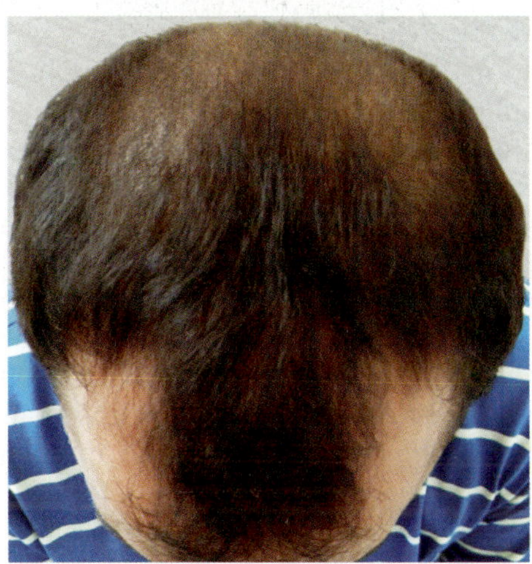

Fig. 1: Thinning of hair and loss of hair is noted mainly over bitemporal and vertex areas—corresponds to grade IV of Hamilton Norwood classification

Q4. What are the etiological factors for androgenetic alopecia?

Ans:
- Genetics—autosomal dominant, polygenic, and inherited
- Systemic hormonal effects—androgens
- Local hormonal effects—increased number of androgen receptors (ARs), functional polymorphisms of the AR, increased local production of DHT (dihydrotestosterone), or reduced local degradation of DHT.
- Role of oxidative stress—direct role in mediating DHT—stimulated TGFβ (transforming growth factor beta) secretion by dermal papilla cells.
- Contact between the arrector pili muscle and the bulge may be required for the reversal of hair follicle miniaturization.
- Hair cycle dynamics—the duration of anagen decreases with each successive cycle with prolongation of telogen.

Q5. What are the trichoscopic findings in androgenetic alopecia?

Ans: Trichoscopic findings (Figs 2 and 3):
- Hair diameter diversity more than 20% (suggestive of miniaturization process)
- Vellus hairs are more than terminal hairs
- Reduction of terminal hairs in follicular units
- Predominance of follicular units with single hair
- Honey comb pigmentation of scalp
- Peripilar sign/peripilar pigmentation
- Yellow dots
- Local atrichia/eraser like areas (mainly seen in female pattern hair loss).

Q6. What are the biopsy findings of androgenetic alopecia?

Ans: Horizontal sections are more helpful for the diagnosis.
- Diagnostic finding:
  - Terminal to vellus-like hair ratio is <4:1 (cf. normal >7:1) and no other pathology is apparent.
- Other findings:
  - Miniaturized hair follicles and enlarged sebaceous glands (looks like biopsy of face!).

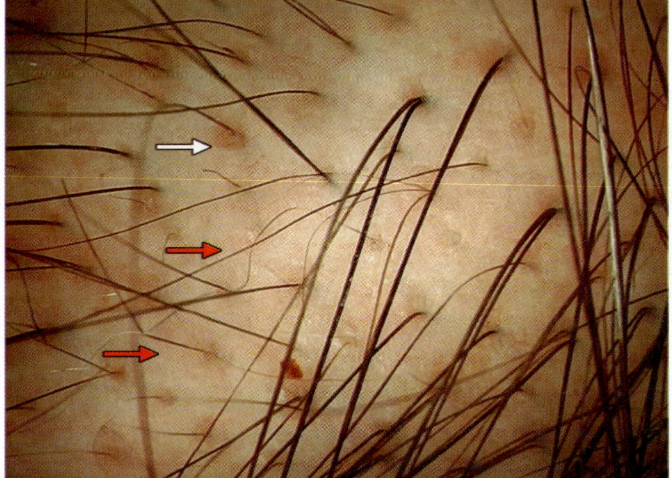

Fig. 2: Trichoscopy shows—hair diameter diversity more than 20% (suggestive of miniaturization process)—notice the difference in diameter of hair fibers
Courtesy: Dr Siddharth Sonthalia

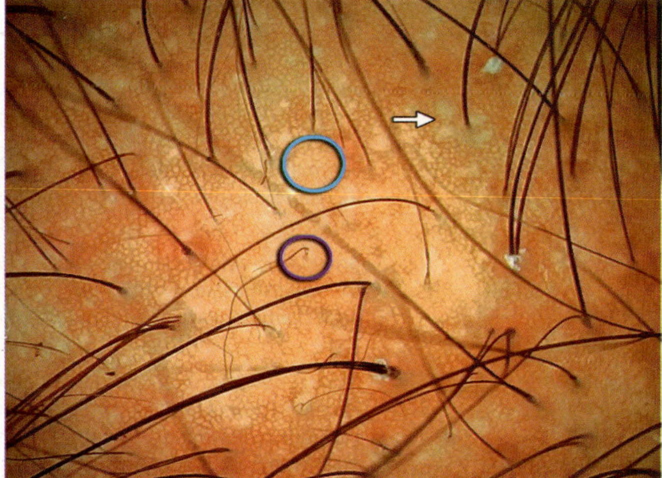

Fig. 3: Dark blue circle—vellus hairs are more than terminal hairs; reduction of terminal hairs in follicular units; predominance of follicular units with single hair. Light blue circle—honey comb pigmentation of scalp. Arrow—yellow dots
Courtesy: Dr Siddharth Sonthalia

- Fibrous tracts or streamers extend from the subcutaneous tissue up the old follicular tract to the miniaturized hair (mark the formal position of the original terminal follicle).
- Arao-Perkins bodies—small clusters of elastic fibers in the neck of dermal papillae may be seen.

Q7. Which of the below statement is true regarding patterned alopecia seen in younger age group?

a. Androgenetic process is not uncommon in adolescent and pediatric population.
b. Individuals without a family history of AGA are at low risk for baldness while men with a history of hair loss in either parent are 2.5 times more likely to have hair loss.
c. Children and adolescents with AGA have a strong genetic predisposition and younger children are more likely to have a family history.
d. There is no approved therapy for AGA in the pediatric population.
e. All the above

Ans: e (All the above)

Patterned alopecia is not uncommon in adolescent population and has also been reported in children as less as 6 years of age. Children and adolescents with AGA are likely to report hair loss in at least one- first or second-degree family member. The clinical patterns of AGA in adolescents are more varied, and girls can have diffuse thinning while males often present with female pattern hair loss (FPHL). Evaluation for hyperandrogenemia is worthwhile in all girls and in boys with diffuse or FPHL and with aberrant pubertal development. Though there is no approved therapy for AGA in pediatric population, topical minoxidil is well tolerated and can be effective at halting AGA progression in adolescents. Finasteride has been tried and found effective for AGA in adolescent boys.

Q8. How do you differentiate male/female pattern hair loss from telogen effluvium and diffuse hair alopecia areata?

Ans: Difference between male/female pattern hair loss from telogen effluvium and diffuse hair alopecia areata is enumerated in Table 1.

Table 1: Male/female pattern hair loss from telogen effluvium and diffuse hair alopecia areata

	Androgenetic alopecia	*Acute telogen effluvium*	*Diffuse alopecia areata*
Clinical presentation	Gradual onset, patterned thinning	Abrupt onset of increased (can be excessive) hair shedding involves entire scalp	Acute onset, marked shedding widespread or may predominantly affect the top of the head and pigmented hairs
Triggering factor	No	Yes	Sometimes
Natural history	Slowly progressive	Self-limited, total recovery usually in 3–6 months	Rapidly progressive (months)
Family history	Usually positive	Negative	Can be seen in 20% of cases
Hair pull	Negative (usually)	Positive	Positive in active stages
Trichogram (hair mount of forcible hair pluck)	Normal anagen: telogen ratio, increased telogen hairs in early cases	Decreased anagen: telogen ratio; (> 20% telogen hairs)	Decreased anagen and slightly increased telogen hairs; increased dysplastic hairs
Dermoscopy	Brown halo at follicular ostium (peripilar signs) and >20% hair shaft diameter variability	Numerous short-tip pointed regrowing hairs, no hair diameter variability	Perifollicular yellow dots (95% of patients), black dots, tapering hairs , exclamation point hairs, broken hairs, and short regrowing hairs
Histology	Normal number of total follicles, increased percentage of miniaturized terminal and vellus follicles, numerous connective tissue streamers, reduced terminal to vellus hair ratio (<4:1 is diagnostic)	Normal total and terminal follicles; increase in telogen hairs to >20%, absence of inflammation and scarring, no vellus or miniaturized hairs	Normal number of total follicles, peribulbar mononuclear cell infiltrate, increased number of miniaturized follicles, increased telogen follicles at the active border

Q9. What are the treatment options in patterned hair loss?

Ans: Treatment options in patterned hair loss are enumerated in Table 2.

In cases of FPHL, the underlying endocrine disturbance needs complete evaluation to determine conditions such as hyperandrogenism, PCOD/PCOS (polycystic ovarian disease/polycystic ovarian syndrome), and hypothyroidism. Antiandrogenic combination oral contraceptives with cyproterone acetate and drospirinone show improvement in FPHL. Rest of the options remain same in both conditions.

Q10. What are the proposed mechanisms of action of minoxidil?

Ans: Minoxidil is converted to minoxidil sulfate, the active form of the drug which opens ATP-sensitive potassium channels in cell membranes, leading to a vasodilatory effect and promotes hair growth. Other mechanisms postulated:

- Decrease in the latent period of the hair cycle (the time between shedding of telogen hair and the onset of the next anagen)
- Blocking EGF (epidermal growth factor)-induced inhibition of hair growth
- Increased expression of vascular endothelial growth factor (VEGF) mRNA in the dermal papillae, indicating its effects in inducing blood vessels
- Activation of cytoprotective prostaglandin synthase-1
- Increased expression of hepatocyte growth factor (HGF) m-RNA(hair growth promoter)
- It increases 17-beta-hydroxylated dehydrogenase activity by almost 40% in dermal papilla cells.
- Binds directly to the AR leading to suppressed AR-related activity and decreased AR protein stability in human hair dermal papilla cells.

Q11. What are the major pharmacological differences between finasteride and dutasteride?

Ans: Major pharmacological differences between finasteride and dutasteride are enumerated in Table 3.

Q12. What are new evolving/experimental therapies for patterned hair loss?

Ans: Evolving therapies:

- Platelet rich plasma
- Microneedling
- Low level laser and 1,550 nm fractional erbium glass laser treatment

Table 2: Treatment options in patterned hair loss

	MPHL	*FPHL*
Topical	• Minoxidil 5-10% • Tretinoin 0.025% • Azelaic acid 5% • Ketoconazole 2%	• Minoxidil 2% • Tretinoin 0.025% • Azelaic acid 5% • Ketoconazole 2%
Systemic	• Antiandrogens • Finasteride • Dutasteride	• Antiandrogens • Finasteride • Dutasteride • Cyproterone acetate • Spironolactone • Flutamide
Surgical	• Hair transplantation • Follicular unit transplantation • Follicular unit extraction	• Hair transplantation • Follicular unit transplantation • Follicular unit extraction
Camoflage	• Hair fibers • Micropigmentation • Wigs, hair pieces	• Hair fibers • Micropigmentation • Wigs, hair pieces

Abbreviations: MPHL, male pattern hair loss; FPHL, female pattern hair loss

Table 3: Major pharmacological differences between finasteride and dutasteride

	Finasteride	*Dutasteride*
Mechanism of action	Selectively inhibits the type 2 isoenzyme of 5α-reductase	Inhibits both type 1 and type 2 isoenzyme of 5α-reductase
Plasma half life	6-8 hours.	4 weeks
Potency		
• Inhibiting type I 5α-reductase	100 times less potent	100 times more potent
• Inhibiting type II 5α-reductase	Three times less potent	Three times more potent
Efficacy	Decrease serum DHT by 70%. In comparison with dutasteride, finasteride reportedly reduces scalp DHT by only 34–41%	Decrease serum DHT by more than 90%
Dose	1 mg/day	0.5 mg/day

Abbreviation: DHT, dihydrotestosterone

- Topical:
  - Bimatoprost, a prostaglandin F-related analog and 0.1% latanoprost
  - Caffeine complex
  - Stemoxydine 5% solution
  - Biomimetic peptides (trifolium pratense flower extract combined with acetyl tetrapeptide-3)
  - Hair stimulating complex (follistatin, Wnt7a, and wound healing growth factors)
  - Melatonin 0.1% solution topically
  - Valproic acid solution 8.3% topically
  - Roxithromycin 5% solution.
- Botox injections of 150 U injected all around the scalp muscle.

CHAPTER 24

Female Pattern Hair Loss

Deepak Vasisht, Kanhaiya Patidar

Case study Female Pattern Hair Loss

Presenting Complaints

Doctor, I am continuously loosing hairs from scalp for last few months, my hair partition has widened and hairs have become sparse.

Setting

Dermatology outpatient department

History of Present Illness

A 42-year-old lady presented with complaints of progressive reduction in hair density on the crown and increase in parting width. She has also noticed that existing hairs are becoming thin and sparse. There is no history of itching, scarring or sudden loss of hairs, hirsutism or acne. She has regular menstrual cycles and no other comorbidity. No history of any illness in recent past.

General and Systemic Examination

No abnormality detected

Dermatological Examination of Scalp

- Diffuse loss of hairs from frontal and occipital region
- Thinning of terminal hairs
- Hair pull test was positive.

Q1. What is the most likely diagnosis?

a. Telogen effluvium
b. Female pattern hair loss
c. Alopecia areata
d. Diffuse alopecia areata
e. Anagen effluvium

Ans: b. (Female pattern hair loss)

Diffuse loss of hair, miniaturization of terminal hairs, absence of patchy loss or scarring—favor diagnosis.

Q2. How many scalp hairs one looses daily?

Ans: Scalp loses around 100 telogen hairs per day normally.

Q3. How do you diagnose female pattern hair loss?

Ans: Female pattern hair loss (FPHL) is diagnosed on clinical grounds. It is a form of nonscarring, patterned hair loss in women characterized by a progressive reduction in hair density on frontal, vertex, and mid scalp, bitemporal and parietal involvement is less common.

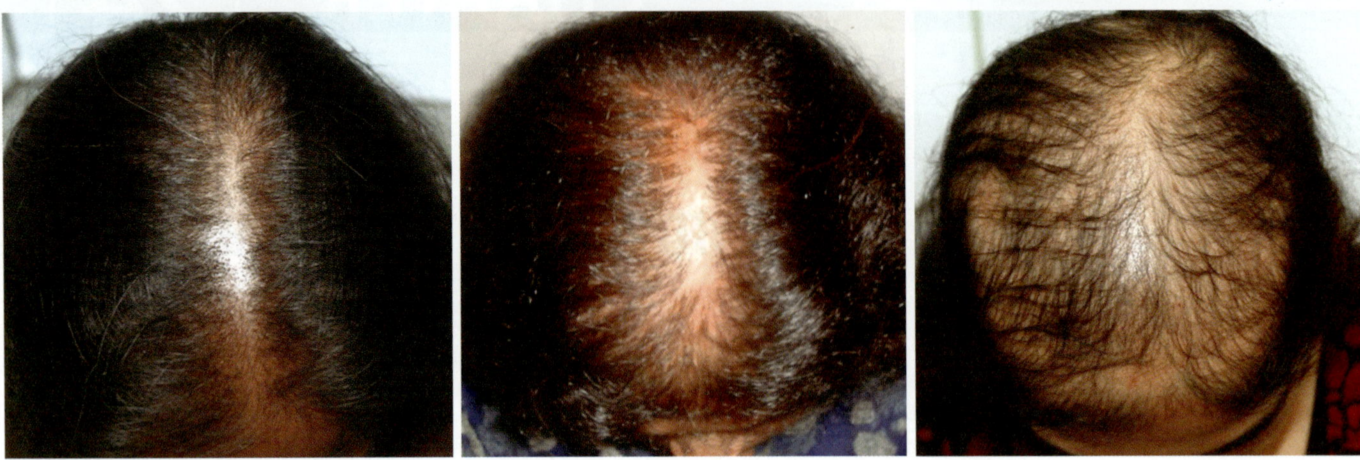

Fig. 1: Ludwig's grading of severity of FPHL—grade I, II, and III

Q4. What are the noninvasive methods to assess the female pattern hair loss?

Ans. Dermoscopy is the mainstay in the diagnosis of FPHL. Others include:

- *Sabouraud's sign*: It is the number of hairs that come out after a gentle traction on hair.
- *Pull-out sign*: It denotes the strength of the hair at the root level.
- *Standardized wash test*: Lady is asked not to wash her hair for 5 days followed by a hair wash with a cotton plug at the drain and collection of all the shedded hair. Then there involves a counting of less than 5 cm and more than 5 cm hair. Less than 5-cm-long hair denotes a telogen hair.
- *Macrophotographic analysis*: Obsolete nowadays.
- *Phototrichogram*: Take close up photographs of the scalp and then analyze qualitatively and quantitatively. This principle is used in folliscope and trichoscan. An area of about 2 cm is trimmed 1 mm short over the area of interest and is photographed using digital photography. One week later same area is rephotographed, serially repeating same trimming and photographing at weekly interval. At the end comparing differentials in growth rates, e.g., hairs not grown, grown less, grown optimally; total number of hairs in that area; hairs missing from the area—this indicates the rate of hair shedding.
- *Traction phototrichogram*: Photographic analysis of hairs pulled out at the gentle traction and recording findings like diameter variability, color, telogen versus anagen effluvium.
- *Trichoscan*: It is an epiluminiscence technique where by an automated computer-based program assesses the various hair-related parameters on a closely trimmed area, e.g., density of hairs per cm^2, vellus hair density per cm^2, terminal hair density per cm^2, the total number of hairs in that area, anagen hairs, telogen hairs, etc. It is a good screening tool as well as an objective way of assessment and documentation.

Q5. What are the dermoscopic findings in patterned hair loss?

Ans: Dermoscopic findings

- Hairs with different caliber reflecting progressive hair miniaturization
- Brown halo, roughly 1 mm in diameter, at the follicular ostium around the emergent hair shaft
- Small bald areas with numerous empty follicles in postmenopausal women
- Scalp pigmentation because of sun exposure.

Q6. How does female pattern alopecia differ from male pattern alopecia?

Ans:

- The progression is slower—possibly due to protective effect of estrogen.
- Hair loss in male begins as frontal recession and occipital baldness whereas in females it is diffuse and does not conform to the traditional patterns of loss in males.
- Hair loss generally worsens following menopause especially at the vertices.
- In men the condition is due to genetic predisposition and is usually age related.
- In women the condition worsens with polycystic ovarian syndrome (PCOS), thyroid disorders, anemia, and chronic illness.

Q7. How common is female pattern alopecia?

Ans: It affects 50% of females by the time they reach 50 years of age.

Q8. How do you assess severity of female pattern alopecia?

Ans: Ludwig classified FPHL into three grades depending on severity as grades I, II, and III (Fig 1).

1. *Type I or mild:* Frontal hairline remains relatively unaffected. Hair loss may occur on the top and front of the scalp. However, such hair loss may be noticeable when the hair is parted down the center of the scalp.
2. *Type II or moderate*: Thinning and shedding with general decrease in volume, and a center part that continues to widen over time.
3. *Type III or severe:* Hair is so thin that it has difficulty camouflaging the scalp, rendering it visible to the naked eye. This may be worsened by a number of factors, including hair miniaturization, progressive thinning, and extensive loss.

Q9. What is the relevance of history in a patient of female pattern hair loss?

Ans. Female pattern hair loss is a visual diagnosis. A complete personal, family, menstrual, and treatment history guides toward the probable cause. Symptoms of androgenization such as oligo- or amenorrhea, infertility of women, acne vulgaris, severe unresponsive cystic acne, hirsutism, galactorrhea, and virilization indicate excess androgens. Chronic illnesses, nutritional alterations, metabolic and endocrinologic alterations, lack of vitamins, and recent surgery help exclude other causes of hair loss.

Q10. How will you investigate a patient of female pattern hair loss?

Ans: Most important is to assess the levels of androgens, which is aided by free testosterone, 5-α-DHT (5α-dihydrotestosterone), DHEA-S (dehydroepiandrosterone sulfate), 17-β-hydroxyprogesterone, prolactin, androstenedione, SHBG (sex hormone-binding globulin), and 3-β-androstanediol glucuronide. Luteinizing hormone (LH), follicle-stimulating hormone (FSH), and the ratio of LH:FSH helps in confirming PCOS. Patients with normal androgen levels should be investigated for TSH (thyroid-stimulating hormone), T4, antimicrosomal and antithyroglobulin antibodies, and ferritin or total iron-binding capacity.

Q11. What are the approaches of female pattern hair loss management?

Ans: Three approaches of FPHL management are:

1. Modification of the androgen action, e.g., spironolactone, cyproterone acetate, finasteride, OCPs (oral contraceptive pills)
2. Modification of the biological response through nonhormonal mechanisms: Topical minoxidil 2%, 5%
3. Hair restoration surgery: FUE (follicular unit extraction), FUT (follicular unit transplant).

Q12. How do you treat female pattern hair loss?

Ans: Patient should be counseled about the natural progression of the disease and the realistic attitude towards the treatment. Treatment only slows the rate of progression of hair loss, rather than promote hair regrowth.

First-line treatment: Minoxidil 2% cutaneous foam preparation gives greater sustained hair growth and

Algorithm 1: Algorithmic approach to a patient with female pattern baldness

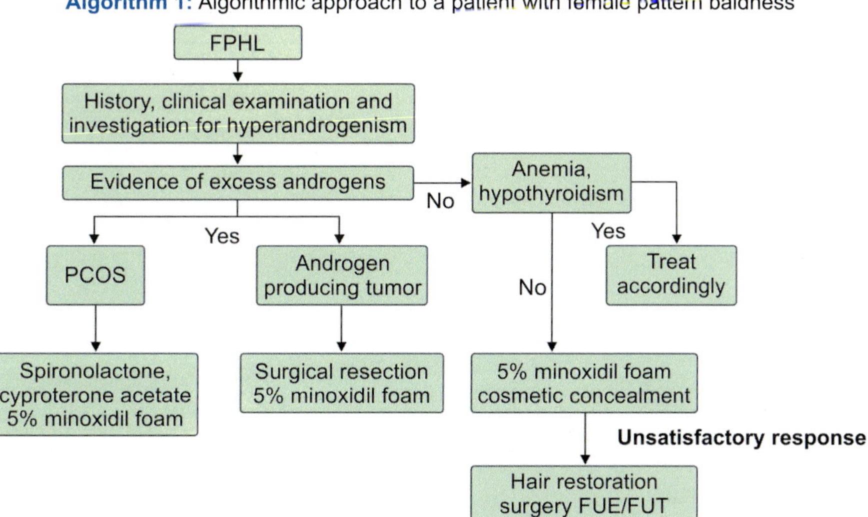

needs to be continued for at least 12 months. Earliest changes in the form of hair fall arrest are noted only after about 8 weeks. Minoxidil lengthens the anagen phase and shortens the resting phase and induces conversion of the miniaturized follicles, to terminal hairs.

Second-line treatment: Antiandrogen therapy is recommended in female patients with hyperandrogenism as a second-line treatment who respond poorly to minoxidil. These drugs inhibit androgen production or its effects, e.g., spironolactone, cyproterone acetate, and flutamide. Spironolactone (an aldosterone antagonist) is the preferred second-line treatment that competitively blocks androgen receptors and weakly inhibits androgen synthesis. It has to be prescribed for at least 6 months for any appreciable hair growth. Flutamide and cyproterone acetate are infrequently used due to lack of data. Finasteride is not recommended in women (Algorithm 1).

Q13. What are the other causes of diffuse hair loss in females?

Ans: Chronic telogen effluvium, diffuse alopecia areata, loose anagen hair syndrome, anagen effluvium, congenital atrichia and hypotrichosis and hair shaft defects.

Q14. What are the characteristic features of chronic telogen effluvium?

Ans: Characteristic features of chronic telogen effluvium include:

- History of generalized abrupt shedding of hair
- Moderate to severe bitemporal recession may be present
- Positive hair pull test all over scalp
- No widening of central parting or miniaturization of hairs as seen in FPHL
- Absence of any other underlying cause
- Histology showing mild increase in telogen hair follicles.

Q15. What is the treatment for chronic telogen effluvium?

Ans: No treatment modality has been specifically proved to improve chronic telogen effluvium. It can spontaneously improve in months. Iron, vitamins especially biotin and minoxidil 2% have been found to improve the condition in various studies.

CHAPTER 25

Trichotillomania

Pallavi Ailawadi

Case study Trichotillomania

Presenting Complaints

Doctor, my daughter has patchy hair loss on her scalp since 6 months.

Setting

Dermatology outpatient department

History of Present Illness

Mother brought her 16-year-old daughter with history of patchy loss of hair over a localized part of scalp since 6 months which has developed gradually over a period of time. History of itching, pain, or other symptoms was absent. Patient denies any history of plucking own hair. However, the parent gives history of noticing occasional hair plucking by the child while she used to study. History of anxiousness, stress, and anxiety episodes for minor issues was present since childhood.

Dermatological Examination

Single to multiple, irregular, bizarre-shaped patches of noncicatricial alopecia is present over the right temporoparietal region of the scalp. Broken hair of uneven length as well as newly growing short hair with tapered ends is seen. No evidence of scaling or inflammation is seen. Hair pull test is negative. No regional lymphadenopathy is present.

Q1. What is your diagnosis?

a. Alopecia areata
b. Trichotillomania
c. Tinea capitis
d. Traction alopecia

Ans: b. (Trichotillomania)

Q2. What is your differential diagnosis?

Ans: The differential diagnosis includes:

- *Alopecia areata*: Well circumscribed round/oval patch of nonscarring alopecia, smooth bald skin, exclamation mark hair/cadaveric hair present, no broken hair/hair of uneven length.
- *Tinea capitis*: Well defined patch of nonscarring alopecia with irregular margins, brokenhair/scaling/erythema/pustules might be present along with regional lymphadenopathy.
- *Monilethrix*: Autosomal dominant inheritance; moniliform hair which is dry, brittle, fragile, and lusterless; shortbroken hair with beading, associated with follicular keratoses; might involve entire body hair.

- *Traction alopecia*: Recession of hairline characterized by a fringe along the hair margin which is the presence of retained hairs along the frontal and/or temporal rim.
- *Temporal triangular alopecia*: Oval-shaped patch of alopecia confined to frontotemporal scalp. Persists through life.

Q3. How do you confirm the diagnosis of trichotillomania?

Ans: Patchy loss of hair in an easily accessible area, with hair broken of different length and no scaling or other signs of inflammation (Fig. 1).

Q4. What is trichotillomania?

Ans: Trichotillomania is characterized by persistent, excessive habitual pulling of one's own hair, resulting in visible hair loss.

Q5. What kind of a disorder is it?

Ans: It is a psychiatric disorder listed in the American Psychiatric Association's *Diagnostic and Statistical Manual of Mental Disorders, Fifth Edition (DSM-5)*, which places trichotillomania in the category of obsessive-compulsive and related disorders.

Q6. What are the diagnostic criteria for trichotillomania?

Ans: The specific *DSM-5* criteria for trichotillomania are as follows:

- Recurrent pulling out of one's hair, resulting in hair loss
- Repeated attempts to decrease or stop the hair-pulling behavior

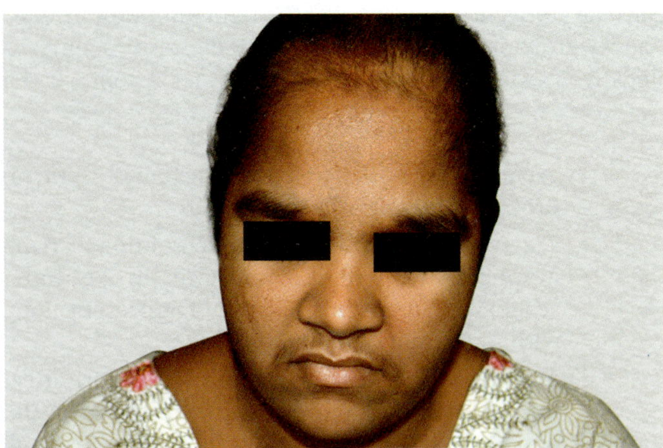

Fig. 1: Trichotillomania manifesting on frontal scalp in this middle-aged lady

- The hair pulling causes clinically significant distress or impairment in social, occupational, or other important areas of functioning.
- The hair pulling or hair loss cannot be attributed to another medical condition (e.g., a dermatologic condition).
- The hair pulling cannot be better explained by the symptoms of another mental disorder (e.g., attempts to improve a perceived defect or flaw in appearance, such as may be observed in body dysmorphic disorder).

Q7. What is the common age of presentation?

Ans: It is seven times more prevalent in children than in adults, with peak prevalence between the ages of 4 and 17 years.

Q8. Are there any gender-based differences in prevalence?

Ans: In all age groups including young children, adolescents, and adults, girls are affected more often than boys. *DSM-5* cites an overall female-to-male ratio of 10:1.

Q9. What is the prognosis of trichotillomania?

Ans: It is a chronic and persistent condition of hair pulling. Children typically have a time-limited disorder with an excellent prognosis, while adolescents and adults have more severe disease with a guarded prognosis.

Q10. Which body part hair is involved in trichotillomania?

Ans: The scalp is the most common area, followed by the eyelashes and eyebrows. Pubic hair and other body parts are less commonly involved.

Q11. What are the common clinical features seen in trichotillomania?

Ans:

- *Hair loss*: Ranges from barely noticeable patches of hair loss to total baldness
- *Hair length*: Short, irregular, and broken
- *Hair regrowth*: Hair of varying lengths may be noted during the regrowing phase
- *Hair abnormalities*: Empty and/or damaged hair follicles; twisted or broken hair of varying length; and wavy, wrinkled, or corkscrew-shaped hair shafts
- Absence of scaling, skin abnormalities, or inflammation
- *Friar Tuck sign*: Areas of hair loss with broken hairs of varying lengths arranged in a circular pattern, with unaffected hairs surrounding the area of

hair loss. (Friar Tuck, friend of Robinhood, had alopecia of vertex with sparing in occipital area—tonsural alopecia.)

- Occasionally, the hair-thinning pattern is not circumscribed and shows only a somewhat deficient volume of hair.

Q12. What are trichophagy, trichotemnomania, and trichoteiromania?

Ans: Trichophagy is the practice of chewing or swallowing of hair that has been pulled out. Trichotemnomania is alopecia occurring when patient cuts his/her hair with scissors, trichoteiromania is the perpetual rubbing of scalp hair that causes hair shaft breakage and then alopecia.

Q13. What is a trichobezoar?

Ans: It is typically found in the stomach and intestines of patients who chew their pulled hairs. These are ball-like aggregations of swallowed hair which are retained within the folds of the gastric mucosa.

Q14. What are the complications of trichobezoar?

Ans: It may give rise to abdominal pain, hematemesis, nausea and vomiting, bowel obstruction, perforation, gastrointestinal bleeding, and pancreatitis or obstructive jaundice.

Q15. How will you investigate a case of trichotillomania?

Ans: In order to confirm the diagnosis of trichotillomania, I would like to do the following investigations:

- Dermoscopy
- Scalp biopsy
- Ultrasonography and computed tomography (CT) may be useful in detecting trichobezoar formation.

Q16. What are the findings in trichotillomania seen on dermoscopy?

Ans: Various findings seen on dermoscopy are decreased hair density, hair broken at different lengths, short hair with trichoptilosis, irregular coiled hair, upright regrowing hair, and perifollicular hemorrhages.

Some findings have been found to be specific to trichotillomania include:

- Flame hair—semitransparent, wavy, and cone-shaped hair residues.
- Hair powder—sprinkled hair residue.
- V sign—two or more hair emerging from one follicular unit which are broken at same length.
- Tulip hair—short hair with darker, tulip flower-shaped ends.
- Hook hair—partially coiled hair.

Q17. What are the findings seen on histopathological examination?

Ans: Multiple sections both transverse and vertical should be taken to view the main findings. The most common findings are empty anagen follicles, increased numbers of catagen follicles, and pigment casts in hair canals along with incompletely keratinized, soft, distorted, and pigmented hair shafts (trichomalacia) and bizarre fractured hair shafts.

Some other findings are:

- *Hamburger sign*: Presence of proteinaceous material and erythrocytes within the vertically oriented split of hair shaft.
- *Zip sign*: Presence of twisted linear pigment in the cortex.
- *Button sign*: Circular, central aggregation of pigment surrounded by the inner root sheath.

Q18. How will you assess the severity of trichotillomania?

Ans: The Trichotillomania Scale for Children (TSC) is a child and parent report that may be used to assess symptom severity and impairment.

- It is a 15 point questionnaire covering three priority domains of trichotillomania psychopathology:
  - Severity (frequency of urges/pulling, duration of pulling episode, number of hair pulled, and controllability of pulling).
  - Distress (emotional responses associated with pulling like guilt, embarrassment, sadness, and self-reproach).
  - Impairment (interference with peer/family relationships, schoolwork, and grooming routine).

It includes five questions from each domain and the level of severity ranges from 0 to 2 for each.

Another scale called Massachusetts General Hospital Hair Pulling Scale (MGH-HPS) is used for psychometric analysis in adults with trichotillomania.

Q19. How will you treat the patient?

Ans: First line of treatment for trichotillomania is behavioral treatment and intervention.

Behavioral interventions

- Habit reversal
- Self-monitoring
- Relaxation training
- Psychotherapy
- Hypnosis
- Elimination of a comorbid behavior.

Pharmacologic therapy.

No pharmacotherapy has been found to be consistently effective in treatment of trichotillomania.

- Primary agents used—selective serotonin reuptake inhibitors like fluoxetine, sertraline, fluvoxamine, escitalopram, and paroxetine.

Other medications that have been used with variable results include:

- Tricyclic antidepressants—amitrypline, clomipramine, desipramine.
- *N*-acetylcysteine
- Dronabinol
- Methylphenidate—trichotillomania patients with comorbid attention deficit hyperactivity disorder (ADHD)
- Oxcarbazepine
- Aripiprazole
- Bimatoprost—madarosis due to trichotillomania.

CHAPTER 26

Cicatricial Alopecia

Savitha AS

Case study 1 Lichen Planopilaris

Presenting Complaints

Doctor, I am losing hair in patches on my scalp for the past 1-year; there is mild itching and burning sensation in the patches.

Setting

Dermatology outpatient department

History of Present Illness

A 30-year-old male presented with progressive patchy loss of hair, which began about 1 year back. There is associated itching and burning sensation in the patches. There is no history of photosensitivity or scaling from the lesions. Few violaceous lesions are present on the lower back since 3 months. No history of pus-filled lesions or application of other medicines.

General and Systemic Examination

No significant findings.

Dermatological Examination

Patchy alopecia is seen in the frontal area. Centers of the patches are violaceous, smooth, and devoid of follicular ostia (Fig. 1). The hairs at the margins can be easily pulled in few areas. There is no scaling or evidence of folliculitis. Hairs on other areas appear normal. No features of follicular plugging or spiny papules. Violaceous papules are seen on the lower back.

Q1. What is your most probable diagnosis?

Cicatricial alopecia due to

a. Lichen planopilaris (LPP)
b. Pseudopelade of Brocq (PPB)
c. Graham-Little syndrome
d. Frontal fibrosing alopecia (FFA)

Ans: a. LPP: Absence of folliculitis, keratosis pilaris and presence of burning and itching sensation with a violaceous hue to the patches is more in favor of LPP.

Q2. How will you diagnose lichen planopilaris on histopathology?

Ans: The histopathological diagnosis of LPP includes:

- Liquefaction degeneration and invasion of the infiltrate into the basal cell layer
- The hair follicles are dilated and filled with a cup-shaped keratotic plug
- Hypergranulosis within the affected infundibula
- A lichenoid lymphocytic infiltrate surrounds the follicle, especially involving the upper portion

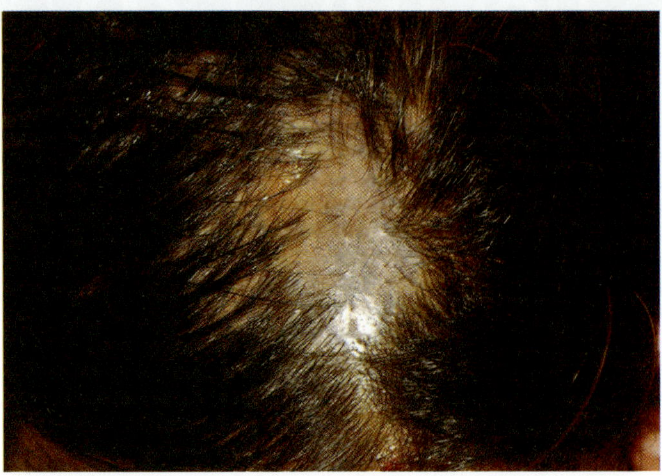

Fig. 1: Violceous alopecic patch with loss of follicular ostia

- Over time, there is flattened epidermis, perifollicular fibrosis with complete disappearance of hair and sebaceous glands, mild perivascular infiltrate and remnants of arrector pili muscles. In the end-stages, loss of elastic fibers results in a superficial dermal wedge-shaped scar.

Q3. What are the findings on immunofluorescence in lichen planopilaris ?

Ans: Direct immunofluorescence shows characteristic pattern of grouped-globular deposition of IgM and fibrinogen adjacent to the follicular epithelium.

Q4. What are the dermatoscopic findings in lichen planopilaris?

Ans: During active LPP trichoscopy shows silvery-white perifollicular scaling with scales entangling hair shafts up to few millimeters above scalp surface, perifollicular inflammation and elongated, concentrically oriented blood vessels. In the fibrotic stage, the dominating features are big, irregular white dots, which merge into milky-red (strawberry ice-cream color) or white areas.

Q5. What are the treatment options for lichen planopilaris?

Ans: Treatment options for LPP are:
- Potent topical (clobetasol propionate twice daily) and intralesional corticosteroids (triamcinolone acetonide 10 mg/cc) in early lesions with active inflammatory changes
- Topical tacrolimus 0.1%
- Antimalarials such as hydroxychloroquine 200 mg bid for 6–12 months.
- Ciclosporin (3–5 mg/kg/day for 3–5 months)
- Mycophenolate mofetil (0.5 g to 1 g bid for up to 6 months)
- Low dose methotrexate.

Q6. What is the classical triad of Graham-Little syndrome?

Ans:
- Cicatricial alopecia of the scalp with prominent follicular plugging
- Keratosis pilaris-like follicular papules
- Loss of axillary and pubic hair.

Q7. How can we differentiate frontal fibrosing alopecia from lichen planopilaris and androgenetic alopecia (AGA) clinically?

Ans: FFA from LPP
- More common in postmenopausal women
- FFA has progressive symmetrical frontotemporal recession
- Skin is pale and shiny in contrast to chronically sun-exposed skin of the upper forehead
- Associated loss of eyebrows is regarded as a helpful diagnostic sign
- FFA is less symptomatic than LPP
- FFA from AGA
- The frontal hairline in FFA recedes in a straight-line rather than bitemporally.

Q8. What are the dermatoscopic findings in frontal fibrosing alopecia ?

Ans: Perifollicular scales, perifollicular erythema, and branching capillaries. In contrast to classic LPP, where the background may be milky-red, in the early fibrotic phase of disease, the background in patients with FFA is always ivory-white.

Q9. What are the clinical features of alopecia in discoid lupus erythematosus (DLE)?

Ans: Lesion is a well-demarcated, dull-red, scaly-macule or -papule, which enlarges into a discoid alopecia patch with erythema and adherent scaling. The removal of scales results in slight bleeding. If scale is lifted intact, conical plugs are seen on under surface—"carpet-tack appearance". Telangiectatic vessels present at the borders and in the center. Other lesions are seen commonly over the scalp, face, and ears.

Q10. What are the histopathology features in discoid lupus erythematosus?

Ans: Thinning and flattening of the stratum malpighii. Funnel-shaped keratotic plugs are found in the follicular openings. Focal basal cell vacuolation is seen. Thickening of the basement membrane zone, pigmentary incontinence, colloid bodies, increased dermal mucin and exocytosis of lymphocytes into the epidermis and follicular epithelium is often present. The infiltrate is usually distinctly patchy and is located mainly in the vicinity of the hair follicles, blood vessels, sebaceous, and eccrine glands, and is composed predominantly of lymphocytes admixed with plasma cells. The infiltrate, by impinging upon the pilosebaceous structures, causes their gradual atrophy and disappearance. Frequently, hydropic changes in the basal layer of the hair follicles are seen, which may have considerable diagnostic value. Diagnostic features on direct immunofluorescence are deposition of IgG, IgM, and C3 in a granular band-like pattern at the dermal interface.

Q11. What are the dermatoscopic findings in discoid lupus erythematosus?

Ans: White patches, keratin plugs, thick arborizing vessels, scattered dark brown discoloration of the skin. Large yellow dots with radial, thin arborizing vessels emerging from the dot referred to, as "red spider in yellow dot" are considered characteristic for DLE. Inactive DLE lesions differ from active lesions by presence of structureless milky-red areas, and lack of follicular orifices.

Q12. Describe the features of pseudopelade of brocq.

Ans: Vertex is primarily involved. Small, round to oval, smooth, soft, atrophic, white or ivory colored alopecic patches appear singly or in small groups which coalesce to form large irregular slightly depressed patches that are frequently compared to "footprints in the snow". The absence of inflammatory signs is characteristic. PPB usually requires 10 or more years before much alopecia appears.

Q13. How is pseudopelade of brocq diagnosed?

Ans: Braun-Falco (1986) proposed the following clinical and histological criteria for making the diagnosis:

- Clinical
  - Irregular but well-defined confluent patches of alopecia
  - Mild perifollicular erythema (early stage)
  - Moderate atrophy (late stage)
  - Long course (>2 years) is frequent
  - Slow progression with spontaneous termination
  - Positive hair pull test during active disease
- Histopathological
  - Absence of marked inflammation except lymphocytic infiltrate around the upper two-thirds of the follicles
  - Prominent perifollicular fibrosis with absence of widespread scarring, i.e. no interfollicular fibrosis
  - Absence of significant follicular plugging
  - Absence or decrease of sebaceous glands
  - Normal epidermis
  - Fibrotic streaks in the subcutaneous tissue.
  - Dense elastic tissue cuffing around fibrous tracts.
- Direct immunofluorescence
  - Negative or at least only IgM.

Q14. How is cicatricial alopecia classified based on cell infiltrate in histopathology?

Ans: Classification of cicatricial alopecia based on infiltrate:

- Lymphocytic
  - DLE
  - LPP
  - Graham-Little syndrome
  - FFA
  - PPB
  - Alopecia mucinosa
- Neutrophilic
  - Folliculitis decalvans
  - Dissecting cellulitis
- Mixed
  - Acne keloidalis
  - Acne necrotica.

Q15. List a few congenital and developmental defects which can present with cicatricial alopecia.

Ans: Aplasia cutis, Conradi-Hünermann disease (chondrodysplasia punctata), incontinentia pigmenti, dystrophic epidermolysis bullosa, keratosis pilaris atrophicans faciei, Darier's disease, epidermal nevus, lamellar ichthyosis, Marie-Unna syndrome, Hallermann-Streiff syndrome, Rapp-Hodgkin syndrome.

Q16. List the infections which can result in cicatricial alopecia.

Ans:
- Fungal infections—kerion and favus
- Viral infections—trigeminal herpes zoster, varicella, and recurrent herpes simplex
- Bacterial infections—lupus vulgaris, carbuncle, deep folliculitis, syphilis (gumma), yaws
- Protozoal—leishmaniasis.

Q17. What are the salient features of central centrifugal cicatricial alopecia (CCCA)?

Ans: Central centrifugal cicatricial alopecia begins as a focus of cicatricial alopecia over the vertex region which gradually spreads centrifugally in a symmetrical manner affecting a large area on the top with extension to the sides of the scalp. The alopecic area shows loss of follicular ostia with usually no signs of inflammation. The most distinctive histological feature of CCCA is premature desquamation of the inner root sheath (IRS) below the isthmus and eccentric thinning of the follicular epithelium.

Case study 2 Folliculitis Decalvans

Presenting Complaints

Doctor, I have loss of hair for the past one year and have noted pus-filled areas on my head.

Setting

Dermatology outpatient department

History of Present Illness

A 32-year-old male presented with pus-filled lesions on the scalp and loss of hair for past 3 years. The lesions are asymptomatic.

Systemic and Dermatological Examination

No significant findings

Dermatological Examination

Alopecia is seen in the occipital area. Center of the lesion is a smooth shiny, atrophic scar. In the margins follicular papules and pustules are seen. There are no sinus tracts.

Q1. What is your most probable diagnosis?

a. Folliculitis decalvans (FD)
b. Tufted folliculitis
c. Dissecting cellulitis
d. Tinea capitis

Ans: a. FD: presence of lesions in the occipital area with the absence of sinus tracts is more in favor of FD.

Q2. What are the histopathological findings in folliculitis decalvans?

Ans: Peri- and intrafollicular infiltrate of mainly neutrophils, also containing lymphoid cells, histiocytes and plasma cells, which are most intense around the upper portion of the follicle. Perifollicular abscess are present, which often contain a good amount of plasma cells. In older lesions, chronic granulation tissue containing numerous plasma cells, lymphoid cells and fibroblasts are seen.

Q3. What are the dermatoscopic findings in folliculitis decalvans?

Ans: Multiple hairs emerging from a single dilated follicular opening. Perifollicular hyperplasia arranged in a starburst pattern. Yellowish tubular scaling (with a collar-like widening at the distal end), crusting, and follicular pustules. In long-lasting lesions white- and milky-red areas lacking follicular openings predominate.

Q4. How will you treat folliculitis decalvans?

Ans: Treatment

- Appropriate antimicrobials can be selected following pus culture and antibiotic sensitivity
- A combination of rifampicin (300 mg bid) for 10 days with cephalexin (500 mg qid) or clindamycin (300 mg bid) or doxycycline (100 mg bid) or clarithromycin or co-trimoxazole for 10 weeks has been found to be beneficial
- Topical antibiotics like clindamycin phosphate 1% solution or gel, mupirocin cream or fusidic acid 1% can be used
- Tar shampoos and topical keratolytics help to remove the scales and reduce tufting.

Q5. What is tufted folliculitis?

Ans: Tufted folliculitis is a variant of FD in which tufts of hair are the cardinal and prominent feature surrounding relatively small patches of hair loss (Fig. 1).

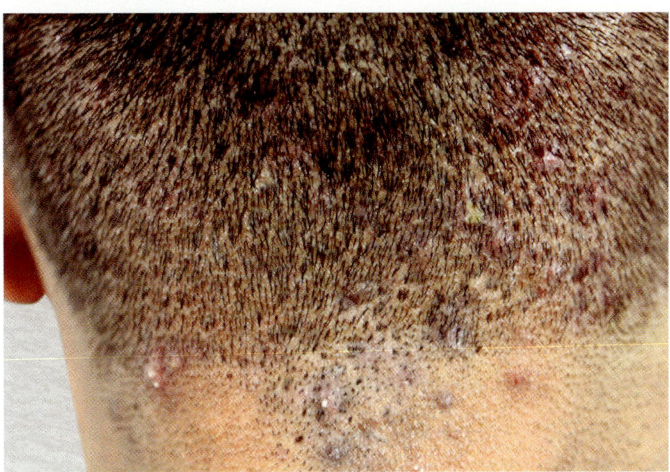

Fig. 1: Tufted folliculitis

Q6. How is folliculitis decalvans differentiated from dissecting cellulitis?

Ans: Dissecting cellulitis starts with painful, indurated, skin colored nodules over the vertex, which later becomes soft and fluctuant. Tubular ridges are formed by coalescence of confluent nodules leading to irregular cerebriform pattern, on a red edematous background. Pressure on one region of the scalp elicits discharge of pus from distant sites. Characteristically, hair is lost from the summits of these inflammatory lesions and retained in the valleys. The condition tends to be chronic with frequent acute exacerbations and ultimately leads to scarring and extensive hair loss.

Q7. What is follicular occlusion tetrad?

Ans: Follicular occlusion tetrad comprises of:

- Hidradenitis suppurativa
- Acne conglobata
- Pilonidal sinus
- Dissecting cellulitis of scalp

Q8. What are the treatment options available for dissecting cellulitis?

Ans: Dissecting cellulitis is a notoriously treatment-resistant disease. Isotretinoin (1–2 mg/kg/day) for 5–6 months may cause significant long-lasting remission. Other treatment options include systemic antibiotics, corticosteroids (intralesional and/or systemic), dapsone and surgical excision with grafting.

Q9. Describe folliculitis keloidalis.

Ans: The early lesions are small, flesh-colored, folliculocentric papules or pustules over the nuchal region and lower occiput. The lesions coalesce to form large nodules, plaques and hypertrophic scar. The histopathology of early lesions is that of folliculitis and perifolliculitis with predominant lymphocytic and plasma cell infiltrate surrounding the lower part of infundibulum and isthmus. Subsequently, there is a variable degree of inflammation around the degenerating follicles, loss of sebaceous glands, destruction of follicles and lamellar fibrosis. In advanced keloidal lesions, there are numerous "naked" hair shafts trapped within a dense fibrotic matrix associated with foreign body granulomatous reaction.

Treatment: Potent topical corticosteroids, antibiotics (topical and oral), intralesional corticosteroids, excisional surgery

Q10. What is acne necrotica?

Ans: Acne necrotica is a severe form of scalp folliculitis. The exact etiology is unknown, although staphylococci are usually cultured from these patients. Papules and pustules evolve to form crusts leaving depressed scars. The condition is chronic and recurrent.

Q11. What is keratosis follicularis spinulosa decalvans (KFSD)?

Ans: KFSD begins in infancy or childhood. Extensive keratosis pilaris first appear on the scalp and later progress to involve eyebrows, eyelids and limbs. Progressive cicatricial alopecia of scalp, eyebrows, and eyelashes is noted. Associated features are palmoplantar keratoderma, punctate corneal epithelial defects, ophthalmitis, photophobia and facial erythema. If it has a more persistent pustular course, it is termed folliculitis spinulosa decalvans.

Q12. What is the end-stage non-specific cicatricial alopecia?

Ans: The early stages of untreated primary cicatricial alopecias like LPP, FFA, PPB, CCCA, and FD can usually be diagnosed based on their distinctive clinical and histopathological features. Overtime these primary cicatricial alopecias ultimately burn out and the characteristic features are no longer present. The end-stage is an irregular area of cicatricial alopecia without follicular ostia and without inflammation.

The histology is variable and non-specific. The features are similar to the late stages of various primary cicatricial alopecias which include:

- Non-specific perifollicular inflammation;

- Mild superficial perivascular infiltrate;
- Depletion or absence of follicles;
- Vertical fibrous tracts as traces of vanished follicles;
- Absence of sebaceous glands;
- Atrophic epidermis, sclerotic dermis; and
- Granulomatous inflammation (rare).

Q13. List any drugs which can cause cicatricial alopecia.

Ans:
- Mepacrine
- Para aminosalicylic acid.

Q14. From which metastasis, primary tumors can cause cicatricial alopecia?

Ans: Metastatic nodules from renal, breast, and lung carcinomas.

CHAPTER 27

Trachyonychia

Nirmal Krishna B

Case study Trachyonychia

Presenting Complaints

Doctor, all my nails are rough and disfigured since childhood.

Setting

Dermatology outpatient department

History of Presenting Illness

An 18-year-old boy presented with complaints that all his nails were rough and disfigured since the age of 5 years. His mother had noticed that all nails developed these changes progressively. There were no other associated symptoms.

General and Systemic Examination

No abnormalities detected

Dermatological Examination

All twenty nails are discolored, thick, and are dystrophic (Fig. 1). No associated hair or skin changes.

Q1. What is the diagnosis?

a. Lichen planus (LP) of nails
b. Psoriatic nails
c. Trachyonychia
d. Pachyonychia congenita nails

Ans: c. Trachyonychia

Q2. What is trachyonychia?

Ans: Trachyonychia derived from the Greek word trakos, meaning rough, is a benign nail disorder characterized by rough nail plate changes involving one, several or all digits.

Q3. How is it otherwise known as?

Ans: It is otherwise known as twenty-nail dystrophy, though all 20 nail involvement is not necessary to make a diagnosis.

Q4. What is the mode of inheritance?

Ans: It has been reported to be transmitted in an autosomal dominant pattern in some families;

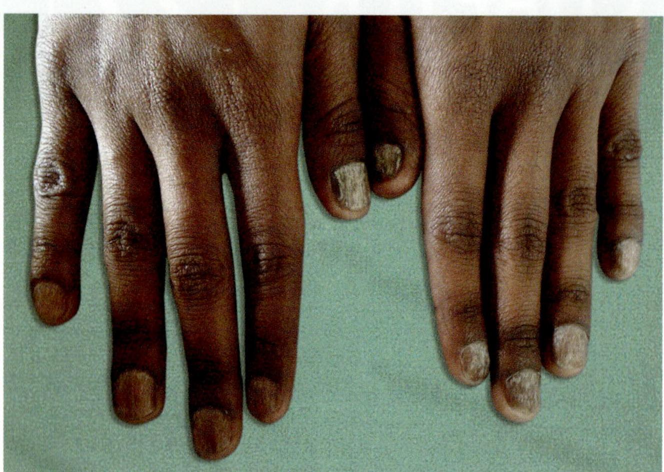

Fig. 1: Dystrophy of all twenty nails

however they are likely due to inheritance of alopecia areata in families.

Q5. Which age group is it common?

Ans: Though the disease can occur at any age, it is more common in children with a peak incidence at the age of 3–12 years.

Q6. What are the clinical types of trachonychia?

Ans: Clinically, trachyonychia can be divided into two main groups: (1) idiopathic trachyonychia and (2) trachyonychia associated with other dermatologic diseases.

Q7. What are the associations of trachyonychia?

Ans: Common associations of trachyonychia are alopecia areata, psoriasis, LP, and vitiligo. Other reported associations include: atopic dermatitis, autoimmune hemolytic anemia, Bart syndrome, congential cutaneous candidiasis, dyskeratosis congenita, graft-versus-host disease, punctate palmoplantar keratoderma, hidrotic ectodermal dysplasia, ichthyosis vulgaris, idiopathic thrombocytopenic purpura, immunoglobulin A deficiency, incontinentia pigmenti, nail-patella syndrome, pachyonychia congenita, pemphigus vulgaris, primary biliary cirrhosis, sarcoidosis, and trauma.

Q8. What is the most common association of trachyonychia?

a. Alopecia areata
b. LP
c. Tinea manuum
d. Psoriasis

Ans: a. Alopecia areata is the most common disease associated with trachyonychia.

Q9. How is lichen planus presenting as trachyonychia different from other usual nail changes due to lichen planus?

Ans: In LP presenting as trachyonychia, nail changes are usually isolated and seldom forms pterygium or cause scarring. It usually resolves spontaneously and portends a benign course.

Q10. What are the clues for clinical diagnosis of trachyonychia?

Ans: Longitudinal ridging and fissuring, longitudinal regular small pits, nail plate thinning, roughness and hyperkeratotic cuticles.

Q11. What are the morphological types of trachyonychia?

Ans: Based on morphology, it is divided into: opaque and shiny trachyonychia, while both can coexist in the same patient.

- In opaque trachyonychia, the nails are opaque, lusterless, rough and surface shows longitudinal ridging the classic sandpaper nails
- In shiny trachyonychia, the nail has multiple small punctuate geometric depressions on a shiny nail plate without obvious nail thinning.

Q12. What is the pathogenesis of trachyonychia?

Ans: Trachyonychia is due to insult to proximal nail matrix keratinocytes resulting in impairment of their maturation and differentiation without interrupting their mitotic activity. Milder intermittent inflammation produces shiny trachyonychia and severe persistent inflammation produces opaque trachyonychia.

Q13. What are the changes seen in histopathology in trachyonychia?

Ans: Three microscopic patterns can be identified namely:

1. Spongiotic
2. Psoriasiform
3. Lichenoid.

The most common feature is being spongiosis with exocytosis of inflammatory cells. This pattern is commonly seen in idiopathic variant and those associated with alopecia areata.

Q14. Is biopsy of nail matrix recommended routinely in trachyonychia?

Ans: Nail biopsy is not recommended to be performed routinely in patients with trachyonychia as the condition is known to resolve spontaneously and never produces nail scarring.

Q15. Is it necessary to treat trachyonychia always?

Ans: About 50% of patients achieve total resolution or marked improvement within the first 6 years regardless of treatment. Hence, a conservative approach including a mild emollient for opaque trachyonychia and cosmetic camouflage with nail lacquers in shiny trachyonychia should be advised and treatments must be given when deemed essential.

Q16. What are the various treatment modalities available to treat trachyonycia?

Ans: There is no single evidence-based treatment for trachyonychia. Treatments should be aimed at treating the associated disease. Various treatment modalities that have been used include:

- Intralesional injection of triamcinolone acetonide into the proximal nail fold at a concentration of 2.5–10 mg/mL
- Topical tazarotene 0.1% gel
- Topical 5-fluorouracil 5% cream
- Psoralen plus ultraviolet A (PUVA)
- Intramuscular triamcinolone acetonide once monthly
- Systemic retinoids-citretin 0.3 mg/kg
- Systemic cyclosporine at a dose of 3 mg/kg/day
- Oral biotin at 20 mg/day
- Oral steroids
- Oral antimalarials (chloroquine phosphate at 250 mg twice daily).

SECTION 6

Disorders of Sweat and Sebaceous Glands

Surajit Gorai

CHAPTER 28

Hyperhidrosis

Eswari L

Case study Hyperhidrosis

Presenting Complaints

Doctor, my palms, soles, and armpits sweat excessively and I am not able to write because my hands are very slippery.

Setting

Dermatology outpatient department

History of Present Illness

A 19-year-old girl presented with complaints of excessive sweating of her palms and soles since the past 1 year. Her hands become very slippery due to which she is not able to write. She also complains of increased sweating in her armpits which drenches her clothing and cause severe embarrassment and discomfort. Her mother and aunt also have similar problems. She does not give history of any triggering factors but she says she is free of the symptoms during sleep.

General Physical Examination and Systemic Examination

No abnormality detected

Dermatological Examination

- Palms and soles are wet and slippery with excessive sweating
- Droplets of sweat can be seen in the axilla (Fig. 1)

Q1. What is the most likely diagnosis?

a. Hyperhidrosis: Primary focal hyperhidrosis
b. Hyperhidrosis: Secondary hyperhidrosis
c. Bromhidrosis
d. Hexsel's hyperhidrosis

Ans: a. Hyperhidrosis: Primary focal hyperhidrosis. Presence of palmoplantar and axillary hyperhidrosis with a positive family history and a chronicity of more than 1 year, with no apparent secondary cause suggest primary focal hyperhidrosis.

Q2. How do you diagnose primary hyperhidrosis?

Ans: Criteria for diagnosis of primary hyperhidrosis are as follows:

- Focal, visible, and excessive sweating of at least 6-months duration without apparent cause.
- At least four of the following:
  - Bilateral and relatively symmetric
  - Impair daily activities
  - At least one episode per week
  - Age of onset less than 25 years

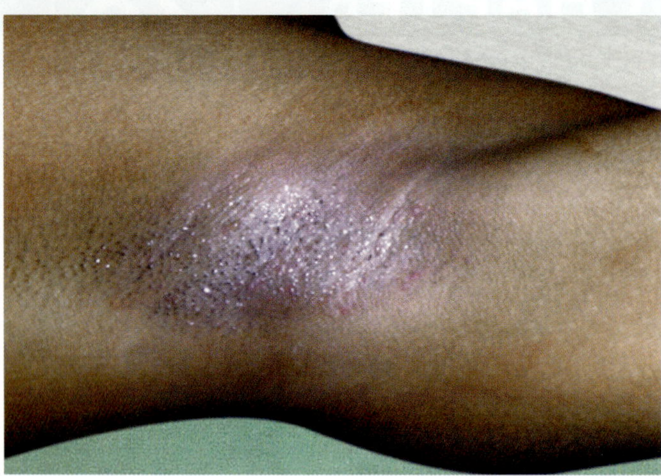

Fig. 1: Hyperhidrosis of the axilla

- Family history of hyperhidrosis
- Cessation of focal sweating during sleep

• Exclusion of secondary causes of excessive sweating

Q3. What are the types of secondary hyperhidrosis?

Ans: Types of secondary hyperhidrosis are:

- *Secondary generalized hyperhidrosis:* Generalized excessive sweating attributable to a definitive underlying medical cause; most commonly used drugs, substance abuse, cardiovascular disorders, respiratory failure, infections, malignancies, endocrine or metabolic disorders, or neurologic disease.
- *Secondary regional hyperhidrosis*
  - Localized anhidrosis with compensatory excessive sweating in other areas.
  - Identification of a definitive underlying cause; most commonly stroke, peripheral nerve damage, spinal cord lesion, neuropathy, or Ross syndrome.
- *Secondary focal hyperhidrosis*
  - Excessive sweating in typical anatomic sites (palms, soles, axillae, or craniofacial) or in a well-defined anatomic distribution (trunk, inguinal folds, buttocks, legs, submammary folds, neck, or wrist).
  - Identification of a definitive underlying cause; most commonly Frey's syndrome, eccrine nevus, social anxiety disorder, neurologic disorder, or tumor.

Investigations should be done to rule out underlying causes of secondary hyperhidrosis in all cases.

Q4. What are the causes of secondary hyperhidrosis?

Ans: Causes of secondary hyperhidrosis are described as:

- *Infective*
  - Acute: viral or bacterial
  - Chronic: Tuberculosis, Malaria, Brucellosis
- *Drug mediated:* Alcohol, cocaine, heroin, Nortriptyline, Pilocarpine, Zinc supplements, ciprofloxacin, Acyclovir, Esomeprazole.
- *Endocrine:* Diabetes mellitus, hyperthyroidism, menopause, pregnancy, Parkinson's disease, neurological disorders, gout, carcinoid syndrome, cardiac failure, cerebrovascular accident, vitiligo, spinal cord injuries, gustatory sweating
- *Non-neural disorders:* Arterial-venous fistula, cold erythema, local heat, Klippel-Trenaunay syndrome
- *Malignancy:* Lymphoma

Q5. How will you assess the degree of impairment in hyperhidrosis?

Ans: The degree of impairment in hyperhidrosis can be assessed as follows:

- Subjective assessment
  - *The dermatology life quality index (DLQI)* is a validated measure that consists of ten questions, each with four possible answers. This simple method assesses the impact of skin disease on quality of life.
  - *The hyperhidrosis disease severity scale (HDSS)* is another measure which was especially designed to evaluate effects of hyperhidrosis in particular on the patient's life. Higher score in this test indicates a greater negative impact on life quality:
    - My sweating is never noticeable and never interferes with my daily activities
    - My sweating is tolerable but sometimes interferes with my daily activities
    - My sweating is barely tolerable and frequently interferes with my daily activities
    - My sweating is intolerable and always interferes with my daily activities.
- Objective assessment
  - *Minor's starch iodine test:* The skin must be clean, shaved, and dry. Iodine solution, 3.5% in alcohol, is applied to the skin area of concern and starch flour is dusted on top. When sweat gets in contact with both substances a violet color will appear as a sign of positive reaction.

The extent and distribution of the hyperhidrosis can then be identified.

- *Gravimetry:* To quantify the amount of sweat, gravimetric is used, mainly for assessing axillary hyperhidrosis. Filter paper will be weighed before and after exposure to axillary skin for a defined time period (60 sec or 5 min). The weight difference quantifies the amount of sweat produced over a period of time (in mg/min). Hyperhidrosis is defined as greater than 50 mg/min/m^2 body surface area.

Q6. An echo-Doppler study found impaired left ventricular filling in a patient with essential hyperhidrosis. What is the reason?

a. Hyperhidrosis is a component of metabolic syndrome
b. Hyperhidrosis patients have hypertension
c. Hyperhidrosis patients have associated cardiac autonomic dysfunction
d. Hyperhidrosis patients have sclerotic valves

Ans: c. Hyperhidrosis patients have associated cardiac autonomic dysfunction because sympathetic fibers to eccrine glands of the palms of the hand arise from stellate and upper thoracic ganglia, which also innervate the heart.

Q7. What are the characteristics of primary versus secondary hyperhidrosis?

Ans: The characteristics of primary versus secondary hyperhidrosis have been described in Table 1.

Q8. What is the underlying pathology of increased sweating?

Ans: The underlying pathology of sweating disorders is not well-understood till now. There is extreme nonthermoregulatory sympathetic stimulation of the sweat glands. Emotional stimuli play an important role. The anterior cingulate frontal cortex seems to be responsible for emotional or sensory stimuli, which then leads to sweating. It is primarily regulated by preoptic-anterior hypothalamus. Patients suffering from palmar hyperhidrosis have a family history, which suggests a genetic component in an autosomal dominant manner with variable penetrance. Other risk factors are still unknown.

Table 1: Characteristics of primary versus secondary hyperhidrosis

Primary hyperhidrosis	*Secondary hyperhidrosis*
• Sweating in a typical distribution • Positive family history	• Onset age is older than 25 years • Unilateral and/or symmetric • Generalized rather than focal • Present even during sleep

Q9. What are the concomitant cutaneous disorders that can be expected in hyperhidrosis?

Ans: Verruca vulgaris, dermatophytosis, candidiasis, dyshidrotic eczema.

Q10. What are the various treatment options in managing hyperhidrosis?

Ans: The various treatment options in managing hyperhidrosis are described as:

- Medical management
  - *Topical:* These agents reduce perspiration by denaturing keratin and thereby occluding the pores of the sweat glands.
  - *Antiperspirants*:
    - 20% aluminum chloride hexahydrate in anhydrous absolute alcohol
    - 2–5% tannic acid solution
    - 5–20% formalin solution
    - 10% glutaraldehyde'
  - Anticholinergics
- Systemic management
  - *Tranquilizers*: Diazepam
  - *Anticholinergics*:
    - Propantheline bromide
    - Glycopyrrolate
    - Oxybutynin
    - Benztropinemesylate
  - *Nonsteroidal anti-inflammatory drugs (NSAIDs):* Indomethacin
  - *Calcium-channel blockers*: Diltiazem
  - *Botulinum toxin*: Since botulinum toxin inhibits the release of acetylcholine not only at the neuromuscular junction, but also in postganglionic sympathetic fibers to sweat glands, it has been found to be useful to treat palmar and axillary hyperhidrosis (Fig. 2).
- Surgical:
  - Sympathectomy
  - Excision of axillary sweat glands
  - Liposuction

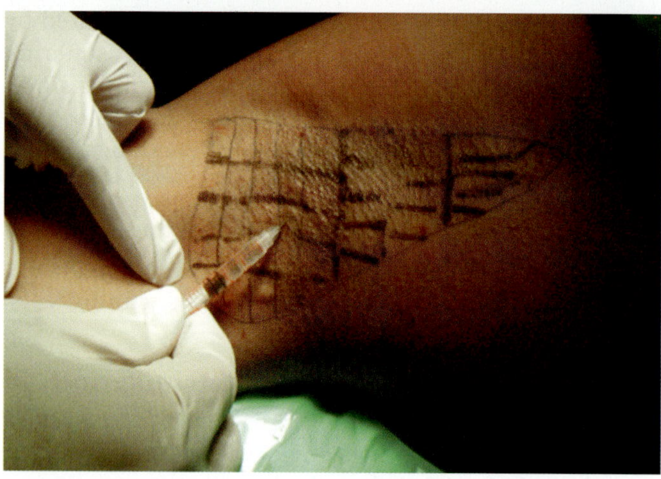

Fig. 2: Intradermal botulinum toxin injection for axillary hyperhidrosis

- Electrical:
  - *Iontophoresis:* It is defined as the introduction of an ionized substance through intact skin by the application of a direct current .It is thought that this form of treatment is effective because it introduces ions of soluble salts and other molecules into the skin, blocking the sweat ducts without damaging the sweat glands; however, this only gives relief for a period of 2-weeks up to 3 months, and then the treatment procedure has to be repeated.

Q11. What is the drawback of systemic anticholinergics?

Ans: Systemic anticholinergics also result in side effects including xerostomia, mydriasis, cycloplegia, and bowel and bladder dysfunction.

CHAPTER 29

Hidradenitis Suppurativa

Nagesh TS

Case study Hidradenitis Suppurativa

Presenting Complaint

Doctor I have painful swellings with pus discharge and scars in the axilla and groin on and off since 2 years.

Setting

Dermatology outpatient department

History of Present Illness

A 25-year-old male presented with episodic painful swellings with pus discharge in the axilla and groin since 2 years. Initially started over the axilla and gradually spread to the other areas. He has had around 5–6 episodes of similar complaints in the last 2 years. The lesions reduce on taking treatment and resolve with residual scarring. No history of fever or joint pains associated with the lesions.

General Physical Examination and Systemic Examination

No abnormality detected

Dermatological Examination

Multiple tender nodules present in both the axilla and groin along with discharging sinuses (Fig. 1). Multiple comedones present in the affected area along with interconnecting scars.

Q1. What is the most likely diagnosis?

a. Hidradenitis suppurativa (HS)
b. Cutaneous tuberculosis
c. Acne conglobata
d. Actinomycosis

Ans: a. Hidradenitis suppurativa (HS)

Q2. Enumerate the criteria to diagnose hidradenitis suppurativa?

Ans: There are three criteria to diagnose HS. All the three should be present for diagnosis:

1. *Characteristic lesions*: Deep-seated painful nodules, pus discharge from sinuses, abscesses, bridging scars, multiple open pseudocomedones.
2. *Typical sites*: Axilla, groin, perineal and perianal region, buttocks, inframammary and intermammary folds.
3. *Chronic and recurrent lesions.*

Q3. Name the synonyms for hidradenitis suppurativa.

Ans: The synonyms for HS are:

- Velpeau disease
- Acne inversa

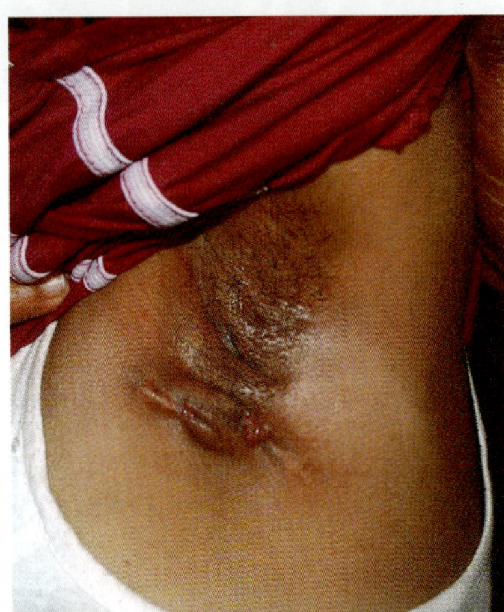

Fig. 1: Multiple nodules and discharging sinuses in the axilla

- Ectopic acne
- Verneuil disease
- Pyoderma fistulans sinifica.

Q4. What are the predisposing factors for hidradenitis suppurativa?

Ans: Obesity, smoking, hormonal influences (female preponderance—premenstrual and postnatal flare-ups and improvement during pregnancy), and certain medications like lithium (induces follicular hyperkeratosis) and sirolimus has been shown to be predisposing factors for HS.

Q5. What is the pathophysiology of hidradenitis suppurativa?

Ans: Initially, HS was considered to be due to involvement of apocrine gland. However, recent studies have shown that follicular occlusion to be the main event in the pathogenesis of HS. The progression of events leading to HS include: hyperkeratosis in the infundibulum (spongiform infundibulofolliculitis) followed by dilatation of the follicles, cyst formation and rupture of the follicle leading to inflammation and fistula formation.

Q6. What are the associated conditions with hidradenitis suppurativa?

Ans: Various diseases have been reported to be associated with HS.

1. HS along with acne conglobata, dissecting cellulitis of scalp, and pilonidal sinus constitute the follicular occlusion tetrad.
2. Inflammatory disorders like Crohn's disease and spondyloarthropathy of axial joints.
3. Syndromes like pyoderma gangrenosum, acne conglobate, and suppurative hidradenitis (PASH), pyogenic arthritis, pyoderma gangrenosum, acne conglobate, and suppurative hidradenitis (PAPASH) and synovitis, acne, pustulosis, hyperostosis and osteitis (SAPHO).
4. Congenital alpha-1 deficiency.

Q7. What are the clinical features of hidradenitis suppurativa?

Ans: As mentioned in the diagnostic criteria, the presence of characteristic lesions at typical sites with a history of chronicity and recurrence is required for the diagnosis of HS.

- The initial lesions are usually dermal or subcutaneous nodules which may persist for duration of 1–2 weeks and which regress later or form abscesses.
- Can form pointing abscesses and rupture to form draining and non-draining sinus tracts.
- The lesions resolve leaving behind bridged- or rope-like scars. Scarring can be hypertrophic or atrophic, contractures can be seen.
- Multiple twin comedones and polyporous comedones can be seen.
- Flexural areas: axilla, inguinal and anogenital regions are commonly affected. Other areas involved include perineal, perianal, gluteal, sub and inframammary areas.
- Manifest as few nodules to multiple abscesses, sinus tracts, contractures and scarring.

Q8. The staging system used for the severity of hidradenitis suppurativa is:

a. Huxley's staging
b. Hurley's staging
c. Henle's staging
d. Breslow's staging

Ans: b. The severity of HS is based on Hurley's staging:

- Stage I: Only recurrent solitary or multiple abscess formation without scarring
- Stage II: Recurrent abscess with sinus tracts and cicatrization
- Stage III: Multiple abscesses, sinus tracts and scarring diffusely involving an entire region
- Other severity assessment methods include hidradenitis severity score (HSS) or modified Sartorius score. The various criteria considered in this score include the number of sites affected, lesions, area-involved and the presence of normal skin.

- Hidradenitis suppurativa clinical response (HiSCR) has been recommended to measure the treatment outcome. It considers more than 50% reduction in the number of inflamed lesions compared to baseline along with the absence of increase in the number of fistulae.

Q9. What are the investigations done in a case of hidradenitis suppurativa?

Ans: The diagnosis of HS is mainly clinical-based on the criteria mentioned earlier. Certain investigations are needed for evaluation and treatment purpose.

- Pus culture and sensitivity can be done from discharge to look for secondary infection and to plan for antibiotic usage.
- Imaging studies like ultrasound and magnetic resonance imaging (MRI) are done if surgical intervention is planned to look for the subclinical extent of the disease.
- Routine blood tests are done to look for conditions like anemia, diabetic status and inflammatory markers.

Q10. What is the differential diagnosis for hidradenitis suppurativa?

Ans: The differential diagnosis for HS depends on the stage of the disease:

- *Early stages*: Furuncle, carbuncle, abscesses, infected cysts (sebaceous cyst). Presence of follicular occlusion triad or tetrad has to be ruled out.
- *Anogenital region*: Cutaneous crohn's disease
- *Late stages*: Cutaneous tuberculosis, actinomycosis, lymphogranuloma venereum, sporotrichosis.

Q11. What are the complications associated with hidradenitis suppurativa?

Ans: Complications associated with HS are:

- Lymphedema due to lymphatic obstruction
- Superinfections
- Fistula formation in gastrointestinal tract (GIT), genitourinary tract—rare
- Squamous cell carcinoma in anogenital disease
- Anemia, hypoalbuminemia can occur as part of chronicity of disease.

Q12. What are the treatment options available for hidradenitis suppurativa?

Ans: The treatment of HS is challenging and depends on the severity of the disease. The aim of the treatment should be achieved to cure and prevent recurrences. The treatment options include:

- *General measures*
  - Local hygiene
  - Weight reduction
  - Cessation of smoking
  - Warm saline compress
  - Wearing loose-fitting clothing
  - Laser hair removal
- *Specific measures:*
  - *Topical therapy:* Clindamycin 1–2%
  - *Systemic antimicrobials:* Tetracycline, doxycycline, clindamycin (300 mg twice daily), rifampicin (300 mg twice daily), moxifloxacin A combination of rifampin-moxifloxacin-metronidazole has been reported to be used for a period of 12–24 weeks in severe stage II and III disease.
  - *Retinoids:* Isotretinoin has been used in doses used for severe acne. Few reports have shown Acitretin to be more effective than isotretinoin.
  - *Anti-inflammatory:* Intralesional corticosteroids like triamcinolone (5 mg/mL) can be used. However it is avoided in the presence of infection. Dapsone (100 mg/day) has been reported to be used for a long-term treatment. Cyclosporine (4.5 mg/kg body weight) and short course of systemic steroids (Prednisolone—0.5–1 mg/kg body weight) have also been used.
  - *Biological agents:* Anti-tumor necrosis factors (TNF)-α agents have been tried in HS. Infliximab and adalimumab are used. Adalimumab with a loading dose of 160 mg and 80 mg at week-2 followed by 40 mg every week for 12 weeks has shown promising results.
- *Surgical treatment:* Include deroofing, incision and drainage, wide excision, electrosurgery, ablative lasers and laser hair removal have all been used in late stages of the disease. Extensive surgery with excision of the entire area involved remains the only option in the end stage of disease.
- *Radiation therapy can also be tried in selected cases to destroy the affected apocrine unit.*

CHAPTER 30

Acne

Shilpa Garg, Priyanka Borde Bisht

Case study Acne

Presenting Complaints

Doctor, I am having multiple large pimples over my face since last 3–4 months. They are painful and some burst to ooze-out pus. Also, they leave behind scars after resolving.

Setting

Dermatology outpatient department

History of Present Illness

A 17-years-old boy presented with complaints of multiple painful skin color to reddish lesions over face mainly on cheeks, forehead and nose since 3–4 months. Some of the lesions are tender and pus-filled. He also complains of excessive oiliness over face. These eruptions resolve over few weeks to months leaving behind ugly scars.

General and Systemic Examination

No abnormality detected

Dermatological Examination:

- Patient has oily skin over the face
- Multiple skin-colored papules, erythematous nodules, and pustules are seen over the face
- Predominant involvement: Cheeks and nose ranging in size from 5 mm to 1.5 cm in diameter (Fig. 1).
- Multiple open and closed comedones are also present especially involving the cheek.
- Multiple cystic, boggy lesions that tend to rupture are also observed.
- Multiple scars are also present.

Q1. What is the most likely diagnosis?

a. Nodulocystic acne
b. Folliculitis
c. Acne fulminans
d. Acne conglobata

Ans: a. Nodulocystic acne: Age of the patient, presence of nodules, pustules, cystic lesions and comedones in the absence of sinuses and systemic findings like fever and joint pain suggest the diagnosis of nodulocystic acne. Recent studies say that since they

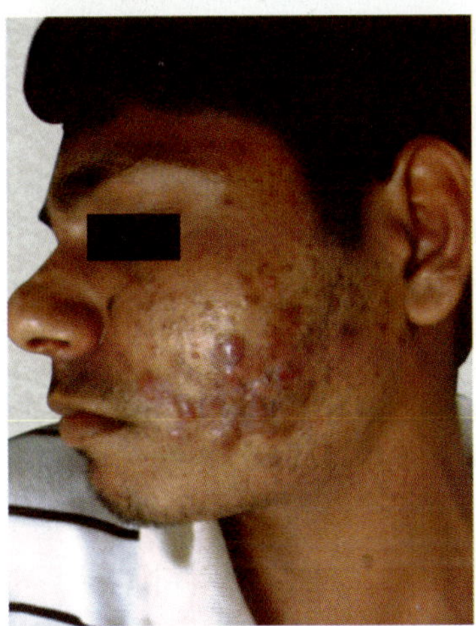

Fig. 1: Multiple nodules and cysts on face

are pseudocysts, it should only be named as severe nodular acne.

Q2. What is the pathophysiology of acne?

Ans: There are four main factors:

1. Follicular epidermal hyperkeratinization causing blockage of the content of sebaceous gland.
2. Excess sebum production
3. Inflammation due to production of free fatty acid from the complex fat of sebum.
4. Increased presence and activity of *Propionibacterium acnes*—an anerobic, gram-positive bacterium (rod) thought to be the normal commensal of skin.

Q3. What are the clinical features of acne?

Ans: Clinical features of acne are:

- Primary site: Face, other sites: back, chest, shoulders
- Appearance: Open or closed comedones, normal pigmented to erythematous papules, pustules and large, tender, fluctuant nodules, rarely cysts.
- Scarring: Atrophic, ice-pick, rolling, box-car and hypertrophic.

Q4. What are the laboratory investigations required in case of acne?

Ans: Laboratory workup is not indicated for the diagnosis of acne. However, hormonal workup is needed in women whose acne has the following features and some other laboratory workup is needed in few severe forms of acne like acne fulminans:

- Patient with late-onset acne (acne tarda)
- Features of hyperandrogenism like hirsutism, androgenetic alopecia, seborrhea, oligo or amenorrhea
- Premenstrual flare of acne
- Acne not responding to conventional therapy
- Acne mostly located on the lower cheeks, jaw and neck.

In females suspected to have hormonal imbalance, the following investigations are indicated:

- Serum-free testosterone, dehydroepiandrosterone sulfate (DHEAS), prolactin, thyroid profile, 17-hydroxyprogesterone, serum-fasting insulin, and free androgen index to be done on day-2 of menstrual cycle.
- Ultrasound pelvis to look for volume of ovary, number of follicles and size of follicles.
- In acne fulminans serum level of vitamin D3, calcium, and other electrolytes should be done.
- Few basic lab parameters also should be checked before starting systemic isotretinoin therapy (Mentioned below).

Q5. What are the complications of acne?

Ans: Complications of acne are:

- Transient macular erythema may persist after resolution of lesions.
- Postinflammatory hyperpigmentation may persist for months in darker skin types after resolution.
- Permanent scarring commonly occurs in this type of acne
- Psychiatric disturbances, social, emotional, psychological impairment may occur.
- With severe forms of acne like acne fulminans there may be persistent bone and joint pain, dyselectrolytemia and erythema nodosum.

Q6. What is the clinical course of acne?

Ans: Clinical course of acne:

- May start as early as 8 years or by 20 years or later
- May persist for several years followed by spontaneous remission, usually clear by early or late 20s
- Course may extend till 3rd or 4th decade
- Flares may be associated with menses, stress, seasonal variation, and lifestyle changes.

Q7. What are grades of acne?

Ans: Acne was graded by many researchers to measure acne severity. But a composite grading system that includes each parameters are still lacking. Simple grading systems that are widely accepted are as follows:

Grade 1: Comedones, occasional papules

Grade 2: Papules, comedones, few pustules

Grade 3: Predominant pustules, nodules, abscesses

Grade 4: Mainly cysts, abscesses, widespread scarring.

Q8. Describe the treatment options available for nodulocystic acne.

Ans: Treatment options for nodulocystic acne are:

- *General Measures:* Treatment of acne should start with education regarding the nature and course of acne, different modalities of treatment and their limitations and likely duration of therapy.
- *Diet:* There is conflicting evidence regarding the role of diet in acne. Until further evidence accumulates, patients are advised to avoid the food which they feel causes exacerbation or development of acne.
- *Medicated face washes:* Medical face washes containing benzoyl peroxide or salicylic acid are advised for patients with oily skin to be used twice daily. Patients with sensitive skin, dry skin and those on oral isotretinoin are advised mild cleansers to avoid irritation to skin.
- *Medications*
  - Grade 1: Topical retinoids (adapalene or tretinoin)
  - Grade 2: Two of topical retinoids or topical antibiotic (clindamycin or nadifloxacin) or benzoyl peroxide
  - Grade 3: Oral antibiotic (doxycycline or azithromycin or minocycline) and topical retinoids and topical antibiotic or benzoyl peroxide or topical azelaic acid
  - Grade 4: Oral isotretinoin and benzoyl peroxide and topical antibiotic
- *Surgical options*
  - Incision drainage or aspiration of pus-filled lesion
  - Intralesional corticosteroids for cysts
  - Cryotherapy

Q9. What are the advantages of using isotretinoin as first-line in nodulocystic acne?

Ans: Isotretinoin is the first drug of choice for the treatment of nodulocystic acne because its use leads to rapid reduction in inflammation, prevention of clinical and psychological scarring, quick improvement in the quality of life and reduction in the risk of depression. The rate of relapse of acne is lowest with oral isotretinoin in comparison to all other available therapies.

Q10. What are the side effects of isotretinoin?

Ans. Side effects of isotretinoin can be divided as:

- *Minor*
  - Dryness especially over lips that indicate effectiveness of treatment. Can be prevented by repeated application of lip emollient
  - Nasal mucosal dryness that may lead to epistaxis. It can be prevented by application of normal saline nasal drop
  - Dry eyes with visual blurring
  - Headache
  - Nausea, vomiting and abdominal pain
  - Increased chance of cutaneous infection
  - Paronychia
- *Severe*
  - Pseudotumor cerebri specially when given with tetracycline group of antibiotics
  - Hyperlipidemia. Regular monitoring is needed
  - DISH- Diffuse interstitial symmetric hyperostosis
  - Teratogenicity.

Q11. What is iPLEDGE?

Ans: It is a mandatory program for isotretinoin distribution in the USA. Idea is to prevent use of the drug during pregnancy due to high risk of teratogenicity. It is a web-based risk management system where a patient has to register herself before getting monthly dose of isotretinoin.

Q12. What are the side effects of topical retinoids and how will you prevent it?

Ans: *Side effects of topical retinoids:*

- Erythema, burning sensation, itching
- Photosensitivity
- Dryness and peeling of skin
- Severe burning, redness with blister formation.

These are all due to allergic or irritant contact dermatitis due to topical retinoids.

Advice for prevention:

- If there is severe reaction then stop application
- Apply at night or do not go out in sun after application
- Apply in a small quantity
- If there is itching or burning then apply it for 30 minutes and then gradually increase it to overnight
- Does not rub the area after application
- Does not apply it over folds.

Q13. What advice will you give for patients on oral isotretinoin?

Ans: Following advice should be given to patients on oral isotretinoin:

- Repeated application of emollient over body and lips.
- Regular monitoring of lipid profile
- Avoid drugs that increase chance of intracranial tension like tetra or doxycycline.
- Avoid pregnancy during or 1 month after stoppage of isotretinoin therapy.
- Use two forms of birth control measures 1-month before, during and 1-month after isotretinoin therapy.

Q14. What are the baseline investigations to be done before starting isotretinoin?

Ans: Few baseline investigations should be done prior to isotretinoin therapy:

- Pregnancy test in women with child bearing potential (Preferably two)
- Complete blood count
- Lipid profile
- Liver function test
- Renal function test

Q15. What are the severe forms of acne?

Ans: The severe forms of acne are

- *Acne conglobata:* One of most severe type of inflammatory acne characterized by multiple nodulocystic lesions with discharging sinuses over face. May affect neck, upper arms and back. Seen in adolescent male. May be a part of follicular occlusion triad that includes hidradenitis suppurativa, dissecting cellulitis of scalp along with acne conglobata.
- *Acne fulminans*: This is the most severe type of acne. Along with inflammatory acne lesions over face, systemic symptoms like fever, arthralgia, myalgia and weakness are usually associated. Facial lesions evolve rapidly to become necrotic and ulcerative. Systemic corticosteroid is the mainstay of therapy here.
- *Acne with solid facial edema (Morbihan syndrome)*: This is a very rare type. Here central middle-third of the face become woody-hard along with inflammatory acne lesions.

Q16. What are the syndromes associated with acne?

Ans: The syndromes associated with acne are

- PAPA: Pyogenic arthritis, pyoderma gangrenosum and acne.
- SAPHO: Synovitis, acne, pustulosis, hyperostosis, osteitis.

In few syndromes with insulin resistance, acne may be the predominant feature like:

- CAH: Congenital adrenal hyerplasia.
- PCOS: Polycystic ovarian syndrome.
- HAIR-AN: Hyper androgenism, insulin resistance and acanthosis nigricans.
- SAHA: Seborrhea, acne, hirsutism, androgenetic alopecia.

CHAPTER 31

Rosacea

Saloni Katoch

Case study Rosacea

Presenting Complaints

Doctor, I have this red rash on my cheeks, forehead and nose that aggravates on going out in the sun since 5 months.

Setting

Dermatology outpatient department

History of Presenting Illness

A 45-year-old female patient presents with complaints of a red rash on the forehead, nose and cheeks since 5 months. She gives history of the rash being associated with burning and stinging sensation. She describes the rash as being mild initially, only present on exposure to sunlight and later progressing to being present all the time. Her face becomes flushed on sun exposure, on taking hot beverages and spicy foods. She has also noticed red pimple like eruptions over cheeks and chin along with some pus-filled lesion over forehead since 3 weeks.

General Physical Examination and Systemic Examination

No abnormality detected.

Dermatological Examination

- Diffuse erythema present over the central face—forehead, nose, cheeks and chin
- Telangiectasias present over the nose and cheeks
- Multiple monomorphic erythematous papules and few pustules present over the forehead, cheeks and chin.

Q1. What is the most likely diagnosis?

a. Acne vulgaris

b. Rosacea

c. Seborrheic dermatitis

d. Lupus erythematosus

Ans: b. Rosacea. The characteristic history of repeated episodes of flushing with sun exposure, hot beverages and spicy food being triggers, progressing to a nontransient erythema primarily of the convexities of the central face is in favor of the diagnosis. Examination findings of erythema, telangiectasia, monomorphic erythematous papules and pustules over the central face, absence of comedones, scaling and scarring and a normal general and systemic examination support the diagnosis of rosacea.

Q2. How do you diagnose rosacea?

Ans: Rosacea is a clinical diagnosis. Guidelines for diagnosis of rosacea as proposed by the National Rosacea Society Expert Committee are as follows:

- Presence of one or more of the following primary features:
  - Flushing (transient erythema)
  - Non-transient erythema (Fig. 1)
  - Papules and pustules
  - Telangiectasia

Graded as absent, mild, moderate or severe (0–3).

- May include one or more of the following secondary features:
  - Burning or stinging
  - Plaque
  - Dry appearance
  - Edema
  - Ocular manifestations
  - Peripheral location
  - Phymatous changes

Graded as absent or present.

Q3. What are the triggers of rosacea?

Ans: The triggers of rosacea are as follows:

- Sun exposure
- Hot beverages
- Spicy foods
- Alcohol consumption especially wine
- Wind blow
- Temperature variation
- Topical irritants like soap and cosmetics
- Emotional disturbances
- Few medications.

Q4. What are the subtypes of rosacea?

Ans: The subtypes of rosacea are as follows:

- *Erythematotelengiectatic*: Flushing, persistent central facial erythema with or without telangiectasia (Fig. 2)
- *Papulopustular*: Persistent central facial erythema with transient, central facial papules or pustules or both (Fig. 3)
- *Phymatous*: Thickened skin, irregular surface nodularities and enlargement, may occur on the nose, chin, forehead, cheeks or ears (Fig. 4)
- *Ocular*: Erythema of the eyelid margin, scaling and crusting. Foreign body sensation, burning or stinging, dryness, itching, photosensitivity, blurred vision, telangiectasia of peripheral sclera or periorbital edema may be present.
- Variants of rosacea
- *Granulomatous*: Yellow brown or red papules or nodules mainly distributed over cheeks and periorificial skin. Granuloma formation is seen on histopathology.

Q5. What are the differential diagnoses of Rosacea?

Ans: Differential diagnosis:

- *Acne vulgaris*: Younger age group, extensive distribution over face, neck and trunk, absence of flushing and telangiectasia, characteristic presence of comedones and seborrhoea
- *Seborrheic dermatitis*: It involves scalp, retro-auricular region, eyelids and nasolabial folds,

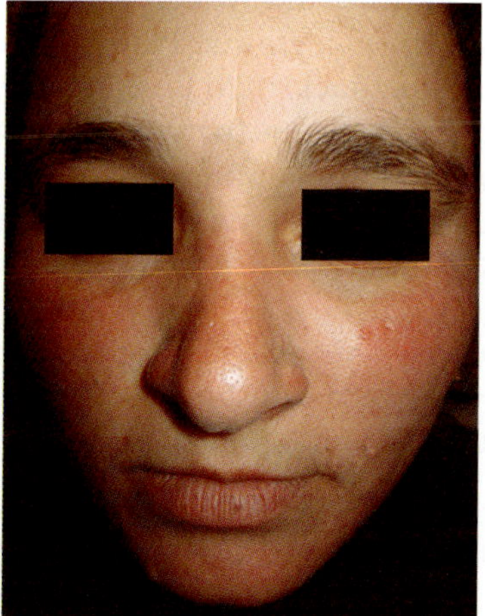

Fig. 1: Nontransient erythema of rosacea
Courtesy: Dr Shashikiran and Dr Nadiga Rajashekhar, JJM Medical College, Davangere, Karanataka, India

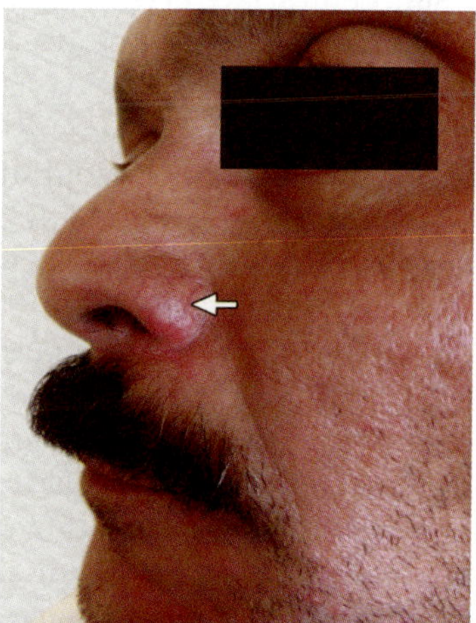

Fig. 2: Erythematotelengiectaticroacea: Telengiectasia seen on the alaenasi
Courtesy: Dr Sneha Gandhi and Dr SB Murugesh, JJM Medical College, Davangere, Karanataka, India

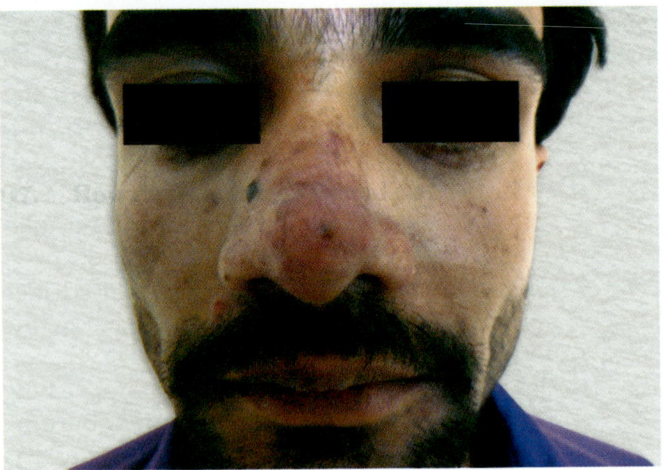

Fig. 3: Papulopustular rosacea: inflammatory papules seen on the central face
Courtesy: Dr Shashikiran and Dr Nadiga Rajashekhar, JJM Medical College, Davangere, Karanataka, India

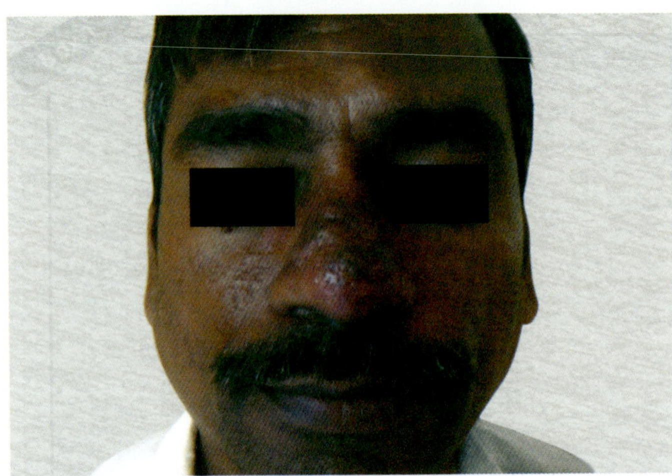

Fig. 4: Phymatous rosacea: large follicular openings with thickened and irregular skin giving rise to the *Peau d'orange* appearance
Courtesy: Dr Sneha Gandhi and Dr SB Murugesh, JJM Medical College, Davangere, Karanataka, India

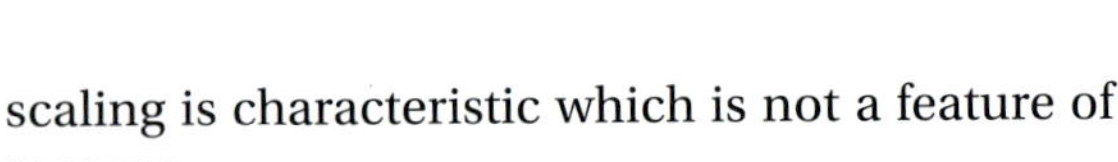

scaling is characteristic which is not a feature of rosacea

- *Lupus erythematosus*: Scarring, scaling and follicular plugging are seen in discoid lupus erythematosus, butterfly erythema of systemic lupus erythematosus is associated with systemic symptoms and lacks pustular lesions
- *Demodicidosis*: Pruritic papular eruptions on the face and neck, skin scrapings demonstrate the demodex mites
- *Perioral dermatitis*: Perioral microvesicles, micropustules, scaling and peeling, affects younger women, central face erythema and inflammatory papules are not features, exacerbates on topical steroid use
- *Topical steroid-induced rosacea like dermatitis*: After long and erroneous use of topical corticosteroids, marked thinning of skin with papulopustules, nodules, atrophy and telangiectasia, withdrawal of steroid causes exacerbation
- *Chronic photodamage*: affects periphery of face and neck, hyperpigmentation and hypopigmentation are seen along with erythema and telangiectasia, unlike rosacea submental sparing is present
- *Lupus pernio*: It can resemble rhinophymatous rosacea, involves the nasal septum as well, lacks the *peau d'orange* surface characteristic of rhinophyma and has multisystem involvement
- *Basal cell carcinoma*: It may mimic or occur in association with rhinophyma, biopsy aids in differentiation.

Q6. What systemic conditions would you like to consider in a patient presenting with episodes of facial flushing?

Ans: Systemic findings:

- *Carcinoid syndrome*: Associated diarrhea, wheezing, weight loss and hepatomegaly. Elevated urinary 5-hydroxyindoleacetic acid confirms diagnosis
- *Connective tissue disorders*: Lupus erythematosus, dermatomyositis
- *Mastocytosis*: Flushing episodes associated with headache, wheezing, palpitations, abdominal pain, diarrhea and syncope
- *Phaeochromocytoma*: Pallor typically present during an attack, mild flushing may rarely occur after the attack due to rebound vasodilation
- *Neurological*: Brain tumors, spinal cord lesions, orthostatic hypotension, migraine headaches, Parkinson's disease and parotid gland injury or surgery
- *Dumping syndrome*: Following gastric surgery, characterized by flushing, sweats, tachycardia and abdominal pain.

Q7. Which drugs can cause flushing?

Ans: Drugs that cause flushing:

- All vasodilator drugs can cause facial flushing like calcium channel blockers, nitrates, nitrites and amiodarone
- Systemic steroids
- Cyproterone acetate

- Tamoxifen
- Cyclosporine
- Metronidazole and cephalosporin antibiotics especially when prescribed in alcoholics
- Alcohol especially wine.

Q8. How would you manage a patient of rosacea?

Ans: Treatment modalities

1. *General measures*: trigger avoidance, broad spectrum sunscreen, cleansing with soap-free cleanser, use of gentle emollient, avoidance of harsh products (astringents, toners, menthol, camphor and sodium lauryl sulfate), facial massage in direction of lymphatic flow (Soybe's technique).
2. *Topical measures*:
   - FDA approved
     - Metronidazole 0.75% gel and 1% cream
     - Azelaic acid 15% gel
     - 10% sodium sulfacetamide with 5% sulfur (cream, suspension, cleanser or lotion)
     - Ivermectin 1% cream (papulopustular rosacea)
     - Brimonidine 0.33% gel (persistent facial erythema)
   - Others
     - Azelaic acid 20% cream, clindamycin 1%, erythromycin 2%, 5% benzoyl peroxide gel, topical retinoids
     - Tacrolimus ointment and pimecrolimus cream (for topical steroid-induced rosacea like dermatitis)
     - 5% permethrin cream, 1% lindane, 10% crotamiton cream (papulopustular rosacea)
     - Methylnicotinamide, oxymetazoline.
3. *Systemic measures*:
   - FDA approved
     - Doxycycline 40 mg once daily for 6–12 weeks
   - Others
     - Tetracycline 500 mg bd
     - Doxycycline 50–100 mg bd
     - Minocycline 50–100 mg bd
     - Azithromycin 250 mg three times weekly
     - Clarithromycin 250–500 mg bd-qd.
   - Other antibiotics
     - Penicillin
     - Erythromycin
     - Amoxicillin
     - Ampicillin
     - Metronidazole
     - Dapsone
   - For flushing
     - Oral contraceptives
     - Amitriptyline
     - Clonidine
     - Pimozide
     - Aspirin
     - Beta blockers
     - Ondansetron
     - COX-2 inhibitors.
   - Others
     - Ivermectin (refractory rosacea)
     - Isotretinoin (phymatous rosacea)
     - Acitretin
     - Ketoconazole
     - Spironolactone
     - Prednisone (rosacea fulminans only).
4. *Laser and light therapy*: To eliminate telangiectasia, reduce erythema, reduce papule and pustule count, extend remission
   - *Short wavelength lasers (superficial vessel destruction)*: Pulsed dye laser, long pulsed dye laser, potassium-titanyl-phosphate laser, diode pumped frequency doubled laser
   - *Long wavelength lasers (deeper and larger vessels)*: Long pulsed alexandrite, diode and Nd:YAG laser
   - Intense pulsed Light (broadband light with filters) and photodynamic therapy.
5. *Surgical modalities*: Advanced phyma treated with surgical debulking and contouring or combination of surgery followed by isotretinoin. Modalities include tangential excision, electrocautery, cryosurgery, dermabrasion and laser ablation.
6. *Ocular rosacea*: Ophthalmology referral, gentle nonmedicated cleanser, sulfacetamide/sulfur cleanser, 10% sulfacetamide ophthalmic ointment and oral tetracyclines.

Q9. What complications can a patient of rosacea develop?

Ans: Complications:

- *Chronic lymphedema*: Coarsening of facial features (leonine facies), chronic upper facial erythematous edema (Morbihan's disease)
- *Ocular complications*: Episcleritis, recurrent chalazion, hordeolum, rosacea keratitis can lead to scarring and corneal perforation.

Q10. What are the key points in the etiopathogenesis of rosacea?

Ans: Etiopathogenetic factors:

- *Vascular hypothesis*: Constitutional predisposition to flushing and blushing, vasomotor lability pronounced during menopause, microcirculatory disturbances
- *Exaggerated innate immune responses*: Increased cathelicidin peptides mediated inflammation of the epidermis
- *Degenerative changes*: Matrix degeneration and connective tissue damage lead to small vessel dilatation with perivascular leakage of inflammatory mediators
- *Helicobacter pylori*: Increased flushing due to vasodilators like nitric oxide, gastrin, TNF-alpha and IL-8 produced by the organism
- *Demodex folliculorum*: Mite living in lumen of sebaceous follicles has been implicated, decrease of papules and erythema with topical metronidazole, benzyl benzoate, crotamiton and permethrin support this view
- Photoaggravation with solar damage to the dermis
- As a part of immune reconstitution inflammatory syndrome
- Common in fair-skinned individuals and is unmasked or induced by chronic repeated trigger exposure.

Q11. What are the stages of rosacea?

Ans: The stages of rosacea are as follows:

- *Pre-rosacea*: Frequent flushing due to triggers
- *Stage 1*: Transient erythema that becomes more persistent, telangiectasia and increased skin sensitivity
- *Stage 2*: Persistent erythema, papules, pustules, edema, enlarged pores and ocular changes
- *Stage 3*: Inflammatory nodules, tissue hyperplasia, fibroplasia and rhinophyma.

Q12. What are the different phymas in rosacea?

Ans: Localized swellings of facial soft tissue develop over many years due to increase in connective tissue, sebaceous gland hyperplasia, ectatic veins and chronic deep inflammation. Most commonly involves the nose.

The following are the different types:

- Rhinophyma (nose)
- Gnathophyma (chin)
- Metophyma (forehead)
- Otophyma (ears)
- Blepharophyma (eyelids).

Q13. Systemic prednisolone can be used in the management of?

a. Erythematotelengiectatic rosacea
b. Rhinophyma
c. Granulomatous rosacea
d. Rosacea fulminans

Ans: d. Rosacea fulminans.

- *Synonym*: Pyoderma faciale, it presents as an acute facial eruption of coalescing nodules, pustules and draining sinuses with pronounced erythema and edema.
- Seborrhoea is a constant feature, significant associations have been reported with pregnancy and inflammatory bowel disease.
- Management includes systemic prednisolone 0.5–1 mg/kg/day initially which is rapidly effective and isotretinoin started concurrently 0.5–1 mg/kg/day over 6–12 months to maintain remission.
- Oral tetracycline, erythromycin, dapsone and azithromycin have also been used.
- Other measures include compresses, topical antibiotics, intralesional steroids and cryotherapy.

SECTION 7

Vascular Disorders

Ananta Khurana

CHAPTER 32

Vasculitis

Resham Vasani, Shreyaswini Pujary, Biju Vasudevan

Case study Vasculitis

Presenting Complaints

Doctor, I have red raised painful lesions on my legs since the past 1 week and they are progressively increasing.

Setting

Dermatology Outpatient Department.

History of Presenting Illness

A 30-year-old female presented with complaints of red raised lesions over the bilateral lower extremities associated with burning sensation since past 1 week. The red lesions were first noticed over the dorsa of both feet associated with fever that was low grade, intermittent and not associated with chills. The patient further developed progressive crops of lesions to involve the bilateral lower extremities, trunk and the upper extremities. There was associated swelling of the feet and pain at the ankle joints making it difficult to walk. The patient gave history of upper respiratory tract infection 5 days before the appearance of symptoms. There were no associated systemic comorbidities or any preceding drug intake. The past, personal and family history was unremarkable.

General Physical Examination

Well oriented to time, place and person.
BMI: 24 kg/m^2, Pulse: 90 BPM, BP: 130/90 mm of Hg.
No pallor, icterus, lymphadenopathy. Bilateral pitting pedal edema present.

Systemic Examination

No abnormality detected.

Dermatological Examination

Lesions are polymorphic in varying stages of evolution distributed on bilateral lower and upper extremities, lower back and buttocks. The lesions do not blanch on diascopy. There are discrete minimally elevated purpuric papules over the dorsa of feet and lower one third of legs (Figs 1A and B) and further extending to involve the thighs (Figs 1C and D). There are interspersed areas of residual hyperpigmentation (Fig. 2). The abdomen shows evidence of koebnerization of lesions along the sites of trauma (Fig. 3).

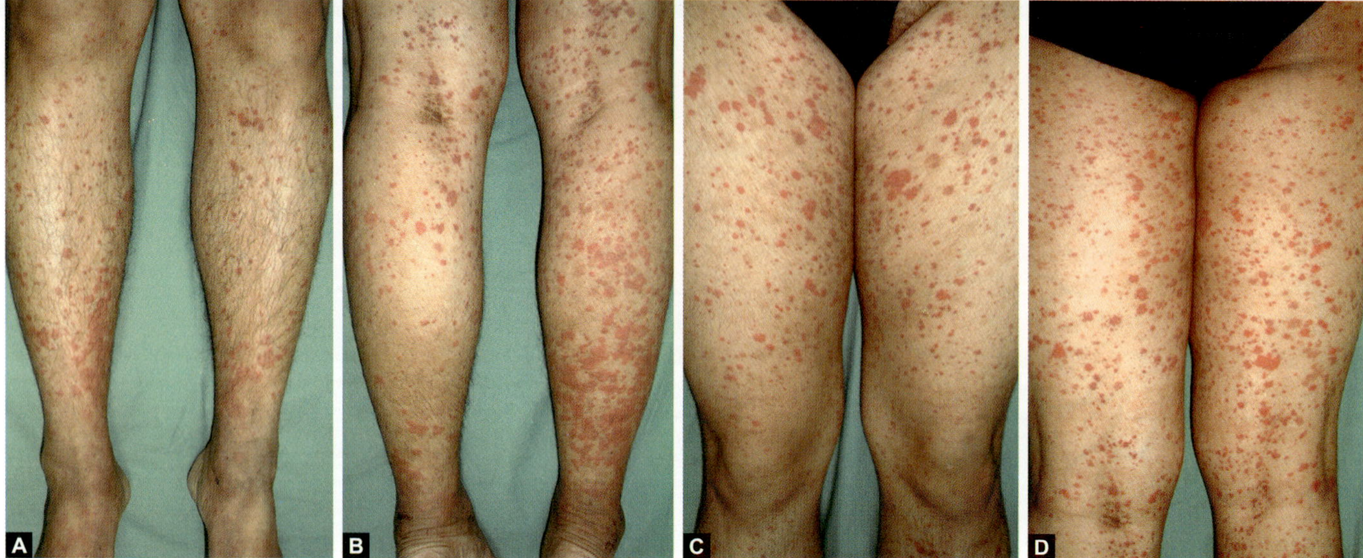

Figs 1A to D: A and B: Discrete purpuric papules over the dorsa of feet and lower one-third of legs; **C and D:** Purpuric papules further extending up to involve the thighs

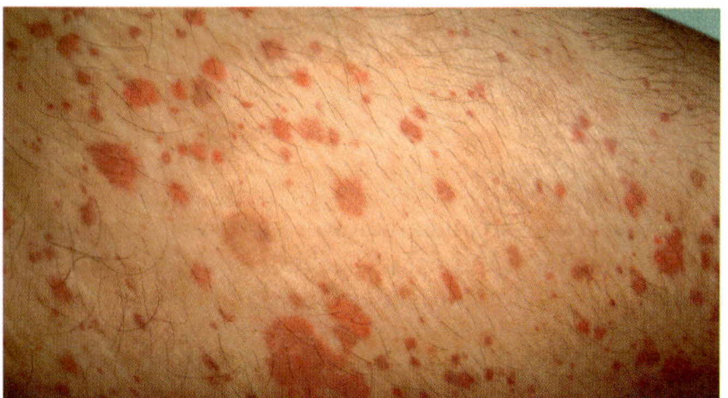

Fig. 2: Interspersed areas of residual hyperpigmentation

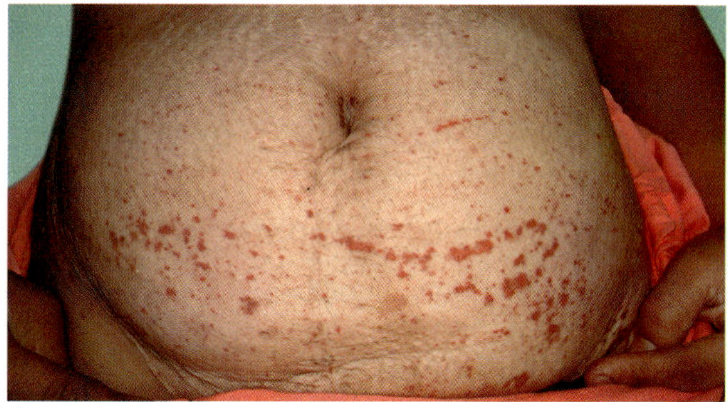

Fig. 3: Abdomen shows evidence of koebnerization of lesions along the sites of trauma

Q1. What is the most likely diagnosis?

a. Cutaneous small vessel vasculitis
b. Henoch-Schönlein purpura (HSP)
c. Urticarial vasculitis
d. Medium vessel vasculitis

Ans: a. Cutaneous small vessel vasculitis (CSVV). The failure to blanch on diascopy identifies purpura. Palpable purpura indicates vasculitis. Upper respiratory tract infection prior to lesions indicates an infectious case. So also, since the patient does not exhibit any other systemic symptoms, though subject to further investigations to rule out systemic involvement, the vasculitis seems limited to the skin and hence, the diagnosis. Cutaneous small vessel vasculitis is essentially a diagnosis of exclusion.

Q2. How can we clinically assess the size of vessels involved in vasculitis?

Ans: Clinical Assessment

- Small blood vessels: Purpuric macules (seen in this case), papules, hemorrhagic vesicles, urticarial plaques. Necrosis is not usually a major feature
- Medium size vessels: Broken livedo pattern, infarction, ulceration, deep nodules
- Large size vessels: Claudication and necrosis.

Q3. Why lower limbs are involved in small vessel vasculitis?

Ans: Increased pressure in venous circulation causes increased blood leakage and purpura. Prolonged standing exaggerates venous hypertension and increased blood leakage and purpura.

Q4. How will you evaluate this patient presenting with cutaneous small vessel vasculitis?

Ans: The aims behind investigating a patient of vasculitis are:

- To establish primary or secondary nature of vasculitis (to r/o rheumatological disease, malignancy, infection)
- Demonstrate presence of vasculitis in internal organs if present
- To confirm the clinical diagnosis in case of doubt.

In acute vasculitis with an obvious infection or a drug trigger, the investigations should be minimal. Hence in this case, where upper respiratory tract infection is an obvious trigger, the investigations can be limited to

- Full blood count: Raised white cells would suggest infection
- ESR: It may be raised in systemic vasculitis, infection and malignancy
- Urinalysis: Hematuria and proteinuria occur in renal involvement
- Urea and electrolytes: Raised creatinine and urea occur in renal involvement
- Liver function: Albumin is low in renal disease
- C-reactive protein: Raised in infections.

Depending on the clinical presentation, the battery of investigations can be extended in selected cases to include the screening tests for infection, malignancy and other systemic inflammatory disease wherever suspected from history and clinical examination (Table 1).

Table 1: Laboratory evaluation of suspected vasculitis

System	*Tests*
Blood	CBC, WBC, platelets, ESR, CRP
Renal	Urine, BUN: Serum creatinine
Liver	LFT, hepatitis B and C antibody, cryoglobulins
Immunologic	Complement, RA, ANA, Anti-dsDNA, ENA, ANCA
Infections	Blood culture; urine culture
Head and Neck	Sinus radiographs and CT
Lungs	Chest X-ray and CT
CVS	ECG, CPK, Echo
Neurologic	Nerve conduction studies
Muscle	EMG, enzymes

Skin biopsy should be done in all cases.

Q5. How does histopathology help in this condition?

Ans: In doubtful cases in order to rule out thromboembolic disorder as a cause of purpura, a tissue biopsy is helpful. Early biopsy is imperative between 18 hours and 48 hours of onset of lesions. In classical CSVV, the cells are predominantly polymorphonuclear leukocytes around and in the walls of the post capillary venules in the superficial dermis. There is associated leukocytoclasis (fragmentation of neutrophils) and fibrinoid deposition in and around the vessel walls, endothelial swelling and extravasation of erythrocytes.

Biopsy helps to define the type of vasculitis, based on vessel type and size, type of reaction (e.g. segmental arteritis in polyarteritis nodosa), infiltrating cells (e.g. prominently eosinophilic infiltrate in drug-induced vasculitides), extent of infiltrate (e.g. pan-dermal small vessel disease in a patient with fever suggests possible sepsis) and may define a specific vasculitis process [e.g. CSVV with vascular IgA deposit determined by direct immunofluorescence (DIF) in HSP].

Direct immunofluorescence is shown to be present throughout the evolution of lesion and, hence, is a useful adjunct in the late stages of the disease. DIF with IgM, C3, fibrin suggests rheumatoid factor associated disease. Strong C3 fluorescence favors Urticarial vasculitis. IgA fluorescence is typical of HSP. Lupus band is suggestive of SLE. Absence of immune reactants in a clinically diagnosed vasculitis is suggestive of ANCA- associated disease.

Q6. What are the pointers in the history or clinical examination you would look out for to suspect systemic involvement in vasculitis?

Ans: The following clues in the history of a patient with cutaneous small vessel vasculitis may point towards a systemic involvement

- Weight loss, fatigue, fever
- Arthralgia, myalgia, arthritis
- Dry eyes, dry mouth
- Red eye, eye pain, vision loss
- Nasal or sinus congestion
- Ear pain

- Oral/nasal ulcers
- Chest pain/dyspnea
- Abdominal pain, blood in feces
- Blackouts, weakness, fits, etc.

Q7. How do you classify vasculitis?

Ans: Vasculitis can be classified as either primary/secondary or incidental.

- Primary vasculitis is where the primary cause is unknown and inflammation is directed primarily at the vessels. It includes, idiopathic cutaneous leucocytoclastic vasculitis and systemic vasculitis such as Wegener's granulomatosis (WG), Churg-Strauss syndrome (CSS), microscopic polyangitis (MPA) and the cutaneous and systemic variants of polyarteritis nodosa (PAN)
- Secondary Vasculitis is an additional manifestation of a systemic multisystem disease as part of connective tissue disorders (CTD), infections, adverse drug reactions (ADRs) or malignancies
- Incidental vasculitis is a localized finding that is a consequence of another pathologic process like typically a necrotizing process such as a traumatic ulceration or diffuse neutrophilic infiltrates due to Sweet's syndrome or pyoderma gangrenosum.
- The most widely adopted classification system is Chapel Hill Consensus System which is based on pathological criteria (Box 1).

Box 1

Classification of cutaneous vasculitis adapted from the 2012 Chapel Hill Consensus nomenclature

1. Single-organ (skin) small vessel vasculitis
   - Cutaneous small vessel vasculitis
   - Urticarial vasculitis
   - Erythema elevatumdiutinum
   - Acute hemorrhagic edema of infancy
   - Recurrent cutaneous necrotizing eosinophilic vasculitis
   - Granuloma faciale
2. Cutaneous vasculitis associated with systemic disease or variable vessel size
   - Behcet syndrome
   - Lupus vasculitis
   - Sarcoid vasculitis
   - Rheumatoid vasculitis
3. Small-vessel immune complex associated vasculitis
   - IgA vasculitis (Henoch–Schonlein purpura)
   - Cryoglobulinemic vasculitis
   - Hypocomplementemic urticarial vasculitis
   - Antiglomerular basement membrane vasculitis (anti-GBM/Goodpasture syndrome)
4. Small-vessel ANCA associated vasculitis
   - Microscopic polyangitis
   - Granulomatosis with polyangiitis (Wegener's granulomatosis)
   - Eosinophilic granulomatosis with polyangiitis (Churg-Strauss syndrome)
5. Medium vessel vasculitis
   - Polyarteritis nodosa
   - Kawasaki disease
6. Large vessel vasculitis
   - Giant cell arteritis
   - Takayasu arteritis

Q8. What is the management of CSVV?

Ans: Since most of the cases of CSVV are self-limiting, a conservative approach is followed.

Specific Treatment:

- Identification of offending antigens and eliminating them by use of antibiotics and antivirals
- Withdrawal of offending drugs in cases of drug induced leukocytoclastic vasculitis
- Environmental chemicals need to be removed whenever implicated in causation
- Treatment of underlying connective tissue disease when found to be positive.

General Measures:

- Bed rest with frequent turning and elevation of lower limbs
- Avoid pressure and use loose clothing
- Avoid preservatives and coloring agents
- Diet rich in vitamin C.

For Symptomatic Relief

Supportive therapy: Use of compression hosiery and elevation of dependent areas, Antihistamines, nonsteroidal anti-inflammatory drugs to decrease the symptoms.

For Skin Lesions Alone

- Pentoxyphylline
- Colchicine
- Dapsone

For Ulcerative Skin Lesions Alone

- Thalidomide
- Low-dose weekly methotrexate
- Prednisolone (dosage of 30–80 mg once daily, tapered over 2–3 weeks).

For Systemic Disease

- Prednisolone
- Azathioprine
- Cyclophosphamide
- Mycophenolate mofetil
- Ciclosporin
- Interferon-α (if hepatitis C-associated)
- Intravenous gamma-globulin
- Extracorporeal immunomodulation

- Infliximab
- Rituximab
- Plasmapheresis.

Q9. What are the features of drug-induced vasculitis?

Ans: Cutaneous small vessel vasculitis is a common presentation of drug-induced vasculitis. Blood and tissue eosinophilia is a common in these cases. Systemic vasculitis can also be seen and renal involvement should be regularly monitored using renal parameters.

Q10. Enumerate the drugs causing vasculitis.

Ans: Penicillins, sulfonamides, quinolones, cephalosporins, minocycline, clindamycin, vancomycin, macrolides, rifampicin, isoniazid, imidazoles, griseofulvin, zidovudine, didanosine, efavirenz, antithyroid (propylthiouracil), analgesics (nonsteroidal anti-inflammatory drugs, COX inhibitors), thiazides, furosemide, anticonvulsants (hydantoins, carbamazepine), phenothiazines, allopurinol, hydralazine, quinidine, thiouracils and colony-stimulating factors.

Q11. Discuss the features of Henoch–Schonlein purpura.

- HSP is defined by the Chapel Hill Consensus Conference as a vasculitis affecting small vessels, involving deposition of IgA immune complexes that characteristically involves the skin, gastrointestinal system and glomeruli with or without arthralgia or arthritis.
- The most common triggering factor for HSP is infection with β-hemolytic streptococci, other pathogens have also been implicated including *Bartonella henselae*, parvovirus B19, *Staphylococcus aureus*, coxsackie viruses, adenovirus, hepatitis A and B viruses.
- The typical findings of HSP are purpura, arthralgia and abdominal pain. The lesions are typically distributed over the extensor aspects of the limbs (especially elbows and knees) and buttocks in a symmetrical fashion, and also seen over the trunk and face. Rarely, only systemic manifestation can occur in the absence of skin disease. Renal involvement with HSP is common, seen in 40–50% of patients; hematuria (gross or microscopic), proteinuria (60%). Gastrointestinal involvement is common (65%), with gastrointestinal bleeding and pain abdomen. Painful arthritis is seen in about 75% of patients, commonly affecting the knees and ankles.
- Management of HSP: HSP is mostly self-limiting and cases with systemic manifestation requires:
  - Systemic corticosteroids in a dose of 1 mg/kg body weight
  - Dapsone 100 mg /day—known to shorten the duration of the disease
  - Cyclophosphamide/cyclosporine/azathioprine can be used as a steroid sparing agents
  - Dipyridamole in patients with progressive renal involvement
  - Intravenous immunoglobulin (IVIG) has a role in halting rapidly progressive nephritis, gastrointestinal and cutaneous disease.

Q12. What are antineutrophil cytoplasm antibodies (ANCA) and which are the ANCA associated vasculitis?

Ans: Antineutrophil cytoplasm antibodies have diagnostic value as well as an important role in the pathogenesis of vasculitis.

ANCA are classified, based on their indirect immunofluorescence (IIF) pattern on ethanol-fixed neutrophils, as C-ANCA (granular cytoplasmic staining with accentuation between the nuclear lobes), P-ANCA (perinuclear and/or nuclear staining) and atypical ANCA (various patterns, including diffuse cytoplasmic and "very perinuclear"). Atypical ANCA are also termed X-ANCA, snowdrift-ANCA or more recently a-ANCA.

C-ANCA associated vasculitis are Wegener's granulomatosis (WG), microscopic polyangiitis (MPA), Churg–Strauss syndrome (CSS).

P-ANCA associated vasculitis are MPA, CSS, WG, ANCA-positive drug-induced systemic vasculitis. Seen in 50% cases of MPA and CSS.

C-ANCA has more specificity and is associated with disease severity (98% specificity in WG, 20% in CSS).

Q13. What is urticarial vasculitis?

Ans: Urticarial vasculitis (UV) is a chronic disease, which presents as urticarial lesions persisting for more than 24 hours and demonstrates purpura and postinflammatory pigmentation, with associated symptoms of burning.

Two types of UV have been described:

- UV associated with hypocomplementemia,
- UV without associated hypocomplementemia (normocomplementemic UV).

Patients with the hypocomplementemic UV have constitutional symptoms such as fever, malaise and myalgia and signs such as lymphadenopathy, hepatosplenomegaly, with associated symptoms like abdominal pain with or without nausea and/or diarrhea, laryngeal edema, dyspnea, chronic obstructive pulmonary disease (COPD), glomerulonephritis, conjunctivitis, uveitis and episcleritis.

Hypocomplementemic UV has features similar to SLE, but manifestations like ocular inflammation, angioedema and COPD distinguish UV from SLE.

Clinical pearls in diagnosis: Wheals lasting for more than 24 hours, associated pain and purpuric lesions.

Q14. What is the management of urticarial vasculitis?

Ans:
- Systemic corticosteroids
- Steroid sparing agents like dapsone (100-200 mg day), colchicine (0.6 mg twice to three times daily) and hydroxy chloroquine (200 mg once to twice daily).
- Mycophenolatemofetil (2 g once daily) as maintenance therapy.

Q15. A 7-month-old infant presents with annular purpuric lesions on the extremities with associated acral edema since 3 days following a bout of upper respiratory tract infection. He also had low grade fever, though was feeding well and was playful. Investigations revealed leukocytosis and marginally raised ESR. Urinalysis, Liver and kidney function tests were normal.

What is the most likely diagnosis in this case?

a. Sweet's syndrome
b. Acute hemorrhagic edema of infancy
c. Acute urticaria
d. Kawasaki disease

Ans: b. Acute hemorrhagic edema of infancy. It is characterized by a dramatic onset of fever, edema with rosette, annular, targetoid shaped purpura, primarily over the face, ears, extremities in a nontoxic infant. It is usually seen in males between 4 months and 24 months of age and follows upper respiratory and gastrointestinal infections, medications or vaccinations. Visceral involvement is rare. It shows spontaneous recovery within 1-3 weeks. Histopathology of this condition shows leukocytoclastic vasculitis (*see* Box 1).

CHAPTER 33

Livedoid Vasculopathy

Aseem Sharma, Biju Vasudevan

Case study Livedoid Vasculopathy

Presenting Complaints

Doctor, I have a 6-year history of developing ulcers over both legs that leave white scars on healing. Because of this, I also have leg and foot pain and am unable to walk for a long period of time. Presently, I am having fresh ulcers since 7 days.

Setting

Dermatology outpatient department

History of Present Illness

A 30-year-old male presented with complaints of multiple ulcers over both legs of 6 years' duration. The patient developed few ulcers on the left foot after prolonged wearing of boots for duration of 07 days (>18 hours/day). He progressively developed similar multiple ulcers over both lower legs and dorsum of feet over a duration of 2 weeks. They were associated with moderate intensity pain and would increase on walking or running and reduce with rest. The ulcers had a waxing and waning course and would generally heal with course of antibiotics and rest. There were no other associated complaints or history of any other risk factors. Presently, I am having fresh exacerbation of lesions since 7 days.

General Physical Examination

Well oriented to time, place and person.
Pulse: 74 BPM, Pedal pulses: Normal, BP: 128/76 mm Hg, No cyanosis or pedal edema, ankle brachial pressure index (ABPI): 0.9 Right, 1.0 Left (within normal range).

Systemic Examination

No abnormality detected.

Dermatological Examination

- Multiple well-defined, non-discharging reticulate ulcers
- Ulceration over both medial and lateral aspects (Fig. 1)
- Multiple atrophic porcelain stellate white scars over the lower limbs (Fig. 2).

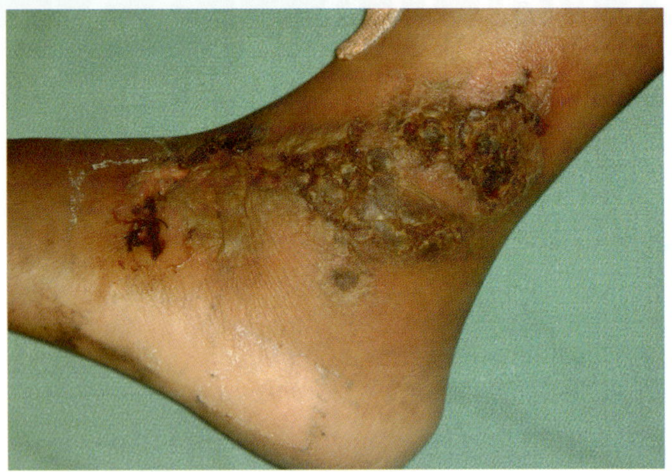

Fig. 1: Multiple reticulate ulcers on lower legs

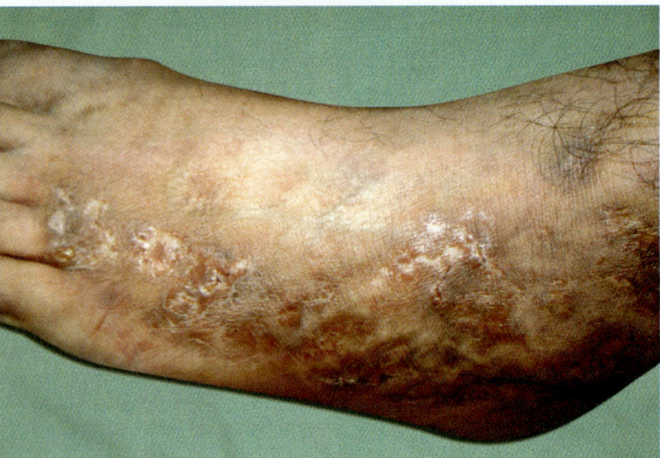

Fig. 2: Atrophic porcelain white scars on foot

Q1. What is the most likely diagnosis?

a. Peripheral vascular disease
b. Chronic venous insufficiency
c. Cutaneous vasculitis
d. Livedoid vasculopathy (LV)

Ans: d. Livedoid vasculopathy: Ulceration over both medial and lateral aspects, with normal pedal pulses, no delay and normal ABPI rules out arterial/venous causes. The ulcers healing with star-shaped atrophic scars, i.e. atrophie blanche (AB) clinches the diagnosis of LV over vasculitis.

Q2. What are the synonyms of LV?

Ans: Segmental hyalinizing vasculitis, livedo reticularis with summer ulcerations, capillaritis alba, and painful purpuric ulcers with reticular patterning on the lower extremities (PPURPLE).

Q3. How do you diagnose LV?

Ans: It is primarily a clinical diagnosis. Laboratory investigations are done to look for etiology and associations, and histopathology for confirmation. Some salient clinical pointers (with case-specific incidence in parenthesis) towards LV include:

- Female sex, 4–5th decade of life (70%)
- Bilateral lower extremity involvement (81%)
- Ulceration involving both medial and lateral aspects (68.9%)
- Atrophie blanche (71.1%)
- Ankle brachial pressure index normalcy (70%).

Q4. What are the biopsy finding characteristics of LV?

Ans: Ulceration stage: There is characteristic occlusion of the capillaries in the upper and middle dermis by fibrin, and thrombus formation can be demonstrated in the vessel walls. However, in comparison to primary vasculitis, there is hardly any perivascular inflammatory infiltrate. When present, infiltrate is predominantly lymphocytic. Extravasation of RBCs can be seen due to vessel destruction, and endothelial proliferation is also present. Neutrophilia or leukocytoclasia is usually absent, which argues against a primary vasculitis.

Atrophie blanche stage: Hyalinization of dermis and capillary walls are seen.

Immunofluorescence: DIF demonstrates deposition of immune complexes, fibrin, and complement in the vessel wall. C3, IgM, IgA, IgG and fibrin in descending order are the commonest components found in the deposits.

Q5. How is it histopathologically different from cutaneous vasculitides?

Ans: LV shows sparse inflammatory infiltrate with fibrin deposition in the vessel lumen with obliteration of the same, rendering it a vaso-occlusive phenomenon whereas vasculitis will show dense, multicellular inflammatory infiltrate with fibrinoid necrosis.

Q6. What specific laboratory investigations will yield an etiology?

Ans: Liver function tests, prothrombin time (PT), activated partial thromboplastin time (aPTT), international normalized ratio (INR)--*prothrombotic state*

Antinuclear antibody (ANA), extractable nuclear antigen profile, antiphospholipid antigen (APLA), lupus anticoagulant (LAC), cardiolipin antigen

(CLA), antineutrophil cytoplasmic antibody (p/c ANCA)--*autoimmunity*

Serum homocysteine, protein C and S estimation, prothrombin and antithrombin III gene test, methyl tetrahydrofolate reductase (MTHFR), factor V Leiden mutation--*procoagulant state.*

Q7. Does imaging have any role in LV?

Ans: Yes. Color Doppler of the arterial and venous systems of both lower limbs is important to rule out pure arterial or venous causes, along with ABPI.

Q8. Discuss the pathogenesis of LV?

Ans: Initially debated to be a form of vasculitis, the pathogenesis includes occlusion of the cutaneous capillary microcirculation leading to thrombosis, ischemia and infarction. The thrombotic effect could result from either defects in the endothelial cell plasminogen activation, platelet dysfunction or enhanced fibrin formation. Pericapillary deposition of fibrin and formation of thrombus act as diffusion barrier, impairing the oxygen supply to tissue causing ischemic infarction. The poorly perfused wound heals even poorly and is unable to induce killing of bacteria by leukocytes, thereby leading to infection. Thus, a vicious cycle of tissue destruction, edema and thrombosis occurs, further diminishing the tissue perfusion.

Q9. What are the systemic manifestations of LV?

Ans: Systemic involvement is not seen in primary LV. However, any associated condition, especially the autoimmune connective tissue disorders and other prothrombotic associations may involve many organ systems, in secondary LV.

Q10. What is the significance of ABPI in LV?

Ans: ABPI is calculated by dividing of systolic pressure of the lower limbs, viz. doralis pedis or tibial arteries by that of the upper limbs/brachial artery. The interpretation is as follows:

- <0.5 Severe arterial insufficiency
- 0.5–0.89 Moderate to mild arterial disease
- 0.9–1.2 Normal range
- >1.2 Calcification

Q11. What is the role of skin oxygen tension (TcPO2) measurement in LV?

Ans: Measuring partial pressure of oxygen by transcutaneous oximetry near site of ulcer can be used as a reliable marker of tissue ischemia and also to see effects of therapy.

Q12. What is the main principle in treating a case of LV?

a. Treatment and prevention of ulceration and scarring
b. Treatment of the underlying cause (if any)
c. Alleviating pain
d. All of the above

Ans: d. All of the above

Q13. Outline the treatment modalities in LV?

Ans: Supportive therapy:

- Counseling
- Avoid temperature extremes
- Avoid smoking, caffeine, emotional and physical stress
- Physical therapy: Compression (etiology-specific)
- Topical therapy: Frequent cleansing and application of emollient, antibiotics, anti-inflammatory agents for leg ulcers

Antiplatelets:

- Aspirin, Dipyridamole, Pentoxiphylline, Buflomedil, Sarpogrelate hydrochloride

Anticoagulants:

- Heparin and newer analogues: Dalteparin-Nadroparin, Rivaroxaban, Fluindione

Fibrinolytics:

- Tissue plasminogen activator (tPA), Stanozolol, Danazol

Immunosuppressants:

- Oral, topical corticosteroids: Short- to long-acting, low- to ultra-potent, azathioprine, colchicine, cyclosporine-A

Anti-inflammatory agents:

- Dapsone, sulfasalazine, hydoxychloroquine

Vasodilators:

- Nifedipine, Cilostazol, Nicotinic acid, Alprostadil (PGE-1), Ketanserin

Nutritional supplements (Nutraceuticals):

- Vitamins B_6 (Pyridoxine), B_9 (Folic Acid), B_{12} (Cynacobalamin) especially for hyperhomocysteinemia

Miscellaneous:

- Intravenous immunoglobulin (IVIg)
- Hyperbaric oxygen therapy (HBOT)

Q14. How does HBOT help in LV?

Ans: HBOT delivers 100% oxygen at high pressures (02–03 ATA) wherein oxygen dissolves 20 times more in plasma, creating a high oxygen gradient across wound site, thus negating tissue ischemic effects by nitric oxide synthesis and increases microvascular hyperperfusion. It also promotes angiogenesis, neovascularization, inhibits collagen formation and bacterial overgrowth, thus promoting healing and preventing recurrences.

Q15. What are the differential diagnoses of LV?

Ans: Livedoid mimickers include:

- Peripheral vascular disease
- Vasculitis, especially polyarteritis nodosa
- Stasis dermatitis
- Systemic lupus erythematosus
- Scleroderma
- Sneddon's disease
- Cryoglobulinemia
- Dego's disease
- Pyoderma gangrenosum
- Rheumatoid arthritis.

CHAPTER 34

Behcet's Disease

Aditi Bhagat, Biju Vasudevan

Case study Behcet's Disease

Presenting Complaints

Doctor, I am getting recurrent ulcers in my mouth since the last 3 years and have recently developed 2 painful ulcers on my genital region since the last 10 days. I also have difficulty in walking due to pain and swelling in my right knee and left ankle since the last 1 month.

Setting

Dermatology outpatient department.

History of Present Illness

A 33-year-old married male, a lawyer by profession was apparently alright 3 years back when he started developing recurrent episodes of painful ulcers in the oral cavity, which lasted for 1–2 weeks, limiting the oral intake and healed without any scarring or discoloration. He had multiple such episodes over the last 3 years with an average of 4–5 episodes per year. He also developed a slow onset pain and swelling in the right knee joint, causing him difficulty in walking. Two weeks later, he developed pain in the left ankle as well. The patient developed two small painful ulcers on his scrotum 10 days back. There was no history of any swelling in the groin, fever, burning micturition or urethral discharge.

General Physical Examination and Systemic Examination

No abnormality detected.

Dermatological Examination

- Multiple, papulovesiculopustular, non-follicular lesions, ranging in size from 2 mm to 4 mm were present over the forearms.
- Oral mucosa: Multiple well-defined small ulcers surrounded by an erythematous border and yellowish floor present on the labial mucosa and dorsal aspect of the tongue (Fig. 1).
- Genital mucosa: Two well-defined tender ulcers with yellowish center, surrounded by a red halo present over the scrotum (Fig. 2). They are not associated with bleeding or purulent discharge.
- Musculoskeletal examination revealed swelling and tenderness over the right knee and left ankle joint. Range of motion could not be assessed due to extreme pain in the involved joints.

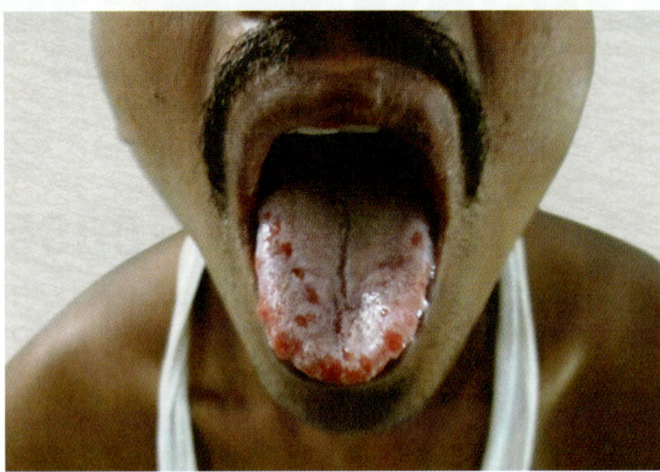

Fig. 1: Multiple oral ulcers

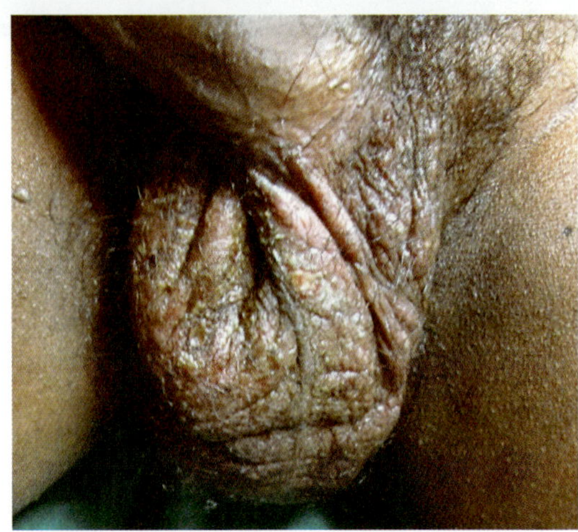

Fig. 2: Scrotal ulcers

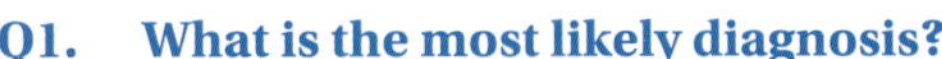

Q1. What is the most likely diagnosis?

a. Behcet's disease
b. Systemic lupus erythematosus
c. PFAPA syndrome
d. Mucous membrane pemphigoid

Ans: a. Behcet's disease: Presence of recurrent oral aphthae of more than three episodes per year which are tender, non-scarring along with tender genital ulcerations on the scrotum, migratory non-deforming oligoarthritis and papulopustular skin lesions in a young male suggests diagnosis of Behcet's or Adamantiades Behcet disease.

Q2. How do you diagnose Behcet's disease?

Ans: There are several diagnostic criteria developed for Behcet's disease. The most commonly used ones are the International Study Group Criteria (ISG) and International Criteria for Behcet's Disease (ICBD). The International Criteria for Behcet's Disease (ICBD) revised in 2010 was found to be more sensitive and specific than the International Study Group Criteria (ISG).

Sign/symptom	*Score*
Oral aphthosis	2
Genital aphthosis	2
Ocular manifestations	2
Skin manifestations	1
Vascular manifestations	1
Central nervous system manifestations	1
Positive pathergy test	1

A patient scoring greater than or equal to 4 points is classified as having BD. Pathergy testing is optional and the primary scoring system does not include pathergy testing. However, where pathergy testing is conducted, one extra point may be assigned for a positive result.

Q3. What is pathergy test?

Ans: Pathergy phenomenon is defined as a state of altered tissue reactivity that occurs in response to minor trauma. Pathergy test (PT) is an easy to perform skin test to look for the pathergy phenomenon. It is performed on the flexor forearm by obliquely inserting a 20- to 22-gauge sterile hypodermic needle to a depth of 5 mm ± an intradermal injection of 0.1 mL of normal saline. A positive reaction is defined as the development of a papule or pustule at the site as observed by the physician at 24–48 hours.

Q4. Which of the following diseases can be diagnosed by pathergy test?

a. Behcet's disease
b. Sweet's syndrome
c. Pyoderma gangrenosum
d. All of the above

Ans: d. All of the above. Other than the above diseases, Pathergy test is also positive in interferon alpha-treated chronic myeloid leukemia patients, inflammatory bowel disease rarely spondyloarthropathies and around 3% normal individuals.

Q5. How will you confirm the diagnosis?

Ans: Diagnosis is made on clinical grounds with the help of the diagnostic criteria. There are no confirmatory laboratory tests to diagnose Behcet's disease.

Q6. What are the various systems involved in Behcet's disease?

Ans: Behcet's disease is a multisystem disorder with vascular, gastrointestinal, neurological, psychiatric, pulmonary, cardiac and renal manifestations. However, other than mucocutaneous involvement, skeletal and ocular systems are the ones that are most commonly affected.

- **Ocular:** Panuveitis, retinal vasculitis, glaucoma, neurovascular lesions, tractional retinal detachment, cystoid macular edema, frosted branch angiitis, conjunctival erosions and ulcerations, and optic nerve atrophy.
- **Joint manifestations:** Characteristic: Asymmetric, sterile, non-erosive, seronegative, oligoarthritis. Most common: Symmetric polyarthritis.
- **Vascular involvement:** Vasculitis, venous thrombosis: Deep veins of the leg, vena cava, hepatic veins (Budd-Chiari syndrome) and cerebral venous sinuses. Arterial involvement: aneurysms, stenosis and thrombosis. Aneurysms: common in abdominal aorta, pulmonary artery and peripheral arteries.
- **Neurological involvement:** Meningoencephalitis, cerebral venous sinus thrombosis, cranial nerve palsies, benign intracranial hypertension, brainstem lesions, pyramidal and extrapyramidal lesions.
- **Gastrointestinal involvement:** Mucosal aphthae, perforation, peritonitis.
- **Cardiac manifestations:** Myocarditis, endocarditis, coronary arteritis, valvular disease.
- **Renal manifestations:** Minimal change disease, proliferative glomerulonephritis, rapidly progressive crescentic glomerulonephritis, amyloidosis.
- **Pulmonary:** Pulmonary vasculitis, pulmonary artery aneurysms.

Q7. What are the differential diagnoses of Behcet's disease?

Ans: Differential diagnosis:

- Oculocutaneous/mucocutaneous syndromes: Erythema multiforme, Stevens-Johnson syndrome, Reiter disease, bullous autoimmune diseases: pemphigus vulgaris, cicatricial mucous membrane pemphigoid, epidermolysis bullosa aquisita, viral infections (herpes, coxsackie, echovirus), syphilis.
- Articulo-mucocutaneous syndromes: SLE, magic syndrome (mouth and genital ulcers with inflamed cartilage), yersiniosis, psoriatic arthropathy.
- Gastrointestinal/mucocutaneous syndromes: Ulcerative colitis, Crohn's disease, tuberculosis, bowel-associated dermatitis: arthritis syndrome.
- Aphthae: Recurrent aphthous stomatitis, cyclic neutropenia, herpes simplex infection.
- Genital ulcers: Herpes genitalis, Lipshutz ulcer.
- Arthritis: Ankylosing spondylitis, juvenile rheumatoid arthritis.
- CNS manifestation: Multiple sclerosis, Neuro-Sweet disease.
- Lung manifestation: Sarcoidosis.

Q8. What are the various mucocutaneous manifestations of Behcet's disease?

Ans: Mucocutaneous manifestations:

- Oral ulcers
- Genital ulcers
- Acneform lesions
- Follicular pustules
- Erythema nodosum like lesions
- Erythema multiforme like lesions
- Sweet's syndrome like lesions.

Q9. What is the treatment of Behcet's disease?

Ans: Treatment depends on whether there is mucocutaneous or systemic involvement. It can be divided into general measures, topical and systemic agents.

General measures:

Bland diet, avoidance of spicy, salty, hard and irritating foodstuff like toast, lemon, tomatoes, spices: chillies, pepper, etc., alcohol, CO_2 holding drinks, toothpaste containing sodium laurel sulfate. Smoking should be avoided as some studies have been found with association between smoking and induction of aphthous ulcers.

Topical agents:

- Caustic solutions like silver nitrate, methyl violet 0.5% (1–2 times/day)
- Antiseptic and anti-inflammatory preparations: 0.1% triclosan mouth washes and in toothpaste, 1–2% chlorhexidine mouth wash, tetracycline mouth wash: 250 mg/5 mL glycerine solution (4–6 times/day)
- Corticosteroids: Triamcinolone mucosal ointment, dexamethasone mucosal paste (4 times day or overnight application), intralesional triamcinolone infiltration 0.1–0.5 mL
- Anesthetics: 2–5% lignocaine, 0.5–1% tetracaine gel or mucosal ointment (2–3 times/day).
- 500 mg of cyclosporine A solution (3 times/day)
- 5 mL of sucralfate suspension (4 times/day)

Systemic agents:

- Methylprednisolone: 1 g/day × 5 days pulsed
- Azathioprine: 2.5 mg/kg/day orally

- Cyclosporine: 10 mg/kg/day
- Mtx (especially in patients with joint pains)
- Infliximab, Etanercept

For oral ulcers and cutaneous lesions:

- Rebamipide: 300 mg/day orally
- Colchicine: 1–2 mg/day orally
- Dapsone: 100 mg/day orally
- Thalidomide: 100 mg/day orally.

Q10. What are the general principles of management of Behcet's disease?

Ans: EULAR recommendations for the management of mucocutaneous lesions:

- The decision to treat skin and mucosa involvement will depend on the perceived severity by the doctor and the patient. Mucocutaneous involvement should be treated according to the dominant or codominant lesions present.
- Topical measures (i.e. local corticosteroids) should be the first line of treatment for isolated oral and genital ulcers.
- Acne-like lesions are usually of cosmetic concern only. Thus, topical measures as used in acne vulgaris are sufficient.
- Colchicine should be preferred when the dominant lesion is erythema nodosum.
- Leg ulcers in BD might have different causes. Treatment should be planned accordingly.
- Azathioprine, IFN-α and TNF-α antagonists may be considered in resistant cases.

CHAPTER 35

Sweet Syndrome

Disha Dabbas

Case study Sweet Syndrome

Presenting Complaint

Doctor, I have developed painful red bumps on my face, arms and back since last 3 days.

Setting

Dermatology outpatient department.

History of Present Illness

A 45-year-old lady presented with complaints of fever and red raised painful lesions over her face, back and arms of 3 days' duration. She is a known case of acute myeloid leukemia and had taken chemotherapy for the same. Presently, she was not on many medications since last 2 years. Fever is high grade and associated with myalgia and arthralgia. No history of oral or ocular mucosal involvement.

General Physical Examination

Well oriented in time, place and person.
Patient is ill-looking.
Pulse: 104 BPM, Temp: 101^0 F.
Pallor: Present.

Systemic Examination

No abnormality detected.

Dermatological Examination

Tender, erythematous papulonodular lesions distributed asymmetrically over face, upper limbs and upper back (Figs 1 and 2). The lesions appear to have vesiculation but are solid on palpation.

Q1. What is the most likely diagnosis?

a. Leukemia cutis
b. Sweet syndrome
c. Cellulitis
d. Drug eruption

Ans: b. Sweet syndrome. Presence of fever, acute onset tender erythematous papulonodular lesions with appearance of pseudovesiculation and history of hematological malignancy points toward the diagnosis of malignancy-associated Sweet syndrome.

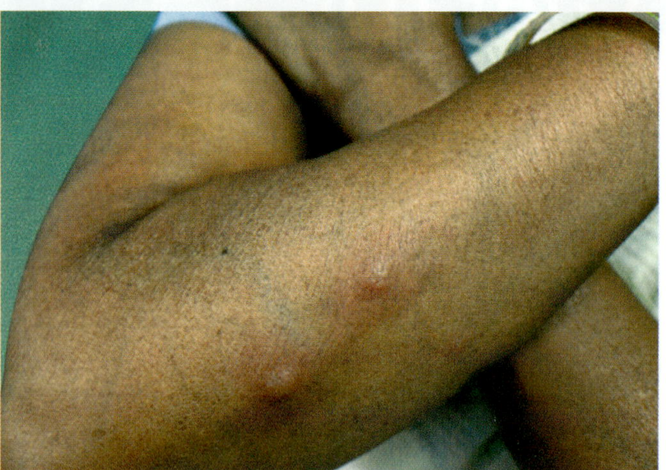

Fig. 1: Multiple erythematous papulonodular lesions on the forearm

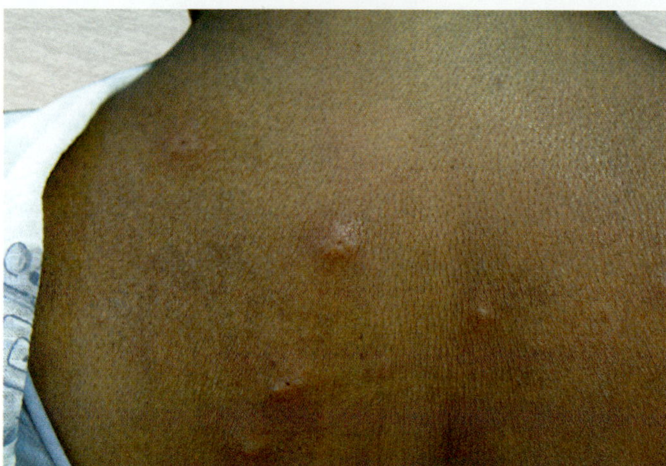

Fig. 2: Multiple erythematous papulonodular lesions on upper back giving a pseudovesicular appearance

Leukemia cutis (usually asymptomatic or with very little pain) would be a probable differential diagnosis and the patient would require a skin biopsy to confirm the same. Absence of a recent history of drug intake precludes the diagnosis of drug eruption or drug-induced Sweet syndrome.

Multiple lesions make cellulitis less likely. Though the histopathological similarity between Sweet syndrome and cellulitis necessitates that infection be ruled out by submitting the sample to bacterial, fungal and mycobacterial culture.

Q2. Sweet syndrome usually occurs in which clinical settings?

Ans: Sweet syndrome occurs in three clinical settings:

a. Classic or idiopathic Sweet syndrome: This is associated with infection (upper respiratory tract or gastrointestinal tract), pregnancy or inflammatory bowel disease. It most commonly occurs in women between 30 and 60 years of age.

b. Malignancy-associated Sweet syndrome occurs in patients with underlying hematologic or solid organ malignancies. The onset or recurrence of Sweet syndrome is associated with discovery or relapse of cancer. There is no female preponderance in these cases. Commonest associated malignancy is acute myelogenous leukemia.

c. Drug-induced Sweet syndrome occurs after initiation of medications, most commonly granulocyte-macrophage colony-stimulating factor (GM-CSF).

Q3. How do you diagnose Sweet syndrome?

Ans: Diagnostic criteria for diagnosis of classic and malignancy-associated Sweet syndrome:

Major:

- Abrupt onset of painful erythematous plaques or nodules
- Histopathologic evidence of dense neutrophilic infiltrate without leukocytoclastic vasculitis.

Minor:

- Fever (>38^{0}C)
- Association with underlying malignancy, inflammatory bowel disease, pregnancy or preceded by upper respiratory infection, gastrointestinal infection or vaccination
- Abnormal lab values (three out of four): ESR (>20 mm/hour), positive CRP, leukocytosis (8,000/mm^3), >70% neutrophils
- Excellent response to treatment with systemic steroid or potassium iodide.

Presence of both major criteria and two of the four minor criteria is required to establish diagnosis.

Drug-induced Sweet syndrome:

- Abrupt onset of painful erythematous plaques or nodules
- Histopathologic evidence of dense neutrophilic infiltrate without leukocytoclastic vasculitis
- Fever (>38^0 C)
- Temporal relationship between drug ingestion and clinical presentation
- Temporally related resolution of lesions after drug withdrawal or treatment with corticosteroids

All five criteria are required for diagnosis of drug-induced Sweet syndrome.

Q4. How will you confirm the diagnosis?

Ans: Diagnosis is based on clinical findings, laboratory parameters and histopathology. Histopathology of skin should be accompanied by bacterial, fungal and mycobacterial stain and culture. Histopathology of lesional tissue reveals diffuse infiltrate of mature neutrophils (so called as acute febrile neutrophilic dermatoses) and edema in papillary and reticular dermis. Leukocytoclastic vasculitis is absent.

Q5. What are the cutaneous manifestations of Sweet syndrome?

Ans: Typical skin lesions are tender, erythematous papules and nodules with appearance of pseudovesiculation. Lesions can merge to form plaques, appear bullous, ulcerative or pustular. Lesions are usually distributed asymmetrically. They resolve spontaneously or after treatment without scarring. Recurrent episodes may occur in one-third to two-third patients. Most common sites of involvement are upper extremities and head and neck region. Pathergy (cutaneous lesions at the site of trauma) can be present.

Q6. What are the various systems involved in Sweet syndrome?

Ans:

System	*Features*
Central nervous system	Acute benign encephalitis, aseptic meningitis, Guillain-Barre syndrome, Neuro-Sweet disease, psychiatric symptoms
Ears	Tender red nodules and pustules in external auditory canal
Eyes	Blepharitis, conjunctivitis, dacryoadenitis, episcleritis, iridocyclitis, peripheral ulcerative keratitis, retinal vasculitis, scleritis
Bone	Acute sterile arthritis, arthralgia, osteomyelitis
Kidneys	Glomerulonephritis, hematuria, proteinuria
Gastrointestinal	Aphthous ulcer, necrotizing ulcerative periodontitis, pancolitis, transaminase elevation
Other	Pleural effusion, aortitis, aortic stenosis, cardiomegaly, heart failure

Q7. What are the drugs associated with Sweet syndrome?

Ans: G-CSF or (GM-CSF) is the commonest agent implicated in causation of Sweet syndrome. Apart from this, other drugs like trimethoprim-sulfamethoxazole, all- *trans* retinoic acid (used in promyelocytic leukemia and the drug ATRA convert leukemic myelocytic cells to mature neutrophils), minocycline, carbamazepine, oral contraceptives, etc. have also been associated.

Q8. What are the malignancies associated with Sweet syndrome?

Ans: Hematologic malignancies: Acute myeloid leukemia (commonest), chronic myeloid leukemia, Hodgkin disease, cutaneous T-cell lymphoma, non-Hodgkin lymphoma.

Non-hematologic malignancies: Carcinoma of genitourinary tract, breast and gastrointestinal tract.

Q9. What is the differential diagnosis of Sweet syndrome?

Ans: *Clinical differential diagnosis:* Drug eruptions, cellulitis, erythema nodosum, leukemia cutis, leukocytoclastic vasculitis, pyoderma gangrenosum, panniculitis, erythema nodosum leprosum (ENL, mainly in Indian scenario), neutrophilic ecrine hidradenitis, subacute lupus erythematosus, granuloma faciale.

Histopathological differential diagnosis: This includes conditions microscopically characterized by neutrophilic infiltration like cellulitis, leukemia cutis, leukocytoclastic vasculitis, pyoderma gangrenosum, granuloma faciale, erythema elevatum diutinum.

Q10. What is the therapeutic mainstay for Sweet syndrome?

a. Cyclosporine
b. Dapsone
c. Systemic steroids
d. Colchicine

Ans: c. Systemic steroids: Prednisolone 1 mg/kg/day, taper over 3–6 weeks or methylprednisolone pulse--1,000 mg/day for 3–5 days.

Identification of underlying disease or drug intake is first step in management of Sweet syndrome. Underlying malignancy requires concurrent treatment alongwith treatment of Sweet syndrome. Ruling out any infectious cause is must before starting treatment, as many infectious diseases can mimic Sweet syndrome, especially erythema nodosum leprosum.

Other first-line therapy includes:

- Potassium iodide: Saturated solution of potassium iodide (1 drop: 50 mg): Start at 3 drops three times a day, increasing by 1 drop three times a day to final dose of 21–30 drops/day
- Colchicine: 0.5 mg three times a day.

Second-line therapies in patients non-responsive or having suboptimal response to first line are:

- Indomethacin: 150 mg once a day
- Cyclosporine: 2–4 mg/kg/day
- Others like clofazimine and dapsone can also be used.

Q11. What are the recent advances in the treatment of Sweet syndrome?

Ans: The future treatment modality may include repertaxin, which inhibits chemokine receptors CXCR1 and CXCR2, thereby inhibiting responses of IL-8 (CXCL8), which is a major activator of neutrophils; other avenues of exploration include development of further inhibitors of IL-8 activated neutrophil chemotaxis, such as thapsigargin. Such approaches may be particularly valuable in those with systemic neutrophilic dermatoses.

Q12. What are the other neutrophilic dermatoses?

Ans: Other neutrophilic disorders include:

- Pyoderma gangrenosum
- Behcet's disease
- Bowel-associated dermatosis arthritis syndrome
- Neutrophilic ecrine hidradenitis
- Neutrophilic dermatosis of dorsal hand.

CHAPTER 36

Leg Ulcer

Neetu Bhari, Sanjay Singh

Case study Leg Ulcer

Presenting Complaints

Doctor, for the past 4 years, I have had a feeling of heaviness along with a dull aching pain in my legs accompanied by occasional swelling that subsides in the morning. There are many itchy, discolored lesions on the legs and last month, I developed a single, mildly painful ulcer over my lower leg.

Setting

Dermatology outpatient department.

History of Present Illness

A 47-year-old woman presented with complaints that for the last 4 years, she has experienced persistent dull aching pain associated with mild swelling, which worsens as the day progresses, in the lower extremities. She has also noticed gradually progressive, mildly itchy, nonhomogenous, brownish discoloration of the skin over the legs. For the past 3½ years, she has noticed progressively increasing multiple asymptomatic tortuous vessels, which become more prominent after prolonged standing or other exertional activities. One month ago, she developed a single, mildly painful ulcer over the right leg. She entered menopause at 45 years of age and has been on hormone replacement therapy (HRT) for the last 2 years. The patient is a school teacher by occupation. Her medical history indicates that she developed tender diffuse swelling in the right calf region during her last pregnancy, which resolved with anticoagulant therapy. There is no history of chronic smoking or alcoholism.

General Physical Examination and Systemic Examination

No abnormality detected.

Dermatological Examination

- Multiple dilated tortuous veins, which engorge on standing
- Hyperpigmentation over lower legs with excoriation marks and eczematous changes at places, more prominent around the ankles
- Single, well-defined, irregular-shaped, 6 × 4 cm shallow ulcer with slight purulent slough at the floor with a sloping margin over lateral aspect of the right leg (Fig. 1)
- Peripheral pulses: Palpable, normal volume and synchronous
- No sensory loss or motor weakness.

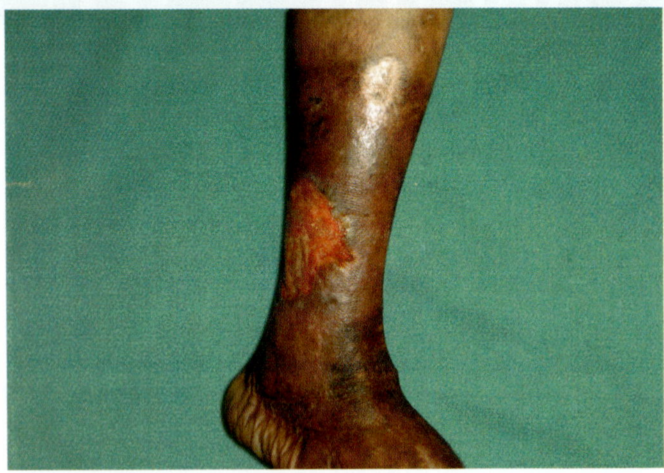

Fig. 1: Single, well-defined, irregular-shaped, shallow ulcer with purulent slough at the floor with a sloping margin over the right lower leg with surrounding hyperpigmentation

Q1. What is the most likely diagnosis?

a. Thromboangiitis obliterans
b. Medium-vessel vasculitis
c. Venous ulcer with stasis dermatitis
d. Diabetic neuropathy with trophic ulcers

Ans: c. Venous ulcer with stasis dermatitis. The presence of multiple tortuous veins, eczematous changes, brownish hyperpigmentation, shallow ulcer in gaiter area with normal peripheral pulses and no sensory and motor loss suggest the diagnosis of venous ulcer with stasis dermatitis.

Q2. How do you diagnose venous ulcer?

Ans: Diagnosis is based on the classical clinical presentation of venous ulcer and supporting examination findings. In general, the venous ulcer is an irregularly-shaped wound, initially superficial but with the potential to deepen, with well-defined borders. The surrounding skin is erythematous or hyperpigmented with variable degrees of induration (acute or chronic lipodermatosclerosis). Yellowish exudate is usually observed. The size and site of ulcers vary, but they usually occur in the distal portion of the lower limbs. Varicose veins and ankle edema are common. A venous ulcer is often not very painful. When the patients have severe pain, one should consider the possibility of other causes of ulceration such as arterial disease.

Q3. How will you confirm the diagnosis?

Ans: Diagnosis is mainly made on clinical grounds. Duplex ultrasonography, magnetic resonance venography and venous plethysmography may be needed to assess the extent and severity of the disease.

Many patients with venous insufficiency have clinically unrecognized chronic recurrent varicose thrombosis due to stasis. Such patients may have elevated levels of D-dimer.

Ulcers with elevated and everted borders, with excessive production of exudate and necrotizing tissue and those that fail to heal should alert the clinician to consider a malignant change. These ulcers should be subjected to histopathological evaluation.

Q4. What are the risk factors for developing venous disease?

Ans: Following are the risk factors for developing venous disease:

- Advanced age
- Female sex
- Family history of leg ulcers
- Obesity
- History of deep venous thrombosis or phlebitis
- Previous serious traumatic leg injury
- Chronic lower extremity edema
- Sedentary lifestyle
- Occupation requiring prolonged long periods of standing
- Oral contraceptive and HRT.

Q5. What is the spectrum of skin manifestations in patients with venous disease?

Ans: The spectrum of skin manifestations in patients with venous disease is listed below:

- Localized edema over bilateral lower legs and feet
- Hemosiderin staining
- Venous eczema
- Venous ulcer
- Corona phlebectatica paraplantaris (starburst of veins radiating distally from the medial malleolus)
- Lipodermatosclerosis (acute and chronic)
- Atrophie blanche.

Q6. What are the complications of chronic venous disease?

Ans: Complications of chronic venous disease are:

- Contact dermatitis
- Ankle joint stiffness
- Fixed plantar flexion
- Periostitis and osteomyelitis
- Malignancy.

Q7. What are the differential diagnoses of a venous leg ulcer?

Ans: Differential diagnoses of venous leg ulcers are:

Common causes:

- Peripheral arterial disease (arteriosclerosis)
- Neuropathy
- Decubitus (pressure)
- Vasculitis (small-vessel leukocytoclastic vasculitis)
- Connective tissue diseases (scleroderma, etc.).

Rare causes:

- Ulcus hypertensivum (Martorell ulcer)
- Infection (mostly *Streptococcus haemolyticus*)
- Clotting disorders
- Hematological disorders (sickle cell anemia, thalassemia, glucose-6-phosphate dehydrogenase deficiency)
- Antiphospholipid syndrome
- Malignancies
- Pyoderma gangrenosum
- Drugs (Hydroxyurea, steroid injection, pentazocine injection).

Q8. Which of the following treatment option for venous disease with ulcer has the highest level of evidence?

a. Compression therapy
b. Leg elevation
c. Aspirin
d. Debridement.

Ans: a. Compression therapy. Compression therapy is the standard of care for venous ulcers and chronic venous insufficiency. Methods include inelastic, elastic, and intermittent pneumatic compression. Compression therapy reduces edema, improves venous reflux, enhances healing of ulcers, and reduces pain. Success rates range from 30% to 60% at 24 weeks, and 70% to 85% after 1 year. After an ulcer has healed, lifelong maintenance of compression therapy may reduce the risk of recurrence. Compression stockings are graded, with the greatest pressure at the ankle and gradually decreasing pressure toward the knee and thigh (pressure should be at least 20–30 mm Hg, preferably 30–44 mm Hg). Compression stockings are removed at night, and should be replaced every 6 months because they lose pressure with regular washing.

Inelastic compression therapy provides high working pressure during ambulation and muscle contraction, but no resting pressure. The most common method of inelastic compression therapy is the Unna boot, a zinc oxide-impregnated, moist bandage that hardens after application.

Unlike the Unna boot, elastic compression therapy methods conform to changes in leg size and sustain compression during both rest and activity.

Q9. What are the other treatment modalities?

Ans: *Leg elevation:* Leg elevation, used in combination with compression therapy, is also considered the standard of care. Leg elevation requires raising lower extremities above the level of the heart, with the aim of reducing edema, improving microcirculation and oxygen delivery, and hastening ulcer healing.

Pentoxifylline: Pentoxifylline (400 mg three times per day) has been shown to be an effective adjunctive treatment for venous ulcers, when added to compression therapy.

Aspirin: Like pentoxifylline therapy, aspirin (300 mg per day) combined with compression therapy, has been shown to improve the ulcer healing time and reduce the ulcer size, compared with compression therapy alone.

Iloprost: Intravenous iloprost, when used with elastic compression therapy, significantly reduces the healing time of venous ulcers.

Skin grafting: Human skin grafting has been used to treat large or refractory venous ulcers.

Q10. What are the other common causes of leg ulcer and how to differentiate from venous ulcers?

Ans: Venous ulcers account for 80% of lower extremity ulcerations. Other common causes of lower extremity ulcers are arterial, neuropathic and pressure ulcers (Table 1).

Q11. What is the characteristic presentation of pyoderma gangrenosum?

Ans: The most common clinical presentation of pyoderma gangrenosum (PG) is an inflammatory papule or pustule that rapidly progresses to a painful ulcer with a violaceous undermined border and a purulent base (Fig. 4). PG may also present with bullous, vegetative, peristomal, and extracutaneous lesions. With the exception of vegetative PG, lesion development is often very rapid and the level of pain is often greater than expected based on the appearance of the ulcer. Vegetative PG begins as a single papule, nodule, or plaque that slowly evolves into a granulomatous or vegetative lesion, which is minimally painful.

Q12. What are the various subtypes of pyoderma gangrenosum?

Ans: The clinical manifestations of PG are variable, and can be divided into four major subtypes: ulcerative (classic) PG (the most common variant), bullous (atypical) PG, pustular PG, and vegetative PG.

Q13. Pathergy test is helpful in the diagnosis of which of the following disorder?

a. Pyoderma gangrenosum

Table 1: Summary of common causes of leg ulcers

Ulcer type	*General characteristics*	*Clinical features*	*Treatment*
Venous	Most common type (80%); women (obese) affected more than men; often occurs in older persons. H/o prolonged standing, worsening of symptoms as day passes.	Shallow, irregular, painful ulcer located over bony prominences, particularly the gaiter area; granulation tissue and fibrin present. Associated findings include edema, venous dermatitis, varicosities, atrophie blanche and lipodermatosclerosis.	Leg elevation, compression therapy, aspirin, pentoxifylline, surgical management
Arterial	Associated with cardiac or cerebrovascular disease. H/o smoking, hyperlipidemia, hypertension, diabetes. Patients may present with claudication, impotence, pain in distal foot.	Ulcers are commonly deep, located over bony prominences, round or punched out with sharply demarcated borders (Fig. 2); yellow base or necrosis; exposure of tendons. Associated findings include abnormal pedal pulses, cool limbs, femoral bruit and prolonged venous filling time.	Revascularization, antiplatelet medications, management of risk factors
Neuropathic	Most common cause of foot ulcers, usually from diabetes mellitus.	Painless ulcer. Usually occurs on plantar aspect of feet in patients with diabetes, neurologic disorders, or Hansen's disease. Associated clinical findings include claw toes, neuropathic (Charcot) arthropathy, and reduced sweating resulting in dry, scaly feet.	Off-loading of pressure, topical growth factors, tissue-engineered skin
Pressure	Usually occurs in patients with limited mobility.	Located over bony prominences (Fig. 3); risk factors include excessive moisture and altered mental status.	Off-loading of pressure; reduction of excessive moisture, shear and friction; adequate nutrition.

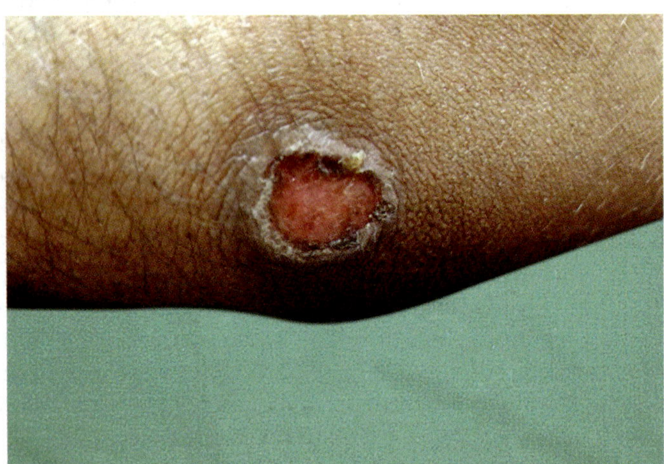

Fig. 2: **Medium-vessel vasculitis:** Punched out ulcers over the lower legs with surrounding erythema

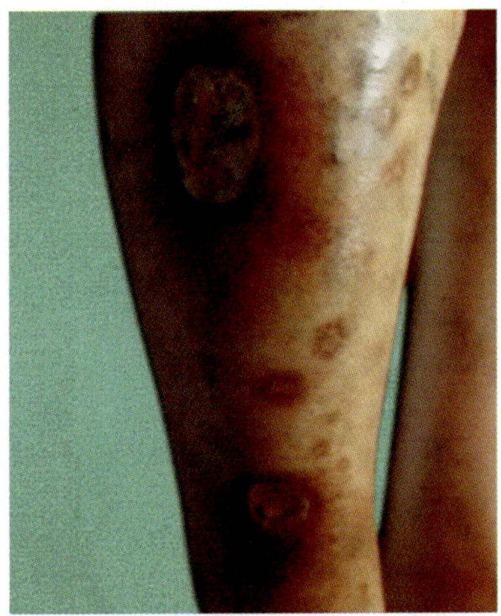

Fig. 3: **Pressure ulcer:** Well-defined punched out ulcer over the elbow

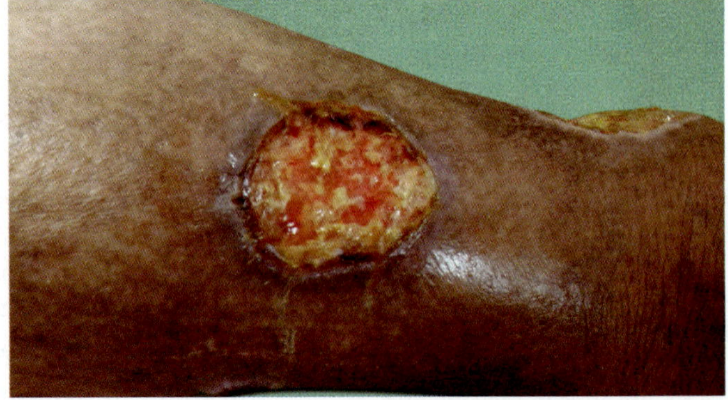

Fig. 4: **Pyoderma gangrenosum:** Punched out ulcer over the lower leg with a violaceous undermined border and purulent base

b. Medium-vessel vasculitis
c. Thromboangiitis obliterans
d. Venous ulcer

Ans: a Pyoderma gangrenosum

Pathergy phenomenon is defined as a state of altered tissue reactivity that occurs in response to minor trauma. It is frequently mentioned in descriptions of the clinical behavior of PG.

Q14. How do you diagnose pyoderma gangrenosum?

Ans: The diagnosis mainly depends on recognition of the evolving clinical features and is supported by histopathology and pathergy test. The histopathologic findings in PG are not specific. Microscopic features of ulcerative PG (most common type) include massive neutrophilic infiltration, hemorrhage, and necrosis of the overlying epidermis. Centrally, at the base or border of the ulcer, the cellular infiltrate is predominantly neutrophilic, often with abscess formation. Moving peripherally, the infiltrate is first mixed, then predominantly lymphocytic as the surrounding erythematous areola is reached and is concentrated about the dermal vessels, both superficial and deep, and there may be endothelial swelling. In some cases, there is definite vascular damage with fibrin deposition in the walls, thrombosis, and extravasation of erythrocytes, but the full picture of vasculitis is generally absent.

Q15. How do you treat pyoderma gangrenosum?

Ans: Pyoderma gangrenosum is managed with a combination of topical and/or systemic therapies that suppress the inflammatory process and wound care measures that optimize the environment for wound healing. PG frequently occurs in association with other medical disorders, most commonly inflammatory bowel disease, hematologic malignancy, and arthritis. Although, the course of the disease does not always parallel PG, treatment of the associated disorder sometimes results in improvement in PG.

First-line therapies:

- Wound management
  - Local care
  - Surgery
- Limited disease
  - Topical corticosteroids
  - Topical calcineurin inhibitors
- More extensive disease
  - Systemic glucocorticoids
  - Systemic cyclosporine

Second line and adjunctive therapies:

- Infliximab
- Other biologic tumor necrosis factor-alpha inhibitors
- Conventional immunosuppressants as azathioprine, methotrexate and cyclosporine
- Dapsone
- Minocycline
- Refractory disease
  - Intravenous immune globulin
  - Alkylating agents.

ACKNOWLEDGMENTS

Dr Mamta Rai, Junior Resident, Department of Dermatology and Venereology, AIIMS, New Delhi, for providing Figures 2, 3 and 4.

SECTION 8

Photosensitive Disorders

Debdeep Mitra

CHAPTER 37

Polymorphic Light Eruption

Anju George

Case study Polymorphic Light Eruption

Presenting Complaints

Doctor, I am having a reddish rash on my upper limbs and upper back since 3 weeks. There is also severe itching and the rash turns more prominent after going outdoors. Last year, at the beginning of summer, I had similar lesions which subsided with creams and few medicines.

Setting

Dermatology outpatient department

History of Present Illness

A 28-year-old lady presented with complaints of itchy, red rashes on both forearms for 3 weeks duration. The lesions initially developed on the back of both hands and later progressed to involve both forearms, arms and upper back. There is history of aggravation of itching and lesions turning more prominent after exposure to sunlight. The patient is an office goer and rides a two-wheeler daily. She also gives history of similar lesions a year ago during summer which subsided with topicals and few systemic medications. There is no history of fever, oral ulcers, joint pains or hair loss. She is not on any regular medications.

General Examination and Systemic Examination

No significant abnormality detected

Dermatological Examination

Multiple discrete and confluent erythematous papules and plaques, the largest measuring 3 × 2.5 cm, distributed on the dorsa of both hands, extensor aspect of forearms (Fig.1), arms and upper back. A few hypopigmented macules and vesicles are also present in the same areas. The lesions are distributed almost bilaterally symmetrically. The unexposed sites are completely spared and all mucosae are normal.

Q1. What is the most likely diagnosis?

a. Subacute cutaneous lupus erythematosus
b. Erythropoietic protoporphyria
c. Polymorphic light eruption
d. Seborrhoeic dermatitis

Ans: c. Polymorphic light eruption (PMLE).

Q2. What is polymorphic light eruption?

Ans: Polymorphic light eruption is an idiopathic endogenous photodermatosis characterized by intermittent polymorphic eruptions ranging from papulovesicular lesions to large plaques, localized predominantly in a photoexposed distribution.

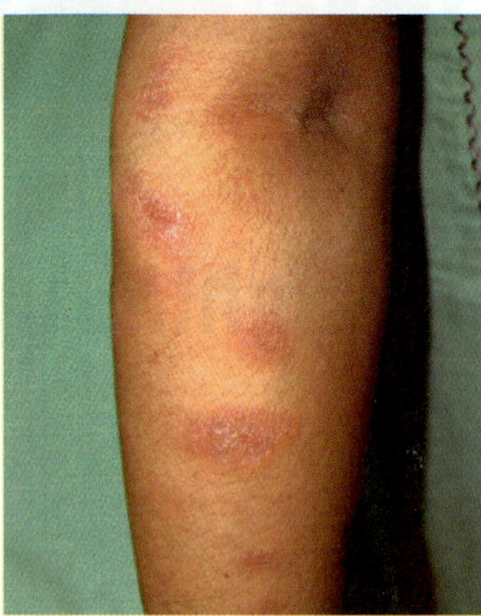

Fig. 1: Multiple polymorphic lesions on the forearm

The eruptions may be induced by sunlight or even artificial ultraviolet (UV) rays.

Q3. Is there any gender predisposition?

Ans: Yes. It mostly affects young women of less than 30 years of age, in temperate regions.

Q4. What is the etiopathogenesis of polymorphic light eruption?

Ans: Etiopathogenesis is as follows:

- There is always a genetic predisposition to develop PMLE. The eruption is hypothesized to be a delayed type hypersensitivity response to an endogenous cutaneous photo antigen. Glutathione depletion in genetically predisposed individuals can lead to free radical-mediated injury and hence development of lesions.
- Another etiological hypothesis is immunosuppression by UV radiation resulting in increased recognition of antigens.
- Ultraviolet radiation induces suppression of the contact hypersensitivity response caused by the release of immunosuppressive cytokines (IL-10) from keratinocytes. Recently, it has been demonstrated that 17β-estradiol in females prevents this UV radiation-induced suppression of the contact hypersensitivity response. This could be the reason why PMLE is more common in females than in males and why the risk decreases in women after menopause.
- The action spectrum is unclear, although it is mostly between 290 nm and 365 nm and rarely visible light. Photoprovocation studies have shown an equal positive response to broadband UVA and narrowband UVB.

Q5. What are the typical affected sites and the nature of onset?

Ans: The typical sites affected are the nasal bridge, malar region of cheeks, chin, back, sides and 'V' area of neck, dorsal aspect of hands, feet and extensor aspect of extremities. The lesions occur mostly on sun exposed sites, however a few exposed sites may be spared. Rarely, it may involve covered areas as well. Pruritus almost always occurs within minutes of exposure and the rash within minutes to hours. Thereafter, it may last for days or even weeks if exposure continues.

Q6. What does the term 'polymorphic' imply?

Ans: The lesions vary in morphology from erythematous macules, papules, papulovesicles to large plaques. However, a single morphology predominates in a given individual and the same type of lesions may recur each year. Lesions of different morphologies may also be present in the same individual at different sites.

Q7. What is hardening effect?

Ans: The lesions develop mostly in early summer or spring and gradually improves as summer progresses. This is known as the hardening effect.

Q8. Which of the following is a variant of polymorphic light eruption?

a. Actinic prurigo
b. Juvenile spring eruption
c. Solar urticaria
d. Hydroa vacciniforme

Ans: b. Juvenile spring eruption. Other entities are idiopathic photodermatosis besides PMLE. The variants of PMLE include:

- *Juvenile spring eruption*: Occurs in epidemics and affects young boys. Vesicular lesions appear on the sun-exposed helices of ears.
- *Photosensitive lichenoid eruption*: Presents as micropapular lichen nitidus like lesions or lichen planus like lesions on upper extremities and neck with relative sparing of face.
- Rarely, the PMLE rash may become generalized due to autosensitization.
- Secondary eczematization and lichenification are also observed.

Q9. Name the other idiopathic photodermatoses?

Ans: Actinic prurigo, hydroa vacciniforme, solar urticaria and chronic actinic dermatitis.

Q10. What are the differentials to be considered?

Ans: The differentials to be considered are:

- Systemic lupus erythematosus (SLE)
- Erythropoietic protoporphyria
- Light-exacerbated seborrheic and atopic eczema
- Erythema multiforme
- Solar urticarial.

Q11. How will you differentiate polymorphic light eruption from similar other conditions and what are the disease associations, if any?

Ans: Differentiating features:

- *Systemic lupus erythematosus:* Circulating antinuclear antibody and anti-double stranded DNA titers are needed to rule out SLE. In addition, SLE presents with constitutional symptoms, arthralgia, oral mucosal lesions, malar/discoid rash, vasculitic lesions and frequently systemic manifestations. But, it should be noted that lupus erythematosus may also precede or coexist with PMLE.
- *Porphyria:* Estimation of blood, urinary and stool porphyrin concentrations may be required. Erythropoietic protoporphyria presents with painful lesions and raised red blood cell protoporphyrin concentrations.
- *Direct immunofluorescence:* Negative in PMLE
- *Light-exacerbated seborrhoeic and atopic eczema:* Differentiated by the characteristic eczematous clinical and histological features, along with the distribution of lesions at typical sites.
- *Erythema multiforme:* Distinguished by its clinical features, characteristic histology and association with a precipitating agent.
- *Solar urticaria:* Characteristic rapid onset (5–10 minutes) after exposure, short total duration of lesions (1–2 hours) and different lesional morphology.
- Recent evidence suggests that PMLE may be associated with thyroid function disorders and vice versa. Hence, a thyroid function testing is advised in all cases of PMLE and patients should be clinically examined for features of thyroid disorder.

Q12. How will you confirm the diagnosis of polymorphic light eruption?

Ans: Few measures to confirm the diagnosis:

- The diagnosis is mostly based on the history and clinical findings.
- Skin biopsy for histopathological examination: Even though histology is useful, it is not fully diagnostic. Epidermis shows variable spongiosis. Dermis shows perivascular and periadnexal lymphocytic infiltration with edema, often extending deep into the dermis in older lesions.
- *Photoprovocation test*: There is no standard protocol for a photoprovocation testing and it is difficult to reproduce the lesions. Repeated UV radiation exposures are required rather than a single exposure.

Q13. How will you treat a case of polymorphic light eruption?

Ans: Treatment procedures:

- Photoprotection is the mainstay of treatment and patient should be advised to minimize sun exposure.
- Broad spectrum sunscreens, use of wide-brimmed hats, umbrellas and protective clothing is essential.
- In mild cases, topical moderately-potent steroids and antihistamines may be adequate.
- In severe cases, a short course of oral prednisolone in tapering doses may be tried.
- In moderate to severe cases, hydroxychloroquine, beta-carotene and omega-3 fatty acid supplements are used.
- Narrowband UVB and psoralen plus ultraviolet light (PUVA) therapy have been found to be helpful in recurrent episodes.
- Other drugs tried in severe recalcitrant cases include azathioprine, thalidomide and cyclosporine.
- Topical immunomodulators like calcitriol (1,25-dihydroxyvitamin D) and its analogs such as calcipotriol have been tried as a prophylactic measure in patients with PMLE.

CHAPTER 38

Xeroderma Pigmentosum

Maheshwari NS

Case study Xeroderma Pigmentosum

Presenting Complaints

Doctor, my daughter has developed black spots all over the face since 5 years. She also complains of burning sensation over the face for 2 years.

Setting

Dermatology outpatient department

History of Present Illness

A 7-year-old girl born from second degree consanguineous marriage (Fig. 1) was brought by her parents to the pediatric dermatology department with history of black spots all over her face for 5 years and burning sensation over the face and hands because of which she refuses to go out in the sun. Both symptoms are insidious in onset and gradually progressive.

General Physical Examination

Short statured, conscious, irritable due to photophobia

Systemic Examination

Central nervous system: No ataxia/hyporeflexia
No sensorineural deafness

Ophthalmological Examination

Normal vision with conjunctival xerosis, no corneal opacity

Dermatological Examination

- Generalized xerosis
- Freckles all over the face, upper limbs, trunk and lower limbs (Figs 2 and 3)
- Face: Telangiectasia, atrophic macules giving mottled appearance
- Hyperpigmented scars over nose
- A single-pigmented lesion with rolled out edges present over left temple, suggestive of basal cell carcinoma
- Normal oral cavity and mucosa
- Normal nails.

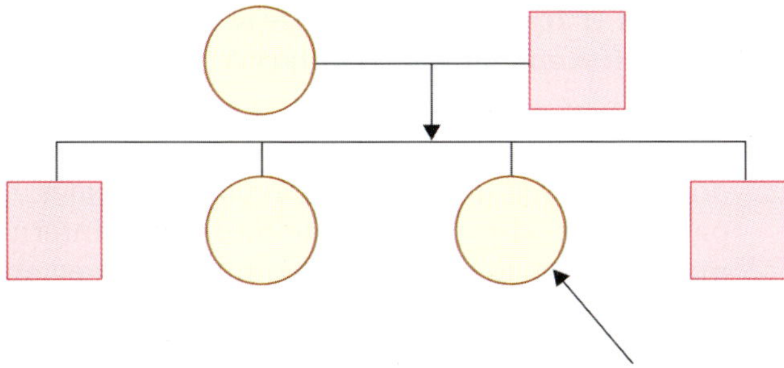

Fig. 1: Pedigree chart

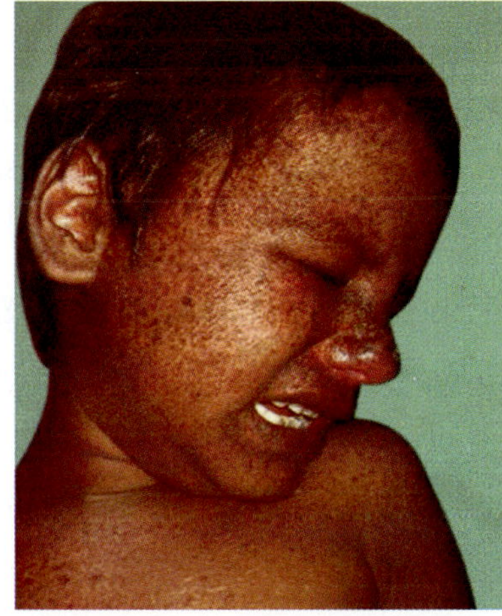

Fig. 2: Early freckling with atrophic hypopigmented macules. Girl is irritable due to photophobia. Normal hair and teeth can be seen

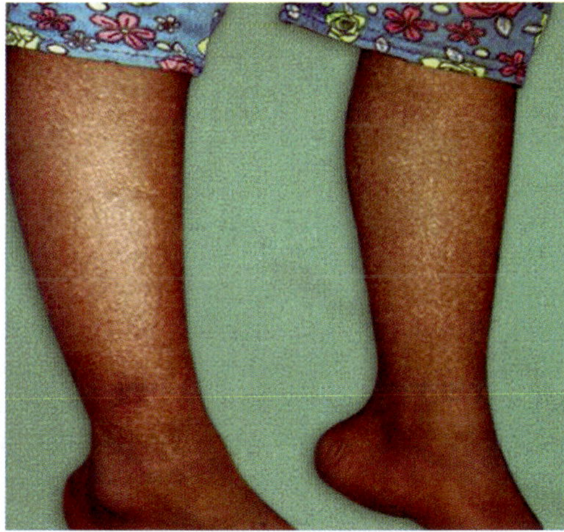

Fig. 3: Severe pigmentary changes over the nonexposed lower limbs

Q1. What is the most likely diagnosis?

a. Xeroderma Pigmentosum
b. Bloom syndrome
c. Cockayne syndrome
d. Ataxia telangiectasia

Ans: a. Xeroderma pigmentosum (XP)

Presence of early onset of photosensitivity, freckles, photophobia and carcinoma are suggestive of XP.

Q2. What is the mode of inheritance of xeroderma pigmentosum?

a. Autosomal dominant
b. Autosomal recessive
c. X-linked dominant
d. X-linked recessive

Ans: b. Autosomal recessive.

Q3. What is the pathology in xeroderma pigmentosum?

a. DNA repair defect
b. Abnormal DNA helicase function
c. Absence of X chromosome
d. Absence of Y chromosome

Ans: a. DNA repair defect

There is a defect in the nucleotide-excision-repair (NER) pathway, responsible for the removal and replacement of damaged DNA. This results in diminished DNA repair in the cells exposed to the ultraviolet (UV)-B range of sunlight.

Q4. Mention the types of xeroderma pigmentosum.

Ans: Xeroderma pigmentosum A to G.

- Cutaneous manifestations are severe in XP-A, XP-C, XP-D, and XP-G.
- Neurological manifestations are seen mostly among XP-A and XP-D, occasionally among XP-C, and XP-G.
- Clinical features are mild in XP-E and XP-F.

Q5. Enumerate the cutaneous manifestations in xeroderma pigmentosum.

Ans: Cutaneous manifestations in XP:

- Photosensitivity
- Freckles
- Lentigines
- Mottled hypo- and hyperpigmentation
- Atrophy, blisters and scarring
- Telangiectasia
- Early onset of malignancies like basal cell carcinoma, squamous cell carcinoma, actinic keratosis, fibroxanthoma, melanoma, keratoacanthoma.

Q6. What are the neurological features seen in xeroderma pigmentosum?

Ans: Microcephaly, developmental delay, hyporeflexia, cerebellar ataxia, mental retardation and sensorineural deafness. In patients with XP-A, neurological manifestations appear early, before the age of 7 years, whereas in XP-D, these are late in onset, beyond the age of 7 years.

Q7. What are the ocular manifestations xeroderma pigmentosum patients can present with?

Ans: Ocular manifestations are present in 80% patients with XP and include photophobia, conjunctival xerosis, recurrent conjunctivitis, and freckle-like pigmentation in the bulbar conjunctiva.

Photodamage leading to scarring of the eyelids, loss of eyelashes, symblepharon, and ectropion. Other changes include vascular pterygium, corneal opacities, ocular keratoacanthoma, and epithelioma of the eyelids.

Q8. Is it mandatory to perform skin biopsy? What are the histopathological findings to expect in xeroderma pigmentosum?

Ans: No, it is not mandatory to do skin biopsy as it is more of a clinical diagnosis. Histopathological examination shows flattened epidermis with irregular proliferation of rete pegs, heavily laden with pigment. Basophilic degeneration of dermal collagen, solar elastosis, and increased vascularity can be seen.

Q9. How do you confirm xeroderma pigmentosum?

Ans: Demonstration of the DNA repair defect is confirmatory for diagnosis. The unscheduled DNA synthesis assay following UV-irradiation of skin fibroblasts, lymphocytes, or epidermal cells in culture is the standard diagnostic method.

Q10. Is it possible to diagnose xeroderma pigmentosum prenatally?

Ans: Yes, DNA repair defects are also demonstrable in amniotic fluid cells. DNA analysis of trophoblast cells, polymerase chain reaction and alkaline comet assay are the other methods of prenatal diagnosis. Successful prenatal carrier detection for XP-A is possible by a DNA-based study of chorionic villus cells.

Q11. What is the course and prognosis of xeroderma pigmentosum?

Ans: There are no means to prevent freckling or the occurrence of malignancies except avoidance of sun exposure. Early death results from metastatic malignancies. Two-thirds of the patients die before 20 years of age. Milder cases may survive longer. Other causes of morbidity and mortality are recurrent infections and neurological complications.

Q12. Why is it important to follow up xeroderma pigmentosum patients regularly?

Ans: The risk of developing basal cell carcinoma and squamous cell carcinoma is 2500 times that of normal population and of melanoma 1000-fold greater. XP patients are also more prone to develop internal malignancies including brain, lungs, kidney and gastrointestinal tract. Hence, proper education of the parents and regular follow up is a must.

Q13. How do you counsel the patient?

Ans:
- Strict lifelong sun protection, including total sun avoidance, application of sunscreens that protect throughout the UVB and UVA spectrum, UV shields over windows, sun-protective clothing, broad-brimmed hats, and sunglasses.
- Annual examination of skin to detect early malignancies
- Ophthalmological examination every 6 months.

Q14. How do you treat cutaneous premalignant lesions?

Ans:
- Cryosurgery
- Topical 5-fluorouracil
- Imiquimod application
- Intralesional interferon alpha
- Ingenol mebutate
- Topical diclofenac
- Surgical removal
- Oral isotretinoin (1 mg/kg body weight per day) can reduce the incidence of cutaneous malignancies in patients.

Q15. What is the enzymatic treatment for xeroderma pigmentosum?

Ans: We know that the basic defect in XP is nucleotide excision repair leading to a deficient repair of the DNA damaged by UV radiation. So repairing DNA damage after UV exposure is a definite treatment option. T4 endonuclease V, a repair enzyme in experimental studies has been shown to repair the cyclobutane pyrimidine dimers resulting from DNA damage. This DNA repair enzyme can be delivered by specifically engineered liposomes into the skin and repair the defect. It may become an important treatment option in the future.

Q16. Which are the other DNA repair disorders?

Ans: The other DNA repair disorders are:
- Bloom syndrome
- Ataxia telangiectasia

- Cockayne syndrome
- Fanconi's anemia
- Rothmund-Thomson syndrome
- Werner's syndrome
- Progeria
- Trichothiodystrophy.

Q17. What is De Sanctis-Cacchione syndrome?

Ans: It is a subset of XP with distinct features like microcephaly, dwarfism, severe mental retardation, deafness, hypogonadism, shortening of tendo-Achilles, and neurological features like chorea athetosis and cerebellar ataxia.

CHAPTER 39

Porphyria

Ananta Khurana

Case study Porphyria

Presenting Complaints

Doctor, I develop blisters over my hands and forearms since 6 years. The wounds that develop heal slowly leaving discoloration and scars. Off late, I have noted excessive long hair on my face and small elevated lesions over hands.

Setting

Dermatology outpatient department

History of Present Illness

A 50-year-old man presented with complaints of blistering over the dorsa of hands and forearms since 6 years. He also complains of shearing of skin following friction or mild trauma over these areas. The wounds so formed heal very slowly leaving scars and often become infected. The patient has also noticed excessive hair growth on his face since 2 years. He does not have any history of eye problems or similar lesions over any mucosa. He has noticed that his urine often has a reddish brown tinge on standing.

He has been an alcoholic since the age of 30 years. No other family member has similar complaints. He does not give any history of sudden attacks of fever, abdominal pain and neurological features. He is not on any drug therapy.

General Physical Examination

- Well-oriented to time, place and person
- Body mass index: 30 kg/m^2, pulse: 80 bpm, blood pressure: 130/85 mm Hg

Systemic Examination

Hepatomegaly is present.

Dermatological Examination

- The dorsa of hands show vesicles, a single large hemorrhagic bulla, erosions and pigmentary changes (hypo and hyper).
- Numerous milia and scarring can be appreciated over the dorsa of hands and forearms.
- Lanugo like hypertrichosis is seen over the periorbital, temporal and malar regions.
- Severe elastosis and sclerodermoid changes are present over the face.

Q1. What is the most likely diagnosis?

a. Epidermolysis bullosa acquisita
b. Porphyria cutanea tarda
c. Bullous pemphigoid
d. Pseudoporphyria

Ans: b. Porphyria cutanea tarda (PCT).

Q2. How will you investigate the patient and confirm your diagnosis?

Ans: *Bedside:* Urine (and occasionally the skin lesions) fluoresce red with a Wood's lamp.

Biochemical tests to demonstrate increased porphyrins:

- Most commonly used: Fresh random urine (light-protected sample): Quantitative porphyrin analysis demonstrates elevated uroporphyrin I/ uroporphyrin III ratio.
- Stool samples (used less commonly): Increased isoporphyrin and hepatocarboxyl porphyrin III
- Plasma: Fluorescence emission peak at 620 nm.

Investigations for the predisposing condition:

- Full blood count
- Liver function tests
- Kidney function tests
- Blood sugar
- Screening for hepatitis A, B and C
- Serum ferritin
- Serum iron and iron binding capacity
- Abdominal ultrasound
- Liver biopsy (if indicated).

Histopathology and immunofluorescence

- Lesional skin biopsy shows subepidermal separation, minimal inflammatory infiltrate (bland bullae), and protuberance of rigid dermal papillae into blister cavity (festooning).
- Caterpillar bodies are the diagnostic histopathological finding in PCT. These are linear eosinophilic periodic acid-Schiff-positive globules in the epidermis overlying subepidermal bullae of PCT. They contain degenerating keratinocytes, colloid bodies, and basement membrane bodies.
- Direct immunofluorescence shows immunoglobulin G, immunoglobulin M, fibrinogen, and complement in the basement membrane and around vessels of the upper dermis.

Q3. What are porphyrias?

Ans: Porphyrias are a group of disorders due to enzyme deficiencies which affect the metabolism of porphyrins. Porphyrins are intermediate molecules in the heme synthesis pathway, involving eight dedicated enzymes (Fig. 1). A defect in the pathway leads to build up of these toxic precursors leading to the typical clinical findings.

Q4. How do you classify porphyrias?

Ans: Classification of porphyrias:

- Porphyrias are classified into two categories based on whether the porphyrins build up in the liver (Hepatic porphyrias) or bone marrow (Erythropoietic porphyrias).
- Hepatic porphyrias are further divided into acute and chronic subtypes.
- Hepatic porphyrias generally have secondary factors (e.g. drugs, infections, hormones, alcohol, fasting) which increase the demand for heme and thus trigger the disease.
- Acute hepatic porphyrias [Acute intermittent porphyria, variegate porphyria (VP), hereditary coproporphyria (HCP), and aminolevulinic acid (ALA) dehydratase-deficient porphyria] present with episodes (acute attacks) of abdominal or neurological symptoms caused by a genetic predisposition with a secondary metabolic trigger. VP and HCP are associated with PCT like skin findings in 60–80% and 5–20% cases respectively.
- Porphyria cutanea tarda is the only chronic hepatic porphyria. PCT may be familial (type I), with an autosomal dominant inheritance of the defective Uroporphyrinogen III decarboxylase (UROD) gene, or acquired (sporadic or type II). However, a secondary event is required to trigger both forms. Thus, PCT is a multifactorial disease, common associations being alcoholism, exogenous hormones, iron overload, hepatitis C, human immunodeficiency virus, drugs, diabetes, dialysis-dependent renal failure and hepatocellular carcinoma.
- Erythropoietic porphyrias include erythropoietic protoporphyria (EPP), congenital erythropoietic porphyria, and X-linked dominant protoporphyria.

Q5. What are the major cutaneous clinical presentations of porphyrias?

Ans: Cutaneous lesions develop in one of the two following forms:

1. *Bullous type:* Skin fragility in sun exposed regions, mostly on the back of the hands. Tense blisters and erosions may develop in the same distribution. Over time, scarring, hypo-and hyperpigmentation and milia develop at sites of healed erosions. Facial hypertrichosis, sclerodermoid changes and

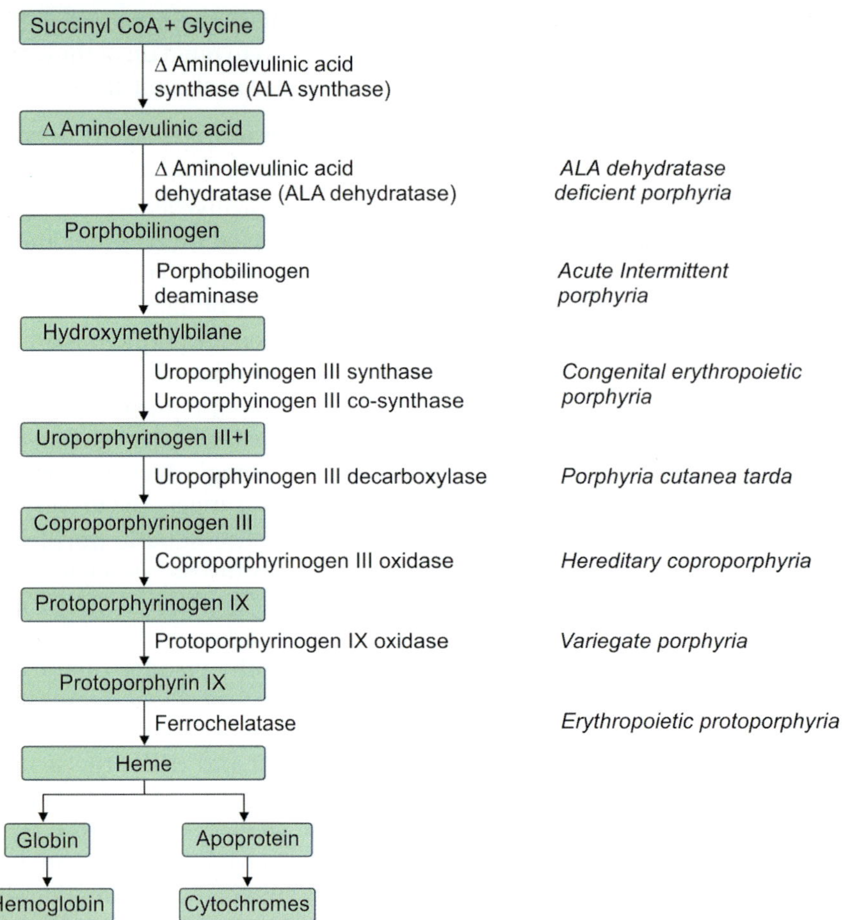

Fig. 1: Heme biosynthetic pathway (The disease associated with each enzyme deficiency is mentioned on the right side in italics)

pseudorhagades often develop later (Figs 2 and 3). The disease is worse in summers, although the patients are generally not aware of the induction of lesions following irradiation, as the onset is delayed (delayed phototoxic reaction).

This type of presentation develops with accumulation of the water soluble porphyrins (formed in the early and middle steps of the pathway), which diffuse in the skin up to the dermoepidermal junction, causing phototoxic effects in the upper dermis. The presentation is classical of PCT, but the rarer VP and HCP also present in the same way on skin.

2. *Immediate painful photosensitive type:* Rapid onset of intense stinging and burning pain in the skin following sun exposure (immediate phototoxic reaction). Edema and erythema may be present. The attacks last for 2–3 days and are unresponsive to analgesia except cold water and cold air. This type is classical of EPP, wherein the more lipophilic protoporphyrin accumulates in the erythrocytes. Diffusion is limited to the endothelial cells and as a result, the phototoxic

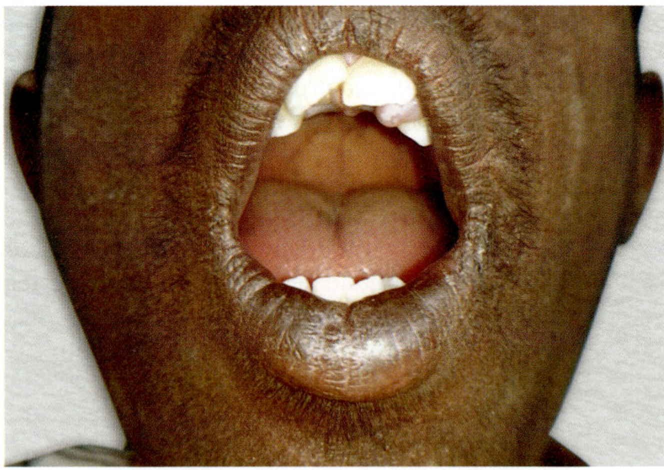

Fig. 2: Pseudorhagades and hypertrichosis in a case of porphyria cutanea tarda

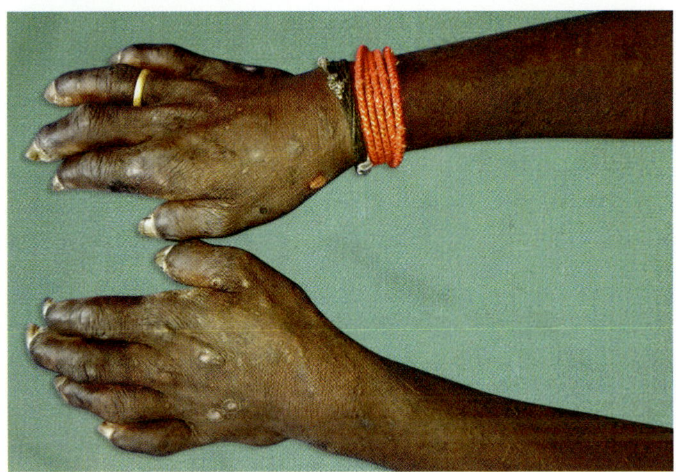

Fig. 3: Sclerodermoid changes

reaction causes endothelial necrosis in the upper dermis, producing the typical presentation.

Q6. What are the features of an "acute attack"?

Ans: Acute attack in porphyria:
- The most common feature is severe abdominal pain, generally accompanied by nausea and vomiting.
- Motor neuropathy in the form of muscle weakness to generalized paralysis, cranial nerve involvement and bulbar involvement leading to respiratory depression.
- Hypertension and tachycardia are often present; obstipation and even paralytic ileus may develop.
- Water and electrolyte disturbances, especially hypomagnesemia and hyponatremia
- Psychiatric symptoms ranging from depression and apathy to agitation and psychosis.

Q7. Do relatives need testing in porphyria?

Ans: Among the porphyrias which can present to a dermatologist with cutaneous features, genetic testing to detect an underlying defect is indicated in VP and HCP, as relatives may inherit the gene (and thus be at risk of acute attacks) without skin changes.

Q8. What are the treatment modalities available for different porphyrias?

Ans: Treatment modalities:
- *Photoprotection*: Excess porphyrins are catalyzed and produce singlet oxygen molecules upon skin exposure to visible light (predominantly wavelengths of 400–410 nm–the Soret band), as well as four additional absorption bands of decreasing intensity in the range of 500–700 nm. Consequent oxidative damage leads to clinical symptoms. Thus, photoprotection is central to the management of cutaneous porphyrias. Only physical sunscreens containing zinc oxide (preferable) or titanium dioxide are effective in protecting against higher than 400 nm wavelengths. Additional protection in UVA spectrum is also desirable as wavelengths as low as 360 nm can also cause phototoxicity. Photostable UVA filters are effective in this regard. Physical measures including UV protection factor clothing, eyeglasses and window films need to be stressed upon as well.
- *Additional treatment in porphyria cutanea tarda:*
  - Avoidance of exacerbating factors
  - Low dose chloroquine or hydroxychloroquine
  - Phlebotomy
  - Iron chelation
  - Vitamin E
  - Management of the coexisting liver disease.
- *Additional treatment in EPP*:
  - Afamelanotide
  - Beta-carotene
  - Phototherapy
  - Cysteine and N-acetylcysteine
  - Monitoring for liver disease
  - Liver transplantation
  - Bone marrow transplantation
  - Pain management.

Q9. What are the factors which can trigger or aggravate porphyrias and hence should be avoided?

Ans: Factors triggering and aggravating porphyria:
- Sunlight
- Pregnancy
- Menstruation
- Alcohol
- Smoking
- Surgery
- Low carbohydrate diet or fasting
- High dietary iron
- Drugs: Barbiturates, chloroquine, dapsone, estrogens, griseofulvin, heavy metals, metoclopramide, phenytoin, progestins, rifampicin, sulfonamides.

SECTION 9

Sexually Transmitted Disorders

Malcolm Pinto

CHAPTER 40

Genital Ulcer

Ankur Talwar

Case study Genital Ulcer

Presenting Complaints

Doctor, I have developed multiple painful sores on my penis since the past 5 days after contact with my girlfriend.

Setting

Dermatology outpatient department.

History of Present Illness

A 28-year-old unmarried man presented with complaints of multiple ulcers on the genitalia since past 5 days. The lesions started as small raised lesions which gradually eroded on the surface and progressed to the present size. He admitted to having regular unprotected sexual contact with his girlfriend since the past couple of years. The last such exposure was around 1 week prior to the onset of lesion. He had no other sexual partners. The patient complained of severe pain in the lesions and also reported discharge of foul smelling purulent material. There were no other systemic complaints.

General Physical Examination and Systemic Examination

No abnormality detected.

Dermatological and Venereological Examination

- Multiple small oval to round ulcers are present on the glans penis and undersurface of prepuce measuring 1–1.5 cm in diameter (Fig. 1).
- The ulcers have an ill-defined, serpiginous border and friable base; covered with necrotic, purulent exudates.
- On palpation, the ulcers were extremely tender and non-indurated.
- Right-sided inguinal lymphadenopathy was present and was mildly tender.

Q1. What is the most likely diagnosis?

a. Syphilis
b. Chancroid
c. Herpes genitalis
d. Granuloma inguinale

Ans: b. Chancroid

The lesion of chancroid is often termed as a soft chancre because it is not indurated. Ulcers may be single or multiple. The ulcers are extremely painful and deep with irregular, ragged margins. The ulcer base is composed of malodorous yellow-gray exudates.

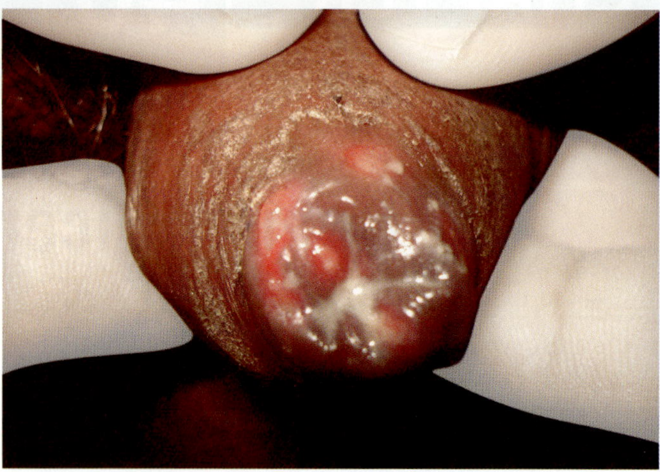

Fig. 1: Multiple non-indurated irregular ulcers on prepuce

Q2. What is the incubation period of different sexually-transmitted infections?

Ans: The incubation period of different sexually-transmitted infections is mentioned in Table 1.

Q3. Describe the lymph node involvement in chancroid?

Ans: Painful, usually unilateral, regional lymphadenopathy occurs in approximately 50% of patients. This is more commonly seen in men. Of patients with lymphadenitis, 25% may have progression to a suppurative bubo, which may rupture spontaneously and ulcerate. If untreated, chronic draining sinuses may follow.

Q4. What are the different types of ulcers which can occur in chancroid?

Ans: Types of chancroid ulcers:

- Transient chancroid
- Dwarf chancroid
- Follicular chancroid
- Giant chancroid
- Pseudogranuloma inguinale
- Mixed chancroid
- Papular chancroid
- Transient chancroid
- Phagedenic chancroid.

Table 1: Incubation period of different sexually-transmitted infections

Sexually-transmitted disease	*Incubation period*
Chancroid	5–14 days
Syphilis	9–90 days
Herpes genitalis	2–7 days (for primary herpes)
Granuloma inguinale	1–180 days
Lymphogranuloma venereum	3–30 days

Q5. What is phagedenic chancroid?

Ans: In a minority of patients with chancroidal ulcers, superinfection with fusospirochetal organisms may occur leading to deep, necrotic, and gangrenous ulcers. The infection rapidly spreads to subcutaneous and deeper tissues, leading to rapid destruction of the external genitalia.

Q6. Describe the typical syphilitic chancre.

Ans: Syphilis presents as a single ulcer (chancre) in 70% of cases. The chancre begins as a raised, firm, red papule which erodes to create an ulcerative crater within the papule, with slightly elevated edges around the central ulcer. The edge and base of the ulcer have a button-like consistency on palpation. The lesion is characteristically painless.

The primary lesion is usually associated with regional lymphadenopathy that may be unilateral or bilateral. Inguinal adenitis is usually discrete, firm, mobile, and painless, without overlying skin changes.

Q7. What are the basic investigations warranted in an undiagnosed case of genital ulcer disease?

Ans: The basic investigations include:

- Herpes simplex virus (HSV) type-specific serology (both HSV 1 and 2 preferably)
- Syphilis serology should include a nontreponemal test like venereal disease research laboratory or rapid plasma reagin
- Enzyme-linked immunosorbent assay (ELISA) for human immunodeficiency virus
- Hepatitis B surface antigen, anti-hepatitis C virus
- Gram's stain of smear prepared from base of ulcer
- Bacterial culture (where facilities are available).

Q8. What are the Centers for Disease Control and Prevention guidelines for treatment of chancroid?

Ans: Centers for Disease Control and Prevention (CDC) recommends one of the following antibiotic options:

- Azithromycin: 1 g orally (PO) as a single dose
- Ceftriaxone: 250 mg intramuscularly as a single dose
- Erythromycin base: 500 mg PO 4 times daily for 7 days
- Ciprofloxacin: 500 mg PO twice daily for 3 days

Azithromycin and ceftriaxone as single-dose treatments have the advantage of observed compliance.

Q9. Describe the typical lesion in granuloma inguinale?

Ans: Granuloma inguinale usually presents with large, usually painless, expanding, suppurative ulcers. The ulcers have clean, friable bases with distinct, raised, rolled margins and have a tendency to bleed easily. The ulcers are "beefy red" and slowly expand centrifugally, eventually becoming more granulomatous with serpiginous borders. They are commonly located on the shaft of the penis, labia, or perineum. Autoinoculation is a common feature, resulting in lesions on adjacent skin.

Q10. What are the Centers for Disease Control and Prevention guidelines for treatment of granuloma inguinale?

Ans: The guidelines are as follows:

Recommended regimen

- Azithromycin 1 g orally once per week or 500 mg daily for at least 3 weeks and until all lesions have completely healed.

Alternative regimens (one of)

- Doxycycline 100 mg orally twice a day for at least 3 weeks and until all lesions have completely healed
- Ciprofloxacin 750 mg orally twice a day for at least 3 weeks and until all lesions have completely healed
- Erythromycin base 500 mg orally four times a day for at least 3 weeks and until all lesions have completely healed
- Trimethoprim-sulfamethoxazole one double-strength (160 mg/800 mg) tablet orally twice a day for at least 3 weeks and until all lesions have completely healed.

Q11. What is the management of antiviral resistant herpes simplex virus?

Ans: All acyclovir-resistant strains are also resistant to valacyclovir, and most are resistant to famciclovir. Foscarnet (40–80 mg/kg IV every 8 hours until clinical resolution is attained) is often effective for treatment of acyclovir-resistant genital herpes. Intravenous cidofovir 5 mg/kg once weekly might also be effective. Imiquimod is a topical alternative.

Q12. Which of the following is not a suppressive regimen for recurrent herpes genitalis?

a. Acyclovir 400 mg twice a day
b. Famciclovir 500 mg twice a day
c. Valacyclovir 500 mg per day
d. Valacyclovir 1000 mg twice a day

Ans: b. Famciclovir 500 mg twice a day.

Famciclovir is given in dosage of 250 mg twice a day for suppression of recurrent herpes episodes. Acyclovir, famciclovir, and valacyclovir appear equally effective for episodic treatment of genital herpes, but famciclovir appears somewhat less effective for suppression of viral shedding.

Valacyclovir 1000 mg is preferred in individuals with very frequent recurrences (>10 episodes/year) while 500 mg per day suffices in individuals with infrequent recurrences.

Q13. What is Lipschutz ulcer?

Ans: Lipschutz ulcer is an acute non-venereal vulvar ulcer which is now also known as "ulcus vulvae acutum". It has been described as occurring predominantly in young girls of 14–20 years; 70% of the cases being virgins. In most cases, the ulcer is located on the inner aspect of labia minora, labia majora, introitus, external urethral orifice or posterior commissure. The ulcers may be one to many in number. They are extremely tender to touch with sharp edges and yellow base with minimum slough. Inguinal lymph nodes are usually enlarged.

Q14. How do we differentiate various genital ulcers?

Ans: Various genital ulcers can be understood with the help of Table 2.

Q15. What are the complications of chancroid?

Ans: Phimosis, paraphimosis, urethral fistula and phagedenic ulcer.

Table 2: Various genital ulcers

	Lesions	*Tenderness*	*Edge*	*Base*	*Lymphadenopathy*
Syphilis	Usually single	None	Indurated	Clean	Indolent
Chancroid	Usually multiple	Marked	Soft	Dirty	Tender, fluctuant, usually unilateral
Herpes	Multiple	Marked	Soft	Clean	Tender, bilateral
Donovanosis	Multiple	None	Serpiginous, may be white	Beefy red, granulation tissue	Erosive lesions overlying nodes
Lymphogranuloma venereum	Single	None	Soft	Eroded papule	Prominent, tender

CHAPTER 41

Inguinal Bubo

Samujjala Deb

Case study Inguinal Bubo

Presenting Complaints

Doctor, I have a swelling in my right groin which has been slowly increasing in size over the last 1 month.

Setting

Dermatology outpatient department.

History of Present Illness

A 28-year-old unmarried man, presented to dermatology outpatient department with complaints of a painless swelling over the right groin, progressively increasing in size. Of late the patient was experiencing mild pain while walking. He had history of unprotected sexual exposure to a commercial sex worker about a month prior to onset of swelling. He did not remember developing any eruptions or lesions on his genitalia. For the last 1 week he was suffering from fever which was associated with sweating along with chills and rigor. He complained of loss of appetite and generalized weakness.

General Physical Examination

- Well oriented to time, place and person
- Body mass index: 24 Kg/m^2
- Pulse: 90/min
- Temperature (oral): 101.4° F

Systemic Examination

No abnormality detected.

Dermatological Examination

- Diffuse swelling over the right inguinal region (Fig. 1) on inspection with a stretched and shiny appearance of the skin
- On palpation the swelling was mildly tender with a fluctuant feel. There was matting of the superomedial and lateral group of inguinal lymph nodes. The swelling did not increase on coughing while transillumination revealed no fluid.
- The femoral group of lymph nodes was also enlarged leading to the appearance of a groove in the right inguinal region.
- The genitalia was normal on inspection and there was no discharge.

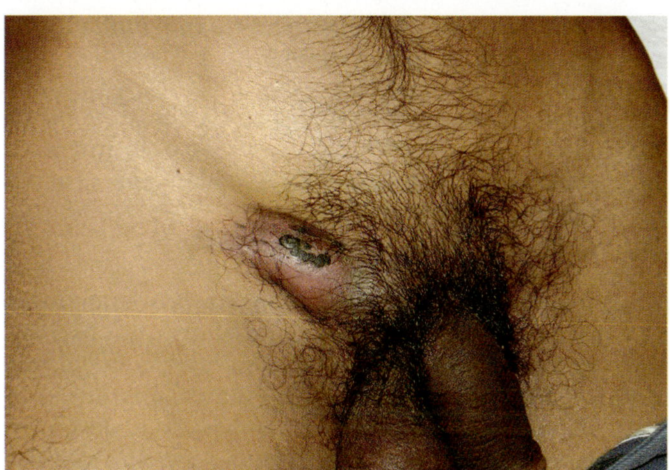

Fig. 1: Inguinal bubo on the right

Q1. What is the most likely diagnosis?

a. Lymphogranuloma venereum (LGV)
b. Chancroid
c. Donovanosis
d. Syphilis

Ans: a (Lymphogranuloma venereum)

Presence of a painless inguinal swelling without history of any ulcer or discharge from the genitalia following unprotected sexual exposure is suggestive of LGV.

Q2. How do you diagnose lymphogranuloma venereum?

Ans: Diagnosis of LGV can be made by taking a thorough history, clinical examination and ruling out the differentials.

Laboratory tests which help in establishing a clinical suspicion are mild leukocytosis with increased eosinophils and monocytes, which is seen in the early stage of inguinal bubo.

Laboratory diagnosis of LGV can be made with:

- Positive serology for *Chlamydia trachomatis* via
  - Nucleic acid amplification test
  - Complement fixation
  - Microimmunofluorescence
- Polymerase chain reaction
- Culture on cell lines.

Q3. What are the other possible differentials?

Ans: The other clinical conditions that may result in inguinal bubo are sexually transmitted infections, chancroid, cutaneous tuberculosis, scrofuloderma, filariasis and malignant metastasis.

Q4. What is the causative agent of lymphogranuloma venereum?

Ans: Lymphogranuloma venereum or LGV is a sexually transmitted infection caused by *Chlamydia trachomatis* serovars L1, L2 and L3 which preferentially affects the lymphatic system. *Chlamydia spp.* are Gram negative and intracellular obligate parasites.

Q5. What are the epidemiological features of lymphogranuloma venereum?

Ans: More common in men with a ratio of 5:1 but long-term complications are more severe in women (ulcerations, genital hypertrophy, rectal strictures). It can be transmitted through the non-sexual routes as well. Vertical transmission does not occur but baby may get infected while passing through the birth canal. LGV has an incubation period of around 3–30 days.

Q6. What are the clinical stages of lymphogranuloma venereum?

Ans: The clinical spectrum of LGV can be divided into three stages: primary stage, secondary stage (inguinal stage) and tertiary stage (complications).

- The primary stage is usually never noticed in the patients and it may be a papule, vesicle, erosion or ulceration at the site of inoculation.
- The secondary stage or the inguinal stage is the commonest clinical presentation in men. Women may present with genito-anorectal syndrome and homosexual men with anorectal syndrome.
- Tertiary stage: It includes all complications of LGV.

Q7. What are the complications of lymphogranuloma venereum?

Ans: Complications:

- Complications in LGV can be myriad due to the extensive involvement and destruction of the lymphatics. The presentations are varied based on the anatomical differences in the lymphatic drainage of the male and female genitalia.
- Males: Ram horn penis and saxophone penis. Rare: Strictures of the urethra, prostatitis, seminal vesiculitis and epididymo-orchitis.
- Females: Chronic edema of the vulva leads to enlargement with development of a condition known as *esthiomene*.
- Involvement of the rectum and anal canal in either sex can lead to development of strictures. Carcinoma of the rectum has been reported to occur in rectal strictures.

Q8. What is inguinal syndrome?

Ans: Inguinal syndrome is the inflammatory swelling of inguinal lymph nodes and their corresponding tributaries and branches. It is the commonest manifestation of LGV in men. It is usually unilateral and can be bilateral in one-third of cases.

Initially painless, the swelling becomes progressively painful with difficulty in walking. The skin overlying the bubo changes from shiny to stretch and finally violaceous before it becomes thickened and rugose while becoming fixed to the underlying lymph nodes and finally ruptures.

There is accompanying fever and constitutional symptoms like chills, rigor, arthralgia, myalgia along with loss of appetite and weakness which may precede or accompany the bubo. There is subsidence of these symptoms once the bubo ruptures.

The inguinal group of lymph nodes commonly undergoes suppuration with softening and rupture. Suppuration occurs as multiple foci with discharge of thick, grayish-white gluey pus. These sinuses may become secondarily infected, persist for months or finally undergo resolution. Bilateral involvement may result in gradual development of genital elephantiasis.

Q9. What are the possible sequelae of inguinal bubo?

Ans: Inguinal adenitis may soften and suppurate (60–70% cases), undergo spontaneous resolution (25–30%) or persist as a stationary mass (5%).

Q10. What is esthiomene?

Ans: This is the development of elephantiasis with chronic genital ulceration of the vulva due to inflammation and infection of the lymphatics draining this area.

The sites affected are the inner surface of the labia, fourchette, urethral orifice, root of the clitoris and the peri-anal area. The lesions are initially soft and smooth which become verrucous and mammillated leading to masses of hypertrophic tissue barricading the introitus. Ulcers if occur are chronic, non-healing and debilitating. Further involvement leads to formation of strictures in the urethral and vaginal mucosae. Perforating ulcers may lead to rectovaginal, urethrovaginal, cervicovaginal or vulval fistulae.

Q11. What is saxophone penis?

Ans: If there is chronic bilateral inguinal adenitis, penile and scrotal elephantiasis can occur. If the penis becomes solidified it is called ram rod penis. When it becomes twisted and curved, it appears like a saxophone, and hence the name. Sometimes subcutaneous swelling may develop along the dorsal lymphatics of the penis leading to lymphangitis. These are known as bubonuli.

Q12. What is triple syndrome?

Ans: When esthiomene occurs in association with strictures and changes in the rectum, anal canal, it is known as triple syndrome.

Q13. What is pseudobubo?

Ans: Pseudobubo is seen in donovanosis or granuloma inguinale caused by Calymmatobacterium granulomatis. Lymphatic involvement is not seen in donovanosis. The bacteria migrate from regional lymph nodes to overlying skin and form abscess leading to subcutaneous swellings. These subcutaneous swellings may be seen in inguinal region which can be easily mistaken for classical bubo of LGV. The term pseudobubo is used because there is no regional lymphadenitis. On Wright or Giemsa stain, Donovan bodies can be demonstrated.

Q14. How is inguinal bubo of chancroid different?

Ans: Chancroid is the second most important cause for inguinal bubo. It is caused by *Haemophilus ducreyi*. Here the incubation period in very short with a definitive history of an exquisitely painful ulcer over the genitalia following exposure. The bubo is commonly unilateral and tender. Matting of lymph nodes is less commonly seen. The swelling is unilocular and ruptures to form ulcers which heal with less scarring.

On laboratory examination, characteristic Gram negative coccobacilli are seen in typical "school of fish" or "railroad track" or "fingerprint" appearance. *H. ducreyi* can be isolated from the lesions on culture.

Q15. What is Groove sign of Greenblatt?

Ans: The femoral group of lymph nodes can be enlarged along with the inguinal group in about 20% of cases. When this is separated by the Poupart's ligament, a groove is produced which is considered to be pathognomonic of LGV.

Q16. What is Parinaud's syndrome?

Ans: This is one of the extracutaneous manifestation of LGV infection. It occurs due to autoinoculation in the eye leading to the development of unilateral follicular conjunctivitis along with regional lymphadenopathy.

Q17. What are the other cutaneous manifestations of LGV?

Ans: The various cutaneous manifestations in LGV include:

- Transient generalized exanthema

- Papular/papulonodular lesions, erythema nodosum or erythema multiforme
- Cutaneous photosensitivity causing itchy, papular and papulovesicular lesions in sun-exposed parts (Sonck solar dermatitis)
- Ulcerative lesions along the course of the affected lymphatics.

Q18. What is the treatment for inguinal bubo?

Ans: Inguinal bubo can be treated as a part of syndromic management as per the NACO guidelines. The goals of treatment are to kill the causative organism and render the patient non-infectious, to provide symptomatic relief and to prevent/minimize the complications.

- If lymphogranuloma venereum is the cause for the inguinal bubo treatment can be given with the following:
  - 1st line—Doxycycline 100 mg bid orally for 3 weeks or
  - 2nd line—Erythromycin base 500 mg qid orally for 3 weeks (pregnant women and nursing mothers, children less than 8 years of age and patients sensitive to doxycycline)
- For LGV proctocolitis—Empiric therapy with doxycycline (100 mg orally twice daily for 7 days) plus ceftriaxone (250 mg stat IM). If diagnosis confirmed, to continue doxy for 14 more days.

Other drugs that have been used for the treatment LGV are –

- Azithromycin 1 g orally one dose with doxycycline 100 mg bid for 7 days
- Minocycline 300 mg initially followed by 200 mg orally bid for 10 days
- Rifampicin 450 mg orally on empty stomach od for 10 days.

The treatment is same for HIV infected individuals except duration of treatment will be longer.

Q19. What is syndromic management for inguinal bubo?

Ans: Syndromic management of sexually transmitted infections is an approach to treat a patient on the basis of the presenting symptoms or syndromes without waiting for the etiological confirmations.

It has its own merits and demerits which are beyond the scope of discussion of this chapter.

The National AIDS Control Organization guidelines for syndromic management of inguinal bubo is given in Flowchart 1.

Q20. What is partner management for inguinal bubo?

Ans: All partners of the patient who have been in contact within the last 2 months must be treated for both LGV and chancroid. Treatment should include azithromycin 1 g single dose orally along with doxycycline 100 mg orally twice daily for 7 days. Counsel, educate the patient along with referral for voluntary counseling for HIV, syphilis and Hepatitis B. A return visit should be scheduled after 7 and 21 days.

Q21. What are the surgical methods for management of inguinal bubo and its complications?

Ans: Fluctuant buboes can be treated with hot fomentation followed by aspiration and drainage with a wide bore needle from a non-dependent part of the bubo. Strictures arising as a complication of LGV infection can be progressively dilated using Hegar's dilators. Strictures of the vulva, penis, scrotum, esthiomene and genital elephantiasis can be managed by reconstructive surgeries.

Flowchart 1: Management in inguinal bubo

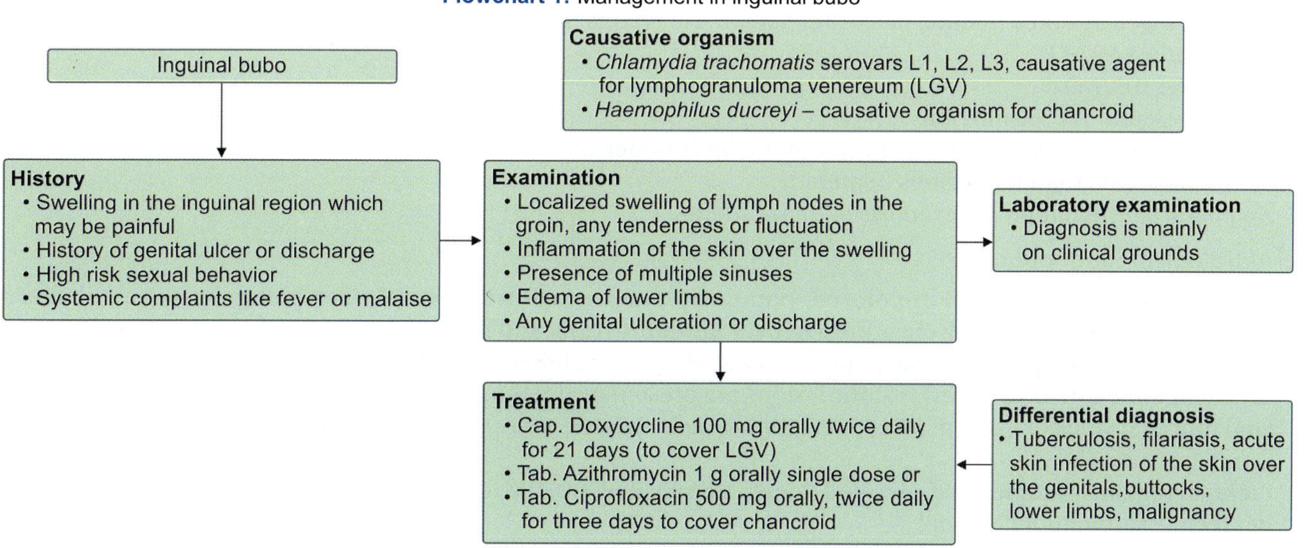

CHAPTER 42

Secondary Syphilis

Ankan Gupta

Case study Secondary Syphilis

Presenting Complaint

Doctor, I have a flaky red eruption over my trunk, palms and soles since the last 10 days.

Setting

Dermatology outpatient department.

History of Presenting Illness

A 42-year-old unmarried man presented with history of a generalized red scaly rash over the trunk and proximal limbs including the palms and soles for 10 days. There was no history of fever, photosensitivity, oral or genital lesions, joint pains, groin swelling, any neuropsychiatric symptoms or ocular redness. Patient gives history of two regular male sexual partners in the previous 6 months, and reported inconsistently protected oral and anal sex with both and a recent occurrence of similar generalized cutaneous lesions in one of them. There was no history of similar skin lesions, genital ulceration, or history suggestive of other sexually transmitted infections like genital growths or discharge in the past. There was no history of chronic cough, weight loss, jaundice, recurrent upper respiratory tract infection (URTI) or diarrhea. Patient was a postgraduate, working in entertainment industry and was addicted to alcohol, smoking tobacco and marijuana.

General Physical Examination

The patient is well oriented in time, place and person. He is conscious, well built and cooperative.

- Temperature: 99.6° F
- Pulse rate: 102/min
- Blood pressure: 100/60 mm Hg.
- Multiple, non-tender, mobile, firm, discrete lymph nodes of size 1–2 cm are felt in occipital, cervical, axillary, epitrochlear and inguinal regions bilaterally.
- No pallor, icterus, clubbing, cyanosis or pedal edema.

Dermatological Examination

- A bilaterally symmetrical skin-colored, papulosquamous rash with each lesion being discrete and sharply demarcated, measuring 0.5–2 cm is present over the entire trunk and flexures of arms. There is complete sparing of face and lower limbs. Deep dermal tenderness was elicitable in few lesions using back of a pin. Multiple, non-tender, erythematous, corn-like hyperkeratotic lesions are present over palms and soles (Fig. 1).
- Oral mucosa: Single, raised, fissured, flat topped, moist papule over right angle of mouth.
- Genitals: Normal.
- Perianal region: Multiple, pale, elevated, moist, sharply demarcated flat topped papules present
- Per rectal examination: Normal

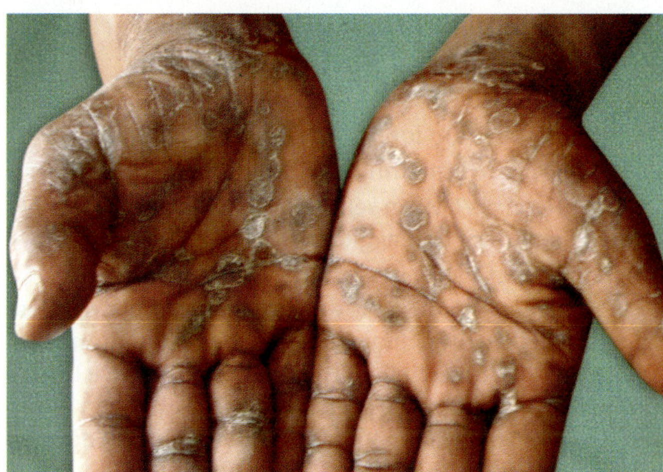

Fig. 1: Hyperkeratotic well-defined lesions on the palms

Q1. What is the first step in the management of this patient?

a. Performing a skin biopsy
b. Administration of intravenous antibiotics
c. Examination of the partner
d. Investigating for sexually transmitted infections (STIs) and HIV

Ans: d. (Investigating for STIs and HIV).

Although all the options are correct but the next best step would be to first establish the diagnosis by sending for a non-treponemal test and HIV-ELISA.

Q2. What important points in history can point towards the diagnosis of syphilis?

Ans: Presence of recent onset generalized psoriasiform rash involving the trunk, palms and soles, high promiscuity, absence of photosensitivity and history of similar lesions in partner point towards the diagnosis of secondary syphilis.

Q3. What are the other examination findings, likely to be seen in a case of secondary syphilis?

Ans: Clinical features in syphilis are unpredictable and can mimic any cutaneous disease and systemically can affect any organ. The cutaneous features include:

Corona veneris: A row of papules seen along the hairline on the forehead with sparing of face.

Generalized rash: Apart from the papulosquamous rash seen in this patient, macular, papular, pustular and rarely follicular, lichenoid (which can be pruritic), lenticular (which may involve face), bomb-shell or corymbose, annular and nodular (mimicking erythema nodosum leprosum) rash may also be seen.

Leukoderma syphiliticum: Also known as the 'necklace of Venus' signifies a resolving rash which has left behind depigmented patches, present over upper trunk.

Mucosa: Serpiginous ulcers, known as *"snail-track" ulcers,* are classically seen although the cutaneous syphilitic rash is seen intraorally too. Condyloma lata as classically described in the patient's perianal region.

Scalp: "Moth eaten" alopecia wherein irregular, non-scarring, patchy alopecia mostly at the margins and rarely in beard and eyebrows is classically seen in secondary syphilis. Telogen effluvium may coexist rarely.

Nails: Pitting, onycholysis, onychodystrophy, Beau's lines.

Systemic features

- *Constitutional symptoms:* Malaise, fever, nausea
- *Central nervous system:* Especially in people living with HIV and AIDS (PLHA) early neurosyphilis may be seen which is now considered to be a component of secondary syphilis rather than tertiary syphilis.
- Transaminitis
- Glomerulonephritis
- *Ocular symptoms:* Uveitis, iritis, iridocyclitis.

Q4. What is lues maligna?

Ans: An explosive, widespread or malignant form of secondary syphilis which starts as a prodrome and is followed by papulopustular cruptions that rapidly transform into necrotic, sharply demarcated ulcers with hemorrhagic brown crusts organized in rupoid layers. It is characterized by a very high venereal disease research laboratory (VDRL); rapid plasma regain (RPR) titer, Jarisch-Herxheimer reaction on treatment and a dramatic response to therapy (Fischer's criteria).

Q5. How will you manage this case?

Ans: Management:

- Confirm the diagnosis
  - Dark ground microscopy: Clean one of the condyloma lata with saline gauze and squeeze to produce a serous exudate which may be seen under a dark ground microscope to look for the characteristic 'cork-screw' movement of treponemes.
  - Direct fluorescent antibody test.
  - Gene PolA PCR or multiplex PCR positivity will prove beyond doubt the diagnosis of syphilis.
  - Non-treponemal and treponemal tests: See Case 2.
  - A skin biopsy would also aid the diagnosis and would show lymphocyte and plasma cell rich

infiltrate in papillary dermis extending onto the deep dermis. Few epithelioid granulomas may be seen too.

- Investigate for other STIs
  - Blood borne virus screen [human immunodeficiency virus (HIV), hepatitis B virus (HBV), and hepatitis C virus (HCV)].
  - IgM for herpes simplex or polymerase chain reaction.
  - Gram stain for chancroid.
  - Candidial scraping.
  - Urine routine examination for urethritis.
  - Complement fixation test or latex agglutination test for gonorrhea.
  - Enzyme immune assay for chlamydia trachomatis.
- Treat the patient
  - Benzathine penicillin 2.4 MU single dose intramuscularly OR Aqueous. Procaine penicillin 60,000 units intramuscularly every day for 10 days.
  - If the patient is allergic to penicillin, doxycycline 100mg twice daily orally for 14 days.
  - If doxycycline is contraindicated (e.g. pregnancy), though not relevant in this patient, penicillin desensitization can be done. Other alternatives though less effective, would include ceftriaxone 1 g intravenously twice daily for 5–10 days, erythromycin 2 g daily orally in four divided doses, azithromycin 500 mg orally once daily for 7–10 days and amoxicillin 2 g single twice daily with probenecid 0.5 g twice daily for 3 weeks.
- Counsel the patient about the illness, its implications, safe sex practices, condom use and chances of relapse of the rash.
- Partner tracing and treatment: Every partner during last 90 days and partners before 90 days who have positive serology are to be treated.
- Follow-up with VDRL titers at 1, 3, 6 and 12 months. Fourfold fall in titers at the end of 6 months in early syphilis and six months in late syphilis signifies cure. Failure of titer to fall should prompt cerebrospinal fluid examination. Fourfold rise in titer suggests reactivation or reinfection.

The patient recovered after management with above modalities. 10 weeks later, he had to undergo blood tests before he had to travel abroad for work purposes. His blood tests revealed VDRL positivity and was not being allowed to travel abroad, in spite of the fact that he was completely fit.

Q6. What is the next best step in the management of this patient?

a. Repeat VDRL
b. Retreat him for Syphilis
c. Declare him unfit for travelling
d. Repeat VDRL in serial dilution and do treponema pallidum hemagglutination (TPHA)

Ans: d (Repeat VDRL in serial dilution and do TPHA)

A reactive VDRL test without titers is meaningless as smaller titers may be seen in normal population as well. Biologically false positive (BFP) reaction to non-treponemal tests like VDRL may be seen in

- Certain genetically labile individuals who develop BFP after a URTI, LRTI, vaccination
- Pregnancy
- Infections like leprosy (more in lepromatous pole), tuberculosis, malaria, rickettsial infections, trypanosomiasis, leptospirosis, measles, infectious mononucleosis, etc.
- Connective tissue diseases like lupus erythematosus, rheumatoid arthritis, sarcoidosis
- Hodgkin's lymphoma
- Miscellaneous: Prolonged ether anesthesia.

A titer of more than or equal to 1:16 for VDRL in the absence of rash or greater than or equal to 1:8 in presence of cutaneous features would be suggestive of syphilis.

Treponemal tests like TPHA, fluorescent treponemal antibody-absorbed (FTA-ABS) are specific and become reactive earlier than non-treponemal tests but they persist for years, probably lifelong and hence can be used as screening for syphilis and not for measuring the disease activity or response to treatment. A fourfold fall in titers by 6 months is considered as adequate treatment response in early syphilis and 12 months in late syphilis.

Q7. What are the serological tests used in diagnosis of Syphilis? Explain the algorithm for diagnosis (Fig. 2).

Ans: Serological tests in syphilis are of two types:

1. Non-treponemal tests
   - VDRL
   - RPR
   - Toluidine red unheated serum test (TRUST)
2. Treponemal tests
   - TPHA
   - FTA-ABS
   - Microhemagglutination test for antibodies to Treponema pallidum (MHA-TP)

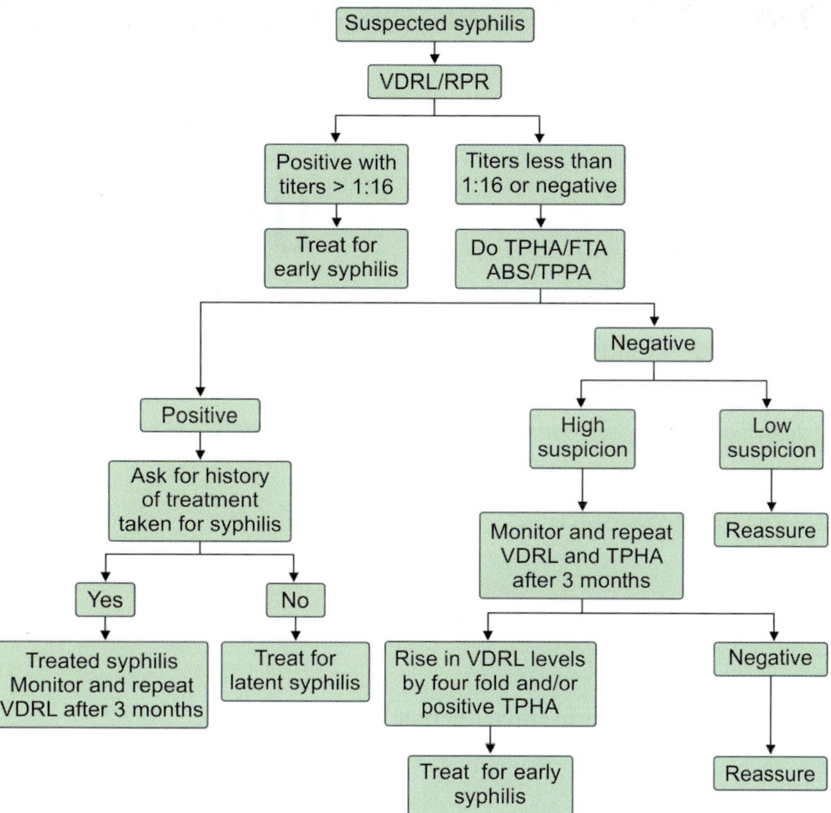

Fig. 2: Algorithm for diagnosis of syphilis

- Treponema pallidum particle agglutination assay (TP-PA)
- Treponema pallidum enzyme immunoassay (TP-EIA).

Q8. What is the treatment protocol for syphilis?

Ans: Treatment protocol:

a. Primary, secondary and early latent syphilis: Benzathine penicillin G 2.4 million units IM in a single dose (Children: Benzathine penicillin G 50,000 units/kg IM).
b. Tertiary and late latent syphilis: Benzathine penicillin G 7.2 million units total, administered as 3 doses of 2.4 million units IM each at 1-week intervals.
c. Neurosyphilis: Aqueous crystalline penicillin G 18–24 million units per day, administered as 3–4 million units IV every 4 hours or continuous infusion, for 10–14 days.
d. With HIV: no change in protocol.

CHAPTER 43

Urethral Discharge

Malcolm Pinto

Case study Urethral Discharge

Presenting Complaints

Doctor, I have yellowish discharge in my urine since the past 4 days.

Setting

Dermatology outpatient department.

History of Present Illness

A 28-year-old male presented with complaints of yellowish urethral discharge of 4 days duration. Initially he developed burning micturition which was followed 12 hours later by foul smelling yellowish discharge from urethra which continued to be present till the day he visited the hospital. He also gave history of sexual contact with a commercial sex worker 3 days prior to the onset of symptoms.

General Physical Examination and Systemic Examination

No abnormality detected.

Dermatological Examination

- Erythema of the urethral meatus with foul smelling, mucopurulent discharge from urethra (Fig. 1)
- No inguinal lymphadenopathy
- Per rectal examination was normal.

Q1. What is the most likely diagnosis?

a. Syphilis
b. Chancroid
c. Gonococcal urethritis
d. Non-gonococcal urethritis

Ans: c. (Gonococcal urethritis)

Presence of foul smelling, mucopurulent, urethral discharge and dysuria in the background of a short incubation period in a patient with high risk exposure clinches the diagnosis.

Q2. What are the different sites for specimen collection in a patient with gonorrhea?

Ans: Sites for specimen collection

- Heterosexual men: Urethral swab, first void urine
- Homosexual men: Urethral, rectal, oropharyngeal swab
- Women: primary site: endocervical canal
- Women: secondary site: urethra, vagina, rectum, oropharynx
- Disseminated infection: Blood culture.

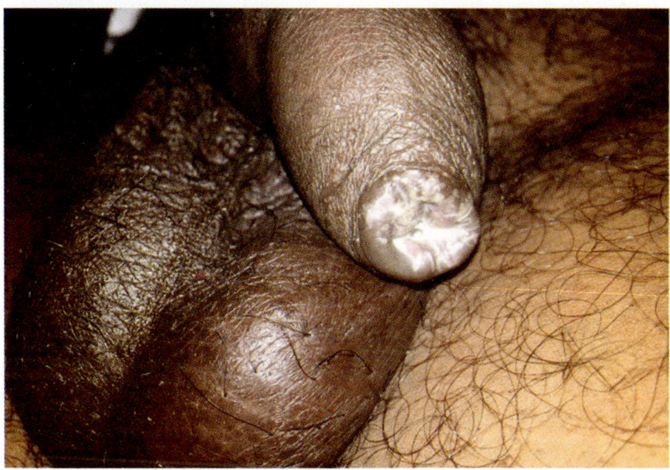

Fig. 1: Discharge from urethra

Table 1: Differentiation between gonococcal and nongonococcal urethritis

Parameter	*Gonococcal urethritis*	*Nongonococcal urethritis*
Incubation period	2-6 days	1-5 weeks with peak at 2-3weeks
Onset	Abrupt	Gradual
Constitutional symptoms	Fever, malaise	Absent
Discharge	Profuse, purulent and yellowish green	Scanty, mucoid or mucopurulent
Dysuria	Intense burning sensation	'Smarting' feeling in the urethra on passing urine

Q3. Describe the procedure of sample collection in a patient with urethral discharge.

Ans: The procedure is well described in Flowchart 1:

In women: Urethra is massaged against the pubic symphysis from its proximal end towards the meatus if no pus is visible.

Q4. Define urethritis.

Ans: Urethritis is the response of the urethra to inflammation of any etiology characterized by the physical finding of urethral discharge and laboratory findings of increased number of polymorphonuclear leukocytes (PMNL (number of PMNL) on Gram stain of a urethral smear or in the sediment of the first-voided urine.

Q5. List the organisms producing urethritis.

Ans: Gonococcal urethritis: *Neisseria gonorrhoeae.*

Non-gonococcal urethritis: *Chlamydia trachomatis, Trichomonas vaginalis, Mycoplasma genitalium, Ureaplasma urealyticum,* Herpes simplex virus (HSV) types 1 and 2, Adenovirus

Q6. How do you differentiate between gonococcal and nongonococcal urethritis?

Ans: Differentiation is given in Table 1.

Q7. How will you confirm the diagnosis of gonococcal urethritis?

Ans: Confirmation:

Gram stain of urethral discharge: Gram negative, encapsulated, diplococci (kidney-shaped cells with adjacent sides flattened) within PMNL.

Culture media (Gold Standard):

- Transport media: Stuart medium
- Non-selective media: Chocolate agar
- Selective media: Modified Thayer-Martin, modified New York City, Martin-Lewis, Chacko-Nair medium
- Presence of CO_2-enriched medium is very important.
- Colony morphology: Pathogenic strains: Small (0.1–1 mm diameter) translucent, nonpigmented to brownish colonies with fine granular surface.

Flowchart 1: The procedure of sample collection in a patient with urethral discharge

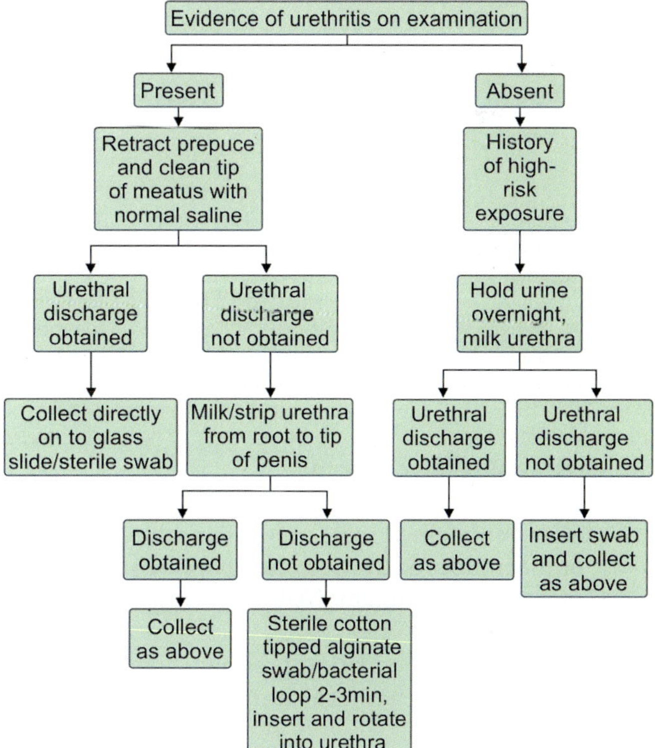

Biochemical test: Oxidase test positive: Purple staining.

Carbohydrate utilization test: Gonococci produce acid from glucose

Molecular diagnostic methods: Nucleic acid amplification test (NAAT), nucleic acid hybridization (NAH).

Q8. How will you confirm the diagnosis of non-gonococcal urethritis?

Ans. (A) Chlamydia

Specimen collected: Urethral exudates for gram staining.

For culture: A fiber-tipped swab with shaft made of inert material, from endocervix in females; or endourethal swabs (passed at least 5 cm into the urethra in males).

Specimens need to be transported in special transport media cooled by liquid nitrogen unless processed within 2 hours.

Gram stain	*Giemsa-Romanowsky stain*	*Cell line culture*	*DNA probes*	*PCR/ Ligase chain reaction (LCR)*
Absence of intracellular gram-negative diplococci	Inclusion (elementary) bodies within infected cells	McCoy cells (mouse fibroblasts) pretreated with idoxuridine, HeLa cells are used	These are less sensitive than culture	These are amplified DNA tests and are more sensitive than culture

(B) Genital Mycoplasma

M. genitalium is related to persistent or recurrent NGU after treatment of male urethritis with tetracyclines or macrolides and is detected more frequently from men with symptomatic NGU than those men without symptoms.

Specimen collected: Urine, prostatic secretions, blood (liquid specimen) on calcium alginate or polyester-tipped swabs.

Culture	*Serology*	*Polymerase chain reaction (PCR)*
Shepard's 10B broth and A8 agar Colony morphology: Urease-negative, fried egg appearance	Metabolism-Inhibition assays or ELISA	Sequence detection: MgPa adhesin gene of M. genitalium 16S rRNA gene PCR assays Transcription-mediated amplification (TMA) assay targeting the 16S rRNA

(C) Trichomoniasis

Per speculum examination	*Wet mount*	*Culture*
Cervix: Punctuate hemorrhages (strawberry cervix) Greenish-yellow foamy discharge in the vagina	Motile trichomonads with characteristic flagella and undulating membrane with jerky motility when examined with light microscopy under low power	Diamond's medium. Modified Feinberg-Whittington medium

(D) Adenoviral infection: Evaluate for adenoviral etiology in all cases of dysuria, scant discharge in addition to meatitis and/or conjunctivitis or recent sexual contact with partners with signs of acute upper respiratory infections. PCR assay is helpful.

Q9. What are the challenges in the existing routine diagnostic tests in a patient presenting with urethral discharge?

Ans:

Gonorrhea	*Chlamydia*	*Mycoplasma infections*	*Trichomoniasis*
Gram stain: Lower sensitivity (40–60%) in females	Stains (Giemsa, Machiavello-Giminez): Low sensitivity and specificity	Culture: Low sensitivity, time consuming	Wet mount microscopy: 50% sensitivity
Culture: Technically demanding, fastidious nature of gonococcus	Tissue culture (McCoy cell) gold standard: Technically demanding		Culture:Low sensitivity, technically demanding
Direct immunofluorescence (DIF), Enzyme immunoassay (EIA), Serology: Poor sensitivity and specificity	Antigen detection assays (DIF, EIA), Antibody detection (solid phase ELISAs): Poor sensitivity and specificity		

Q10. What are the applications of molecular diagnostic methods in a patient presenting with urethral discharge?

Ans: 1. Gonorrhea

Nucleic acid amplification test (NAAT): Sensitivity of NAAT (95%) is superior to culture, especially for rectal and pharyngeal swabs. Only NAAT for urethral swab is presently Food and Drug Administration (FDA), USA approved.

Nucleic acid hybridization (NAH)

Multiplex PCR. Advantages: Faster availability of results in <24 hours.

2. Chlamydia

   NAH: PACE 2 test (Probe Assay Chemiluminescence Enhanced) is a commercially available non-isotopic DNA probe for the detection of specific parts of r-RNA of *C. trachomatis* in the endocervical and urethral specimens.

   NAAT: This technique reduces the need for strict transport and storage of specimens, is highly sensitive and specific with freedom to use a wide variety of specimen types and can also be combined for the detection of *N. gonorrhoeae.*

Q11. What are the complications of urogenital gonorrhoea?

Ans: *Local complications: Males:* Epididymitis, lymphangitis, penile edema, periurethral abscess, prostatitis, phimosis, paraphimosis, tysonitis, littritis, cowperitis, seminal vesiculitis, trigonitis, watering-can perineum, sterility.

Females: Bartholin abscess, lymphangitis, skeinitis, parametritis, infertility, Pelvic inflammatory disease-salpingitis, pelvic abscess, pyosalpinx.

Systemic complications: Disseminated gonococcal infection- arthritis, tenosynovitis, endocarditis, myocarditis, hepatitis, pyelonephritis, Fitz Hugh-Curtis syndrome, septicemia.

Q12. Mention the pharmacological management of a patient with urethral discharge.

Ans:

Regimes	*(A) Uncomplicated gonococcal infections of urethra*	*(B) Complicated gonorrhea*	*(C) Chlamydial infections in adolescents and adults*
Recommended	Ceftriaxone 250 mg IM in a single dose PLUS Azithromycin 1g orally in a single dose	Ceftriaxone 1 g IM or IV every 24 hours PLUS Azithromycin 1 g orally in a single dose	Azithromycin 1 g orally in a single dose OR Doxycycline 100 mg orally twice a day for 7 days
Alternate	Cefixime 400 mg orally in a single dose PLUS Azithromycin 1 g orally in a single dose		Erythromycin base 500 mg orally qid for 7 days OR Erythromycin ethyl succinate 800 mg orally qid for 7 days OR Levofloxacin 500 mg orally od for 7 days OR Ofloxacin 300 mg orally bd for 7 days

Management of Sex Partners

Recent sex partners (i.e. persons having sexual contact with the infected patient within the 60 days preceding onset of symptoms) should be referred for evaluation, testing, and presumptive dual treatment.

Q13. Syndromic management in urethral discharge comprises treating the following microbes?

Flowchart 2: Approach: Syndromic management of urethral discharge

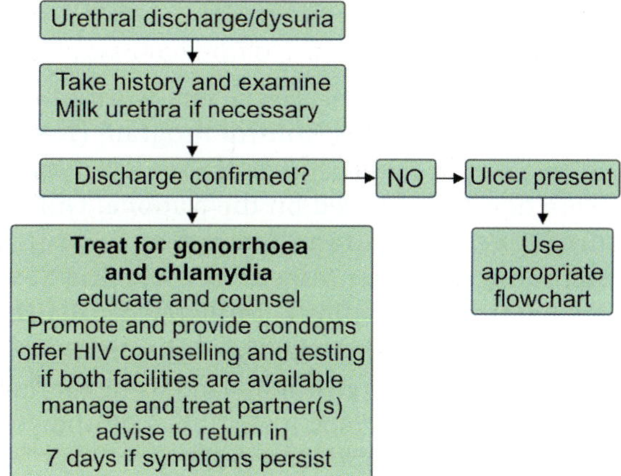

a. *Neisseria gonorrhoeae* and *Treponema pallidum*
b. *Chlamydia trachomatis* and *Mycoplasma genitalium*
c. *Neisseria gonorrhoea* and *Chlamydia trachomatis*
d. *Chlamydia trachomatis* and Herpes simplex virus-2

Ans: c. *Neisseria gonorrhoea* and *Chlamydia trachomatis*

Syndromic management refers to the approach of treating STI symptoms and signs based on the organisms most commonly responsible for each syndrome (Flowchart 2). For urethral discharge, it comprises of treating the patient for *Neisseria gonorrhoeae* and *Chlamydia trachomatis.* This leads to immediate treatment of the most important possible causative agents as mixed infections occur frequently in STI/RTI. This approach effectively treats cases in settings with limited or no laboratory facilities and quickly renders the patient non-infectious.

Q14. Name the color of the pre-packed STI/RTI kit used in the management of urethral discharge?

a. Yellow
b. Red

c. Green

d. Gray

Ans: c. Gray

Seven pre-packed STI/RTI kits were proposed under National Aids Control Program (NACP) III for syndromic management of STIs/RTIs. These kits were developed based on the National Guidelines on Prevention, Management and Control of Reproductive Tract Infections including Sexually Transmitted Infections, Ministry of Health and Family Welfare, August 2007.

Urethral discharge is managed using Kit number 1 which is gray in color. It has Tab. Azithromycin 1 g (1) and Tab. Cefixime 400 mg (1).

Various pre-packed STI/RTI kit used in syndromic management.

Kit No.	*Color*	*Indication*
1	Gray	Urethral discharge, cervicitis, anorectal discharge, painful scrotal swelling
2	Green	Vaginal discharge
3	White	Genital ulcer disease- Non Herpetic
4	Blue	Genital ulcer disease- Non Herpetic (Penicillin sensitive)
5	Red	Genital ulcer disease- Herpetic
6	Yellow	Lower abdominal pain
7	Black	Inguinal bubo

Q15. What is persistent and recurrent NGU?

Ans: Persistent NGU, when symptoms do not resolve following treatment, occurs in 15–25% of patients following initial treatment of acute NGU. Recurrent NGU is empirically defined as the recurrence of symptomatic urethritis occurring 30–90 days following treatment of acute NGU and occurs in 10–20% of patients.

Q16. What is the criteria for treatment failure in gonococcal urethritis?

Ans: Patients with gonorrhea should be retested 3 months after treatment.

Gonorrhea treatment failure should be suspected if:

- Symptoms remain for more than 7 days after initial antibiotic treatment with Kit 1 regimen (Cefixime 400 mg + Azithromycin 1 g)
- The patient remains positive for one of the following tests for *N. gonorrhoeae*
  - Presence of intracellular Gram-negative diplococci on microscopy taken at least 72 hours after completion of treatment; or
  - Isolation of *N. gonorrhoeae* by culture taken at least 72 hours after completion of treatment
  - Denies sexual contact during the post-treatment follow-up period.

CHAPTER 44

Vaginal Discharge

Anju George

Case study Vaginal Discharge

Presenting Complaints

Doctor, I am having severe itching in my genitalia and a burning sensation while passing urine since1week. I have observed that my underclothes are frequently getting stained with a whitish discharge.

Setting

Dermatology outpatient department.

History of Present Illness

A 32-year-old married lady presented to the dermatology outpatient department with complaints of pruritus in the genitalia along with dysuria of 1 week duration. She also complains of increased discharge per vagina, frequently staining her underclothes. The discharge is white, thick without any foul smell. She denies any extramarital contacts and her spouse is apparently symptom free. Last contact with spouse was 2 weeks ago, which was unprotected. Her menstrual cycles are regular. She has one child and currently she is on oral contraceptive pills (OCPs). There is no history of fever, abdominal pain, oral or genital ulcers, or similar complaints in the past.

General and Systemic Examination

No abnormalities detected.

Dermatological Examination

Examination of the genitalia revealed oedema and erythema of both labia majora and minora. Per speculum examination was painful and showed a thick curdy white discharge coating the vaginal walls, extending to the fornices. Cervix appears healthy. Rest of the dermatological examination was within normal limits

Q1. What is the most likely cause?

a. Bacterial vaginosis
b. Vulvovaginal candidiasis
c. Trichomoniasis
d. Gonorrhea

Ans: b. Vulvovaginal candidiasis. The diagnosis is based on the symptoms, thick curdy white discharge and intake of OCPs, all of which makes the patient more susceptible to candidial infection.

Q2. What are the characteristics of normal vaginal discharge?

Ans: A normal vaginal discharge is white, non-homogenous and floccular, with pH < 4.5. Microscopic examination reveals vaginal epithelial cells and large rods representing gram-positive lactobacilli which are normal inhabitants.

Q3. When should you suspect a vaginal infection and what are the common causes of vaginal discharge?

Ans: A spontaneous complaint of abnormal vaginal discharge (in terms of quantity, color or odour) is most commonly a result of a vaginal infection. It may be due to infectious and non-infectious causes.

- The three most common infectious causes of vaginal discharge are bacterial vaginosis (BV), trichomoniasis or trichomonal vaginitis (TV) and vulvovaginal candidiasis (VVC). *Neisseria gonorrhoeae* and *Chlamydia trachomatis* mostly cause cervical infection, which can manifest as vaginal discharge. The clinical detection of cervical infection is difficult because a large proportion of women with gonococcal or chlamydial cervical infection are asymptomatic. The symptom of abnormal vaginal discharge is highly indicative of vaginal infection, but poorly predictive for cervical infection.
- Rare infectious causes: Rarely *staphylococcus aureus, streptococcal sp., H. ducreyi, C. granulomatis, T. pallidum*, HSV, varicella zoster virus, enterobius sp., can produce vaginitis and may present with vaginal discharge. It may, in rare cases, be caused by mucopurulent STI-related cervicitis.

Q4. What are the non-infectious causes of vaginal discharge?

Ans:
- Traumatic: Due to foreign bodies
- Allergic and irritant: Depilatories, detergents, douches, spermicides, suppositories, condoms, menstrual pads
- Miscellaneous: Atrophic vaginitis, lichen sclerosus et atrophicus.

Q5. How will you approach a case of vaginal discharge and enumerate the basic investigations?

Ans:
- A detailed history is essential including menstrual history, obstetric history and sexual history
- Examination of external genitalia followed by a per speculum examination using a sterile Cusco's speculum. Note the color, amount, consistency and odour of the discharge. Look for whether the discharge is from the vagina or cervix (vaginal discharge/ cervicitis), cervical erosions and evidence of cervicitis
- Bimanual examination to elicit cervical motion tenderness or lower abdominal pain
- A provisional clinical diagnosis can be made based on the history, associated symptomatology and clinical examination
- The basic investigations to be done include determination of pH, a potassium hydroxide (KOH) test, microscopic examination of fresh samples of the discharge (wet smear examination), Gram stain and culture
- HIV counselling and testing should also be offered if both facilities are available.

Q6. What is the importance of pH examination of vaginal discharge?

Ans: The pH of the vaginal secretions can be determined by narrow-range pH paper; an elevated pH (i.e. ≥ 4.5) is common with BV or trichomoniasis.

Q7. What is wet mount examination and what is its significance?

Ans: As pH testing is not highly specific, the discharge should be further examined microscopically. Specimens for the wet smear examination are taken from the posterior fornix with a sterilized cotton swab and diluted with one or two drops of 0.9% normal saline solution on a clean glass slide. A coverslip is placed and it is examined microscopically under low and high power. Wet mount testing can detect trichomoniasis and bacterial vaginosis.

- A diagnosis of trichomoniasis is made if the wet mount shows pear-shaped organisms with characteristic jerky movements (motile flagellate organisms or trichomonads).
- The presence of clue cells points to a diagnosis of bacterial vaginosis. Clue cells are vaginal epithelial cells with granular surface and obscured borders due to adherent coccobacilli.

Q8. What is the significance of KOH mount examination?

Ans: A drop of 10% KOH is added to the vaginal secretions taken on a clean glass slide and mounted with a cover-slip. Candidal organisms can be identifed as highly refractile, round or oval budding yeast cells (hyphae or blastospores). A fishy odour of vaginal discharge before or after addition of 10% KOH suggests bacterial vaginosis (i.e. the whiff test or amine test). It is not a sensitive test as a similar odour may be seen in trichomoniasis also.

Q9. Will a negative wet mount and KOH examination rule out infection?

Ans: No. The absence of trichomonads in saline or fungal elements in KOH samples does not rule out these infections as the sensitivity of these tests is low.

Q10. What is the role of a Gram stain in diagnosis?

Ans: A Gram-stained smear of the discharge should be examined for the following:

- Intracellular Gram-negative diplococci-gonococcal infection
- Clue cells–Bacterial vaginosis
- Gram-positive pseudohyphae with budding yeast cells- candidal infection.

Q11. In which of the following conditions is the normal vaginal lactobacilli replaced by anaerobic organisms?

a. Vulvovaginal candidiasis
b. Trichomoniasis
c. Chlamydial infection
d. Bacterial vaginosis

Ans: d. Bacterial vaginosis

Bacterial vaginosis is a polymicrobial clinical syndrome resulting from replacement of the normal hydrogen peroxide producing Lactobacillus sp. in the vagina, with high concentrations of anaerobic bacteria (e.g. Prevotella sp. and Mobiluncus sp.), *G. vaginalis*, Ureaplasma, Mycoplasma, and numerous fastidious or uncultivated anaerobes.

Q12. What are the risk factors associated with bacterial vaginosis?

Ans: Multiple male or female partners, a new sex partner, douching, lack of condom use, use of IUCDs and lack of vaginal lactobacilli are the risk factors for developing infection. Women who have never been sexually active are rarely affected. Nonetheless, women with BV are at increased risk for the acquisition of some STDs (e.g., HIV, *N. gonorrhoeae*, *C. trachomatis*, and HSV-2), complications after gynecologic surgery, complications of pregnancy, and recurrence of BV.

Q13. How will you diagnose BV?

Ans: Diagnosis:

- A diagnosis can be made based on the clinical criteria known as Amsel's Diagnostic Criteria, by a Gram stain or by demonstrating clue cells on wet mount examination
- A Gram stain is used to determine the relative concentration of lactobacilli, gram-negative and gram-variable rods and cocci (i.e. *G. vaginalis*, Prevotella, Porphyromonas, and peptostreptococci), and curved gram-negative rods (i.e. Mobiluncus) characteristic of BV. It is considered to be the gold standard laboratory method for diagnosing BV.
- Culture of *G. vaginalis* is not specific and does not have much utility as a diagnostic tool.
- Cervical Pap tests are also not recommended in the diagnosis in view of their low sensitivity and specificity.

Q14. What is Amsel's diagnostic criteria for diagnosis of BV?

Ans: The criteria requires three of the following symptoms or signs:

- Homogeneous, thin, white discharge that smoothly coats the vaginal walls
- Clue cells (e.g. vaginal epithelial cells studded with adherent coccoobacilli) on microscopic examination
- pH of vaginal fluid >4.5 or
- A fishy odor of vaginal discharge before or after addition of 10% KOH (i.e. the whiff test).
- Detection of three of these criteria has been correlated with results by Gram stain.

Q15. What is Nugent score?

Ans: This is a scoring system to diagnose BV based on Gram staining of vaginal smears. It is considered to have superior reproducibility and sensitivity compared to Amsel's criteria. The score ranges from 0 to 10 and is calculated as follows:

- Presence of large gram-positive rods (lactobacillus-morphotypes; decrease in lactobacillus, scored as 0 to 4)
- Small gram-variable rods (*G.vaginalis* morphotypes; scored as 0 to 4)
- Curved gram-variable rods (Mobiluncus sp. morphotypes; scored as 0 to 2)
- A score of 7 to 10 is consistent with BV.

Q16. What are the other diagnostic tests for BV?

Ans: Other diagnostic tests for BV:

- Affirm VP III: A DNA hybridization probe test that detects high concentrations of *G. vaginalis*
- OSOM BV Blue test: Detects vaginal fluid sialidase activity
- Proline aminopeptidase card test: For the detection of elevated pH and trimethylamine. However, it is not recommended as it lacks sensitivity and specificity
- Recent evidence suggests that PCR can be tried for the detection of a variety of organisms associated with BV, but a thorough evaluation of its clinical

utility is still underway. Detection of specific organisms might be predictive of BV by PCR.

Q17. What is the pregnancy outcome in a case of BV?

Ans: Premature rupture of membranes, preterm labor, preterm birth, intra-amniotic infection, and postpartum endometritis have been associated with symptomatic BV in some observational studies.

Q18. How do you treat a case of bacterial vaginosis?

Ans:
- Metronidazole 500 mg orally twice a day for 7 days OR
- Tinidazole 2 g orally once daily for 2 days OR
- Tinidazole 1 g orally once daily for 5 days OR
- Clindamycin 300 mg orally twice daily for 7 days OR
- Clindamycin ovules 100 mg intravaginally once at bedtime for 3 days
- Metronidazole gel 0.75%, one full applicator (5 g) intravaginally, once a day for 5 days OR
- Clindamycin cream 2%, one full applicator (5 g) intravaginally at bedtime for 7 days.

Q19. Will lactobacillus replacement therapy help in the treatment of BV?

Ans: Many trials have been done to evaluate the clinical and microbiologic efficacy of using intravaginal lactobacillus formulations to treat BV and restore the normal flora. But there is no proven evidence to suggest lactobacillus formulations or probiotics as an adjunctive or replacement therapy in women with BV. More studies are needed to gain good insight into these treatment options.

Q20. What is the classical presentation of trichomoniasis?

Ans: TV is characterized by discharge that is diffuse, malodorous, yellow-green with or without vulvar irritation. Local pain and abnormal vaginal bleeding due to co-existing cervicitis may also occur. However, most infected persons (70–85%) have minimal or no symptoms, and untreated infections might last for months to years.

Q21. What is the cause for the yellowish green color of discharge?

Ans: The color is due to the myeloperoxidase pigment in the polymorphonuclear leukocytes.

Q22. What is colpitis macularis?

Ans: In trichomonal infection, the cervix appears erythematous with punctuate hemorrhages and erosions. This is known as colpitis macularis or 'strawberry' cervix.

Q23. Are there any risks in pregnant women with TV?

Ans: In pregnant women the infection is associated with adverse pregnancy outcomes like premature rupture of membranes, preterm delivery, and delivery of a low birth-weight infant.

Q24. How will you confirm the diagnosis of TV?

Ans: Wet mount examination may help in the diagnosis as already described above. pH will be >4.5. Diagnosis is confirmed by culture of the protozoan, which is 100% specific.

Q25. Name the media used for culture of the organism?

Ans: Feinberg-Whittington medium, modified Diamond medium and Kupferberg medium are the common media used for culture.

Q26. What are the newer molecular detection methods in trichomoniasis?

Ans:
- OSOM trichomonas rapid test: An antigen-detection test using immunochromatographic capillary flow dipstick technology
- Affirm VP III: A DNA hybridization probe test that evaluates for *T. vaginalis*, *G. vaginalis*, and *Candida albicans*.

These tests have been FDA approved for detection of trichomonas vaginalis in vaginal secretions.

Q27. What are the treatment regimens for trichomonal vaginitis?

Ans: *Recommended Regimen*
- Metronidazole 2 g orally in a single dose OR
- Tinidazole 2 g orally in a single dose.

Alternative Regimen
- Metronidazole 500 mg orally twice a day for 7 days.

Q28. How will you classify vulvovaginal candidiasis?

Ans:

Uncomplicated VVC	*Complicated VVC*
Sporadic or infrequent VVC	Recurrent VVC
Mild to moderate VVC	Severe VVC
Likely to be due to *C. albicans*	Non C. albicans candidiasis
VVC in non-immunocompromised women	VVC in uncontrolled diabetes, debilitation, immunosuppression and pregnant women

Q29. What is the usual clinical presentation in VVC?

Ans: Severe vulvar pruritus, dysuria, dyspareunia, discharge, pain, swelling, and redness are the chief presenting complaints. Clinical signs include vulvar edema, fissures, excoriations, and thick white curdy or cottage cheese-like vaginal discharge.

Q30. How do you confirm the diagnosis of VVC?

Ans: The diagnosis can be made when either (a) a wet preparation (saline, 10% KOH) or Gram stain of vaginal discharge which demonstrates budding yeasts, hyphae, or pseudohyphae or (b) a culture or other test yields a positive result for a yeast species. Diagnosis is confirmed by culture on Sabouraud's agar. Vaginal pH is usually normal (<4.5).

Q31. Enumerate the treatment regimens for uncomplicated VVC as recommended by CDC?

Ans: *Over-the-Counter Intravaginal Agents*:

- Clotrimazole 1% cream 5 g intravaginally daily for 7–14 days OR
- Clotrimazole 2% cream 5 g intravaginally daily for 3 days OR
- Miconazole 2% cream 5 g intravaginally daily for 7 days OR
- Miconazole 4% cream 5 g intravaginally daily for 3 days OR
- Miconazole 100 mg vaginal suppository, one suppository daily for 7 days OR
- Miconazole 200 mg vaginal suppository, one suppository for 3 days OR
- Miconazole 1,200 mg vaginal suppository, one suppository for 1 day.

Oral Agent:

- Fluconazole 150 mg orally in a single dose.

Q32. How will you manage a pregnant lady with vaginal discharge?

Ans: Follow the same protocol of examination and investigations to arrive at the diagnosis.

- Pregnancy and BV: Treatment is recommended for all symptomatic pregnant women. Metronidazole 500 mg orally twice a day or metronidazole 250 mg orally thrice a day for 7 days can be used
- Pregnancy and TV: Symptomatic pregnant women, regardless of pregnancy stage, should be tested and considered for treatment. Metronidazole 2 g orally in a single dose may be given
- Pregnancy and VVC: Only topical azoles applied for 7 days, are recommended for use among pregnant women.

Q33. What will be your line of management if an HIV positive patient presents with vaginal discharge?

Ans: Investigations as mentioned before. Treatment is as follows:

- HIV and BV: Occurs with a higher frequency. Treatment is the same for HIV positive and negative patients
- HIV and TV : It has been suggested that to improve cure rates, trichomoniasis coexisting with HIV infection should be treated with metronidazole 500 mg orally twice daily for 7 days (rather than with a 2 g single dose of metronidazole)
- HIV and VVC: Symptomatic VVC is more frequent in women with HIV infection and also correlates with the severity of immunodeficiency. Studies have shown that therapy for uncomplicated and complicated VVC in women with HIV infection should not differ from that for seronegative women.

Q34. How will you differentiate the three common causes of vaginal discharge.

Ans:

Disease	*Bacterial vaginosis*	*Trichomoniasis*	*Vulvovaginal candidiasis*
Etiology	*Gardnerella vaginalis, Mycoplasma hominis*, Prevotella sp., Mobiluncus sp., Ureaplasma	*Trichomonas vaginalis*	*Candida albicans* and other yeasts
Symptoms	Foul smelling vaginal discharge	Diffuse malodorous yellow-green discharge, local pain, irritation, abnormal vaginal bleeding	External dysuria and vulvar pruritus, pain, swelling and redness
Clinical findings	No signs of inflammation	Erythema of vulva and vagina, raised punctuate erythema of cervix and upper vagina (strawberry cervix)	Vulvar edema, fissures, excoriations
Nature of discharge	Homogeneous, thin, white discharge that smoothly coats the vaginal walls	Copious, frothy, malodorous, yellowish green	Thick, curdy white discharge
pH	>4.5	>4.5	<4.5
Diagnosis	Clue cells in gram stain and wet mount examination, positive whiff test on addition of 10% KOH.	Motile trichomonads on wet mount with leucocytes and confirmed by culture.	Presence of hyphae or blastospores on a KOH mount; confirmed by culture.

Q35. What is the syndromic treatment for vaginal infection recommended by WHO?

Ans: In a case of vaginal infection, WHO recommends therapy for *T. vaginalis* PLUS therapy for bacterial vaginosis and, where indicated,therapy for *C. albicans* infection.

CHAPTER 45

Genital Warts

Amina Asafiya

Case study Genital Warts

Presenting Complaints

Doctor, I have multiple growths on my genitalia since 3 months. They do not cause me any discomfort but they are slowly increasing in number and size.

Setting

STD Clinic.

History of Present Illness

A 30-year-old male, unmarried, driver by occupation, presented to the STD clinic with complaints of asymptomatic skin colored growths over the external genitalia since 3 months. Initially they were few in number, smaller in size and gradually progressed to the present size. On enquiry he gives history of unprotected penovaginal sexual contact with multiple partners with the last exposure being 2 weeks ago. He gives history of alcohol abuse. No history of oral/anal intercourse.

General Physical Examination and Systemic Examination

No abnormality detected.

Dermatological Examination

- Multiple, soft, pink to skin colored papules with a warty surface present on the coronal sulcus and the undersurface of the prepuce (Fig. 1)
- Rest of the external genitalia : No abnormality detected
- Perianal examination and Per rectal examination: No abnormality detected.

Q1. What is the most likely diagnosis based on history and physical examination?

a. Pearly penile papules

b. Genital warts

c. Skin tags

d. Molluscum contagiosum

Ans: b. Genital warts. Asymptomatic soft, skin colored warty papules with the background of high risk behavior suggests that the most likely diagnosis is genital warts. It is sexually transmitted and caused by the human papillomavirus (HPV). The average incubation period is 3- 8 months.

Q2. Describe the basic structure of Human Papillomavirus.

Ans: Structure:

- Unenveloped double stranded DNA virus, > 100 different genotypes are present.
- Family: Papovaviridae

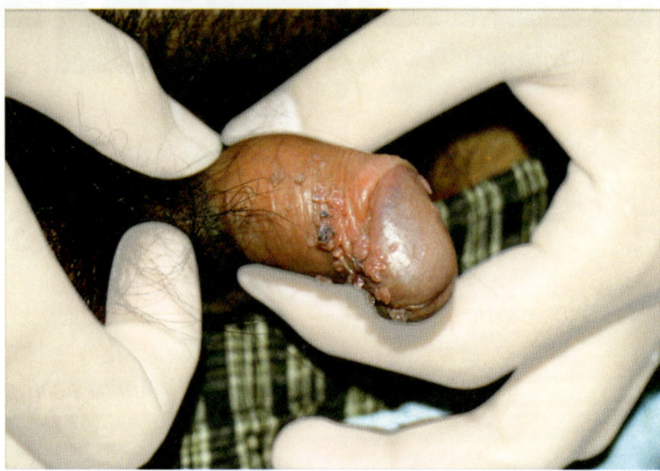

Fig. 1: Multiple, soft, pink to skin colored papules with a warty surface present on the coronal sulcus and the undersurface of the prepuce

- 55 nm size, 7.2–8.0 Kbp
- Outer coat –
  - 72 pentameric capsomers
  - Major and minor capsid proteins arranged on a skewed icosahedral lattice
- Genes are distributed into :
  - Early (E_1-E_7): Regulation of viral DNA replication and transcription, involved in oncogenic transformation (E_6, E_7)
  - Late (L_1-L_2): Encode major and minor capsid protein
- Alpha-papillomavirus: Responsible for cutaneous and mucosal HPV
- Beta-papillomavirus: Responsible for epidermodysplasia verruciformis.

Q3. Which is the most common HPV strain causing genital warts?

a. HPV 18
b. HPV 16
c. HPV 33
d. HPV 6 and 11

Ans: d. HPV 6 and 11—approximately 90%.

Q4. Describe the oncogenic potential of various HPV types.

Ans: Oncogenic potentia:

- Low/no oncogenic risk - HPV 6, 11, 42, 43, 44
- Intermediate risk - HPV 31, 33, 35, 51, 52
- High risk
  - HPV 16, 18, 45, 46
  - HPV 16 is most oncogenic.

Q5. What are the morphological types of genital warts?

Ans: There are four morphological types of genital warts:

1. Condylomata acuminata: Cauliflower shaped, occur on moist surfaces
2. Smooth papular warts:1-4-mm, skin-colored, dome-shaped papules
3. Keratotic genital warts: Thick, horny layer, resemble common warts or seborrheic keratosis
4. Flat warts: Flat to slightly raised, flat-topped papules.

Q6. What are the differential diagnoses for a genital wart?

Ans: Differential diagnosis:

- *Normal anatomic structures:* Pearly penile papules, Vestibular papillae, Sebaceous glands
- *Acquired conditions:* Bowenoid papulosis, condyloma lata, Molluscum contagiosum, Crohn's disease, Seborrheic keratosis, Lichen planus, Lichen nitidus, Skin tags, Melanocytic nevi, Pseudoverrucous papules, Condyloma lata, Bowenoid papulosis, Vulvar intraepithelial neoplasia (in women), Buschke-Lowenstein tumor.

Q7. What is the histopathology of a genital wart?

Ans:

- Minimal hyperkeratosis
- Papillomatosis
- Acanthosis
- Elongation of rete ridges
- Mitotic figures
- Most characteristic: Areas of epithelial cells showing distinct perinuclear vacuolization-Koilocytes
- Viral antigen can be demonstrated in nuclei of cells in stratum granulosum.

Q8. How do you diagnose a case of genital warts?

Ans: Diagnosis is mainly on clinical grounds:

- Speculum examination: To look for vaginal and cervical warts
- Subclinical infections: acetic acid (3–5%) is applied on the suspicious areas for 5–10 minutes. Neoplastic and dysplastic tissues turn white
- Biopsy: Not indicated routinely

- Meatoscopy/proctoscopy: To look for intraurethral and perianal warts.
- Serology: Limited value
- HPV DNA detection: Southern blot hybridization, dot blot, in situ hybridization and PCR
- Detection and typing of HPV
- Serology to look for other STD is must. HIV, hepatitis B and hepatitis C, VDRL in self and partner.

Q9. What are the treatment options available for genital warts?

Ans: Topical (As per CDC guidelines – patient applied and physician office treatment)

- Podophyllotoxin 0.5% solution/0.15% cream: Applied with cotton swab twice daily for 3 days followed by 4 days of no therapy. Total of 4 cycles
- Podophyllin: Applied by the physician using cotton tipped swabs once/twice a week upto 6 weeks
- Imiquimod 5% cream: 3 times/week upto 16 weeks, area washed with soap and water 6–10 hours after application
- 5- Fluorouracil : Applied once/twice per day
- Sinecatechins 15% ointment: Derived from the leaves of green tea (*Camellia sinensis)*, applied 3 times/day upto 250 mg per application

Destructive and surgical:

- Trichloroacetic acid: 80 - 90% solution used
- Cryotherapy: At weekly intervals
- Electrosurgery
- Scissor excision
- CO_2 laser

Systemic:

- Interferons.

Q10. A primigravida with 35 weeks of gestation presents to the OPD with an asymptomatic mass in the groin which is increasing in size during pregnancy. On examination, well defined, hyperpigmented plaque with a verrous surface present over the left labia majora with multiple discrete warty papules in the vicinity.

Which of the following is contraindicated in the management of this patient?

a. Liquid nitrogen
b. Trichloroacetic acid
c. Electrocautery
d. Podophyllin

Ans: d. Podophyllin is contraindicated due to its potential teratogenicity. Other options including laser ablation are safe in pregnancy.

Genital warts grow rapidly in pregnancy due to depressed immunity and increased vascularity.

- Indication for cesarean section: Extensive vaginal or introital warts which block the birth canal.
- Perinatal transmission can give rise to laryngeal papillomatosis- Juvenile Onset Recurrent Respiratory Papillomatosis (JORRP).

Q11. Which are the vaccines available against HPV?

Ans:

	Bivalent vaccine (Cervarix)	Quadrivalent vaccine (Gardasil)
FDA Approval	2009 for females	2006- females, 2009- males
Antigens	HPV 16, 18	HPV 6,11,16,18
Route of administration	Intramuscular	Intramuscular
Schedule	0.5 ml at 0,1 and 6 months	0.5 ml at 0, 2 and 6 months
Cost	Costly	Cheaper
Prevents	Anogenital cancers, subset of head and neck cancers	Anogenital cancers, subset of head and neck cancers. Anogenital warts and laryngeal papillomas

Vaccines are effective when all doses are administered before sexual contact

Recommended for 11–12-year-old girls.

Q12. Does vaccination provide immunity after acquiring the infection?

Ans: HPV vaccines provide protection against new infections but have no effect on the clinical disease in those who have already acquired the infection with the vaccine HPV types.

Q13. How will you counsel a patient with t genital warts regarding treatment and prevention of transmission?

Ans: Counseling:

- Patients should be educated about the cause, treatment options and complications of genital warts such as malignancy in those infected with high risk types.
- Female patients should be advised about the need for regular cervical cytology screening.
- Recurrence is common in the first 3 months after treatment.
- Use of barrier protection is advised till the successful treatment completion.

CHAPTER 46

Human Immunodeficiency Virus Infection

Shekhar Neema

Case study HIV Infection

Presenting Complaints

Doctor, I have a white-colored lesion on the side of my tongue for the last 3 months and I feel that I have also become thinner since the same duration.

Setting

Dermatology outpatient department (OPD).

History of Present Illness

A 28-year-old married male presented to the dermatology OPD with complaints of a white-colored asymptomatic lesion on the tongue for the last 3 months. He also gave history of losing 6 kg of weight in the last 3 months. There was no history of diarrhea, fever or any other systemic complaints. He gives history of multiple, unprotected sexual exposure to commercial sex workers 2 years ago. He is a nonsmoker and does not consume alcohol.

General Physical Examination

- Body mass index (BMI): 17 kg/m^2
- Pulse: 80 beats/min
- Pallor: Present
- Generalized lymphadenopathy: Present.

Systemic Examination

No abnormality detected.

Dermatological Examination

White-colored, vertically-ripped plaque on lateral aspect of tongue (Fig. 1). Right great toe nail-appears white proximally.

Q1. What is the most likely diagnosis?

a. Squamous cell carcinoma (SCC) of oral cavity
b. Human immunodeficiency virus (HIV)
c. Diabetes
d. Lymphoma

Ans: b. HIV. Oral hairy leukoplakia and proximal subungual onychomycosis in a sexually active male with history of unprotected sexual exposure is a strong indicator towards presence of underlying HIV infection.

Q2. How do you diagnose HIV infection?

Ans: An HIV infection can be diagnosed by detection of either antigen or antibody in the blood of an infected individual.

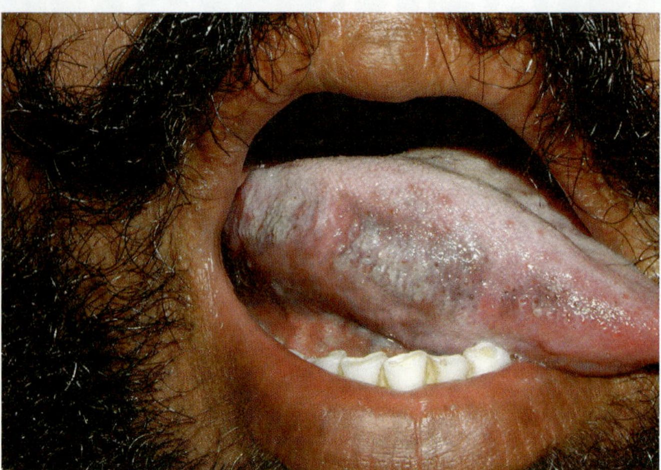

Fig. 1: Rippled white lesions along lateral margin of tongue

Detection of antibody: It is more commonly performed in routine clinical practice. Tests can also be classified as screening and confirmatory tests.

- Screening tests are those which are inexpensive and have higher sensitivity. Available screening tests are:
  - Enzyme-linked immunosorbent assay (ELISA): Most widely used, takes about 3 hours.
  - Rapid test: It takes less than 30 min to give result. It is more expensive than ELISA; however, it is easy to perform and interpret, e.g. immunoblot assay.
  - Simple test: Easy to perform, takes approximately 30 minutes, e.g. particle agglutination tests.
- Confirmatory test (Western blot assay): Highly-specific and sensitive. However, it is very expensive, requires expertise and can give indeterminate result.

Due to nonavailability and high cost incurred on confirmatory test, a strategy is adopted where ELISA by different methods to confirm the diagnosis of HIV infection.

In symptomatic individuals, two out of three tests performed is considered positive for HIV infection. In asymptomatic individuals, all three tests need to be positive for a confirmed diagnosis. Indeterminate test result is confirmed by Western blot method.

Since HIV is associated with social stigma and has profound impact on life of individual, it is mandatory that pretest counseling and posttest counseling is done before and after performing these tests.

Q3. What is window period?

Ans: Window period is the period during which presence of HIV infection cannot be determined by available tests. It depends on test performed. Minimum window period for antibody-based test is 22 days. P_{24} antigen detection reduces window period to 16 days and HIV polymerase chain reaction (PCR) reduces it to 11 days.

Q4. What are the cutaneous manifestations of HIV infection?

Ans: An HIV infection starts with acute retroviral infection, followed by asymptomatic stage, early symptomatic and late symptomatic stage. Cutaneous manifestation of HIV infection depends on the stage of HIV infection.

Acute retroviral syndrome: Patient presents with skin rash which can be morbilliform or papulosquamous. Patients can have generalized lymphadenopathy and other constitutional features like fever and headache. It can be indistinguishable from other viral exanthema.

Symptomatic stage: Cutaneous manifestation depends on etiology and can be classified as infectious, inflammatory or malignant (Table 1).

Apart from these lesions, cutaneous manifestations can occur as a part of immune reconstitution inflammatory syndrome (IRIS) and adverse cutaneous drug reactions (ACDRs).

- *Immune reconstitution inflammatory syndrome*: Paradoxical worsening of symptoms after institution of highly-active antiretroviral therapy (HAART) regimen. It occurs more commonly when HAART is administered in presence of high viral load and low CD4 count. IRIS can present as herpes zoster, herpes simplex, molluscum contagiosum (MC) and tuberculosis (TB) to name a few condition.
- *Adverse cutaneous drug reaction*: Cutaneous ACDRs are common after institution of antiretroviral therapy (ART). Hypersensitivity reactions can occur to nevirapine, efavirenz, abacavir or amprenavir. Lipodystrophy can occur with protease inhibitors (PIs) or nucleoside reverse transcriptase inhibitors (NRTIs). Zidovudine can result in longitudinal melanonychia or trichomegaly.

Q5. How will you manage patients with HIV infection?

Ans: After confirmation of diagnosis, evaluation is performed to rule out underlying opportunistic infections and presence of coinfection. CD4 count is done to know degree of immune suppression. Test performed are: Complete blood count (CBC), renal function test and liver function test (LFT), chest X-ray and Mantoux to rule out TB, venereal disease research laboratory (VDRL), hepatitis B surface

Table 1: Classification of cutaneous manifestation of HIV infection

	Infections
Bacterial	• *Staphylococcus aureus:* Increased incidence • Increased incidence of MRSA • TB: Increased incidence of TB • Atypical mycobacterial infections: *Mycobacterium avium-intracellulare* • Bacterial STI: Gonorrhea, syphilis, chancroid—more common and atypical • Bacillary angiomatoses
Fungal	• Dermatophytosis: Extensive, recurrent • Proximal subungual onychomycosis • Candidiasis: Oropharyngeal, esophageal, disseminated • Invasive fungal infection: Histoplasmosis, cryptococcosis, aspergillosis, penicilliosis, coccidioidomycosis
Viral	• Molluscum contagiosum (MC) 2 virus more common, genital and facial molluscum in adults • HPV infection: Genital warts, extensive warts mimicking EDV, oral warts • Oral hairy leukoplakia: EBV associated • Herpes zoster: multidermatomal (>2 non-contiguous dermatome), disseminated (>20 lesions outside primary dermatome), chronic • Herpes simplex: Herpes genitalis
Parasitic	• Leishmaniasis: Recurrent infection and more difficult to treat • Norwegian scabies, demodicosis
	Inflammatory
Pruritic conditions	• Papular pruritic eruption of HIV: Late symptomatic stage, CD4 < 50 cells/μL • Eosinophilic folliculitis: CD4 < 125 cells/μL, folliculocentric erythematous papules above nipple line, peripheral eosinophilia • Xerosls, Ichthyosls
Papulosquamous	• Psoriasis: Difficult to treat, higher incidence of arthritis • Reactive arthritis
Others	• Seborrheic dermatitis: The most common cutaneous manifestation • Photosensitivity, pigmentary disorders (Addisonian pigmentation, melanonychia), trichomegaly, alopecia
	Malignancy
	• HPV-induced neoplasia: SCC of cervix, anogenital area, penis • Non-Hodgkin β cell lymphoma, Hodgkin disease, primary CNS lymphoma • Kaposi sarcoma, increased incidence of SCC and Merkel cell carcinoma

Abbreviations: MRSA, methicillin-resistant *Staphylococcus aureus*; TB, tuberculosis; STI, sexually-transmitted disease; EDV, epidermodysplasia verruciformis; EBV, Epstein-Barr virus; HPV, human papillomavirus; CNS, central nervous system; SCC, squamous cell carcinoma

antigen (HBsAg) and anti-hepatitis C virus (HCV), ultrasound of abdomen, blood sugar and lipid profile.

When CD4 count is less than 350 cells/μL, HAART is started. Available HAART drugs are given in Table 2.

Goal of treatment:

- Clinical: Prolongation of quality of life
- Virological: Effective viral suppression
- Immunological: Immune reconstitution, prevention of drug toxicity and transmission of HIV infection.

Initiation of ART:

- CD4 count less than 350 cells/μL
- Clinical stage III/IV illness, irrespective of CD4 count
- HIV TB coinfection
- HIV: Hepatitis B virus (HBV)/HCV coinfection
- Pregnant females for prevention of transmission
- Postexposure prophylaxis (PEP).

Pretreatment adherence counseling and treatment of any active opportunistic infection (OI) is must before starting OI.

Regimen:

- Regimen I: Zidovudine, lamivudine, nevirapine; hemoglobin (Hb) > 9 g/dL and not on anti-tuberculosis therapy (ATT)
- Regimen II: Tenofovir, lamivudine, nevirapine; Hb < 9 g/dL and not on ATT
  - Patient on concomitant ATT: Replace nevirapine by efavirenz

- Patient with HBV/HCV coinfection and pregnant women: Tenofovir, lamivudine, efavirenz is first-line therapy
- Patient who develops toxicity to nevirapine or efavirenz or develops immunological or virological failure: Regimen to be given is zidovudine/tenofovir + Lamivudine + Lopinavir/ritonavir or atazanavir/ritonavir
- Nevirapine is introduced as "Lead-in Period"; 200 mg once a day for 2 weeks followed by 200 mg twice daily. It prevents cutaneous and hepatic adverse effect.

Table 2: Highly-active antiretroviral therapy (HAART) drugs

Class	*Drugs*	*Adverse effects*
NRTI	Zidovudine, lamivudine, stavudine, abacavir	Zidovudine: Bone marrow suppression Stavudine: Pancreatitis, lipodystrophy, lactic acidosis Abacavir: Hypersensitivity reaction
Newer NRTI	Apricitabine, elvucitabine, amdoxovir	
Nucleotide reverse transcriptase inhibitor	Tenofovir	Deranged renal function
NNRTI	Nevirapine, efavirenz	Nevirapine: DHS, SJS-TEN, hepatitis Efavirenz: Neuropsychiatric side effects
PI	Lopinavir, ritonavir, indinavir, nelfinavir	Insulin resistance, dyslipidemia, lipodystrophy Indinavir: Nephrolithiasis
Newer PI	Atazanavir, tipranavir, darunavir	
Newer ART classes		
CCR5 receptor inhibitor	Aplaviroc, maraviroc, vicriviroc	
Fusion inhibitor	Enfuvirtide, sifuvirtide	
Integrase inhibitor	Raltegravir, elvitegravir, dolutegravir	
Pharmacokinetic enhancers	Cobicistat	
HIV maturation inhibitor	Bevirimat	

Abbreviations: NRTI, nucleoside reverse transcriptase inhibitor; NNRTI, non-nucleoside reverse transcriptase inhibitor; PI, protease inhibitor; DHS, drug hypersensitivity syndrome; SJS, Stevens-Johnson syndrome; TEN, toxic epidermal necrolysis; ART, antiretroviral therapy; CCR5, C-C chemokine receptor type 5

Q6. How do you follow up these patients?

Ans: Patients with HIV infection can be followed up as described in Table 3.

Q7. What is postexposure prophylaxis (PEP)?

Ans: Exposure refers to exposure to potential bloodborne pathogens (HIV, HBV and HCV).

- First aid: Wash with soap and water, antiseptics not to be used. In case of mucous membrane exposure, irrigate with plenty of water.
- Assessing risk of exposure: First dose to be given within 72 hours.
  - Mild exposure: Mucous membrane/non-intact skin with small volume
  - Moderate: Mucous membrane/non-intact skin with large volume, percutaneous injury with solid needle
  - Severe: Percutaneous exposure with large volume (>18 G needle)
- PEP drug (Table 4).

Table 3: Follow up of HIV infection

Day 0: Baseline	CBC, urea, creatinine, LFT, HBsAg, anti-HCV, VDRL, Mantoux test, USG abdomen, blood sugar, lipid profile, CD4 count
Day 15 and 1 month and 3 months	CBC: Patient on zidovudine LFT: Nevirapine, atazanavir Urea, creatinine: Tenofovir
6 months and repeat every 6 months	CBC, urea, creatinine, LFT, blood sugar, lipid profile, CD4 count
Viral load	Ideally before starting therapy and 6 monthly, not a part of National Programme
Resistance studies	Ideally before initiation of therapy Immunological or virological failure—before starting second-line regimen

Abbreviations: CBC, complete blood count; LFT, liver function test; HBsAg, hepatitis B surface antigen; HCV, hepatitis C virus; VDRL Venereal Disease Research Laboratory; USG, ultrasonography.

Table 4: Postexposure prophylaxis (PEP) drug regimen

Exposure	*HIV positive*		*Status unknown*
	Asymptomatic	*Symptomatic*	
Mild	Consider 2-drug* PEP	Start 2-drug* PEP	No or 2-drug*
Moderate	Start 2-drug*	Start 3-drug†	No or 2-drug*
Severe	Start 3-drug†	Start 3-drug†	No or 2-drug*

*Two drug regimen: Zidovudine/stavudine + Lamivudine.
†Three drug regimen: Zidovudine/stavudine + Lamivudine + Lopinavir/ritonavir.

Postexposure prophylaxis to be given for 28 days and monitoring includes CBC and LFT at 14 days and 28 days, ELISA for HIV at 3 months and 6 months.

Use of barrier contraceptive is essential for 6 months.

Q8. What are the candidates for HIV vaccines?

Ans: The candidates for HIV vaccines are:

- Live-attenuated vaccine
- Whole-inactivated vaccine
- Subunit vaccine
- Synthetic vaccine
- Naked vaccine
- Live recombinant vector vaccine
- Prime boost vaccine.

SECTION 10

Leprosy

Tanmay Padhi

CHAPTER 47

Borderline Tuberculoid Leprosy

Akshi Bansal

Case study Borderline Tuberculoid Leprosy

Presenting Complaints

Doctor, I have been noticing three to four light-colored numb patches over my body since past 6 months.

Setting

Dermatology outpatient department.

History of Present Illness

A 16-year-old male patient, hailing from Bihar, presented with complaints of numb light-colored patches over body. Initially the patient noticed a solitary light-colored flat numb lesion on his right arm 6 months ago and subsequently developed few more lesions. There is no history of associated weakness of muscles or deformities.

General and Systemic examination

Normal.

Dermatological Examination

- Four hypopigmented patches distributed asymmetrically on back, right upper limb and right cheek, varying in size from the smallest 1 cm × 1 cm lesion on back to the largest of 4 cm × 5 cm size on right arm (Fig. 1).
- The patches were well defined with regular-to-irregular border at places, dry and alopecic. A smaller macule of 0.5 cm size was present near the lower border of the patch on right arm (satellite lesion).
- Patches revealed sensory loss to temperature, fine touch and pin-prick sensation.
- Motor examination was normal.
- Right ulnar was enlarged but nontender.

Q1. What is the most likely diagnosis?

a. Hansen's disease: Borderline tuberculoid (BT)
b. Cutaneous leishmaniasis
c. Lupus vulgaris
d. Tinea corporis

Ans: a. Hansen's disease: Most likely BT type. Presence of well-defined hypopigmented, hypoesthetic macules and patches less than 10 in number, satellite lesion and asymmetrically enlarged peripheral nerves suggest diagnosis of BT leprosy.

Q2. How will you confirm the diagnosis?

Ans: Diagnosis of leprosy is based on presence of one or more of the three classical cardinal signs:

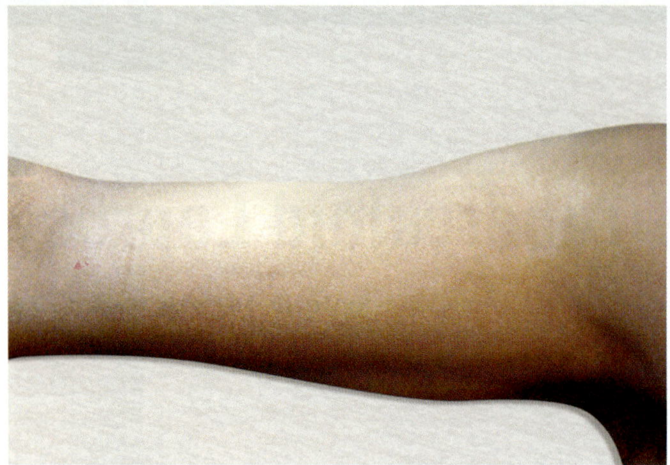

Fig. 1: Large hypopigmented patch on right arm

a. Hypopigmented or erythematous skin lesions with definite loss/impairment of sensations
b. Involvement of peripheral nerves, as demonstrated by definite thickening with sensory impairment
c. Skin smear positive for acid-fast bacilli (AFB).

Laboratory evaluation is required mainly to clear the doubts arising in clinical examination, to classify the patient and to know about the degree of infectivity of patient.

Q3. What are the investigations that can be done to confirm diagnosis?

Ans: Investigations that can be done to confirm diagnosis:

- Routinely done:
  - Slit-skin smear
  - Skin biopsy
- Done in doubtful cases:
  - Nerve biopsy and ultrasonography (USG) of nerves to study nerve involvement
  - Histamine test, pilocarpine sweat test: To check loss of sweating
- Rarely done:
  - Polymerase chain reaction, anti-phenolic glycolipid 1 antibody test: To detect small amount of bacilli in doubtful cases like indeterminate leprosy.

Q4. What are bacterial index (BI) and morphological index (MI) in slit-skin smear?

Ans: Bacterial index and MI in slit-skin smear:

- Bacterial index in slit-skin smear is described in Table 1.
  - G is added to the entry if globi are present.
  - Approximately 100 fields per smear are examined.

Table 1: Bacterial index: Graded 0–6+

Grade	Result
0	No bacilli in 100 fields
1+	1–10 bacilli in 100 fields
2+	1–10 bacilli in 10 fields
3+	1–10 bacilli on average in each field
4+	10–100 bacilli on average in each field
5+	100–1000 bacilli on average in each field
6+	>1,000 bacilli on average in each field

  - In paucibacillary leprosy, the bacterial index is "0".
  - In multibacillary leprosy, it is more than or equal to 1.
- Morphological index: The percentage of solid-staining bacilli in a stained smear is referred to as MI. The total of the MIs for all sites divided by the number of sites gives the average MI for the body. A decreasing MI implies successful treatment. The criteria for calling the bacilli solid rods are:
  - Uniform staining of the entire organism
  - Parallel sides
  - Rounded ends
  - Length 5 times that of the width.

Q5. How will you classify the disease?

Ans: Classification of leprosy:

- Ridley-Jopling classification:
  - Tuberculoid (TT) leprosy:
    - One to five well-defined hypopigmented anesthetic patches
    - Loss of sweating, loss of hair
    - ± Local nerve enlargement
  - Borderline TT (BT) leprosy:
    - 5–20 hypopigmented hypoesthetic lesions
    - Satellite lesions characteristic
    - Asymmetrical enlargement of nerve trunks
  - Borderline-borderline (BB) leprosy:
    - Very unstable
    - Inverted saucer-shaped lesions: Many in number
    - Lesions show tendency towards symmetry
    - Multiple nerves enlarged asymmetrically
  - Borderline lepromatous (BL) leprosy:
    - Multiple infiltrated plaques and hypoesthetic macules
    - Nerves enlarged bilaterally almost symmetrically

- Lepromatous leprosy (LL):
  - Leonine facies
  - Earlobe infiltration
  - Multiple nerves enlarged
  - Glove and stocking anesthesia
  - Systemic involvement including eyes, kidneys, testes.
- World Health Organization (WHO) classification of leprosy:
  - Paucibacillary: Less than or equal to five lesions, negative smear at all sites
  - Multibacillary: More than five lesions, positive smear at any site

The Ridley-Jopling classification is recommended for use in research while the WHO classification is used for field diagnosis and treatment in view of its simplicity and ease in training field workers in its usage.

Q6. Briefly explain the pathogenesis of skin and nerve lesions in BT leprosy.

Ans: Pathogenesis of skin and nerve lesions in BT leprosy:

- *Mycobacterium leprae* have a predilection for neural tissue and upon entry into the body, are engulfed by the Schwann cells
- Bacilli multiply within Schwann cells and slowly destroy them; the process being slow because of 12–13 days taken by each bacillus to divide into two
- Bacilli liberated by effete Schwann cells enter neighboring Schwann cells, leading to intraneural spread of infection until the infection is "recognized" by the immune system
- There is infiltration of lymphocytes, histiocytes (macrophages), few epithelioid cells and giant cells into the nerve with formation of granuloma and subsequent destruction of nerve fibers resulting in anesthesia and/or muscle weakness, depending upon the type of nerve involved
- In BT leprosy, this cellular response is less focal and destructive, and bacilli may be found in the affected nerve, though in few numbers.
- Clinical evidence of nerve damage whether sensory or motor may precede skin lesions by months to years
- When bacilli escape from the nerve into surrounding skin, a skin lesion develops at that site, and a biopsy of the lesion will reveal presence of granuloma in foci surrounding neurovascular and appendageal elements which results in diminished sweating and hair growth in the lesions.

Q7. Enumerate the differential diagnosis for hypopigmented macular lesions in this patient?

Ans: Differential diagnosis for hypopigmented macular lesions:

- Hansen's disease
- Postinflammatory hypomelanosis: History of preceding primary dermatosis, no hypoesthesia or nerve thickening
- Vitiligo: Milky-white macules without any trophic or sensory changes
- Pityriasis versicolor: Presence of fine, powdery scales; scrapings show Malassezia furfur in spaghetti and meatball appearance on KOH (potassium hydroxide) mount
- Lichen sclerosus et atrophicus: Hypopigmented and mildly atrophic plaque with no hypoesthesia or nerve thickening
- Morphea: Indurated, occasionally raised plaque with purplish edges
- Post-kala-azar dermal leishmaniasis: Presence of noduloplaques, papules and nodular infiltration along with hypopigmented macules; presence of Leishman Donovan (LD) bodies on Giemsa stain.

Q8. What are histopathological features of BT leprosy?

Ans: Histopathological features:

- Thinning of epidermis with occasional flattening of rete ridges
- Multiple epithelioid cell granulomas composed of giant cells and moderate number of lymphocytes seen in all the layers of dermis
- Giant cells are typically non-descript and are more of foreign body type than Langhans
- Nerves typically are markedly swollen with granuloma and lymphocytes infiltrating the perineurium causing slight lamination, but they are always identifiable
- AFB: Rarely seen (BI = 0–2.5^{+}).

Q9. What are the major peripheral nerves affected in leprosy? What are the factors that determine nerve damage?

Ans: Major peripheral nerves most frequently affected in leprosy are the ulnar, median, lateral popliteal, posterior tibial and facial nerves. The sites of predilection are at their most superficial and cooler sites where they are also prone to trauma.

- Ulnar nerve: Upper arm, just below the elbow
- Median nerve: At wrist, behind flexor retinaculum
- Radial nerve: Upper arm in radial groove
- Lateral popliteal nerve: Behind knee as it winds around the neck of fibula

- Posterior tibial nerve: Below and behind medial malleolus at ankle
- Factors which determine the nerve damage are:
  - Immune status of patient
  - Presence of skin lesions overlying nerve trunks
  - Reactions, especially type 1.

Q10. Earliest sensation to be lost in Hansen's disease is:

a. Pain
b. Cold
c. Touch
d. Hot

Ans: b (Cold). Cold sensation is the first to be lost in leprosy. Nerve function impairment resulting damage to nerves could be autonomic, sensory or motor; depending on the type and severity of nerve involved.

Q11. Enumerate the causes of palpably enlarged nerves.

Ans: Causes of palpably enlarged nerves:
- Physiological: Strenuous physical exercises, wrestlers
- Pathological:
  - Leprosy
  - Amyloidosis
  - Sarcoidosis
  - Neurofibromatosis
  - Guillain-Barre syndrome
  - Refsum's disease
  - Hereditary sensorimotor neuropathy (HSMN) I (Charcot-Marie-Tooth disease)
  - HSMN III (Dejerine Sotta's disease)
  - Tubercular nerve abscess
  - Cysts and trauma.

Among these, leprosy, primary amyloidosis, HSMN I and III, and sarcoidosis, are associated with some neurological deficit.

Q12. What is the natural course of BT Hansen's disease?

Ans: Instability is the predominant characteristic of BT leprosy. Patients who are untreated or inadequately treated may downgrade towards the lepromatous pole, may finally lose all capacity to respond, and become truly lepromatous; but with some clinical features such as thick, asymmetrical nerves that hint towards their former state. Such patients are classified as having subpolar lepromatous disease.

Other patients, even without treatment, may reverse or upgrade with their disease becoming more tuberculoid in appearance.

Q13. How do you differentiate between TT and BT leprosy?

Ans: Difference between TT and BT leprosy is described in Table 2.

Q14. How will you manage this case?

Ans: Management of BT leprosy:
- Chemotherapy: 6 months
- Rifampicin: 600 mg once a month, supervised
- Clofazimine: 300 mg once a month, supervised; and 50 mg daily, self administered
- Dapsone: 100 mg daily, self administered.

Table 2: Difference between TT and BT leprosy

Parameters	*TT*	*BT*
Skin lesions	1–3	3–10
Borders	Well defined, uniform margins	Margins well defined at few areas, poor at few areas. Satellite lesions seen
Sensation	Anesthesia usually	Hypoesthesia usually
Nerve	Usually single, localized nerve to patch	>1 nerve may be involved asymmetrically
Acid-fast bacilli (AFB)	0	1–2+
Lepromin test	++	+
Histology	Well-defined epithelioid cell granuloma, complete destruction of nerves and appendages	Well-defined granulomas (epithelioid cells, giant cells, destruction of nerves and appendages)

CHAPTER 48

Lepromatous Leprosy

Mary Thomas

Case study Lepromatous Leprosy

Presenting Complaints

Doctor, I have developed raised patches and swellings on my body and painless wounds on my hands and feet. My nose is stuffy and bleeds occasionally. My hands and feet feel cold and numb.

Setting

Dermatology outpatient department

History of Present Illness

A 56-year-old man presented with complaints of multiple raised lesions on the face and body since 2 months. He also developed multiple ulcers on the hands and feet. He has noticed stuffiness of the nose with occasional epistaxis. He complained of numbness and occasional tingling over his hands and feet.

General Physical Examination

Leonine facies present.

Systemic Examination

The cardiovascular, respiratory and central nervous system examination is within normal limits. Abdominal examination reveals mild painless hepatosplenomegaly and examination of genitourinary system reveals testicular atrophy.

Dermatological Examination

Multiple, smooth, firm, skin-colored nodules distributed symmetrically surrounded by infiltrated skin seen on the face, trunk and limbs (Fig. 1). Painless enlargement of bilateral ulnar, median, radial cutaneous, common peroneal and posterior tibial nerves. Glove and stocking anesthesia.

- Eyes: Madarosis, corneal pannus, corneal anesthesia.
- Ears: Infiltration of the earlobes.
- Hands: Tapering digits with dry, lusterless nails.
- Feet: One well-defined dry ulcer on the ball of the foot. Multiple callosities on the pressure points of hands and feet

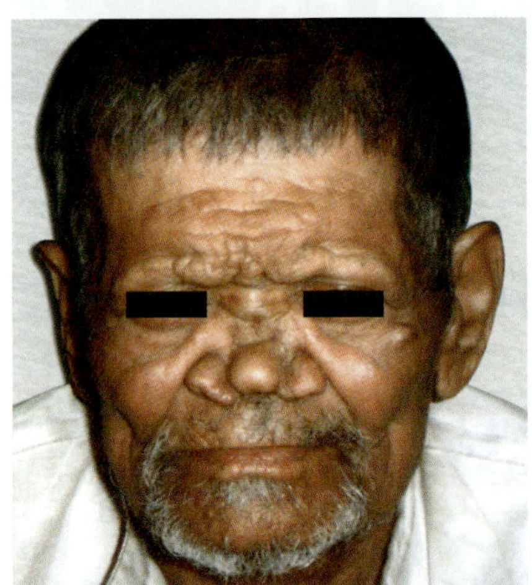

Fig. 1: Multiple nodules on face with leonine look

Q1. What is the most likely diagnosis?

a. Lepromatous leprosy
b. Borderline tuberculoid leprosy
c. Sarcoidosis
d. Leishmaniasis

Ans: a. Lepromatous leprosy. Presence of leonine facies, multiple nodules on the body, glove and stocking anesthesia, diffuse thickening of nerves points towards diagnosis.

Q2. Describe the histopathology of lepromatous leprosy.

Ans: There is an extensive cellular infiltrate that is almost invariably separated from the flattened epidermis by a narrow Grenz zone. The infiltrate causes destruction of the cutaneous appendages and extends into the subcutaneous fat. In florid lesions, the macrophages have an abundant cytoplasm and contain a mixed population of solid and fragmented bacilli. Epithelioid cell granulomas may be absent. Lymphocyte infiltration is not prominent but plasma cells may be present.

The important difference between BL and LL is that in BL the lymphocytes are more prominent and there is some evidence of poorly-defined macrophage granulomas. Acid-fast bacillus (AFB) may be present.

Q3. Enumerate the systemic involvement in lepromatous leprosy.

Ans: Systemic involvement in lepromatous leprosy is described in Table 1.

Table 1: Systemic involvement in lepromatous leprosy

System	*Involvement*
Larynx	Thickening of the laryngeal mucosa and fibrosis of the vocal cords leading to hoarseness of voice
Bones, joints, muscles	Bone cysts, enlarged nutrient foramina, aseptic necrosis, dactylitis, periostitis. Neurotrophic atrophy of the phalanges and metatarsals leading to a sucked candy stick appearance on X-ray and shortening of the fingers and toes. Charcot joints
Testes	Atrophy, impotence
Breast	Gynecomastia in men
Skull	Atrophy of the anterior nasal spine. Collapse of the nasal bridge. Saddle nose deformity. Loosening of upper central incisors or all the four incisors
Reticuloendothelial system	Generalized lymph node enlargement
Abdomen	Hepatosplenomegaly
Kidney	Glomerulonephritis, interstitial nephritis and pyelonephritis. Renal amyloidosis

Q4. What is the Lepromin test?

Ans: Skin test with lepromin is the only in vivo immunological skin test used as an aid to the classification and prognosis of leprosy.

- First described by Mitsuda in 1919
- This test used intradermal injection of a lepromin (Dharmendra or Mitsuda antigen), to classify the stage of leprosy based on the lepromin reaction (Fernandez or Mitsuda reaction); it differentiates tuberculoid leprosy, in which there is a positive delayed reaction at the injection site, from lepromatous leprosy, in which there is no reaction (a negative test result) despite the active *Mycobacterium leprae* infection.

Q5. What is histoid leprosy?

Ans: Histoid leprosy is an uncommon variant of lepromatous leprosy.

- It is characterized by discrete shiny, succulent, globular, firm nodules and papules (button-like lesions) on normal appearing skin.
- It occurs in lepromatous patients who relapse after dapsone monotherapy, in the presence of dapsone resistance or at times de novo.
- Reactions are very rare in this form of leprosy.
- *Histopathology:* It is a well-formed lesion surrounded by a pseudocapsule. Epidermal atrophy, subepidermal Grenz zone, spindle-shaped histiocytes and many macrophages in the dermis along with other inflammatory cells are present. The spindle-shaped cells are arranged in an intertwining pattern resembling a fibrohistiocytic tumor.

Q6. What is Lucio leprosy?

Ans: Lucio leprosy is also known as diffuse lepromatous leprosy or "pretty leprosy" (lepra bonita).

- Clinical variety of lepromatous leprosy
- First described by Lucio and Alvarado in 1852 and re-identified by Latapí in 1936
- Common in Mexico (23% leprosy cases) and in Costa Rica
- This condition is characterized by:
  - Diffuse infiltration of all the skin which never transforms into nodule
  - Complete alopecia of eyebrows and eyelashes and body hair
  - Anhidrotic and dysesthesic zones of the skin
  - Peculiar type of lepra reaction named Lucio's phenomenon/necrotic erythema.

Q7. Leonine facies is seen in all except:

a. Leprosy
b. Chronic actinic dermatitis
c. Atopic dermatitis
d. Leishmaniasis

Ans: c. Atopic dermatitis. Leonine facies is due to diffuse infiltration of the skin of forehead, chin, nose and ears. It can be seen in: Leprosy, chronic actinic dermatitis, leishmaniasis, mycosis fungoides and sarcoidosis.

Q8. What are the differential diagnoses of nerve involvement in Leprosy?

Ans: Differential diagnoses of nerve involvement in leprosy are described in Table 2.

Q9. Enumerate the regimen for the treatment of Leprosy.

Ans: The Government of India [National Leprosy Eradication Programme (NLEP)] made the following recommendations for the treatment of leprosy for control/eradication purposes to be adopted uniformly by the country:

- Fixed drug therapy (FDT) for multibacillary (MB) leprosy: All MB cases may be put on 12 months of standard MB-MDT (multidrug therapy). These patients after release from treatment will be kept under surveillance for 5 years.
- FDT for paucibacillary (PB) leprosy: All PB cases will be treated with 6 months of standard World Health Organization (WHO) PB-MDT and thereafter released from treatment. They should be kept under surveillance for 2 years.
- The recommended drugs are:
  - MB-MDT (adult):
    - Rifampicin 600 mg once a month supervised
    - Clofazimine 300 mg once monthly supervised and 100 mg on alternate days or 50 mg once daily self administered
    - Dapsone 100 mg once monthly supervised with 100 mg daily self administered
  - PB-MDT (Adult):
    - Rifampicin 600 mg once a month supervised
    - Dapsone 100 mg once monthly supervised with 100 mg daily self administered.

Table 2: Differential diagnoses of nerve involvement in leprosy

Type of involvement	*Diseases*
Palpable nerve thickening without anesthesia	Excessive muscle development, pachydermoperiosteitis
Palpable nerve thickening with regional anesthesia	Amyloidosis, Dejerine Sotta's neuropathy, endotoxic polyneuritis, Charcot Marie tooth disease
Regional anesthesia without palpable nerve thickening	Syringomyelia, tabes, compression neuropathy, hereditary sensory radicular neuropathy, congenital indifference to pain, hysteria

Q10. What is A-MDT?

Ans: A-MDT stands for "Accompanied MDT". The patient is provided the full supply of MDT at the time of diagnosis. A person close to or important to the patient assumes the responsibility of helping the patient complete his treatment.

Q11. What is U-MDT?

Ans: U-MDT stands for "Uniform MDT". All patients, irrespective of their clinical and bacteriological status, are provided with the following for 6 months under supervision:

- Rifampicin 600 mg once a month supervised
- Clofazimine 300 mg once monthly supervised and 100 mg on alternate days or 50 mg once daily self administered
- Dapsone 100 mg once monthly supervised with 100 mg daily self administered

U-MDT will over-treat PB leprosy patients and under-treat MB patients, especially those with a high initial bacillary index (BI).

Q12. What are the other alternate drug regimens in leprosy?

Ans: Other alternate drug regimens:

- Multibacillary (MB) cases:
  - Rifapentine 900 mg/rifampicin 600 mg + Moxifloxacin 400 mg + Clarithromycin 1000 mg/minocycline 200 mg once monthly: 12 months.
  - ROM: Rifampicin 600 mg, ofloxacin 400 mg, minocycline 100 mg once monthly: 12 months.

- RMM: Rifapentine 600 mg, moxifloxacin 400 mg, minocycline 100 mg once monthly: 12 months.
- Rifampicin 600 mg + ofloxacin 400 mg + clofazimine 100 mg + minocycline 100 mg once a week: 6 weeks.

- Paucibacillary (PB) cases:
  - Single dose of ROM or RMM for all PB cases
  - 4-week rifampicin 600 mg + Ofloxacin 400 mg daily
  - Once a month ROM for 6 months.

Q13. What is relapse?

Ans: The Guide to Leprosy Control (1988) defined a case of relapse as "a patient who successfully completes an adequate course of MDT, but who subsequently develops new signs and symptoms of the disease either during the surveillance period (2 years for PB and 5 years for MB leprosy) or thereafter".

Becx-Bleumink lists several criteria for relapse, which include:

- New skin lesions
- New activity in previously existing skin lesions
- Bacteriological index 2+ or more in two sets of skin smears
- New nerve function loss
- Histological evidence of relapse in skin or nerve biopsy.

It is relatively easy to recognize relapse in MB cases as compared to PB cases where it can be mistaken for a late reversal reaction.

The WHO has estimated a risk of relapse rate of 0.77% for MB and 1.07% for PB patients 9 years after stopping MDT. Predisposing factors for relapse include persisters, inadequate or irregular therapy, monotherapy, high initial BI, lepromin negativity, HIV infection and multiple lesions.

Q14. What is the grading system for deformities in Leprosy?

Ans: Nerve function impairment is the major cause of deformities in Leprosy.

The WHO deformity grading:

- Hand and feet:
  - Grade 0: No anesthesia, no visual deformity or damage
  - Grade 1: Anesthesia present, but no visible deformity or damage
  - Grade 2: Visible deformity or damage present
- Eyes:
  - Grade 0: No eye problem due to leprosy; no evidence of visual loss
  - Grade 1: Eye problem due to leprosy present.

Q15. What are the vaccines in Leprosy?

Ans: Vaccines in leprosy include:

- BCG (Bacillus Calmette-Guerin)
- HKML/HKML-A (heat-killed *M. leprae*)
- Mw (*M. welchii*)
- *M. vaccae*
- ICRC.

Q16. Enumerate the immunoprophylaxis in leprosy.

Ans: Immunoprophylaxis in leprosy is described in Table 3.

Q17. What are the newer diagnostic modalities for the diagnosis of leprosy?

Ans: Newer diagnostic modalities for the diagnosis of leprosy are described in Table 4.

Table 3: Immunoprophylaxis in leprosy

Type	*Examples*
Antigenically-related mycobacteria with shared antigens	BCG, HKML, Mw, ICRC, *M. vaccae*, *M. Habana*, *M. gordonae*, *M. phlei*
Drugs	Levamisole, corticosteroids, zinc, clofazimine, colchicine, thalidomide, cyclosporine A
Other immunomodulators	Lawrence transfer factor, cytokines (IFN-γ/IL-2), acetoacylated M. leprae, delipidified cell components of *M. leprae*, soluble protein cell wall components, isolated cell wall core antigen

Abbreviations: BCG, Bacillus Calmette-Guerin; HKML, heat-killed *M. leprae*; Mw, *M. welchii*; IFN-γ, interferon-gamma; IL-2, interleukin-2.

Table 4: Newer diagnostic modalities for the diagnosis of leprosy

Type	*Test*
Serological testing	PGL-1, ML0405, ML2331, LID-1, IFN-γ
Immunohistochemical reaction	S100, heat-shock proteins, e.g. 35 kDa and 65 kDa, antibodies against lipoarabinomannan and PGL-1 glycolipids, anti-BCG antibody
Molecular identification of *M. leprae* bacillus	PCR

Abbreviations: PGL-1, phenolic glycolipid 1 antigen; LID-1, leprosy IDRI diagnostic 1; IFN-γ, interferon-gamma; BCG, Bacillus Calmette-Guerin; PCR, polymerase chain reaction.

CHAPTER 49

Type 2 Lepra Reaction

Tanmay Padhi

Case study Type 2 Lepra Reaction

Presenting Complaints

Doctor, I have painful red swellings over my trunk and limbs since last 3 days. I also have fever and pain in the joints.

Setting

Dermatology outpatient department

History of Present Illness

A 46-year-old man presented with complaints of episodic appearance of painful red swellings over the face, trunk, both upper and lower limbs since last 6 months accompanied by low-grade fever and painful joints. He also gives a history of being treated at the local government hospital with multidrug therapy for last 4 months which he stopped on his own when the swellings started appearing. He lives in a slum and one of his immediate neighbor was also taking multidrug therapy around a year back.

General Physical Examination

- Temperature: 100.4°F
- Pulse: 96 beats/min
- Respiratory rate: 16 breath/min
- Pallor: Mild
- Bilateral inguinal lymph nodes: Enlarged and tender.

Systemic Examination

- Bilateral wrist, knee and ankle joints: Swollen and tender.
- Conjunctiva: Congested.
- Testicles: Enlarged and tender.

Dermatological Examination

Diffuse erythematous patches with almost merging margins present over the trunk and extremities. Many of the lesions appear shiny and infiltrated. Small nontender infiltrated nodules present over the earlobes and upper back and thighs. Painful larger and tender subcutaneous nodules present over the face, neck, trunk and bilateral upper and lower limbs (Fig. 1). Diffuse swelling of fingers and toes. Definite loss of sensation present over some of the larger erythematous patches and also over the hands and feet.

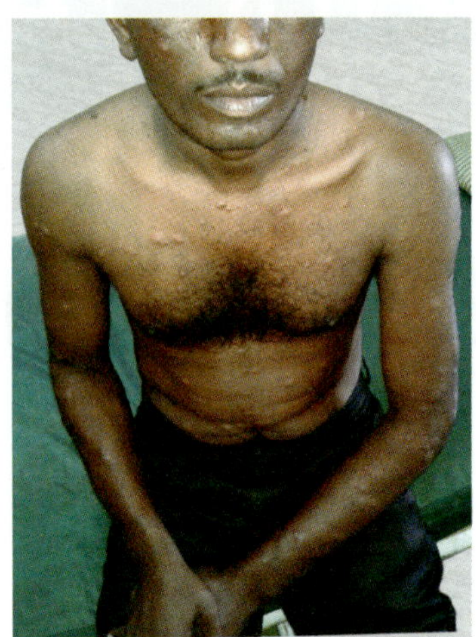

Fig. 1: Multiple tender nodules on the body

Q1. What is the most likely Diagnosis?

a. Erythema nodosum
b. Type 2 lepra reaction
c. Systemic lupus erythematosus (SLE)
d. Sarcoidosis

Ans: b. Type 2 lepra reaction; definite loss of sensation, erythematous infiltrated patches and nodules and sudden onset of tender subcutaneous nodules in the setting of systemic features such as fever and arthralgia point towards the diagnosis of type 2 lepra reaction.

Q2. How do you diagnose type 2 lepra reaction?

Ans: In the setting of leprosy, if a patient presents with sudden onset of erythematous evanescent subcutaneous nodules with or without systemic features such as fever and arthralgia; it points towards type 2 lepra reaction.

Q3. How will you confirm the diagnosis?

Ans: Diagnosis is made on clinical grounds. Investigations such as slit-skin smear and biopsy are required for confirmation. Sometimes, diagnostic procedures may be required to find out any underlying infection or to rule out other dermatological conditions such as erythema nodosum, tuberculosis or SLE.

Q4. What do you mean by REACTIONS in leprosy and what are the other types of lepra reactions?

Ans: Reactions in leprosy are immunologically-mediated episodes of acute inflammation which interrupt the otherwise chronic course of the disease. There are three types of reactions:

1. Type 1 lepra reaction suggests sudden appearance of the features of acute inflammation over existing lesions of leprosy or appearance of new lesions with or without the features of neuritis. It is usually seen along the borderline spectrum of the disease and is rare along the lepromatous pole. It can again be subdivided into upgrading or downgrading types depending on the increase or decrease in host immunity contributing to its appearance.
2. Type 2 lepra reaction is also known as erythema nodosum leprosum (ENL) as its principal dermatological manifestation is erythema nodosum. It is often accompanied by systemic features such as fever, arthralgia, epididymo-orchitis, conjunctivitis, myalgia, lymphadenopathy, hepatitis and glomerulonephritis.
3. There is a third type of reaction known as Lucio phenomenon, which is seen almost exclusively in the diffuse non-nodular form of lepromatous leprosy called Lucio leprosy. It presents with irregular-shaped ulcers and is characterized by invasion of *Mycobacterium leprae* into the vascular endothelium.

Q5. What are the precipitating factors and risk factors for type 2 lepra reaction?

Ans: Precipitating and risk factors:

- High-bacillary index (BI > 4+)
- Lepromatous pole
- Underlying infection
- Physical and mental stress
- Pregnancy.

Q6. What are the dermatological manifestations of type 2 lepra reaction?

Ans: Type 2 lepra reaction, apart from the classical nodular lesions, may present in a variety of morphological patterns, such as:

- Vesiculobullous form
- Ulcerative form
- Necrotic form
- Chronic panniculitis.

Q7. What are the systemic associations of type 2 lepra reaction?

Ans: Systemic associations of type 2 lepra reaction include:

- Musculoskeletal system:
  - Swelling, pain, tenderness of joints
  - Osteoperiostitis
  - Osteoporosis
  - Synovitis and bursitis
  - Acute myositis

- Gastrointestinal system:
  - Ulceration and perforation of hard and soft palates
  - Hepatitis, hepatomegaly
- Respiratory system:
  - Epistaxis, turbinate hypertrophy, perforation of nasal septum
  - Epiglottitis, vocal cord palsy
- Genitourinary system:
  - Hematuria, granular cast in urine
  - Glomerulonephritis
  - Amyloidosis
  - Epididymo-orchitis.

Q8. Are there any clinical tests to diagnose type 2 lepra reaction?

Ans: Clinical tests to diagnose type 2 lepra reaction include:

- Ryrie's test: Stroking the sole with a knee hammer causes burning pain
- Elli's test: Squeezing the wrist causes disproportionately severe pain.

Q9. What are the hematological and biochemical investigations recommended in type 2 lepra reaction?

Ans: Hematological and biochemical investigations include:

- Complete blood count
- Erythrocyte sedimentation rate (ESR), C-reactive protein
- Liver function tests
- Kidney function tests
- Urinalysis.

Q10. What are the differential diagnoses of type 2 lepra reaction?

Ans: Differential diagnoses of type 2 lepra reaction include:

- Erythema nodosum due to other causes, i.e. Streptococcal infection, tuberculosis, etc.
- Panniculitis
- Cutaneous tuberculosis, i.e. erythema induratum
- Vasculitis, i.e. polyarteritis nodosa, giant cell arteritis
- Adverse cutaneous drug reactions, i.e. potassium iodide
- SLE
- Sarcoidosis.

Q11. What are the complications of type 2 lepra reaction?

Ans: Complications arising out of the disease:

- Glomerulonephritis, renal amyloidosis and renal failure
- Superadded infections and septicemia in ulcerative and necrotic variants
- Hepatitis and hepatic failure
- Neuritis, deformities and disabilities

Complications arising due to treatment of the disease:

- Cushingoid habitus, striae
- Reactivation of latent tuberculosis
- Fluid electrolyte imbalance
- Gastritis, peptic ulcer
- Diabetes mellitus, insulin resistance
- Anemia, pancytopenia.

Q12. What are the principles of treatment of type 2 lepra reaction?

a. Treatment of leprosy
b. Treatment of precipitating factors
c. Treatment of reaction
d. Treatment of complications
e. All of the above

Ans: (e) All of the above.

Q13. How to approach a patient of type 2 lepra reaction for treatment?

Ans: A patient of type 2 lepra reaction for treatment can be approached through following process:

- Treatment of leprosy:
  - All cases of type 2 lepra reactions who have not started or completed multidrug therapy (MDT) should be advised to continue MDT.
  - Cases of high BI (>4+) may be advised to continue MDT for one more year depending on the clinical activity of the lesions
  - Family members and household contacts should be encouraged to get examined for presence of leprosy and treated if found to be having the disease
- Treatment of precipitating factors:
  - Underlying infections such as mouth cavity infections, malaria, lymphatic filariasis, enteric fever should be looked for and treated with appropriate antibiotics
  - Cause of immunosuppression, such as diabetes, human immunodeficiency virus (HIV) infection, tuberculosis, should be identified and treated
  - Psychiatric referral should be made for mental stress

- Treatment of reaction:
  - Rest
  - Anti-inflammatory and analgesics
  - Corticosteroids (prednisolone 0.5 mg/kg): World Health Organization (WHO) dosing schedule
  - Methylprednisolone pulse
  - Thalidomide: 100 mg QID for a week, TDS for 1 months, BD for 1 month and so on
  - Antineutrophilic agents, such as colchicine, clofazimine, chloroquine
  - Immunosuppressants, such as cyclosporine, methotrexate, azathioprine, cyclophosphamide
  - Newer and experimental agents, such as infliximab
- Treatment of complications:
  - Dialysis for renal failure
  - Management of steroid-induced diabetes with insulin or oral hypoglycemic agents
  - Management of fluid electrolyte imbalance with salt restriction, potassium supplementation and regulated fluid intake
  - Management of reactivated tuberculosis with antitubercular therapy.

Q14. What are the dosage and duration of steroid therapy in type 2 lepra reaction?

Ans: Prednisolone should be started with 0.5–1 mg/kg/day usually in a single morning dose till all the features of acute inflammation subside. It should be tapered slowly, usually in decrements of 5–10 mg every week over 6–8 weeks. In recurrent ENL, a low maintenance dose of 5–10 mg for another few weeks may be needed after the subsidence of lesions.

Table 1: Type 2 lepra reaction

Mild:	NSAIDs, chloroquine, colchicine	
Severe:	Prednisolone, clofazimine: 100 mg TDS-month, gradually tapered-off, Thalidomide: 100 mg 4 times daily, DCP pulse, azathioprine	Newer drugs: Leukotriene inhibitors, revlimid/actimid, infliximab Other experimental drugs: Pentoxifylline, cyclosporine A, plasma exchange, methotrexate, mycophenolate mofetil

Abbreviations: NSAIDs, nonsteroidal anti-inflammatory drugs; DCP, dexamethasone-cyclophosphamide pulse

Q15. When to think of thalidomide in treating type 2 lepra reaction?

Ans: In male patients and females who are past the child-bearing age, thalidomide should be the first choice if available and affordable. In all others, it should be considered in recurrent ENL not responding to corticosteroids or those who are steroid dependent.

Q16. What other drugs are used to treat type 2 lepra reaction?

Ans: Other drugs used to treat type 2 lepra reaction (Table 1) are:

- Clofazimine in higher dosage, i.e. 100 mg 3 times daily
- Chloroquine 250 mg 3 times daily gradually tapered to twice and once daily
- Methotrexate: 15 mg/week dose
- Pentoxifylline 400 mg 3 times daily
- Etanercept 50 mg twice weekly.

CHAPTER 50

Type 1 Lepra Reaction

Harish Shetty, Mary Thomas

Case study Type 1 Lepra Reaction

Presenting Complaints

Doctor, I have noticed that my leprosy patches have become angrier looking and raised since 1 week. I also feel a sense of warmth over them.

Setting

Dermatology outpatient department.

History of Present Illness

A 35-year-old male diagnosed as borderline tuberculoid (BT) Hansen's disease on multibacillary-multidrug therapy (MB-MDT) since past 5 months came with complaints of redness, swelling and pain in the existing skin lesions and appearance of new skin lesions since past 1 week. History of associated fever with swelling over hands and feet and pain behind the right elbow was also present.

General and Systemic examination

Temperature: 100.2°F. Rest: Normal.

Dermatological Examination

Multiple well-defined tender erythematous plaques of varying sizes ranging from 2 cm × 2 cm to 3 cm × 5 cm are present over the trunk and extremities (Fig. 1). Right ulnar nerve is enlarged and tender on palpation. Right common peroneal nerve and left great auricular nerves are also enlarged, but nontender.

Q1. What is the most likely diagnosis?

a. Type 1 lepra reaction (reversal reaction)
b. Type 2 lepra reaction
c. Relapse of leprosy
d. Erysipelas

Ans: a. Type 1 lepra reaction (reversal reaction). Sudden onset of signs of inflammation in the existing skin lesions along with neuritis in a known case of Hansen's disease on treatment suggests the diagnosis of type 1 reaction (T1R).

Q2. Type 1 reaction is seen commonly in which type of leprosy?

Ans: Type 1 reactions are usually seen in borderline spectrum of Hansen's disease [BT, mid-borderline or borderline-borderline leprosy (BB) and borderline lepromatous leprosy (BLL)]. Amongst

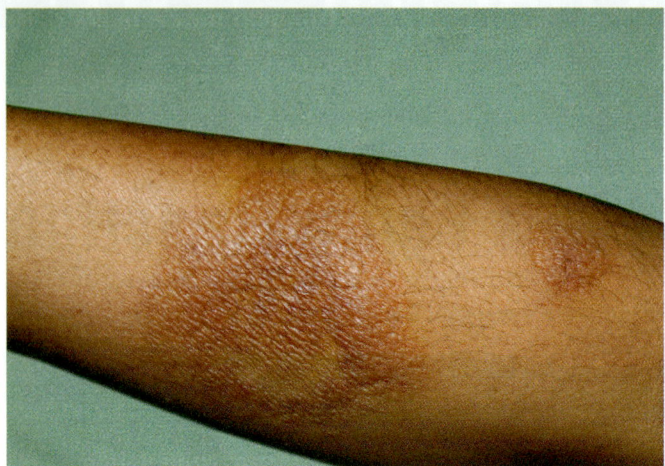

Fig. 1: Erythematous annular raised plaque on forearm

this group BLL and BB patients are at highest risk.

Q3. What is the time of onset of T1R?

Ans: Usually, they occur during the first 6 months of the start of MDT but longer intervals have been noted in patients in BLL spectrum.

Q4. What are the risk factors for developing T1R?

Ans: Risk factors for developing T1R:
- Borderline spectrum
- Females
- Puerperium
- Older age groups
- Multiple patches and multiple nerve involvement
- Large patch overlying a joint, large facial patches and lesions near eyes are at risk of developing ophthalmic complications when in reaction
- Patients who are on MDT
- Hepatitis B or C infections.

Q5. What are the clinical features of T1R?

Ans: The clinical features of T1R are:
- Signs of inflammation in the existing skin lesions and sometimes appearance of new skin lesions
- Necrosis and ulceration of skin lesions can be seen in severe cases
- Edema of face and extremities
- Severe neuritis presenting as pain and tenderness of nerves, palsy of affected areas such as wrist drop and foot drop and very rarely nerve abscess
- T1R can be sometimes present as "silent neuritis" with progressive loss of function but without signs of inflammation.

Q6. What are the histopathological findings of T1R?

Ans: Lymphocytic infiltration with extracellular edema in and around epithelioid cell granulomas. Inflammatory edema and infiltration within the nerves result in pain and functional loss.

Q7. What is the immunological basis of T1R

Ans: Characteristic immunological features of T1R are increased cell-mediated response (type 4). Cytokine responses are of Th-1 type with influx of CD4 T cells into the granuloma with increased expression of interferon-gamma (IFN-γ), interleukin-2 (IL-2) and tumor necrosis factor (TNF) leading to increased lymphocytic infiltration in skin and nerves. A recent study in Brazil has shown that plasma levels of CXCL10/IP-10 [C-X-C motif chemokine 10 (CXCL10)/interferon gamma-induced protein 10] and IL-6 were found to be elevated in T1R which may serve as potential laboratory marker tools.

Q8. What are the criteria for diagnosing T1R?

Ans: Criteria for clinical diagnosis of T1R have been proposed by Naaf's et al.:
- Major: Preexisting and/or new skin lesions become showing signs of inflammation.
- Minor:
  - One or more nerves become tender and may be swollen
  - Crops of new (painless) lesion may appear
  - Sudden edema of face and extremities
  - Recent loss of sensation in hands and feet or signs of recent nerve damage in an area supplied by a particular nerve.

Presence of 1 major or at least 2 minor criterion [without signs of erythema nodosum leprosum (ENL)] is required for the diagnosis of T1R.

Q9. What are the differential diagnoses of T1R?

Ans: The differential diagnosis of T1R includes:
- Relapse
- Acute urticaria
- Erysipelas
- Insect bite
- Cellulitis.

Q10. What are the differences between T1R and T2R?

Ans: The difference between T1R and T2R has been described in Table 1.

Q11. How would you treat T1R?

Ans: Treatment of T1R has been described in Table 2.
- 40 mg once a day × 14 days.

- 30 mg once a day × 14 days.
- 20 mg once a day × 14 days.
- 15 mg once a day × 14 days.
- 10 mg once a day × 14 days.
- 5 mg once a day × 14 days.

Q12. How will you manage neuritis?

Ans: Neuritis is an emergency. Management includes:

- Nonsteroidal anti-inflammatory drugs (NSAIDs): Aspirin, paracetamol
- Codeine compounds
- Steroids
- Intraneural injections (lignocaine, hyaluronidase and hydrocortisone)
- Surgical decompression.

Table 1: Differences between T1R and T2R

T1R	*T2R*
Occurs both in PB and MB leprosy	Occurs in MB cases
Appears due to sudden change in CMI	Appears due to antigen-antibody (humoral immune) reaction
Existing lesions suddenly become red, swollen, tender and warm	Eruption of red, tender, painful, tiny nodules (ENL) in groups commonly on face, arms, and legs. They subside within few days without treatment but reappear in crops
Other organs not affected	Other organs, such as eye, bones, liver, testis, kidney, and spleen, may be involved
Fever and weakness only in severe forms	Complaints like fever, joints pains are common
Occurs within 6 months of starting treatment	Occurs after 6 months of starting treatment
Treated with prednisolone	Treated with thalidomide, prednisolone and clofazimine

Abbreviations: T1R, type 1 reaction; T2R, type 2 reaction; PB, paucibacillary; MB, multibacillary; CMI, cell-mediated immunity.

Table 2: Treatment of T1R

Types of reaction	*Treatment*	*Other drugs*
Treatment of mild T1R	Daily aspirin or paracetamol for a few weeks	
Treatment of severe T1R	Prednisolone, *analgesics	Methotrexate, cyclosporine A, azathioprine, mycophenolate mofetil

*Schedule for prednisolone therapy for adult patients as per World Health Organization (WHO)

SECTION 11

Pigmentary Disorders

Divya Gorur K

CHAPTER 51

Melasma

Siddharth Sonthalia, Deepashree Daulatabad

Case study Melasma

Presenting Complaints

Doctor, I have been noticing these brownish spots of pigmentation on my cheeks and nose for the past 2 years. The spots were initially lighter in color and much smaller, but have become larger and darker over the past few months. They appear darker when I go out in the sun.

Setting

Department of dermatology and sexually transmitted diseases, outpatient unit.

History of Present Illness

A 28-year-old married Indian lady, presented with complaints of developing brown-colored spots of pigmentation over both the cheeks and nose for the past 2 years. The patient first noticed much smaller, ill-defined and light brown-colored spots over her cheeks during the eighth gestational month of her second pregnancy. The spots gradually but progressively increased in number, became larger and darker and started involving other parts of the face. There are no complaints of lesional erythema, itching, burning or photosensitivity. No preceding history of topical or oral medications or frequent use of facial cosmetics.

General Physical Examination and Systemic Examination

No abnormality detected.

Dermatological Examination

- Fitzpatrick skin type IV.
- Multiple hyperpigmented macules present over malar area, nose, forehead and upper lips in a bilaterally symmetrical pattern (Fig. 1).
- The macules are light-to-dark brown in color, with a nonhomogenous pigmentation with well-demarcated margins, without any visible erythema or papulopustules.
- No pigmentation of the ocular or oral mucosa seen.

Q1. What is the most likely diagnosis?

a. Melasma
b. Exogenous ochronosis
c. Acquired bilateral nevus of Ota-like macules (ABNOM or Hori's nevus)
d. Lichen planus pigmentosus

Ans. a. Melasma.

Melasma is an acquired disorder of symmetrical hyperpigmentation that most commonly affects the Fitzpatrick skin type III–VI. It presents as

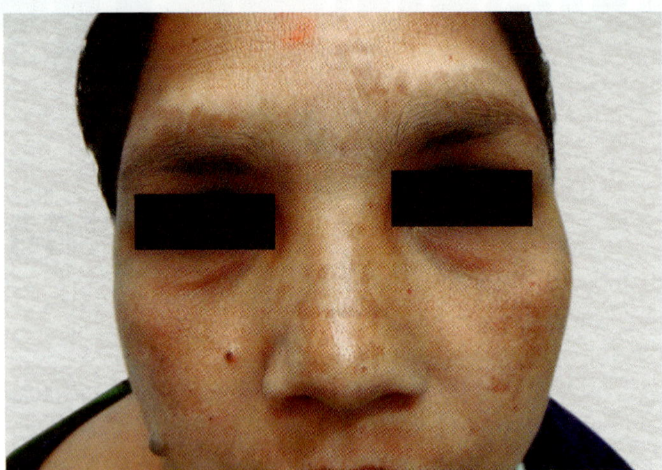

Fig. 1: Hyperpigmented (brown areas) symmetrically for forehead, nose, cheeks and upper lip

light-to-dark brown to muddy brown macules of hyperpigmentation over the face mostly over the malar regions, forehead and chin, typically in a symmetrical pattern.

Q2. What do you understand by "Chloasma"?

Ans. Chloasma is derived from the Greek word chloazein, meaning to be green. This term is equated to "mask of pregnancy". Whereas the term melasma, comes from the Greek melas, meaning black. These terms are often used synonymously. The term chloasma or mask of pregnancy gained popularity owing to frequent onset or worsening of melasma during pregnancy. However, the term melasma is a better term that circumscribes its typical clinical features and includes all underlying initiating or exacerbating factors such as sun exposure, hormonal imbalance, etc.

Q3. What factors have been implicated in the etiopathogenesis of melasma?

Ans. The following risk factors have been implicated in the development and/or exacerbation of melasma:

- Genetic predisposition
- Exposure to light—typically the ultraviolet spectrum, but also includes the visible light and infrared radiation
- Pregnancy
- Exogenous hormones (i.e. oral contraceptives and hormone replacement therapy) have been suggested to be contributory in around a quarter of the affected women
- Vascular factors—increased vascularity and heightened response of cutaneous vasculature of the face to sun exposure
- Phototoxic medications including cosmetics
- Thyroid disorders.

Q4. What are the different types of melasma?

Ans. Melasma can be classified into different types based on different parameters:

Depending on the distribution of patches, melasma can be of three types:

a. *Centrofacial*: This is the most common pattern involving the forehead, cheeks, nose, upper lip, or chin
b. *Malar*: Involving the cheeks and nose mainly
c. *Mandibular*: Involving the skin overlying ramus of the mandible.

Depending on the depth of pigment and Wood's lamp examination, melasma has traditionally been classified into:

- *Epidermal*: Herein, melanin deposition is mainly confined to the basal and suprabasal layers of epidermis. On Wood's lamp examination, accentuation of the pigmentation is observed.
- *Dermal*: This type of melasma has superficial and deep perivascular melanophages in the dermis with noticeably less prominent epidermal pigmentation. No accentuation of pigment is noted with Wood's lamp examination.
- *Mixed*: Deposition of melanin occurs both in epidermis and dermis; hence accentuation is confined to few areas.

However, as per the latest evidence gathered from specialized investigational techniques like in vivo reflectance confocal microscopy (RCM), it has been proven that this traditional depth-based classification of Sanchez et al. lacks credence, since all melasma is essentially *mixed*.

Q5. What are the differential diagnoses of melasma?

Ans. The clinical differentials include:

- Solar lentigines
- Ephelides (Freckles)
- Postinflammatory hyperpigmentation
- Riehl's melanosis (pigmented contact dermatitis)
- Lichen planus pigmentosus and toxic melanoderma
- Pigmentary demarcation lines—type F and G
- Drug-induced facial hyperpigmentation
- Facial acanthosis nigricans
- Frictional melanosis
- Maturational hyperpigmentation
- Nevus of Ota
- Acquired bilateral nevus of Ota-like macules (Hori's nevus)
- Exogenous ochronosis.

Q6. How do you assess the severity of melasma?

Ans. The most commonly used scoring system used for melasma is the "Melasma Area and Severity Index" proposed by Kimbrough-Green et al. It is calculated by dividing the face into four areas: the forehead, right malar area, left malar area and chin. Each area is weighted depending on its surface area contribution to the face such that the forehead, right malar area and left malar area are 30% each, and the chin is 10%. Scoring for darkness of pigment (D) when compared with normal skin and homogeneity of the pigment (H) in the specified area is then performed. A numerical value for area of involvement, ranging from 1 (<10%), 2 (10–29%), 3 (30–49%), 4 (50–69%), 5 (70–89%) or 6 (90–100%) is assigned. The total score is calculated as follows:

- The range of score is 0 to 48.

Other means of assessing severity include:

- Melasma severity score
- Colorimetry
- Mexametry.

Q7. How do you assess the impact of melasma on quality of life?

Ans. The most commonly used tool for assessment of quality of life in patients with melasma is the MELASQoL. This scale has been developed as an improvement over the earlier QoL evaluation methods like SKINDEX-16 and skin discoloration evaluation questionnaire. MELASQoL highlights the three life domains most adversely affected by melasma (social life, recreation/leisure and emotional well-being). It is a 10-question scale that asks patients to rate how they feel about each issue on a scale of 1 (not bothered at all) to 7 (bothered all the time); with the final score varying from 10 to 70 with a higher score indicating a worse quality of life related to melasma.

Q8. Which investigations may help in the diagnosis and/or treatment of melasma?

Ans. The diagnosis of melasma is primarily clinical and seldom requires any invasive investigation like a skin biopsy to differentiate it from a simulating facial melanosis. However, the role of noninvasive evaluation tools is being increasingly recognized with pertinent details given here.

- *Dermoscopy*: It demonstrates presence of light to dark brown diffuse reticular pigmentation with sparing of follicular openings and often the presence of predominant telangiectasias. Annular, honeycomb and arcuate structures may also be observed. Dermoscopy is helpful in assessing the severity of melasma, noninvasive differentiation from other facial melanoses, appreciation of its vascular component and as a pre- and post-treatment comparison tool.
- In vivo RCM
- *Histopathology*: Melasma is characterized by: (1) melanin deposition in basal and suprabasal keratinocytes; (2) highly dendritic (branched) deeply pigmented melanocytes; (3) melanin in the dermis within melanophages, and (4) solar elastosis with elastic fiber fragmentation.

Q9. What are the treatment options of melasma?

Ans. Melasma tends to be a highly recalcitrant condition that invariably recurs on discontinuation of the treatment. However, the pigmentation can be rendered lighter, and the effect may be maintained to variable degrees by employing various topical and/or oral treatment regimes as well as physical procedures.

General measures: These include sun protection, regular use of a broad-spectrum sunscreen, *discontinuation* of hormonal contraception, gentle and mildly exfoliating cleanser, and moisturizer for dry skin. Cosmetic camouflage (make-up) is invaluable to disguise the pigment and should be offered to every patient with conspicuous lesions, during the treatment and if treatment fails.

***Specific Interventions*:**

Topical agents:

- Tyrosinase inhibitors: Hydroquinone (2–4%), low potency steroids like hydrocortisone, mequinol, azelaic acid, arbutin and deoxyarbutin, licorice extract, rucinol, resveratrol, 4-hydroxy-anisole, 2,5-dimethyl-4-hydroxy-3(2H)-furanone, N-acetyl glucosamine, ascorbic acid and glutathione
- Reduction in melanosome transfer: Retinoids and soybean trypsin inhibitor
- Inhibition of melanosome maturation: Arbutin and deoxyarbutin
- Stimulation of keratinocyte turnover: Retinoids (tretinoin—0.25%)
- Interaction with copper: Kojic acid (2%) and ascorbic acid (10–25%)
- Inhibition of protease activated receptor 2: Soybean trypsin inhibitor
- Inhibition of plasmin: Tranexamic acid (3–5%)
- Reduction of alpha-melanocyte-stimulating hormone-induced melanin production: Beta-carotene
- Various combinations of the above agents, like the Kligman's formula, modified Kligman's formula

(containing hydroquinone, a mild-mid potency steroid and 0.25% tretinoin), etc.

Oral agents: Various inhibitors of tyrosinase and agents modifying the vascular component of melasma have been used. These include:

- Oral antioxidants: Proanthocyanidin (75–150 mg/day), combination anti-oxidants containing various concentrations of vitamin C, vitamin E, beta-carotene, copper, selenium, etc.
- Oral tranexamic acid: 250–500 mg twice-a-day for 3–6 months
- Oral glutathione: It is being increasingly used, but how effective it really is, needs confirmation. If given, then a dose of at least 250–500 mg twice-a-day, preferably in combination with alpha-lipoic acid and vitamin C, can be administered for 3–6 months.

Chemical peels:

- Glycolic acid
- Lactic acid
- Salicylic acid
- Trichloroacetic acid
- Tretinoin
- Mandelic acid
- Phytic acid
- Jessner's peel—traditional as well as modified.

Lasers and light devices:

- QS Nd:YAG (neodymium-doped yttrium aluminum garnet) laser 1,064 nm (low fluence mode)—laser toning
- Combination of QS Nd:YAG laser toning and fractional CO_2 laser
- Intense pulsed Light (IPL)
- Combination of IPL with QS Nd:YAG laser toning.

Q10. Which of the following describes the correct combination of the original triple combination for melasma suggested by Kligman?

a. 2% HQ + 0.05% RA + 0.01% fluocinolone acetonide
b. 2% HQ + 0.05% RA + 0.01% dexamethasone
c. 5% HQ + 0.1% RA + 1% hydrocortisone
d. 5% HQ + 0.1% RA + 0.1% dexamethasone

Abbreviations: HQ, hydroquinone; RA, retinoic acid or tretinoin

Ans. d. 5% HQ + 0.1% RA + 0.1% dexamethasone.

Q11. All of the following statements pertaining to melasma are true except:

a. Sun exposure is the most important avoidable risk factor for the pathogenesis of melasma
b. Both the genders are almost equally affected
c. Hormonal treatments such as oral contraceptive pills containing estrogen and/or progesterone are contributory in around a quarter of the affected women
d. Centrofacial pattern is the most common clinical pattern of melasma

Ans. b. Both the genders are almost equally affected.

CHAPTER 52

Diffuse Facial Pigmentation

Vinitha Varghese

Case study — Diffuse Facial Pigmentation

Presenting Complaints

Doctor, I have increasing pigmentation on my face since 1 year.

Setting

Dermatology outpatient department.

History of Present Illness

A 55-year-old lady presented with brownish gray pigmentation over the face since 1 year. She gave a history of applying a particular cosmetic cream for the past 2 years.

General Physical Examination and Systemic Examination

No abnormality detected.

Dermatological Examination

A diffuse brownish hyperpigmentation was seen over the forehead and malar regions (Fig. 1). Her blood investigations including total counts, liver and renal function, thyroid function tests were within normal limits.
Histopathology showed liquefaction degeneration of the basal layer of the epidermis with a perivascular and superficial dermal infiltrate along with pigmentary incontinence.

Q1. What is the diagnosis?

a. Ashy dermatoses
b. Riehl's melanosis
c. Poikiloderma of Civatte
d. Exogenous ochronosis

Ans. b. Riehl's melanosis.

Q2. What are the causative factors of facial hyper-pigmentation?

Ans. Genetic and racial factors are important, the increased pigmentation occurring more frequently in those with dark skins, especially those of Middle Eastern or Asian descent. Endocrine factors play a major role in melasma and are implicated to some degree in other melanoses. External agents (light and photodynamic chemicals) are essential factors in the occupational melanoses but are also implicated in photocontact dermatitis (Riehl's melanosis), erythromelanosis and Poikiloderma of Civatte. Other unknown factors are certainly involved, and wide individual variation in susceptibility must be postulated. Cosmetics may occasionally cause facial melanosis. Facial melanosis, of course, may also be a conspicuous feature of Addisonian pigmentation.

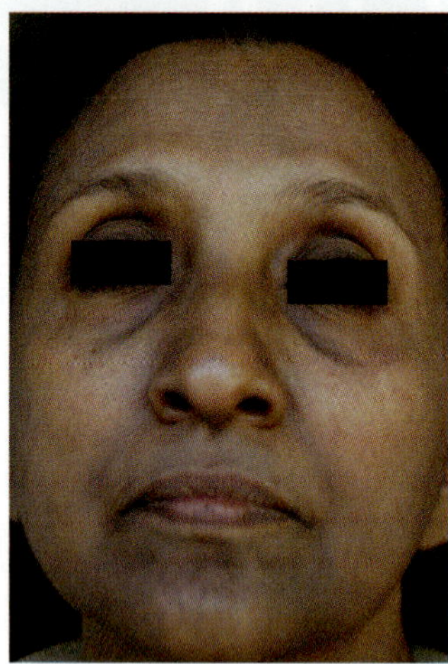

Fig. 1: Diffuse pigmentation over face

Q3. What is pigmented cosmetic dermatitis?

Ans. It is otherwise known as Riehl's melanosis. This is a facial melanosis resulting from phototoxic reaction to skin contact with photoactive agents. Tar derivatives and fragrances are suspected to be the cause. Brownish-gray pigmentation develops quite rapidly over the greater part of the face but is more intense on the forehead and temples.

Smaller pigmented macules, often perifollicular, lie beyond the indefinite margin. The pigmentation may extend to the chest, neck and scalp, and occasionally involves the hands and forearms.

Q4. Which condition presents with mottled pigmentation on face and neck?

Ans. This condition is known as Poikiloderma of Civatte. Poikiloderma of Civatte presents as mottled pigmentation (atrophy, telangiectasia, hyper- and hypopigmentation) which typically appears on the sides of the face and neck and on the upper anterior chest with sparing of submandibular and submental areas (photoprotected areas) after years of repeated ultraviolet (UV) exposure. Milder forms are common and few patients seek medical advice. The condition is mostly asymptomatic, although some patients experience itching, burning and flushing.

Q5. What are the presenting features of erythromelanosis follicularis?

Ans. The condition is characterized by a triad of hyperpigmentation, follicular plugging and erythema with or without telangiectasia, affecting the lateral aspects of the cheeks and in some cases the neck. It has been suggested that it is a subtype of keratosis pilaris. A background of reddish brown pigmentation and telangiectasia is studded with pale follicular papules. The hairs are lost from the majority of affected vellus hair follicles but terminal hair follicles of the scalp and beard are less conspicuously affected. The pigmentation involves the skin in front of, beneath and behind the ear, extending to the side of the neck. It spreads slowly, is persistent and is not influenced by treatment. The distribution and lack of clinical follicular keratosis or scarring readily distinguish erythromelanosis from other forms of keratosis pilaris and from other facial melanoses.

Q6. What are the differential diagnoses of erythromelanosis follicularis?

Ans. The differential diagnoses include:
- Keratosis pilaris and its variants
- Keratosis pilaris rubra
- Melasma
- Poikiloderma of Civatte
- Corticosteroid-induced rosacea
- Actinic telangiectasia.

Q7. Which are the conditions in which patient has multiple small pigmented brownish macules on the face?

Ans. The differentials in this case are ephelides (freckles), lentigines, café au lait macules (CALMs).

Q8. How will you differentiate between the above conditions?

Ans. Differences between freckles, lentigines and CALMs have been listed in Table 1.

Q9. What are the conditions where there is perioral pigmentation?

Ans. The conditions where perioral pigmentation is characteristically seen include peribuccal pigmentation of Brocq and postinflammatory pigmentation of perioral dermatitis. Peribuccal pigmentation of Brocq occurs predominantly in middle aged women: a photodynamic substance in cosmetics is probably responsible. It is clinically characterized by diffuse brownish red pigmentation that occurs symmetrically around the mouth but spares a narrow perioral ring. The erythema may fluctuate but the pigmentation is persistent. It may extend up to the center of the face to forehead, angle of jaw and temples.

Q10. What are pigmentary demarcation lines?

Ans. Pigmentary demarcation lines are abrupt transition lines between hyperpigmented skin and lighter

Table 1: Difference between freckles, lentigines and CALMs

Freckles	*Lentigines*	*CALMs*
Increase in melanin (Hypermelanotic)	Increase in melanocytes (Hypermelanocytic)	Increase in melanin (Hypermelanotic)
Round to oval, ill defined, hyperpigmented macules	Well-defined hyperpigmented macules	Well-circumscribed, uniformly light to dark brown macule or patch
Trigger/aggravating factor: Sun exposure/UV exposure	Not aggravated by UV exposure	Not aggravated by UV exposure
Responds to Sunscreens	No response	No response
In Lentigines and CALMS when they are familial, congenital, multiple or have systemic features—syndromic associations are seen unlike freckles.		

areas. These lines coincide with cutaneous nerve distribution. Facial PDF are classified as F, G and H.

Line F represents an inverted cone-shaped hyperpigmented patch, extending from lateral part of the orbital rim and pointing inferiorly or inferolaterally.

- Line G represents two inverted cones with a rim of normal pigmentation in between forming a W-shaped patch.
- Line H is a linear hyperpigmented patch extending from lateral corners of mouth.

Q11. Which are the conditions characterized by persistent slate-gray color over the face?

Ans. The two important conditions are lichen planus pigmentosus (LPP) and erythema dyschormicum perstans (Ashy dermatosis). Clinically, ashy dermatosis is characterized by progressive macules of varying shades of gray, there may initially be signs of inflammation with a red, slightly raised and palpably infiltrated margin which eventually coalesce over extensive areas of the trunk, limbs and face. Against the general grayish background are macules of hypomelanosis or hypermelanosis. The condition is persistent and slowly extends. The lesions are mostly asymptomatic, although some patients may experience mild pruritus. Mucous membranes are spared. LPP presents as macules over face, neck, upper limbs but may be more widespread and involves the intertriginous areas predominantly. Histopathology of LPP shows relatively flat epidermis with the loss of rete pattern, focal basal cell vacuolization with necrotic keratinocytes, Civatte bodies, dermal melanophages, and sparse lymphohistiocytic infiltrate.

Q12. Enumerate the drugs causing facial melanosis and their clinical presentation.

Ans. Drugs have been enumerated in Table 2.

Q13. What is exogenous ochronosis?

Ans. Exogenous ochronosis is the discoloration of the skin after topical use primarily of hydroquinone, but may also be caused by the use of phenol or resorcinol. It is characterized by gray-brown or blue-black macules in the skin in contact with hydroquinone, normally

Table 2: Drugs causing facial melanosis with clinical presentation

Drugs	*Clinical presentation*
Amiodarone	Slate-gray or purple discoloration of photo-exposed areas due to accumulation of amiodarone and lipofuscin in dermal macrophages. Dose/duration dependent effect
Chloroquine	Bluish gray macular to diffuse pigmentation due to complexes of melanin, hemosiderin and mepacrine, in combination with sulfur. Involves nail bed, palate and bleaches hair
Clofazimine	Initially red, then violaceous brown diffuse pigmentation due to drug accumulation
Anticonvulsants	Melasma like/diffuse brown, post-exanthematous discoloration (hydantoin, phenytoin barbiturates)
Psychotropic drugs	A blue-gray pigmentation of the sun-exposed areas (trifluoperazine, imipramine, chlorpromazine)
Tetracycline (minocycline, doxycycline-rarely)	Well-circumscribed blue-gray macules located respectively in areas of acne scars (type I), at sites of previous inflammation, distant from sites of active inflammation or infection and sun exposed areas (type II), or on the vermilion of the lower lip (type IV). Type III is known as the "muddy skin syndrome" and is characterized by diffuse symmetrical brown-gray discoloration with a tendency to photo-aggravation
Cytotoxic drugs	Bleomycin causes flagellate pigmentation (busulfan, doxorubicin, bleomycin, hydroxyurea)

the face, neck, back and the extensor surfaces of the limbs. No hyperpigmentation of cartilage, sclerae or conjunctivae occurs.

Q14. Enumerate the endocrine causes of diffuse pigmentation which may have facial melanosis as a component?

Ans. Addison's disease. The discoloration in Addison disease is typically diffuse with accentuation in sun-exposed areas. It is also accentuated in the flexures, at sites of pressure and friction, and in the creases of palms and soles. Normally pigmented areas, such as the nipples and genital skin, darken. Pigmentation of the buccal mucous membrane is often present, and the conjunctival and vaginal mucous membranes may also be involved. Addisonian pattern of pigmentation may also be seen in Acromegaly, Cushings syndrome, following adrenocorticotropic hormone administration, hyperthyroidism and vitamin B12 deficiency. In addition, in hyperthyroidism, the eyelids are occasionally conspicuously pigmented (the Jellinek sign). Some patients show melasma-like rather than diffuse pigmentation.

Q15. Are there any infective causes of facial melanosis?

Ans. Yes. Post chikungunya pigmentation has been reported from several parts of India. The most common cutaneous manifestation of chikungunya is an erythematous maculopapular rash. An asymptomatic, brownish-black pigmentation, predominantly involving the centrofacial area, in form of freckle-like macules or slate-colored pigmentation is not uncommon. This may persist for about 3–6 months after the infection. Other patterns of pigmentation observed include melasma-like pigmentation over the face, periorbital melanosis, and a flagellate pattern of pigmentation on the face and extremities.

Table 3: Treatment options for facial melanosis

General measures:
- Photoprotection and sunscreens
- Lifestyle modifications
- Avoidance of aggravating factors

Topical skin lightening agents:
- Kligman regimen
- Hydroquinone
- Topical steroids
- Retinoids
- Glycolic acid creams
- Kojic acid
- Niacinamide
- Mequinol
- Arbutin
- Ascorbic acid
- Liquorice
- N-acetyl-4-S-cysteaminylphenol

Other agents: N-acetyl glucosamine, thioctic acid (alpha-lipoic acid), gentisic acid, soybean extract, and paper mulberry extract.

Physical therapies:
- Chemical peels
- Lasers

Q16. What are the treatment options for a patient with facial melanosis?

Ans. Treatment options for a patient with facial melanosis have been listed in Table 3.

CHAPTER 53

Reticulate Pigmentary Disorders

Samipa S Mukherjee

Case study Reticulate Pigmentation

Presenting Complaints

Doctor, I am having pigmentation of the axilla and groins since teenage. It is progressively increasing and is not improving with any topical medications.

Setting

Dermatology outpatient department.

History of Present Illness

A 32-year-old female born to nonconsanguineous parents, presented with pigmentation of axilla and groins, with no family history or affection of any sibling in the family with similar complaints. The lesions were first noted in the axilla as multiple dark brown dots during early teenage which progressively increased to involve the neck, area below breasts, trunk, proximal arms and front surface of elbows. There were no aggravating or alleviating factors.

General Physical Examination and Systemic Examination

No abnormality detected.

Dermatological Examination

- Reticulate pigmentation over the axilla, groin, neck, inframammary folds, proximal arms, antecubital fossa (Fig. 1).
- Acneiform perioral pits.
- Comedo-like papules on the neck and axilla.
- Epidermal cysts.

Q1. What is the most likely diagnosis?

a. Acropigmentation of Kitamura
b. Dowling Degos disease (DDD)
c. Dyskeratosis congenita
d. Dermatopathia pigmentosa reticularis

Ans. b. Dowling Degos disease. The presence of progressive reticulate flexural pigmentation, acneiform perioral pits, comedo-like papules on the neck and axilla with epidermal cysts lead to the diagnosis of DDD. It is mainly a clinical diagnosis.

Q2. How do you confirm the diagnosis of Dowling Degos Disease?

Ans. Confirmation of the diagnosis can be done on histopathology which shows the characteristic finding of an atrophic epidermis with long, narrow, branched rete ridges that intertwine at their bases

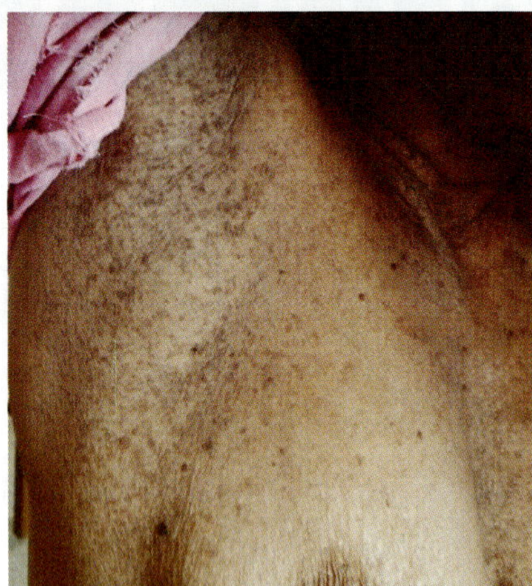

Fig. 1: Hyperpigmented macules in the axilla (*Courtesy*: Dr Rashmi Sarkar)

("antler-like" appearance). Increased melanin in the basal membrane and dilated follicles with cysts can also be seen.

Q3. What are the variants of Dowling Degos Disease?

Ans. Variants of Dowling Degos Disease include:

- *Haber's syndrome*: It is a disorder characterized by pigmented keratotic papules on the axilla, neck, and torso with pitted scars on the face and persistent facial erythema.
- *Galli-Galli disease*: It is essentially an acantholytic variant of DDD.
- *Pigmentatio reticularis faciei et colli*: It is possibly a variant of DDD which presents with hyperpigmentation of the face and neck with multiple epidermoid cysts.

Q4. How do you classify reticulate pigmentary disorders?

Ans. It is classified based on the regional distribution of lesions.

- *Facial involvement*:
  - Haber's syndrome
  - Cantu syndrome
  - Mende's Da Costa syndrome
  - Naegeli-Franceschetti-Jadassohn (NFJ) syndrome
- *Generalized*:
  - Dyschromatosis universalis hereditaria
  - Dyskeratosis congenita
  - Dermatopathia pigmentosa reticularis
  - NFJ syndrome
  - Pruritus pigmentosa
- *Acral*:
  - Acropigmentation of Dohi
  - Acropigmentation of Kitamura
  - Heterochromia extremetarum
- *Flexural*:
  - Dowling Degos disease
  - Galli-Galli disease
  - Confluent reticulate papillomatosis.

Q5. What are the clinical features of acropigmentation of Kitamura?

Ans. Acropigmentation of Kitamura generally presents by the second decade of life. It is characterized by sharply demarcated, slightly depressed blackish brown macules over the dorsum of hands and feet with presence of small pits on the palms causing a break in the epidermal ridge pattern. Eventually the extensors of limbs, neck and upper trunk may also get involved.

Q6. How does acropigmentation of Kitamura differ from acropigmentation symmetrica of Dohi?

Ans. For difference between acropigmentation of Kitamura and acropigmentation symmetrica of Dohi, see Table 1.

Q7. What are the various associations of dyschromatosis universalis hereditaria?

Ans. Associations of dyschromatosis universalis hereditaria include:

- Coxa valga
- Nerve compression
- Small stature
- High tone deafness

Table 1: Acropigmentation of Kitamura and acropigmentation symmetrica of Dohi

	Acropigmentation of Kitamura	*Acropigmentation symmetrica of Dohi*
Course	Gradually progressive	Nonprogressive
Clinical features	Sharply demarcated, slightly depressed blackish brown macules	Hypo-/hyperpigmented macules
Pitting	Small pits in palms causing break in epidermal ridge	No pits
Extent	Involves dorsum of hands, feet, neck, face and trunk with extensors of limbs	Involves dorsal and ventral aspects of hands and feet, proximal limbs and face but trunk is spared

- Photosensitivity
- Neurosensory hearing defect.

Q8. What is the inheritance of dyskeratosis congenita?

a. X-linked dominant
b. Autosomal dominant
c. Autosomal recessive
d. X-linked recessive

Ans. d. It is predominantly X-linked recessive inheritance.

Q9. What is the classical triad of dyskeratosis congenita?

Ans. Classical triad of dyskeratosis congenita includes:

- Abnormal nails
- Reticular skin pigmentation
- Oral leukoplakia and associated with very high risks of developing aplastic anemia, myelodysplastic syndrome, leukemia, and solid tumors.

Q10. What are the extracutaneous manifestations of dyskeratosis congenita?

Ans. The extracutaneous manifestations are:

- Extensive caries
- Aplastic anemia
- Bleeding problems and purpura
- Esophageal diverticuli with dysphagia
- Retardation of growth
- Hypogonadism
- Mental retardation.

Q11. Define the dyspigmentation patterns (coexistent hypo-/hyperpigmentation)?

Ans. Dyspigmentation patterns:

- Mottled pigmentation: Refers to a blotchy pattern/patchy appearance with different shades of color both hyper and/or hypopigmentation with the individual lesions having various sizes.
- Dyschromatosis: Term used for disorders with "freckle like" hypo- and hyperpigmented macules of small and irregular shape.
- Reticular: Refers to net "like" or "lacy" regularly spaced ring/partial rings with sparing of intervening skin.
- Reticulate hyperpigmentation: Hyperpigmented ephelides-like lesions, which have varying degrees of pigment and have indistinct borders, can be both congenital and acquired.
- Poikilodermatous: It is characterized by atrophy, macular or reticulate pigmentation and telangiectasia.

Q12. What is the treatment option for Dowling Degos Disease?

Ans. As Dowling Degos disease is a genetic disorder, there is no curative treatment. The results are usually not satisfactory. However, topical corticosteroids, depigmenting agents (hydroquinone, azelaic acid), topical tretinoin/adapalene, systemic retinoids and Er: YAG laser pulse energy have been used.

CHAPTER 54

Pigmented Purpuric Dermatoses

Indrashis Podder, Biju Vasudevan

Case study Pigmented Purpuric Dermatoses

Presenting Complaints

Doctor, I have developed these darkish, asymptomatic rashes over both my lower legs for the last 8 years. Initially only a few rashes were present, however they have been increasing lately.

Setting

Dermatology outpatient department.

History of Present Illness

A 42-year-old healthy lady, a traffic sergeant by profession presented with the complaints of developing asymptomatic darkish, flat lesions over both her lower extremities for the last 8 years with mild itching occasionally. The lesions have gradually increased in number over the years. These rashes are distributed over the lower part of her legs (mainly around her ankles), no lesion is present above the knee. She also reported recurrent episodes of bilateral leg swelling especially in the evenings which resolved after few hours of rest.

General Examination

Alert, conscious, co-operative.
Pulse rate: 70 beats/min. Peripheral pulses: felt, normal in volume and character, no varicosities noted. Mild pedal edema present.

Systemic Examination

Within normal limits.

Dermatological Examination

- Multiple, well-defined, pinpoint violaceous to hyperpigmented macules; few of them coalescing to form larger patches (Fig. 1).
- The patches are studded with pin-head sized red puncta *(cayenne paper appearance)*
- Distributed over both lower legs, around the ankles.
- Hair, nail, mucosa normal.

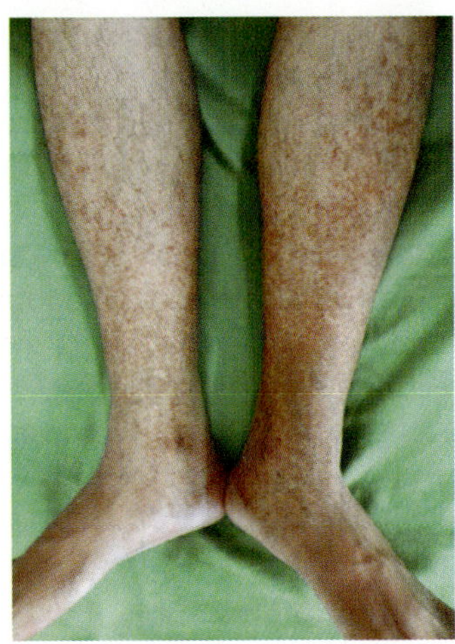

Fig. 1: Multiple hyperpigmented macules on both legs

Q1. What is the most likely diagnosis?

a. Stasis dermatitis
b. Schamberg's disease
c. Contact dermatitis
d. Angioma serpiginosa

Ans: b. Schamberg's disease—a variant of pigmented purpuric dermatoses (PPD).

Q2. What are the points in favor of your diagnosis?

Ans: The points in favor of diagnosis are:

- Typical clinical appearance *(cayenne paper appearance);* localized to the lower part of legs (mostly around the ankles), asymptomatic, absence of lesion above the knees.
- History of prolonged standing (traffic sergeant by occupation) and recurrent episodes of bilateral leg swelling suggesting peripheral pooling of blood.
- Discrete lesions with no evidence of active dermatitis (stasis dermatitis usually presents with diffuse and extensive involvement along with features of dermatitis viz. pruritus etc.).

Q3. How will you confirm your diagnosis?

Ans: Although, clinical picture is sufficient to make the diagnosis, a histopathological examination (HPE) can help to confirm the diagnosis. A lower limb Doppler ultrasound may be needed to assess the status of blood flow and to rule out valvular/perforator incompetence of veins and deep vein thrombosis.

Q4. What are the different clinical variants of pigmented purpuric dermatoses?

Ans: The different clinical variants of pigmented purpuric dermatoses (PPD) are given here:

- Schamberg's disease (progressive PPD)
- Majocchi's disease (purpura annularis telangiectodes) (ring-shaped lesions)
- Pigmented purpuric lichenoid dermatosis of Gougerot and Blum
- Eczematoid-like purpura of Doucas and Kapetanakis (scaly lesions)
- Lichen aureus (usually present with a solitary lesion)
- Itching PPD (disseminated pruriginous angiodermatitis)
- Granulomatous PPD
- Segmental PPD
- Pigmented purpuric dermatoses/mycosis fungoides overlap

Q5. Which variant of PPD occurs most frequently?

a. Lichenoid variety of Gougerot and Blum
b. Eczematoid variant of Doucas and Kapetanakis
c. Schamberg's disease
d. Majocchi's disease

Ans: c. Schamberg's disease (~50% cases of PPD)

Q6. Name some drugs which have been implicated to cause PPD.

Ans: Some of the important drugs which have been reported to cause PPD are given here:

- Nonsteroidal anti-inflammatory drugs
- Diuretics (furosemide)
- Glipizide
- Captopril
- Carbamazepine
- Chlordiazepoxide
- Medroxyprogesterone
- Nitroglycerine
- Amlodipine
- Topical 5 fluorouracil and eutectic mixture of local anesthetics (EMLA).

Q7. Describe in brief the HPE findings in a typical case of PPD.

Ans: The HPE finding of such a case is given here:

Epidermis: Usually unremarkable, occasionally slight acanthosis and/or basal layer degeneration may be found.

Dermis: Perivascular lymphocytic infiltration, extravasation of red blood cells and hemosiderin laden macrophages are usually found.

Special stains: Perls staining demonstrates hemosiderin deposition in the dermis, more superficially that helps to differentiate from stasis dermatitis.

Q8. What is the dermoscopic finding in PPD?

Ans: Coppery background with discrete red dots and globules.

Q9. How will you manage this patient?

Ans: *General measures*:

- Proper counseling regarding the benign nature of the disease, very less likelihood to progress proximal to the knees (trunk and upper limb involvement is extremely rare).
- To take measures to avoid pooling of blood in the dependent parts (lower limbs while standing) like avoidance of prolonged standing, foot end elevation during sleep, etc.
- Supportive stockings should be worn at all times.

Specific measures:

- *Topical therapies*:
  - Topical corticosteroids (medium to high potency) for 2 weeks. Triamcinolone acetonide spray may also be tried
  - Topical calcineurin inhibitors (tacrolimus and pimecrolimus)
- *Systemic therapies*:
  - Pentoxifylline (400–800 mg/day) (acts by inhibiting T-cell adherence to endothelial cells and keratinocytes thereby minimizing inflammation)
  - Oral bioflavonoids (Rutoside 50 mg twice daily) and ascorbic acid (Vitamin C 500 mg twice daily)
  - Aminaphtone 75 mg twice daily, this drug used in stasis purpura, also found to improve Schamberg's disease
  - Anecdotal reports of efficacy: Calcium dobesilate, griseofulvin, colchicine, minocycline, methotrexate and cyclosporine.

Other modalities:

- Phototherapy (narrowband ultraviolet B)
- Photochemotherapy (psoralen combined with ultraviolet A, photodynamic therapy)
- 10% thioglycolic acid peeling: A hemosiderin solubilizing substance, peeling done weekly once for 5–6 sessions
- Advanced fluorescence technology (a method of delivering an intense beam of fluorescent light) has shown favorable results
- 595 nm vascular laser.

Q10. What is the prognosis of this condition?

Ans: It has a benign, chronic, relapsing and remitting course. Spontaneous remission may also occur.

CHAPTER 55

Vitiligo

Debdeep Mitra, Ajay Chopra, Krishna Talukdar

Case study Vitiligo

Presenting Complaints

Doctor, I have these milky white patches on my body since 6 months.

Setting

Dermatology outpatient department.

History of Present Illness

A 58-year-old male presented with white patches on the body since 6 months. The lesions were insidious in onset and gradually progressive. To start with, there were few small lesions over the face. Gradually, the lesions increased in size and number to involve the trunk and limbs as well.

General and Systemic Examination

No abnormality detected.

Dermatological Examination

Multiple depigmented macules on the trunk, face and limbs (Fig. 1). All the macules have a scalloping border. Few white hairs are found in the patches.

Q1. What is the diagnosis?

a. Nevus depigmentosus
b. Albinism
c. Vitiligo
d. Pityriasis alba

Ans. c. Vitiligo. The history and clinical examination findings point toward the diagnosis.

Q2. What is vitiligo?

Ans. Vitiligo is a disorder of pigmentation in which melanocytes in the skin are destroyed. As a result, depigmented macules appear on the skin in different parts of the body. Similar patches also appear on both the mucous membranes and the retina. The hair that grows on areas affected by vitiligo sometimes turns white known as leukotrichia.

Q3. What is the prevalence and is there any sex predilection in vitiligo?

Ans. Vitiligo affects approximately 0.5–1% of the population, with an average age of onset at about 24 years. Its prevalence appears to be equal between men and women and there is no difference in the rate of occurrence according to skin type or race. It

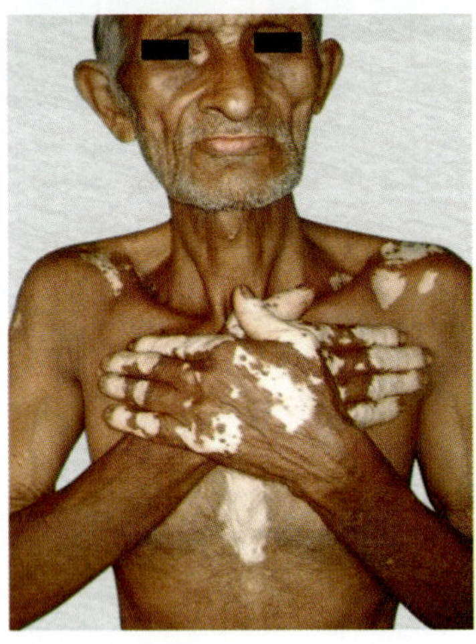

Fig. 1: Multiple depigmented macules on the dorsum of hands and neck

is however more visible in patients with darker skin types due to the contrast.

Q4. How do we classify vitiligo?

Ans. The classification of vitiligo has been proposed by Picardo and Taieb as per Table 1.

Q5. What is the differential diagnosis of vitiligo?

Ans. Following are the conditions which present with depigmented or hypopigmented macules other than vitiligo:

Table 1: Classification of vitiligo

Type of vitiligo	*Subtypes*	*Remarks*
Nonsegmental vitiligo (NSV)	Focal, mucosal, acrofacial, generalized, universal	Subtyping may not reflect a distinct nature, but useful information for epidemiologic studies
Segmental vitiligo (SV)	Focal, mucosal, unisegmental, bisegmental or multisegmental	Further classification according to distribution pattern possible, but not yet standardized
Mixed (NSV + SV)	According to severity of SV	Usually the SV part in mixed vitiligo is more severe
Unclassified	Focal at onset, multifocal asymmetrical nonsegmental, mucosal (one site)	

- Inherited or genetically induced hypomelanoses (usually present at birth)
  - Piebaldism
  - Tuberous sclerosis
  - Ito's hypomelanosis
  - Waardenburg's syndrome
  - Hermansky-Pudlak syndrome
  - Menkés syndrome
  - Ziprkowski-Margolis syndrome
  - Griscelli's syndrome
- Postinflammatory hypomelanoses
  - Related to an increased epidermal turn over
    - Psoriasis
    - Atopic dermatitis
  - Related to an acute lichenoid/cytotoxic infiltrate with pigment incontinence
    - Lichen sclerosus et atrophicus
    - Toxic drug reaction
- Paramalignant hypomelanoses
  - Mycosis fungoides
  - Melanoma-associated depigmentation
- Parainfectious hypopigmentation
  - Pityriasis versicolor
  - Leprosy
  - Leishmaniasis
  - Onchocerciasis
  - Acquired macular hypomelanosis
- Post-traumatic leukoderma
  - Postburns
  - Postscars
  - Occupational and drug-induced depigmentation
  - Phenolic-catecholic derivatives
  - Systemic drugs (chloroquine, fluphenazine, physostigmine and imatinib)
  - Topical drugs (imiquimod, long-term use of topical steroid).

Q6. What are the clinical features of the various inherited or genetically-induced hypomelanosis conditions?

Ans. The clinical features have been listed in Table 2.

Q7. What are the various etiological factors for vitiligo?

Ans. It still remains unclear what causes damage or death to the melanocytes and there are many potential pathophysiological theories involving autoimmune, neural, autocytotoxic, biochemical, oxidative stress, melanocytorrhagy, and decreased melanocyte survival hypotheses.

Table 2: Clinical features of various inherited/genetically-induced hypomelanosis conditions

Disorder	*Clinical presentation*	*Transmission/diagnosis*
Piebaldism	White forelock, anterior body midline depigmentation, bilateral shin depigmentation	Autosomal dominant. Skin biopsy: usually, absence of c-kit protein immunostaining in melanocytes Molecular analysis of c-KIT gene or SNA1 gene
Tuberous sclerosis	Small or larger (ash-leaf) white spots, seizures; other usually later cutaneous symptoms (shagreen patches, angiofibromas, etc.)	Autosomal dominant; brain imaging; cardiac and renal imaging Molecular analysis of TSC1 and 2
Ito's hypomelanosis	Blaschkolinear distribution, unilateral or bilateral of hypopigmented streaks	Sporadic chromosomal or genetic mosaicism (blood or skin cells)
Waardenburg's syndrome (type I)	White forelock, hypertelorism, deafness (variable according to genotype) Possible association to congenital megacolon (Hirschsprung's disease)	Autosomal dominant. Genetic testing according to phenotype (several clinical variants and six possible causative genes mutated)
Hermansky-Pudlak syndrome (type 1)	Diffuse depigmentation pattern, eye pigment dilution, hemorrhagic diathesis	Autosomal dominant, genetic heterogeneity (eight possible causative genes). Molecular testing possible according to ethnic background and phenotype
Menkès syndrome	Hair and body diffuse pigment dilution; Pili torti; Neurodegenerative changes	X-linked recessive ATP7A gene mutations; affects cupper dependent enzymes. Molecular testing possible
Ziprkowski-Margolis syndrome	Iris heterochromia, depigmentation (diffuse) + hyperpigmented macules can remain, neurosensorial deafness	Described in Israel in one family. X-linked recessive Mapped to Xq26.3–q27.1
Griscelli's syndrome (type 1)	Silvery hairs usually diffuse liver enlargement and symptoms related to immunodeficiency	Autosomal recessive, three types corresponding to three different causative genes Molecular testing possible

Q8. What is double strike hypothesis in vitiligo?

Ans. In 2010, Michelsen presented a consolidated set of theses which explain the pathomechanisms of vitiligo- and melanoma-associated hypopigmentation. The main thesis is the double strike hypothesis, i.e. vitiligo is caused by at least two different major pathomechanisms: an antibody-based pathomechanism and a T-cell-based pathomechanism. The antibody-based pathomechanism is dominant in diffuse vitiligo, while the T-cell-based pathomechanism is dominant in localized vitiligo.

Q9. How do we assess the stability in vitiligo?

Ans. The stability in vitiligo can be assessed by:

- *History of progression*: Absence of new lesions in last 12 months
- *Extension of old lesions*: No extension of preexisting lesions in last 12 months'
- *Absence of Koebnerization*: No depigmented macules at healed trauma sites
- Vitiligo Disease Activity (VIDA) score of 0 or -1
- Minigrafting or test grafting to see surgical outcome at a test patch
- Biochemical, serological, microscopic and ultrastructural correlates.

Q10. What are the various scoring systems in vitiligo?

Ans. Scoring systems in vitiligo are:

VIDA: This is a six-point scale for assessing vitiligo activity. Scoring is based on the individual's own opinion of the present disease activity over time. Active vitiligo involves either expansion of existing lesions or appearance of new lesions. Grading is as follows:

- VIDA score +4: Activity of 6 weeks or less duration
- VIDA score +3: Activity of 6 weeks to 3 months
- VIDA score +2: Activity of 3–6 months
- VIDA score +1: Activity of 6–12 months
- VIDA score 0: Stable for 1 year or more
- VIDA score -1: Stable with spontaneous repigmentation since 1 year or more.

A low VIDA score indicates less activity.

Vitiligo area severity index (VASI): The percentage of vitiligo involvement is calculated in terms of hand units. One hand unit (which encompasses the palm plus the volar surface of all digits) is approximately equivalent to 1% of the total body surface area. The degree of pigmentation is estimated to the nearest of one of the following percentages:

- 100%—complete depigmentation, no pigment is present
- 90%—specks of pigment present
- 75%—depigmented area exceeds the pigmented area
- 50%—pigmented and depigmented areas are equal
- 25%—pigmented area exceeds depigmented area
- 10%—only specks of depigmentation present. The VASI for each body region is determined by the product of the area of vitiligo in hand units and the extent of depigmentation within each hand unit measured patch.

Total body VASI = ∑ All body sites (hand units) × (residual depigmentation).

Q11. How do we diagnose vitiligo?

Ans. Table 3 shows the diagnosis of vitiligo.

Q12. What are the treatment options for vitiligo?

Ans. In the assessment steps and before starting treatment, it is important to consider the age of the patient, duration of the disease, the course of the disease (progressive, regressive or stable during the last 12 months), type or subtype of vitiligo (as some types or subtypes may necessitate specific treatment approaches), associated diseases in particular autoimmune diseases, previous medication and if possible the psychological profile of the patient or Global Quality of Life QoL assessment.

Table 3: Diagnosis of vitiligo

To confirm the diagnosis	Punch biopsy from lesional and nonlesional skin. Other tests if needed (mycology, molecular biology to detect lymphoma cells, etc.)
If diagnosis is certain	Antithyroid peroxidase, antithyroglobulin antibodies, thyroid stimulating hormone and other tests if needed to assess thyroid function or diagnosis (e.g. antithyroid stimulating hormone receptor antibodies if Grave's disease) Additional autoantibodies (only if patient's history, family history, and/or laboratory parameters point toward strong risk of additional autoimmune disease), endocrinologist/immunologist advice if multiple autoimmune syndrome detected

- *Medical therapy*:
  - Topical corticosteroids
  - Topical calcineurin inhibitors
  - Oral steroid mini-pulse therapy
  - Biologics and immunosuppressants: Tumor necrosis factor-alpha antagonists, cyclosporine, azathioprine and methotrexate
  - Oral antioxidants:
    - Ginkgo biloba
    - Alpha lipoic acid
    - Vitamin C
    - Vitamin E
    - Polyunsaturated fatty acids
    - Zinc
    - Polypodium leucotomos
  - Topical antioxidants:
    - Catalase
    - Superoxide dismutase
- *Light-based therapy*:
  - Narrow band ultraviolet B therapy (NBUVB)
  - Photochemotherapy with psoralen and ultraviolet A radiation (PUVA)
  - Photochemotherapy with khellin plus UVA (KUVA)
  - Photochemotherapy with L-phenylalanine (L-phe) (PAUVA)
  - 308 nm Monochromatic Excimer laser (MEL)
  - Bioskin is a new device which transmits a focused 311-nm UVB radiation
  - Helium neon (HeNe) laser emits 632.8 nm radiation and is used for the treatment of segmental vitiligo.
- *Surgical therapy*: Limited to cases stable for 12 months or more
  - Primary excision and suturing
  - Suction blister grafting
  - Split-thickness skin grafting
  - Punch grafting
  - Autologous melanocyte suspension transplant
  - Autologous culture melanocyte transplant
- *Adjunct therapy*:
  - Camouflage:
    - Temporary such as, make up (compact, liquid and stick foundation, etc.)
    - Semipermanent, such as self-tanning agents
    - Permanent, such as micropigmentation and tattoos

Flowchart 1: Treatment protocol for vitiligo

First line therapy
Initial presentation

Recommended: Topical steroids (IA) and in combination with topical vitamin D3 analogues (IB) Alternative: topical calcineurin inhibitors (IIA), systemic steroids (IIB), topical L-phenylalanine (IIB) topical antioxidants and mitochondrial stimulating cream (IB), natural sunlight with PO khelin (IIA)

Rapidly progressive vitiligo? Consider short course of systemic steroids. (IIB)

Recalcitrant lesions on extremities? Consider Tacrolimus at night under occlusion (IIB)

Second line therapy
Recalcitrant vitiligo

Recommended: NBUVB with calcineurin inhibitors (IB)
Alternative: adjunct NBUVB therapy with PO antioxidants (IB), systemic steroids (IIB), or popolypodium leucotomous (IB). Adjunct UVA therapy with psoralen (IIA), systemic steroids (IIB) topical vitamin D3 analogues (IB), PO khelin (IIB), PO L-phenylalanine (IIB), or topical L-phenylalanine (IIB)

Third line therapy
Vitiligo unsuccessfuly treated with total body phototherapy

Recommended: 308 nm LASER with topical steroids (IB)
Alternative: Adjunct 308 nm LASER with topical steroids (IA)

Fourth line therapy
Vitiligo recalcitrant to first, second and third line therapy

Recommended: Suction blister graft (III), split thickness graft (III), autologous melanocyte transplant (IB) (Only if the lesions are stable more than 12 months)

Special population, segmental vitiligo: Treatment as above, consider helium neon laser as third line therapy (IIB)

Special population, generalized vitiligo: Treatment as above, consider depigmentation agents for recalcitrant cases

Camouflage and psychotherapy should be offered to patients at all stages of treatment

Abbreviations: Level IA; Recommendation based on evidence from at least one meta-analysis of randomized control trials, Level IB; Recommendation based on evidence from at least one randomized control trial, Level IIA; Recommendation based on evidence from at least one controlled study without randomization, Level IIB; Recommendation based on evidence from at least one other type of experimental study, Level III; Recommendation based on evidence from nonexperimental study, such as comparative studies, correlation studies and case control studies, Level IV; Recommendation based on evidence from expert committee reports or opinions or clinical experience of respected authorities or both

- Depigmentation:
  - Monobenzone ethyl ester of hydroquinone
  - Q-switch ruby laser
  - Q-switch Alexandrite laser
  - Combination between topical methoxyphenol and Q-switched ruby laser
  - Psychotherapy
- Alternative and herbal treatment, e.g.: Placentrex® which is a topical human placental extract.

Q13. What is the treatment protocol for vitiligo?

Ans. The treatment protocol for vitiligo has been described in Flowchart 1.

SECTION 12

Psoriasis and Related Disorders

Anupam Das

CHAPTER 56

Psoriasis Vulgaris

Bhushan Madke

Case study Psoriasis Vulgaris

Presenting Complaints

Doctor, I have these red-colored flaky lesions on my knees, elbows, lower back and abdomen since past 2 years. My scalp is also getting too much of dandruff these days. I have noticed that these skin lesions get worse during winter months.

Setting

Dermatology outpatient department.

History of Presenting Illness

A 46-year-old man, presented with complaints of multiple red-colored raised flaky lesions on knees, elbows and lower back since past 2 years. He also complains of excessive flakiness of his scalp skin. There is history of aggravation of skin lesions during winter season. Past history is positive for hypertension, diabetes mellitus and coronary heart disease.

General Physical Examination

Well oriented to time, place and person.
Weight: 90 kg, Height: 5'4", BMI: 30.90 kg/m^2.

Systemic Examination

Abdominal obesity is present with girth of 42 inches.
No other systemic abnormality is detected.

Dermatological Examination

- Well-defined erythematous scaly plaques on knees, elbows and presacral area (Figs 1 and 2)
- Extensive scaling of scalp extending beyond the hair margins
- Initially scales came off and then punctate bleeding spots were visible on doing Grattage test.

Q1. What is the most likely diagnosis?

a. Psoriasis vulgaris
b. Nummular eczema
c. Pityriasis lichenoides chronic
d. Seborrheic dermatitis

Ans: a. Psoriasis vulgaris. The classic distribution of erythematous scaly plaques with lesions extending beyond hair margin on scalp and winter exacerbation points toward the diagnosis.

Q2. What are your differential diagnoses?

Ans: Nummular eczema, chronic lichenified eczema, pityriasis rubra pilaris, psoriasiform sarcoidosis, psoriasiform lichen planus, secondary syphilis, parapsoriasis, pityriasis lichenoides chronica,

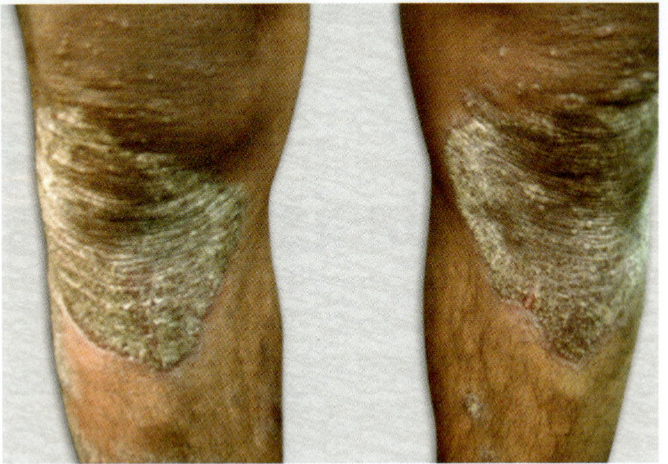

Fig. 1: Well-defined erythematous scaly plaques on knees

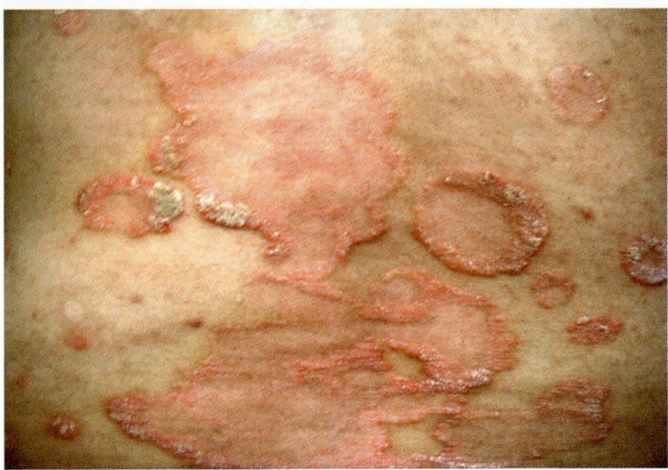

Fig. 2: Similar lesions on lower back

mycosis fungoides plaque stage and reactive arthritis skin lesions.

Q3. How do you diagnose psoriasis?

Ans: Psoriasis can be diagnosed mostly on clinical grounds. It is characterized by well-defined erythematous papules and plaques on extensor aspect of body parts. The pinpoint bleeding is known as 'Auspitz sign'. Where doubt exists, a histopathology will confirm the diagnosis.

Q4. What are the histopathological features of psoriasis?

- Hyperkeratosis and parakeratosis
- Munro's microabscesses in the stratum corneum (collection of neutrophils)
- Hypogranulosis
- Spongiform pustules of Kogoj
- Elongated rete ridges with a camel foot like appearance
- Suprapapillary thinning
- Dilated and tortuous capillaries.

Q5. Is any medical history important?

Ans: History of recurrent tonsillitis (aggravates psoriasis or can initiate a variant known as guttate psoriasis). History of diabetes mellitus [diabetic patients have nonalcoholic steatohepatitis and methotrexate (MTX) therapy can aggravate fatty liver, diabetes mellitus in psoriasis have higher risk of metabolic syndrome], history of smoking (psoriasis and smoking have synergistic adverse effect on cardiovascular system).

Q6. What personal history is important in a patient of psoriasis?

Ans: Alcohol intake, type A personality, presence of stress, any blood transfusion in past (risk of viral hepatitis), high-risk sexual behavior (HIV aggravates psoriasis).

Q7. What are type I and type II psoriasis?

Ans: Henseler and Christophers have identified two ages of onset:

- Type I occurring at or before the age of 40 years and associated with HLA-Cw*0602 allele
- Type II, presenting after the age of 40 years, with a distinct peak at 55–60 years and not associated with MHC gene.

Q8. How do you classify psoriasis?

Ans: Psoriasis can be classified on the basis of morphology of lesions and site:

Morphological classification

- Chronic plaque psoriasis
- Guttate psoriasis
- Annular psoriasis
- Pustular (localized and generalized)
- Erythroderma
- Follicular
- Lichenoid
- Rupoid
- Ostraceous
- Verrucous.

Site

- Inverse
- Scalp
- Nail
- Genital
- Palmoplantar

- Mucosal
- Interdigital.

Q9. How would you like to investigate the patient of psoriasis and what is the rationale of doing these investigations?

- Complete hemogram for baseline counts [methotrexate (MTX) therapy can affect blood counts]
- Liver function test (MTX is contraindicated in liver failure, hepatitis). Serum albumin is required to predict MTX toxicity
- Renal function test (MTX is excreted via kidney, elderly patients have impaired renal function)
- Chest X-ray (to rule out active or latent pulmonary TB as MTX can reactivate latent TB and is contraindicated in active TB)
- Workup for metabolic syndrome (fasting lipid profile)
- Viral markers (active viral hepatitis and MTX can precipitate liver injury)
- HIV (MTX is contraindicated in active HIV infection).

Q10. What are the treatment options available?

Ans: Treatment options include:

Topical

- Emollients
- Corticosteroids
- Dithranol
- *Tars*: coal tar
- Salicylic acid
- *Vitamin D and analogues*: Calcipotriol, calcitriol, tacalcitol
- Tazarotene
- *Calcineurin inhibitors*: Tacrolimus and pimecrolimus.

Phototherapy and photochemotherapy

- Narrow band ultraviolet B
- Excimer laser
- Psoralen plus ultraviolet A (PUVA).

Systemic

- Methotrexate
- *Calcineurin inhibitors*: Cyclosporine
- *Retinoids*: Acitretin, isotretinoin, tazarotene, bexarotene
- *Fumaric acid esters*: Dimethylfumarate and monoethylfumarate
- Hydroxyurea
- Mycophenolate mofetil
- *Retinoic acid metabolism blocking agents*: Liarozole, talarozole
- Leflunomide
- *Thiazolidinediones*: Pioglitazone
- Azathioprine

Biologics

- *Anti-tumor necrosis factor (TNF)-alpha*: Infliximab, etanercept, adalimumab, certolizumab pegol, golimumab
- *Anti-interleukin (IL)-12/23*: Ustekinumab, briakinumab, tildrakizumab
- *Anti-IL-17*: Brodalumab, secukinumab
- *Costimulation inhibitors*: Alefacept
- *Janus kinase inhibitors*: Tofacitinib
- *Phosphodiesterase-4 inhibitors*: Apremilast.

Q11. What are the indications for systemic therapy in psoriasis?

Ans: Indications for systemic therapy in psoriasis are as follows:

- Disease interfering with the quality of life of the patient
- Severe plaque type psoriasis (>10% body surface area involvement or >10 psoriasis area severity index)
- Generalized pustular psoriasis
- Psoriatic erythroderma
- Severe psoriatic arthritis
- Patients refractory to topical therapy
- Patients refractory to phototherapy.

Q12. How do you prescribe methotrexate to a patient of psoriasis?

Ans: Prescription of MTX to a patient of psoriasis:

- Informed consent and thorough counseling
- Advise to strictly use barrier contraception (MTX is present in semen and have abortifacient effect)
- Is patient having any contraindications for receiving MTX?
- MTX can be administered via oral, intramuscular and subcutaneous route
- More commonly, MTX is first given as a test dose to rule out any hypersensitivity or idiosyncratic reactions (MTX-induced pneumonitis)
- MTX can be administered orally as a single dose or either in three divided doses 12-hour apart (Weinstein's regimen).

Q13. Would you like to investigate any other syndrome in this patient?

Ans: As the patient is obese, I would like to assess him for metabolic syndrome. It includes obesity, elevated triglycerides, low high-density lipoproteins (HDL), insulin resistance and hypertension. It is also proposed that the association with metabolic syndrome is stronger for extensive and severe psoriasis. The pathomechanism is attributable to the insulin resistance mediated by TNF-alpha, leptin and adiponectin.

Q14. What are the comorbidities associated with psoriasis?

Ans: Comorbidities associated with psoriasis are as follows:

- Psoriatic arthritis
- Metabolic syndrome
- *Psychiatric*: Depression, anxiety, sexual dysfunction, suicidal tendency
- Diabetes, hypertension, myocardial infarction, dyslipidemia
- Autoimmune diseases
- Inflammatory bowel disease
- Nonalcoholic fatty liver disease
- *Malignancies*: Nonmelanoma skin cancer, lymphoproliferative disorders
- Uveitis
- Chronic obstructive pulmonary disease.

CHAPTER 57

Psoriatic Arthritis

Rajeshwari Dabbas, Ashwani Kumar

Case study Psoriatic Arthritis

Presenting Complaints

Doctor, I have psoriasis since 8 years and pain and swelling of multiple joints since 1 year.

Setting

Dermatology outpatient department

History of Present Illness

A 42-year-old male with psoriasis since 8 years presented with complaints of pain and swelling of multiple joints since 1 year. The joint symptoms had an insidious onset with a gradually progressive course. It started first in the left ankle and later involved the left knee and left wrist. He had early morning stiffness for 2 hours. He also had pain in both heels since 6 months. He had no history suggestive of systemic involvement.

General Physical Examination and Systemic Examination

No abnormality detected

Dermatological Examination

- Multiple, well-defined, erythematous, scaly plaques present on the scalp, back, elbows and legs. Auspitz sign positive. Palms and soles were spared
- Majority of the fingernails showed pitting with subungual hyperkeratosis in few. Toenails showed onycholysis, oil drop sign and subungual hyperkeratosis.

Musculoskeletal Examination

- Gait: Normal
- *Upper limb*: Swelling and tenderness present on the left wrist
- *Lower limb*: Swelling and tenderness present on the left knee and left ankle. Swelling present in the right second toe (dactylitis). Tenderness present at insertion of achilles tendon (bilateral) (enthesitis)
- *Spine*: Normal
- No deformities.

Q1. What is your diagnosis?

a. Rheumatoid arthritis
b. Gout
c. Psoriatic arthritis
d. Seronegative spondyloarthritis

Ans: c. Psoriatic arthritis (PsA). Patient is a known case of psoriasis and has arthritis, dactylitis and enthesitis.

Q2. How do you diagnose psoriatic arthritis?

Ans: Diagnosis is based on history of psoriasis, presence of skin and nail lesions of psoriasis, and clinical criteria for arthritis with usually a negative serological test for rheumatoid factor.

Q3. Which joints are affected in psoriatic arthritis?

Ans: The joints of following region can be affected in psoriatic arthritis—Neck, shoulders, elbows, wrists, fingers and knuckles, base of spine, knees, ankles and toes.

Q4. Which is the commonest type of psoriatic arthritis?

a. Distal interphalangeal (DIP) joint—predominant arthritis
b. Asymmetrical oligoarthritis or monoarthritis
c. Axial disease—predominant arthritis
d. Arthritis mutilans

Ans: a. Asymmetrical oligoarthritis or monoarthritis.

Q5. What are the clinical features of psoriatic arthritis?

Ans: The clinical manifestations of PsA can be divided into:

- *Articular manifestations*—divided into five subtypes
  1. DIP joint —predominant arthritis (10%) (Fig. 1).
  2. Asymmetrical oligoarthritis or monoarthritis (70–80%).
  3. Symmetrical polyarthritis—proximal interphalangeal (PIP) joint predominant arthritis (5–20%)—rheumatoid arthritis (RA) like (Fig. 2).
  4. Axial disease—predominant arthritis (spondylitis and/or sacroiliitis (5–20%).
  5. Arthritis mutilans (rare).
- Other musculoskeletal manifestations
  - Enthesitis
  - Dactylitis
  - Tenosynovitis
  - Peripheral edema.

Q6. What are the different diagnostic and classification criteria in psoriatic arthritis?

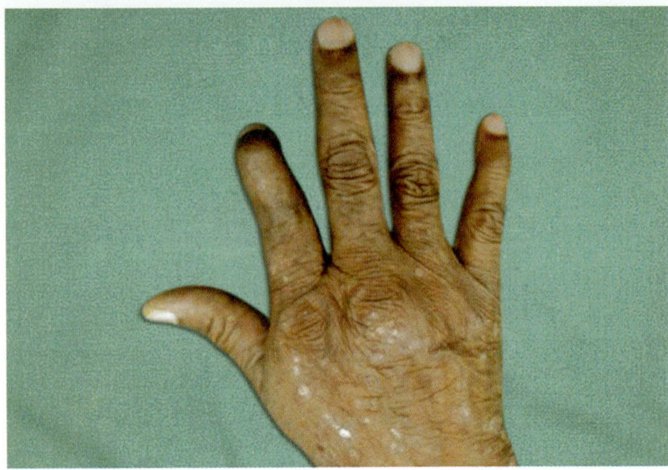

Fig. 1: Synovitis involving distal interphalangeal joints (DIPJs) and dactylitis in a patient with psoriatic arthritis (PsA)

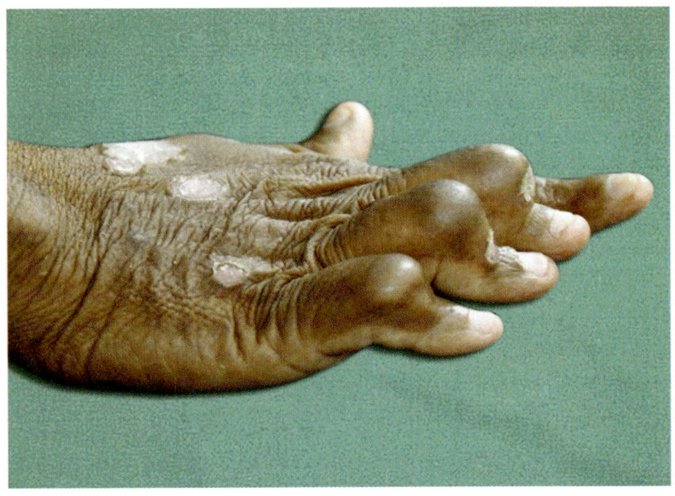

Fig. 2: Boutonniere deformity in a patient with psoriatic arthritis (PsA)

Ans: The original diagnostic criteria of Moll and Wright (1973) are the simplest and the most frequently used. The criteria are:

- An inflammatory arthritis (peripheral arthritis and/or sacroiliitis or spondylitis)
- The presence of psoriasis
- The (usual) absence of serological tests for rheumatoid factor.

Recently, another classification criteria were developed by Taylor et al. in 2006 to ensure uniformity in epidemiological and clinical trials. These are known as the CASPAR (ClASsification criteria for Psoriatic ARthritis) criteria (Table 1). The CASPAR criteria have been evaluated in many studies and their sensitivity and specificity is 91.4% and 98%, respectively.

Table 1: ClASsification criteria for Psoriatic ARthritis (CASPAR) criteria

Category	*Description*	*Points*
Current psoriasis or personal or family history of psoriasis	• Current psoriasis—skin or scalp disease confirmed by rheumatologist or dermatologist • Personal history—obtained from patient, family physician, dermatologist, rheumatologist or other qualified health care provider • Family history—presence of psoriasis in first degree or second degree relative as reported by patient	2 (current) or 1 (history)
Psoriatic nail dystrophy on current examination	Onycholysis, pitting, hyperkeratosis	1
Negative rheumatoid factor	Any method except latex, but preferably enzyme-linked immunosorbent assay (ELISA) or nephelometry, using local laboratory reference range	1
Dactylitis (current or on history as recorded by rheumatologist)	Swelling of an entire digit	1
Radiographic evidence of juxta-articular new bone formation	Ill-defined ossification near joint margins but excluding osteophyte formation on plain X-rays of the hand or foot	1

A patient must have inflammatory articular disease (joint, spine or entheseal) and ≥3 points from the following categories:-

Q7. Is there a relationship between the onset of psoriasis and psoriatic arthritis?

Ans: Most patients with PsA have psoriasis vulgaris. In majority of the patients, onset of psoriasis precedes that of arthritis by approximately 8–10 years. In about 70% of people with PsA, cutaneous psoriasis develops first followed by arthritis. However, in about 15% both arthritis and psoriasis develop simultaneously and in the remaining 15% arthritis may precede the onset of psoriasis.

Q8. What are the characteristic radiological features in psoriatic arthritis?

Ans: The radiological abnormalities typically seen in PsA can be divided into:

- *Peripheral joint features*
  - Destructive changes—erosions, osteolysis. Osteolysis with erosion at the base of adjacent phalanx is known as the "pencil-in-cup deformity". Erosions in PsA involve the PIPJs and DIPJs more commonly with relative sparing of the wrist and MCPJs, unlike RA, where wrists and MCPJs are predominantly involved
  - Proliferative changes—proliferative new bone formation (periostitis) occurs along the shaft of metacarpal and metatarsal bones. When this occurs adjacent to erosion, it is called "whiskering".
- Axial/Spinal features
  - Asymmetric sacroiliitis
  - Paravertebral ossification ("chunky" syndesmophytes)

Q9. Which of the following is an unlikely radiological finding in psoriatic arthritis?

a. DIP joint erosions
b. Periosteal new bone formation
c. Juxta-articular osteopenia
d. MCP joint sparing

Ans: c. Juxta-articular osteopenia.

Q10. What are the differential diagnoses of psoriatic arthritis?

- Rheumatoid arthritis (RA)
- Reactive arthritis (Reiter's disease)
- Gout
- Ankylosing spondylitis (AS)
- Osteoarthritis (OA).

There are some features differentiating psoriatic arthritis from other arthritides which have been described in Table 2.

Q11. How common are autoantibodies in psoriatic arthritis?

Ans: Various autoantibodies may be found in psoriatic arthritis, though they are uncommon. Rheumatoid factor is positive in 5–10% of patients and anti-citrullinated peptide antibodies in 6–10% patients. In addition, up to 10–14% patients may have antinuclear antibodies.

Q12. Are there any predictors for development of psoriatic arthritis?

Ans: Psoriatic features associated with an increased likelihood of developing PsA include nail dystrophy, scalp lesions and intergluteal or perianal psoriasis.

Q13. How does psoriatic arthritis progress?

Ans: Typically, PsA is initially a mild, oligoarticular disease which may become polyarticular with time and

Table 2: Features differentiating psoriatic arthritis from other arthritides

	Psoriatic arthritis (PsA)	*Rheumatoid arthritis (RA)*	*Osteoarthritis (OA)*	*Ankylosing spondylitis (AS)*
Peripheral disease	Asymmetric	Symmetric	Asymmetric	No
Sacroiliitis	Asymmetric	No	No	Symmetric
Stiffness	In morning and/or with immobility	In morning and/or with immobility	With activity	In morning and/or with immobility
F:M ratio	1:1	3:1	1.3:1	1:9
Enthesitis	Common	No	No	Uncommon
Rheumatoid factor positivity	5–10%	~80%	No	No
HLA association	Cw6, B27	DR4	No	B27
Nail lesions	Yes	No	No	No
Psoriasis	Yes	Uncommon	Uncommon	Uncommon
X-ray	Periostitis, osteolysis, erosions (DIPJ), chunky syndesmophytes	Periarticular osteopenia, erosions	Osteophytes	Marginal syndesmophytes

progresses to a severe, erosive condition in at least 20% of patients. Patients who exhibit polyarticular or erosive arthritis at initial presentation tend to have this aggressive course.

Q14. What is the management of psoriatic arthritis?

Ans: *Management*:

Symptomatic treatment

- Nonsteroidal anti-inflammatory drugs (NSAIDs)—useful in treatment of mild PsA and for symptomatic management of pain, inflammatory swelling and morning stiffness. However, NSAIDs must be used judiciously since they can worsen skin lesions. Also, their use is associated with increased cardiovascular risk. Naproxen, therefore, may be the preferable NSAID. However, in case of failure to respond to adequate trial with two different NSAIDs, disease-modifying antirheumatic drugs (DMARD) therapy should be considered.
- Corticosteroids—are often used as short-term therapy. Intra-articular injections may be used in case one or a few joints are involved. Oral corticosteroids are occasionally used for relief of symptoms in patients with polyarthritis or those with inadequate response to NSAIDs. However, they need to be used with extreme caution and tapered very slowly since psoriasis may worsen and sometimes evolve to a more severe pustular form.
- Disease-modifying antirheumatic drugs (DMARDs)
  - Conventional synthetic DMARD (csDMARD)
    - Methotrexate
    - Sulfasalazine
    - Leflunomide
    - Cyclosporine A
  - Targeted synthetic DMARD (tsDMARD)
    - Apremilast
    - Tofacitinib
  - Biological response modifiers
  - Anti-TNF-α agents
    - Etanercept
    - Infliximab
    - Adalimumab
    - Golimumab
    - Certolizumab pegol
  - Anti-IL-12/23 antibody
    - Ustekinumab
    - Guselkumab
    - Tildrakizumab
  - Anti-IL-17 antibodies
    - Secukinumab
    - Ixekizumab
    - Brodalumab
  - Anti T cell agent
    - Alefacept
    - Abatacept.

CHAPTER 58

Pustular Psoriasis

Vinitha Varghese

Case study Pustular Psoriasis

Presenting Complaints

Doctor, I have developed a reddish rash with pus-filled lesions all over my body and I am also running high fever in the evenings.

Setting

Dermatology outpatient department

History of Present Illness

A 42-year-old male presented with acute onset of pustular eruption on an erythematous background, over the neck, trunk, and flexures of the extremities of 1 month duration. The skin lesions were associated with an intense itching and burning sensation. The patient gave a history of intermittent fever with evening rise of temperature associated with chills and rigors. The rise in temperature was also associated with a flare-up of the lesions. He did not give any personal or family history of psoriasis. The patient did not give any history of other systemic illnesses, intake of drug prior to onset of lesions in recent past.

General Physical Examination

Well oriented to time, place and person
BMI—19 kg/m^2, Pulse—100 bpm, Temperature—102°F.

Systemic Examination

No abnormality detected.

Dermatological Examination

Numerous agminate pustules clustered over an erythematous base, coalescing to form bigger sheets of lesions, distributed over the neck, upper part of the chest, upper limbs, abdomen, and back (Figs 1 and 2). Oral mucosa was normal.

Laboratory Investigations

Complete hemogram, liver function tests (LFTs) and renal function tests (RFTs) were within normal limits. Serum calcium and uric acid levels were normal. Gram-stained smear examination of pustular eruptions revealed neutrophils, but no bacteria and the pus culture was sterile.

A histopathological study of the lesional skin revealed parakeratosis, elongation of rete ridges and dermal papillae, along with suprapapillary thinning of epidermis and tortuous capillaries at dermal papillae. Munro's micro abscesses are evident at the lower end of the horny layer.

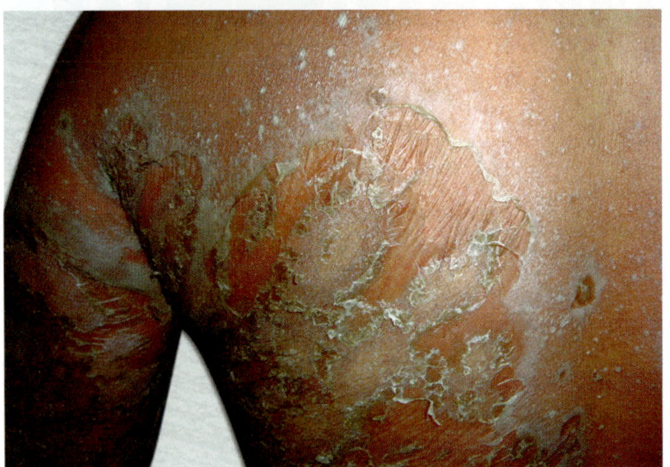

Fig. 1: Coalescing pustules on the back

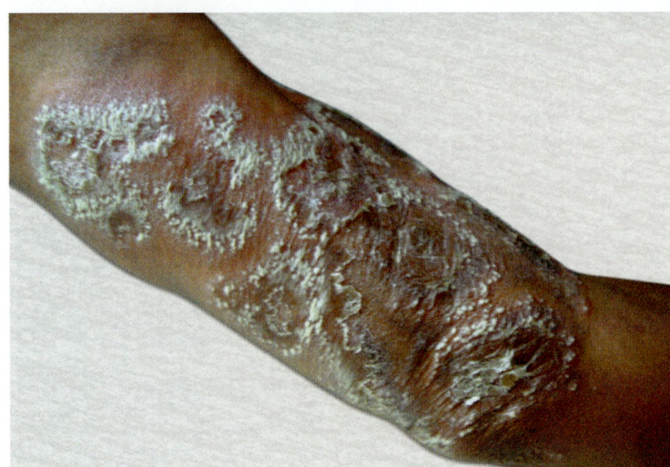

Fig. 2: Clustering of pustules on the upper limb

Q1. What is your diagnosis?

a. Acute generalized exanthematous pustulosis
b. Generalized pustular psoriasis (von Zumbusch type)
c. Staphylococcal scalded skin syndrome (SSSS)
d. Subcorneal pustular dermatosis (SCPD)

Ans: b. Generalized pustular psoriasis (von Zumbusch type). Generalized pustular psoriasis (GPP) can be diagnosed clinically by abrupt onset of fever, malaise and characteristic skin eruption of pustules which coalesce to form lakes of pus appearance.

Histopathological examination is useful for confirmation of diagnosis which shows parakeratosis with Munro's microabscesses, spongiosis, spongiform pustules of Kogoj and elongation of rete ridges. The earliest infiltrate is lymphocytic. Intense papillary and epidermal edema cause spongiosis.

Q2. What are the types of pustular psoriasis? Classify.

Ans: Pustular psoriasis is of two types—localized and generalized

- *Localized*: Palmoplantar pustulosis, acrodermatitis continua of Hallopeau
- *Generalized*: von Zumbusch type, exanthematic type, annular type, impetigo herpetiformis, localized type of GPP.

Q3. What are the clinical features of localized pustular psoriasis?

Ans:

- *Palmoplantar pustulosis*: Erythematous scaly plaques studded with numerous sterile yellow pustules, over the thenar and hypothenar eminences of palms, soles and heels
- *Acrodermatitis continua of Hallopeau*: Chronic pustular lesions at the tips of the digits, preceded by glazed and scaly erythema. Following this, numerous pustules develop and lead to destruction of the nail plate.

Q4. Enumerate the clinical course of lesions in von Zumbusch type. How will you differentiate it from other variants?

Ans: The lesions begin as numerous erythematous tender plaques which become surmounted by pin-head sized pustules which coalesce to form lakes of pus. The patient may have features of systemic toxicity like fever, chills and malaise. The plaques coalesce to give rise to generalized erythema, scaling and crusting. The pustules may dry up in 2–3 days with brown crusts but fresh crop of pustules may erupt on shiny underlying skin. This cycle may be repeated for weeks.

- The other variant exanthematic type usually follows an upper respiratory infection, which begins abruptly on palmoplantar areas and later on spreads to other regions as large areas of erythema and pustules
- Annular variant manifests as annular lesions with erythema, scaling and pustules at the periphery. Systemic symptoms are usually absent
- Impetigo herpetiformis is a variant of GPP seen in last trimester of pregnancy
- Involvement of the oral mucosae is not uncommon. It may present as discrete and confluent denuded areas with white elevated margins, these lesions are known as annulus migrans.

Q5. Annulus migrans is a feature of

a. Generalized pustular psoriasis
b. Reiter's syndrome
c. Acrodermatitis continua of Hallopeau
d. All of the above

Ans: d. All of the above.

Q6. What are the provocative factors of generalized pustular psoriasis ?

Ans: Provocative factors

- Irritant topical therapies like coal tar and dithranol
- Infection
- Pregnancy
- Hypocalcemia
- Withdrawal of systemic steroids
- *Other drugs*: Salicylates, iodide, lithium, phenylbutazone, oxyphenbutazone, progesterone, terbinafine.

Q7. What are the differential diagnosis of generalized pustular psoriasis ?

Ans: The differentials in this case are as follows:

1. Acute generalized exanthematous pustulosis (AGEP) is perhaps the most important differential, occurring as an acute, spontaneously healing reaction to drugs, usually antibiotics.
2. Subcorneal pustular dermatosis (SCPD) can be differentiated from the flexural distribution, seasonal variation and biopsy features.
3. *Migratory necrolytic eruption of glucagonoma*: Wasting, glossitis and anemia seen.
4. Acute pemphigus foliaceus can mimic subacute GPP, but histological and immunofluorescence testing will distinguish the two.
5. Bowel bypass syndrome, Sweet's syndrome and Behçet's syndrome, staphyloderma, rampant impetigo or candidiasis in the immunosuppressed or pustular drug eruption (e.g. caused by halides) should be remembered. Staphylococcal scalded skin syndrome, eosinophilic folliculitis also to be considered.

Q8. What are the complications of generalized pustular psoriasis?

Ans: Complications:

- Hypoalbuminemia may occur because of a sudden loss of plasma protein into the tissues. Hypocalcemia can occur may be as a consequence of the hypoalbuminemia. The consequent oligemia can cause acute and fatal renal tubular necrosis
- There may be evidence of liver damage or even jaundice, perhaps caused by a combination of oligemia, general toxicity and drugs
- Cholestatic jaundice of uncertain pathogenesis, closely related to acute episodes of GPP, has been described
- Deep-vein thrombosis in a leg can cause fatal pulmonary embolism
- Staphylococcal infection may complicate GPP; usually because of nosocomial infections. Inflammatory polyarthritis can occur
- Malabsorption may be a feature of the acute episode and may further contribute to hypocalcemia
- If GPP lasts more than a few days, gross hair loss may follow from all areas of the body. Occasionally, a telogen effluvium follows 2–3 months after the height of the illness
- In the absence of effective treatment, death can occur in the acute stage.

Q9. What are the laboratory findings in generalized pustular psoriasis?

Ans: There may be an absolute lymphopenia at the onset of GPP. A polymorphonuclear leukocytosis quickly follows. Plasma albumin, zinc and calcium may be abnormally low. The erythrocyte sedimentation rate (ESR) is usually raised.

Q10. How will you manage a case of pustular psoriasis?

Ans: Treatment of acute GPP requires hospitalization, elimination of the possible provocative factors, general and supportive measures with topical and systemic drug therapy.

Withdrawal of provocative factors:

Tar or dithranol can be withdrawn abruptly, but massive over dosage with potent topical corticosteroids requires more care. The application of serially diluted topical steroids over several days may be the safest course, and is preferable to substitution of oral or parenteral corticosteroid. Infection, where present, should be treated rigorously with the appropriate antibiotic, usually erythromycin or cloxacillin.

General measures:

- Bed rest, mild sedation with fluid and protein replacement may promote spontaneous reversion to a quieter erythrodermic psoriasis or even psoriasis vulgaris
- Excessive heat loss must be prevented by maintaining an adequate ambient temperature,

avoiding cool draughts of air. A low-reading thermometer is essential
- Fluid intake should be increased so that the daily urine volume remains adequate
- Electrolyte imbalance to be corrected.

Topical therapy:

Often, completely bland creams or lotions are best. Weak corticosteroid creams may be used in subacute forms. Tar and dithranol are contraindicated.

Systemic therapy:
- Acitretin (1 mg/kg/day)
- Methotrexate—0.2–0.4 mg/kg/week
- Cyclosporine—3–5 mg/kg
- Dapsone
- Colchicine
- Biologics—Infliximab, etanercept.

CHAPTER 59

Reactive Arthritis

Suneil Gandhi

Case study Reactive Arthritis

Presenting Complaints

Doctor, I am having a rash over my genitalia, skin rash and pain in both the knees since seven days.

Setting

Dermatology outpatient department

History of Present Illness

Patient was apparently normal 4 weeks ago, when he had unprotected sexual intercourse with a friend. Five days later, he suffered from burning micturition and mild urethral discharge. He immediately consulted a general practitioner for this and was prescribed azithromycin and doxycycline, following which his symptoms subsided.

Seven days ago, he noticed a rash over his penis that was not improving with application of antibiotic cream. He also developed a generalized skin rash and complained of pain in his knee joints, which was gradually worsening. There was no history of any eye disturbance, oral lesions, breathing difficulty, abdominal pain, loose stools or jaundice.

General Physical Examination

A young man, well-built and nourished, oriented to time, place and person. There was no pallor, icterus, cyanosis, clubbing or pedal edema. The inguinal lymph nodes were palpable on both sides, discrete and nontender. There was a slight swelling present around the right knee joint.

Pulse rate: 96 beats per minute, *temperature*: 100 °F, *weight*: 62 kg.

Dermatological Examination

Multiple crusted plaques were present in a generalized distribution over the body (Fig. 1). Multiple, well-defined, nontender, moist erosions with irregular margins were present over the dorsal aspect of the glans penis. They coalesced in a few places to form a circinate pattern (Fig. 2). There was no urethral discharge. There were no lesions in the oral cavity. Hair and nail examination revealed no abnormalities.

Systemic Examination

No abnormalities were detected.

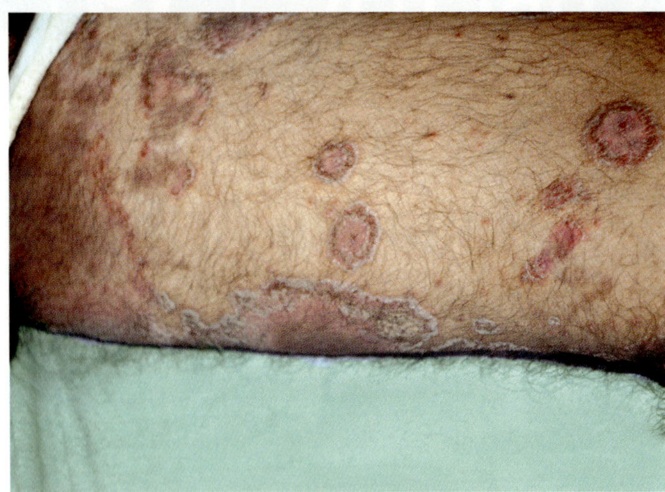

Fig. 1: Multiple crusted plaques were present in a generalized distribution over the body

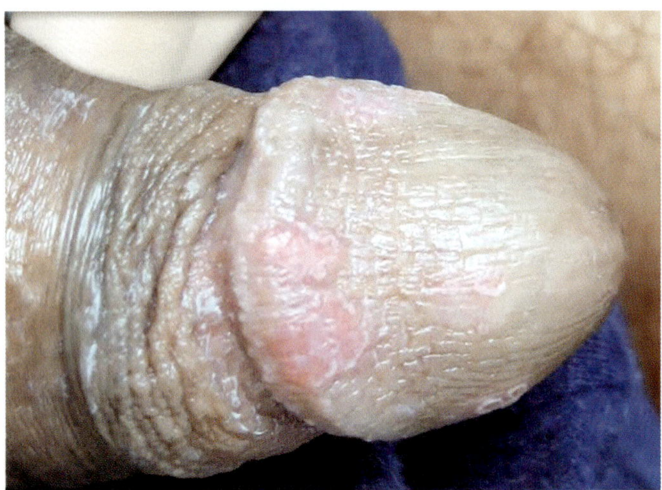

Fig. 2: Multiple, well-defined, non-tender, moist erosions with irregular margins were present over the dorsal aspect of the glans penis. They coalesced in a few places to form a circinate pattern

Q1. What is the most likely diagnosis?

a. Psoriatic arthritis
b. Reactive arthritis
c. Gonococcemia
d. Syphilis

Ans: b. Reactive arthritis. This patient was suffering from characteristic hyperkeratotic skin lesions. Circinate balanitis and arthralgia of the knee joints were the key findings in favor of the diagnosis. Disseminated gonococcal infection can also cause arthritis, but usually affects the small joints of the upper limbs, such as the wrists and fingers, with the exception of fusiform dactylitis, which is more common in reactive arthritis. Polyarthritis, tenosynovitis and laboratory identification of gonococci are other findings that help to differentiate disseminated gonococcal infection from reactive arthritis.

Q2. How do you define reactive arthritis?

Ans: Reactive arthritis is defined as the presence of nonsuppurative polyarthritis lasting more than a month, following a urogenital or enteric infection. It classically presents with the triad of asymmetrical joint pain and swelling, urogenital and ophthalmic manifestations, usually within 4 weeks after infection. Some prefer to describe it as a tetrad, adding the mucocutaneous findings of circinate balanitis and keratoderma blennorrhagicum to the classic triad. However, only one-third of patients present with the full triad of symptoms. This gives rise to the terms, complete and incomplete reactive arthritis.

Q3. What are the criteria for diagnosis of reactive arthritis syndrome?

Ans: The American College of Rheumatology has listed the following criteria:

- Arthritis for greater than 1 month and urethritis (cervicitis) ± conjunctivitis
- Arthritis for greater than 1 month and bilateral conjunctivitis ± urethritis (cervicitis)
- Acute episode of arthritis and conjunctivitis occurring together.

Q4. What are the types of reactive arthritis?

Ans: Types of reactive arthritis are as follows:

- Endemic, usually sexually acquired, more common in adults
- Epidemic, following enteric infection, more common in children

Q5. Which organisms are usually associated with reactive arthritis?

Ans: Organisms associated with reactive arthritis have been discussed in Table 1.

Table 1: Organisms associated with reactive arthritis

Urogenital pathogens	*Enteric pathogens*
Chlamydia trachomatis	*Campylobacter jejuni*
Chlamydia psittaci	*Salmonella typhimurium*
Chlamydia pneumonia	*Salmonella enteritidis*
Ureaplasma urealyticum	*Salmonella paratyphi*
Neisseria gonorrhoeae	*Shigella flexneri*
	Shigella dysenteriae
	Yersinia enterocolitica
	Yersinia pseudotuberculosis

Q6. Which of the following is NOT a manifestation of reactive arthritis?

a. Circinate vulvitis
b. Erythema nodosum
c. Geographic tongue
d. Juxta-articular nodules

Ans: d. Juxta-articular nodules

Q7. What are the mucocutaneous manifestations of reactive arthritis?

Ans: Mucocutaneous lesions occur in up to one-third of patients with sexually-acquired reactive arthritis, but they are less common in reactive arthritis of other causes. Erythema nodosum has been reported in reactive arthritis secondary to Campylobacter, Shigella and Yersinia infection. Juxta-articular nodules are a manifestation of rheumatoid arthritis.

Circinate balanitis is the most common cutaneous manifestation described in up to 40% of men. It can accompany the acute infection or appear afterward. It typically appears as painless, irregular, moist erosions on the glans penis, which coalesce to form a circinate pattern. In uncircumcised males, these lesions evolve to form hard crusts and hyperkeratotic papules. Erosive and circinate vulvitis has been described in females.

Keratoderma blenorrhagicum is seen in up to 15% of patients with sexually-acquired reactive arthritis, and usually appears 1–2 months after the onset of arthritis. They begin as erythematous vesicles and macules that gradually thicken to form papules, pustules and plaques, which resemble pustular psoriasis. These lesions can occur anywhere on the body, but are found most commonly on the feet and the soles can be markedly hyperkeratotic.

Other mucocutaneous manifestations of reactive arthritis

- Erythema nodosum
- Geographic tongue
- Nail dystrophy
- Nail pitting
- Periungual pustules
- Shallow ulcers on the palate, tongue, buccal mucosa, lips, tonsilar pillars or pharynx.

Q8. What are the other systems involved in reactive arthritis?

Ans: Systems involved:

Ocular

- Conjunctivitis (most common, can be bilateral)
- Anterior uveitis (associated with chronic disease)
- Episcleritis
- Scleritis
- Keratitis.

Gastrointestinal

- Abdominal pain
- Diarrhea
- Inflammation resembling inflammatory bowel disease.

Genitourinary

- Urethritis (most common)
- Cervicitis
- Cystitis
- Prostatitis
- Salpingitis.

Cardiac

- Conduction abnormalities (usually transient)
- Myocarditis
- Pericarditis
- Complete heart block
- Acute aortitis.

Musculoskeletal

- Asymmetric oligoarthritis (predominantly of the lower extremity)
- Enthesitis (tendon and ligament insertion site inflammation)
- Sacroiliitis (associated with severe disease)
- Dactylitis (sausage-shaped digits).

Neurological

- Peripheral neuropathy
- Hemiplegia
- Meningoencephalitis.

Others

- Pleuritis
- Pneumonitis
- Thrombophlebitis
- Amyloidosis
- Glomerulonephritis.

On investigating the patient:

Laboratory investigations revealed an elevated total leukocyte count (12,000/mm^3) with the differential count showing 80% neutrophils. The erythrocyte sedimentation rate was 40 mm/hr. Urinalysis showed a 10–20 pus cells. Urine and urethral swab cultures were negative.

Q9. Which laboratory investigations are necessary to diagnose a case of reactive arthritis?

Ans: The diagnosis of reactive arthritis is usually clinical, as no laboratory study or imaging finding is diagnostic. Indicators of inflammation are usually abnormal.

Hematological investigations

- Elevated ESR
- Elevated C-reactive protein
- Mild leukocytosis
- Mild normocytic normochromic anemia.

Microbiology

- Urine analysis for pus cells
- HIV testing in high-risk individuals
- Chlamydia serology
- Cervical or urethral culture in case of urethritis or cervicitis
- Stool cultures if bowel symptoms are present
- Synovial fluid microbiology for leukocytosis and Pekin cells (phagocytized leukocytes)
- Gram stain and culture to rule out septic arthritis
- Antistreptolysin O (ASLO) titer (if poststreptococcal infection is suspected)
- Human leukocyte antigen (HLA) study
- HLA B-27 test.

Q10. What imaging studies are useful for the work-up of a case of reactive arthritis?

Ans: Imaging studies:

X-ray

- Early disease
  - Soft tissue swelling around affected joints
  - Tendon swelling
- Chronic disease
  - Exuberant plantar spurs
  - Bony erosions
  - Adjacent bony proliferation
  - Paravertebral ossification
  - Sacroiliitis
  - Syndesmophytes
- Other imaging studies
  - Whole body scintigraphy (to screen enthesopathy and arthropathy)
  - Magnetic resonance imaging (to detect early sacroiliac involvement and enthesopathy)
  - Ultrasonography (to reveal enthesitis more accurately than physical examination)
  - Electrocardiography (in patients with prolonged course, to rule out conduction disturbances)
  - Echocardiography (to rule out carditis and valvular dysfunction).

Q11. Which of the following tests is most useful to assess the prognosis of reactive arthritis?

a. Complete blood chemistry
b. HLA B-27 testing
c. Radiological imaging of the affected joints
d. Synovial fluid analysis

Ans: b. HLA B-27 testing

Reactive arthritis is usually self-limiting with resolution of symptoms in 3–12 months. Postenteric cases are associated with a better prognosis compared to postvenereal infections. HLA B-27 positive individuals are more likely to have longer disease duration, more extra-articular features, erosive joint damage and higher recurrence rates. The presence of hip-joint involvement, an ESR higher than 30 and unresponsiveness to nonsteroidal anti-inflammatory drugs (NSAIDs) are also associated with a severe outcome or chronic course.

Q12. How do you manage a case of reactive arthritis?

Ans: Treatment of reactive arthritis is aimed at relieving symptoms based on their severity. Most patients have a self-limiting course and just need symptomatic and supportive care. Although microbes are implicated as the triggering agent, antibiotics do not help in altering the course of the disease. Long-term tetracycline therapy has been shown to reduce the total duration of disease in some studies.

Mucocutaneous lesions

- Topical corticosteroids
- Topical salicylic acid for keratotic lesions
- Topical calcineurin inhibitors
- Topical vitamin D analogues
- Methotrexate
- Acitretin
- Cyclosporine
- PUVA therapy.

Arthritis and enthesitis

- Physiotherapy
- NSAIDS
- Intralesional corticosteroids
- Phenylbutazone
- Low-dose prednisolone
- Sulfasalazine
- Methotrexate

- Azathioprine
- Leflunomide
- Infliximab.

Conjunctivitis and uveitis

- Simple eye toilet
- Mydriatics
- Cycloplegics
- Topical corticosteroid drops
- Low-dose prednisolone (for severe cases).

Urethritis and cervicitis

- Antimicrobials based on the causative organism (only helpful in acute cases)
- Tetracycline (for 3 months, is the preferred drug)
- Doxycycline
- Azithromycin

Gastroenteritis

- Antimicrobials based on the causative organism (only helpful in acute cases).

SECTION 13

Other Keratinization Disorders

Saloni Katoch

CHAPTER 60

Pityriasis Rosea

Sriharsha Talabhukta, Anupam Das

Case study Pityriasis Rosea

Presenting Complaints

Doctor, there is a red flaky rash on my trunk since 2 weeks.

Setting

Dermatology outpatient department

History of Present Illness

A 15-year-old female was brought by her parents complaining of a rash on her trunk. The problem started after she had an episode of sore throat 3 weeks back. Initially there was a large red raised flaky lesion on the left side of the trunk. Similar smaller lesions started appearing over the trunk in the next 2 weeks. There was associated mild itching over the lesions.

General Physical Examination and Systemic Examination

No significant abnormality detected.

Dermatological Examination

There was a solitary large oval erythematous scaly plaque measuring 2–5 cm in diameter with a central, wrinkled area, separated from a dark red peripheral zone by fine scales located on the left hypochondrium. The scales were located in the form of a collarette.

There were smaller similar lesions located symmetrically over the trunk, neck and proximal extremities (Fig. 1).

Q1. What is the likely diagnosis?

a. Psoriasis vulgaris
b. Guttate psoriasis
c. Pityriasis rosea
d. Pityriasis lichenoides chronica

Ans: a. Pityriasis rosea. History of sore throat 2 weeks prior, followed by development of a solitary scaly plaque (mother patch) and later similar smaller lesions (secondary lesions) on the trunk points to the diagnosis of pityriasis rosea (PR).

Q2. What is the epidemiology of pityriasis rosea?

Ans: PR has been observed mostly in younger age group between 10 and 35 years although the range varies from 3 months to 83 years.

- It is a typically occurring disorder during the spring and fall. In temperate regions, it is more

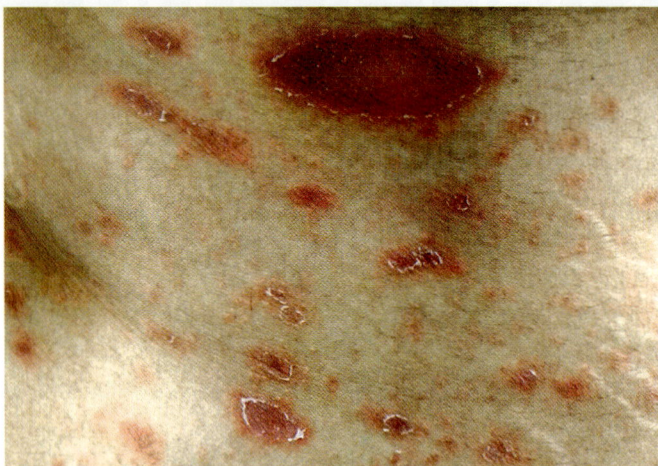

Fig. 1: Characteristic salmon colored herald patch with collarette of scales
Courtesy: Dr Saloni Katoch, Columbia Asia Hospital, Bengaluru

frequent during the winter months. In tropical areas, there may also be some seasonal variation
- Though both sexes seem to be affected equally, it has slightly more predilection toward women
- No racial predominance has been documented.

Q3. What is the etiology of pityriasis rosea?

Ans: Etiology of pityriasis rosea:
- Infection
  - Virus
  - Bacteria
  - Spirochetes
  - Fungi
  - Mycoplasma
  - Gastrointestinal tract parasites
  - Toxic exanthem of occult gastrointestinal infection
- Cell-mediated immune mechanism
- Insect bite
- Isomorphic response
- Drugs
- Autoimmune disease
- Psychogenic cause like stress.

Q4. What is the evidence in support of an infectious etiology in pityriasis rosea?

Ans: Features of the disease that may be related to an infectious etiology include:
- High prevalence in states of altered immunity (pregnancy and bone-marrow transplantation), exacerbation during corticosteroid treatment
- Relation with seasonal variations
- Clustering within families, school children, military bases
- Prodromal symptoms
- The evolution with a primary and multiple secondary lesions (incubation/replication period)
- Primary lesions that could correspond to the site of inoculation
- Self-limiting course
- The rarity of recurrences.

Previous studies have confirmed the possibility of a viral cause with:
- Detection of an elevated erythrocyte sedimentation rate (ESR)
- Lymphocytosis
- Elevation of the serum IgM level
- Cytolysis of keratinocytes adjacent to Langerhans cells causing disintegration of single cells and intracytoplasmic and intranuclear virus-like particles in keratinocyte cultures from lesional skin.

Q5. What is the causal role of herpes viruses in pityriasis rosea?

Ans: PR may be a viral exanthem associated with reactivation of human herpes virus (HHV)-7 or HHV-6 viruses.

Q6. What are the drugs that cause pityriasis rosea like eruptions?

Ans: Various medications including adalimumab, arsenic, imatinib mesylate, allopurinol, ACE inhibitors, barbiturates, clonidine, ketotifen, levamisole, lithium, nonsteroidal anti-inflammatory drugs, omeprazole, metronidazole, isotretinoin, D-penicillamine, gold salts, bismuth and ergotamine are implicated in pityriasis rosea like eruptions.

Q7. What are the clinical features of pityriasis rosea?

Ans: Herald patch (Fig. 1) typically has a flesh-colored central area surrounded by a pink, elevated border with a fine collarette of scales just inside the periphery of the plaque, usually located on the trunk or neck (areas covered with clothing), gradually expands over a few days to become a 2–10 cm single, salmon-colored round or oval patch or plaque.

Typical cases of PR may be preceded by prodromal symptoms including headache, gastrointestinal discomfort, fever, malaise and arthralgias.

From few days to up to 3–4 months after the onset of the herald patch, widespread papulosquamous lesions appear on the body. The rash consists of multiple erythematous scaly plaques smaller than the herald patch distributed in "Christmas or fir tree" pattern, i.e. bilateral and symmetrical, classically arranged with their long axis parallel to lines of cleavage. The secondary rash either resembles the herald patch but smaller in size or small red non-scaly plaques in typical distribution.

Patterns of distribution:

- V-shaped distribution on the upper chest and upper back
- Circumferential pattern around the shoulders and hips
- Transverse pattern on the lower anterior trunk and lower back.

The typical distribution is on the thorax, back, abdomen and proximal extremities. In adults, the face, hands and feet are usually spared.

Pruritus is a relatively common complaint and is severe in 25% of patients. When PR is irritated by water, sweat, or tight clothing, the itching may be more prominent.

Oral and nail involvement is uncommon.

Q8. What are the atypical forms of pityriasis rosea?

Ans: The uncommon variants include papulovesicular, vesicular, urticarial, pustular, purpuric and erythema multiforme like. Unilateral pityriasis has also been reported. Pityriasis circinata et marginata of Vidal, sometimes considered as a special variant of PR, presents with a few large lesions localized to one area of the body.

Q9. What are the differential diagnoses?

Ans: Differential diagnoses of pityriasis rosea:

- *Secondary syphilis*: History of primary chancre, associated features of secondary syphilis, serological tests will confirm diagnosis, absence of herald patch and characteristic Christmas tree pattern distribution of secondary lesions
- *Guttate psoriasis*: Thicker scales, lesions not along skin cleavage lines, histopathology may help to differentiate
- *Pityriasis lichenoides chronica*: Chronic course, more on extremities, biopsy will aid in diagnosis
- *Lichen planus*: Violaceous plane topped papules, absence of herald patch and characteristic collarette of scales, associated nail and oral cavity changes may be present, biopsy will aid in diagnosis
- *Nummular dermatitis*: Absence of collarette of scales, presence of tiny vesicles common
- *Pityriasis versicolor*: Absence of marginal scaling, KOH examination will confirm
- *Tinea corporis*: Scales present at the periphery, KOH examination will confirm diagnosis
- *Pityriasis alba*: Common in children, lesions common on face, hypopigmented patches with dry branny scales
- *Pityriasiform seborrheic dermatitis*: Absence of herald patch, more in the seborrheic areas, dull lesions with greasy scales
- *Drug-induced PR like eruption*: History of drug intake, atypical with larger lesions
- *Others*: Parapsoriasis, erythema dyschromicum perstans.

Q10. How do you diagnose pityriasis rosea?

Ans: Proposed diagnostic criteria for pityriasis rosea are as follows:

A diagnosis of pityriasis rosea can be made if a patient has all the essential clinical features, at least one of the optional clinical features and none of the exclusional clinical features.

Essential clinical features:

- Discrete circular or oval lesions
- Scaling on most lesions
- Peripheral collarette of scaling with central clearance of at least two lesions.

Optional clinical features:

- Truncal and proximal limb distribution with less than 10% of lesions distal to mid-upper-arm and mid-thigh
- Distribution of most lesions along the ribs
- A herald patch (not necessarily the largest) appearing at least two days before the generalized eruption.

Exclusional clinical features:

- Multiple small vesicles at the center of two or more lesions
- Most lesions on palmar or plantar skin surfaces
- Clinical or serological evidence of secondary syphilis, such as generalized lymphadenopathy.

Q11. What are the dermoscopic features of pityriasis rosea?

Ans: Peripheral scaling (so-called collarette of scales) around a diffuse and structureless yellowish center. Dotted vessels may be seen but generally much less evident and fewer in number compared to psoriasis or dermatitis.

Q12. What changes are observed on laboratory investigations?

Ans: The following changes may be observed:
- *Complete blood count*: Leukocytosis, neutrophilia, basophilia, lymphocytosis
- ESR: Elevated
- Increase in total protein, globulins and albumin
- Elevated virus-specific (HHV-6 and HHV-7) serum immunoglobulin M (IgM) and IgG on serology
- Cytolysis of keratinocytes on culture with intra-cytoplasmic and intranuclear virus-like particles
- Plasma viremia has been detected by PCR in some studies.

Q13. What is the histopathology of pityriasis rosea?

Ans: A skin biopsy may not be required as the diagnosis is primarily clinical. The features on histopathology include focal parakeratosis, a reduced granular layer, mild acanthosis and spongiosis and a lymphohistiocytic infiltrate in the superficial dermis. Older lesions have pronounced acanthosis and a deeper dermal component to the infiltrate, difficult to distinguish from psoriasis and lichen planus.

Q14. Double-edged scales are seen in

a. Psoriasis
b. Ichthyosis linearis circumflexa
c. Pityriasis versicolor
d. Erythema annulare centrifugum

Ans: b. Ichthyosis linearis circumflexa.

Q15. What are the different types of scales seen in dermatology?

Ans: The different types of scales are as follows:
- *Furfuraceous*: Loose and fine as in pityriasis versicolor
- *Micaceous*: Silvery parakeratotic scales as in psoriasis
- *Greasy*: Seborrheic dermatitis
- *Ichthyosiform*: Fish scale like as in ichthyosis vulgaris
- *Cornflake like*: Crusting seen in pemphigus foliaceus
- *Double-edged scales*: Patch with advancing double edge of peeling scale, e.g. ichthyosis linearis circumflexa
- *Trailing scale*: Seen trailing at the inner border, e.g. erythema annulare centrifugum
- *Wafer like*: Adherent mica-like scales on lichenoid papules, e.g. pityriasis lichenoides chronica
- *Hystrix-like scale*: Grey brown scaling over verrucous lesions, e.g. ichthyosis hystrix
- *Mauserung desquamation*: Moulting of scales in ichthyosis bullosa of Siemens
- *Coat of armor*: Harlequin ichthyosis
- *Plate like*: Lamellar ichthyosis
- *Oyster like*: Large heaped up scales, e.g. psoriasis
- *Sandpaper like*: Gritty on palpation, e.g. actinic keratosis
- *Erythroderma*: Large plate-like sheets in acute phase, fine and branny in chronic phase.

Q16. How do you treat pityriasis rosea?

Ans: Pityriasis rosea is a self-limiting rash, hence, counseling and patient education are of utmost importance. Uncomplicated cases require no treatment. Pruritus can be managed with mid-potent topical corticosteroids. For patients who experience flu-like symptoms or an extensive skin rash, acyclovir 800 mg (5 times/day) for a duration of 1 week may aid in faster resolution. Phototherapy has also been reported to be beneficial.

CHAPTER 61

Porokeratosis

Aarti Sarda, Abhishek De, Saloni Katoch

Case study Porokeratosis

Presenting Complaints

Doctor, I have this black skin lesion over the left forearm which is progressively increasing in size.

Setting

Dermatology outpatient department

History of Present Illness

A 25-year-old female presented with an asymptomatic, black colored skin lesion on her left forearm since 2 months. She gives history of the lesion being small initially and gradually increasing in size.

General Physical Examination and Systemic Examination

No abnormality detected.

Dermatological Examination

- Solitary annular hyperpigmented plaque present on the left forearm
- The center of the lesion is atrophic while the periphery has a raised hyperkeratotic margin (Fig. 1)
- The raised margin has a depressed furrow running all through its diameter.

Q1. What is your diagnosis?

a. Annular lichen planus
b. Porokeratosis
c. Tinea corporis
d. Erythema annulare centrifugum.

Ans: b. Porokeratosis. The asymptomatic annular plaque with characteristic findings of central atrophy and a raised hyperkeratotic border with a longitudinal furrow are in favor of the diagnosis.

Q2. What is porokeratosis?

Ans: Porokeratosis is a group of hereditary or acquired disorders of epidermal keratinization characterized by keratotic lesions with an atrophic center and a prominent peripheral ridge, the histological hallmark of which is the cornoid lamella.

Q3. Enumerate the different types of porokeratosis.

Ans: Clinically, seven variants have been identified:

1. *Plaque type (classic porokeratosis of Mibelli)*: Usually presents in infancy or childhood, may be familial and inherited as an autosomal dominant trait, characterized by asymptomatic skin colored to brown annular plaques with a raised hyperkeratotic margin with a furrow.
2. *Disseminated superficial porokeratosis*: Autosomal dominant pattern of inheritance, seen in third or fourth decade of life, presents with bilateral

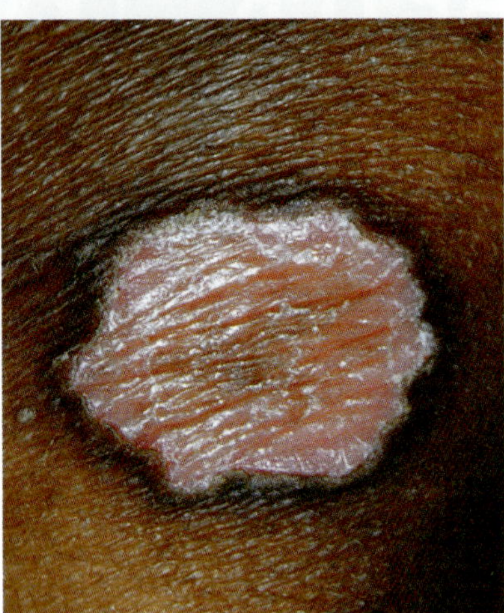

Fig. 1: Solitary plaque with atrophic center and raised hyperkeratotic edge with furrow

symmetrical annular papules on the extremities, sun-covered areas are not spared.

3. *Disseminated superficial actinic porokeratosis (DSAP)*: Most common type, asymptomatic or pruritic, presents with more generalized, bilateral and symmetrical small annular papules in the sun exposed sites with a less evident border, autosomal dominant inheritance.
4. *Linear porokeratosis*: Uncommon variant, presents in early childhood, two clinical variants have been described: (1) unilateral following Blaschko's lines and the rare generalized form, (2) greatest risk of malignant transformation.
5. *Giant porokeratosis*: Rare morphological variant of porokeratosis of Mibelli can present with a diameter of up to 20 cm, predominantly on the lower leg and foot, higher malignant potential.
6. *Porokeratosis palmaris et plantaris disseminata*: Genodermatoses, autosomal dominant inheritance, bilaterally symmetrical small and uniform lesions with prominent hyperkeratosis and furrow, appears on the palms and soles initially, can involve other body parts including mucous membranes.
7. *Punctate porokeratosis*: Characterized by punctate hyperkeratotic lesions on the palms and soles.

Q4. What are the rare variants?

Ans: Hypertrophic, warty-type, porokeratosis ptychotropica, porokeratoma, porokeratotic adnexal ostial nevus and pruritic papular porokeratosis.

Q5. What is CAP syndrome?

Ans: Craniosynostosis, anal anomalies and porokeratosis syndrome.

Q6. What is the etiopathogenesis of porokeratosis?

Ans: The key features are as follows:

- Genetically heterogenous disorder
- Multiple loci identified (DSAP: Chromosomes 12q, 15q and 18p)
- Mutant clone theory: Aneuploidy and chromosomal abnormalities reported in lesional keratinocytes with overexpression of tumor suppressor p53 protein in the cornoid lamella
- Cytogenetic abnormalities in fibroblasts have been reported
- Impaired immunity is permissive and affected keratinocytes have dysplastic potential.

Q7. Describe the histological features of porokeratosis.

Ans: The specimen for biopsy should be taken from the hyperkeratotic ridge. The ridge shows a keratin-filled invagination of the epidermis. The characteristic histopathological feature is the cornoid lamella seen at the edge of the lesion as a column of poorly staining parakeratotic stratum corneum cells. The granular layer is absent below and the underlying keratinocytes are edematous with spongiosis and shrunken nuclei. A moderate dermal lymphocytic infiltrate may be seen under the lamella.

Q8. In which other conditions can cornoid lamella be seen?

Ans: Cornoid lamella can also be seen in viral warts, some ichthyoses, nevoid hyperkeratosis, actinic keratosis, seborrheic keratosis, squamous cell carcinoma, basal cell carcinoma and porokeratotic eccrine nevi.

Q9. What is the malignancy potential of porokeratosis?

Ans: Large lesions have the highest malignancy potential. Malignant change can also occur in long standing lesions of other forms of porokeratosis. Squamous cell carcinoma is the most common malignancy, rarely Bowen's disease or basal cell carcinoma may develop.

Q10. What are the differential diagnoses?

Ans: Granuloma annulare, tinea corporis, actinic keratosis, viral warts, lichen planus, elastosis perforans serpiginosa and inflammatory linear verrucous epidermal nevus (ILVEN).

Q11. Enumerate the treatment modalities in porokeratosis.

Ans: Topical retinoids, calcipotriol, tacalcitol, 5-fluorouracil ointment, imiquimod and systemic retinoids have been tried. Other modalities include cryotherapy, excision, electrodessication and curettage, CO_2 laser, pulsed dye laser therapy and photodynamic therapy.

Q12. All of the following variants of porokeratosis have a risk of malignant transformation except:

a. Porokeratosis of Mibelli
b. Linear porokeratosis
c. Punctate porokeratosis
d. Disseminated superficial porokeratosis

Ans: c. Punctate porokeratosis. Malignant transformation has been described in all variants of porokeratosis except the punctate type.

CHAPTER 62

Perforating Dermatoses

Indrashis Podder

Case study Perforating Dermatoses

Presenting complaints

Doctor, I have developed these itchy, bumpy lesions on both my lower extremities since the last 12 years, which worsen during the winter months.

Setting

Dermatology outpatient department of a tertiary medical center.

History of Present Illness

A 28-year-old lady presented with the complaints of itchy lesions over both her lower extremities for the last 12 years. Her condition worsens during the winter months. Occasionally, she has noted a whitish plug-like material exuding out from these lesions on vigorous scratching. Some of the lesions heal spontaneously over months, leaving behind whitish areas; while new lesions crop up in the vicinity. She reported similar complaints in her mother and aunt. There was no history of any drug intake.

General Physical Examination and Systemic Examination

Within normal limits.

Dermatological Examination

- Papulonodular lesions scattered over the extensor aspect of both lower extremities; measuring approximately 3 mm in diameter (Fig. 1)
- Central umbilication, filled with a keratinous plug
- Some of the lesions were arranged in a linear fashion (Koebner phenomenon) (Fig. 2)
- Hypopigmented, atrophic areas (scars) interspersed between the lesions
- Hair, nail, mucosa → spared.

Laboratory Investigations (Routine Blood Biochemistry)

No abnormality detected.

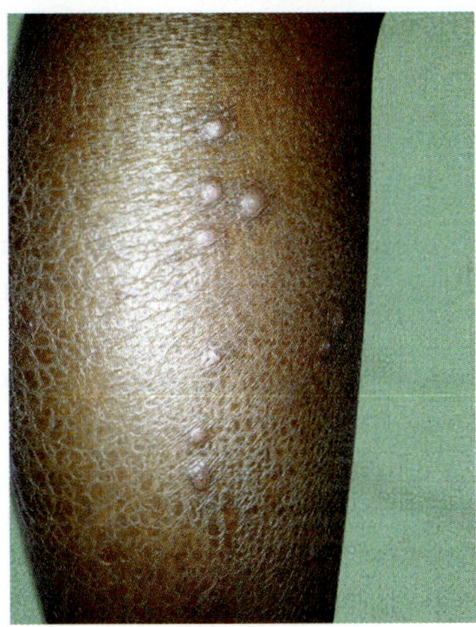

Fig. 1: Papulonodular lesions over the extensor aspect of lower extremities

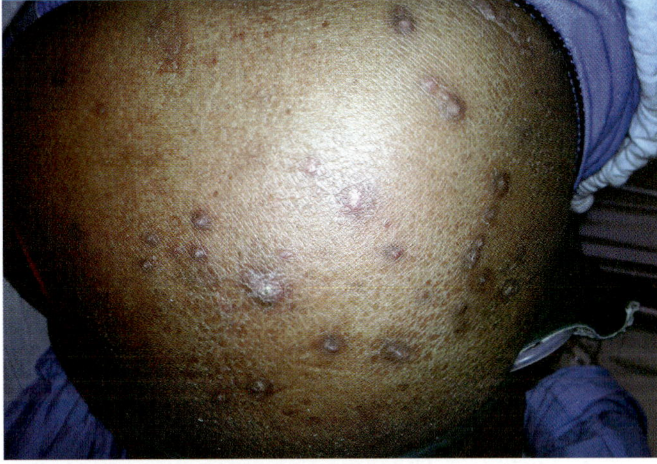

Fig. 2: Central umbilication, filled with a keratinous plug and some of the lesions were arranged in a linear fashion (Koebner phenomenon)

Q1. What is the most probable diagnosis?

a. Molluscum contagiosum
b. Prurigo nodularis
c. Reactive perforating collagenosis
d. Papulonecrotic tuberculid.

Ans: c. Reactive perforating collagenosis.

Q2. What are the points in favor of your diagnosis?

Ans:
- Age of onset → early adulthood
- Positive family history
- Umbilicated papulonodular lesions with a central keratotic plug
- Old lesions heal with scarring
- History of extrusion of whitish material on scratching.

Q3. How will you confirm your diagnosis?

Ans: Although, clinical picture suggests the diagnosis, a histopathological examination (HPE) with special stains (for connective tissue) is necessary to confirm the diagnosis.

Q4. What is the characteristic HPE finding in perforating disorders? What special stain(s) do you think would be helpful?

Ans: The characteristic HPE findings are:
- *Epidermis:* Localized area of hyperkeratosis (keratotic plug); variable parakeratosis; presence of keratotic debris.
- *Dermis:* There is localized collection of altered connective tissue components in the papillary dermis, which is surrounded and engulfed by focal epidermal proliferation; these materials extend through the epidermis into the crusted plaque (transepidermal elimination); early stage → neutrophilic infiltration; late/chronic stage → lymphocytic infiltration (elastosis perforans serpiginosa).

The connective tissue component undergoing transepidermal elimination varies according to the disease (Table 1):

Table 1: Characteristic histopathological examination (HPE)

Name of the perforating disorder	*Perforating substance*
Reactive perforating collagenosis (RPC) (inherited)	Collagen
Elastosis perforans serpiginosa (EPS)	Elastic tissue
Perforating folliculitis	Necrotic material
Acquired perforating dermatoses, viz. Kyrle's disease, acquired RPC, etc.)	Necrotic material, collagen, etc.
Perforating periumbilical calcific elastosis	Calcified elastic tissue

Special stain (s): Some of the common stains used in the laboratory are given below:
- Verhoeff-Van Gieson (VVG) stain (most commonly used) → collagen fibers (red); elastic fibers (black)
- Trichrome stain
- Phosphotungstic acid hematoxylin stain.

Q5. How will you treat a patient with perforating dermatoses?

Ans: The treatment approach of perforating dermatoses are given in Flowchart 1.

Flowchart 1: Perforating dermatoses

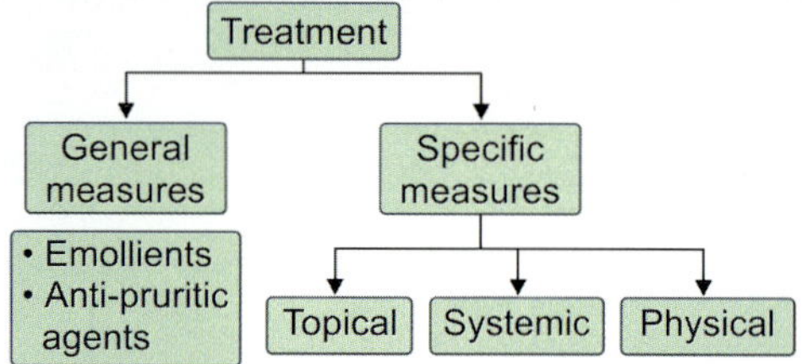

- *Topical Therapy*:
  - Topical retinoids
  - Topical steroid under occlusion
  - Imiquimod.
- *Systemic Therapy*: For extensive cases, not responding to topical medications
  - Oral isotretinoin
  - Methotrexate
- *Physical Modalities:*
  - PUVA (psoralen and ultraviolet A radiation)
  - Laser therapy (Er:YAG, ultrapulsed CO_2, pulsed dye, etc.)
  - Cryotherapy.

Excision and dermabrasion should be avoided as they may worsen the condition.

Q6. What are perforating dermatoses?

Ans: The perforating dermatoses constitute a group of cutaneous disorders characterized by transepidermal elimination of collagen, elastic tissue or necrotic connective tissue from the dermis to exterior, with little or no disruption of the surrounding structures.

Q7. Classify the different types of perforating disorders.

Ans: The important perforating disorders can be classified as:

- According to pathogenesis:
  - Primary perforating disorders
  - Secondary perforating disorders
- According to the mode of occurrence:
  - Familial/Inherited
  - Acquired perforating dermatoses.

Primary perforating disorders: The perforating disorders which occur due to intrinsic defects in the epidermal keratinocytes, hair follicles, collagen or elastic tissue, with transepidermal elimination being the final common pathway. There are mainly four disorders under this category:

1. Reactive perforating collagenosis (RPC).
2. Elastosis perforans serpiginosa (EPS).
3. Perforating folliculitis.
4. Acquired perforating dermatoses/Kyrle's disease.

Secondary perforating disorders: These group of perforating disorders occur due to some underlying cutaneous disorder. There are several cutaneous disorders which may result in secondary perforating disorders. Some of the important ones are mentioned below:

- Perforation of endogenous substances:
  - Chondrodermatitis nodularis helicis
  - Hematomas
  - Perforating pseudoxanthoma elasticum (PXE)
  - Gout
  - Perforating calcinosis
- Perforation of exogenous foreign materials
  - Silica
  - Wood splinters
  - Caustic drilling fluids (petrochemical industry)
- Due to infectious diseases/organisms
  - Chromoblastomycosis
  - Botryomycosis
- Extrusion of neoplastic cells
  - Melanoma
  - Paget's disease
  - Mycosis fungoides.

Familial/Inherited: These group of disorders are often inherited from a family member; onset → childhood. Excepting Kyrle's disease, the remaining three primary perforating disorders are familial.

Acquired perforating dermatoses: These disorders are acquired in the adulthood. There may be several underlying systemic disorders which may result in the development of these acquired perforating disorders. All secondary perforating disorders and Kyrle's disease form this group.

Q8. What is the most common systemic condition to be associated with acquired perforating dermatoses?

a. Chronic renal failure
b. Diabetes mellitus
c. Liver disease
d. Neoplastic disorders

Ans: b. Diabetes mellitus (~11%)

The common acquired perforating dermatoses are given below:

- Acquired RPC
- Kyrle's disease
- Acquired EPS (rare) → may occur due to penicillamine

Table 2: Features of various perforating disorders

Name	*Incidence*	*Onset*	*Usual distribution*	*Lesion morphology*	*Associated disorders*
RPC	Relatively rare	Childhood to adolescence	Dorsal aspect of upper extremities more than lower extremities and trunk	Papulonodules, with central keratinous scale/crust. Koebner phenomenon → +ve	None
EPS	Rare; M >F	Childhood and young adulthood	Neck (nape), cheeks, arms and thighs (symmetrical)	Small, horny umbilicated papules arranged in lines, circles or arcs	PXE, EDS, MFS, OI, Acrogeria and penicillamine therapy
Perforating folliculitis	Common	Young adults	Trunk and extremities	Follicular umbilicated papules/nodules, with keratinous crust	May be associated with ordinary folliculitis with follicular rupture
Acquired	Common	Adults	Lower limbs more than trunk	Pruritic dome-shaped papules with central crust	Long standing DM and renal failure on hemodialysis
Perforating periumbilical calcific elastosis	Very rare; black women	Adults	Abdomen and periumbilical	Periumbilical keratotic papules and plaques	Multiparity

Abbreviations: RPC, reactive perforating collagenosis; EPS, elastosis perforans serpiginosa; PXE, pseudoxanthoma elasticum; EDS, Ehlers–Danlos syndrome; MFS, Marfan syndrome; OI, Osteogenesis imperfecta; DM, diabetes mellitus

- Perforating periumbilical calcific elastosis.

In penicillamine-induced cases of EPS, elastic fibers may have a characteristic *bramble bush* or *lumpy bumpy* appearance.

Q9. Briefly discuss the differentiating features of various perforating disorders.

Ans: The differentiating features of various perforating disorders are described in Table 2.

CHAPTER 63

Pityriasis Rubra Pilaris

Ruby Venugopal, Biju Vasudevan

Case study Pityriasis rubra pilaris

Presenting complaints

Doctor, my face and body has become red and flaky since the last 3 weeks.

Setting

Dermatology outpatient department

History of present illness

A 32-year-old male presented with history of progressive reddish discoloration of skin of 3 weeks duration followed by flaking on body of 1 week duration. Symptoms began as spots of redness along the hairline on the forehead which slowly increased in size and merged with each other to form bigger areas of redness on face, neck and trunk. Over the next week, these lesions became flaky and continued to progress to involve the entire trunk and limbs. The lesions had a mild burning sensation. He also gave history of diffuse flaking over scalp, thickening of skin of palms and soles and swelling of extremities. There was no history of any preexisting skin disease, use of drugs, systemic symptoms or high-risk sexual behavior.

General Physical Examination

- Well oriented to time, place and person
- Body mass index: 29.5 kg/m^2
- Pulse: 80 BPM
- B/L pitting pedal edema, swelling of hands.

Systemic Examination

No abnormality detected.

Dermatological Examination

- Diffuse involvement of face, neck, trunk and extremities in the form of blanchable erythema (BSA 70–80%) (Fig. 1). Follicular papules found scattered in the erythematous regions (Fig. 2)
- Islands of sparing
- Diffuse branny scales along with collarette of scales involving scalp, face, neck, trunk
- Thickening of skin over dorsal and palmar/ plantar aspects of hands and feet (Fig. 3).

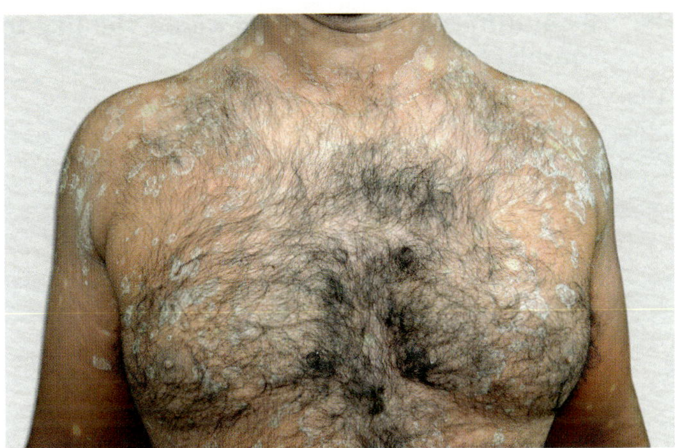

Fig. 1: Extensive scaling of the trunk with few islands of sparing

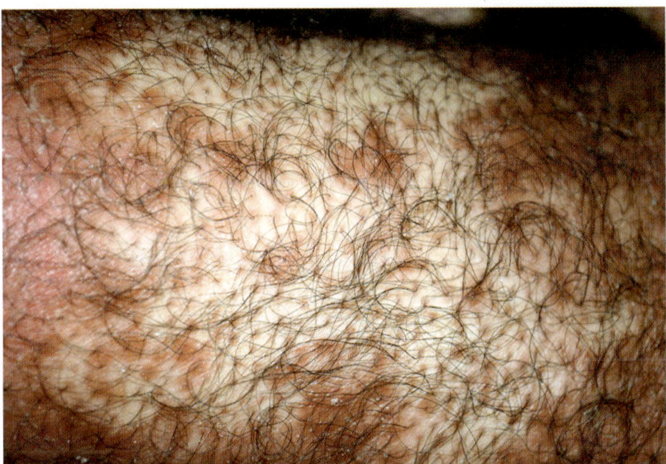

Fig. 2: Few areas of trunk showing the follicular erythematous papules

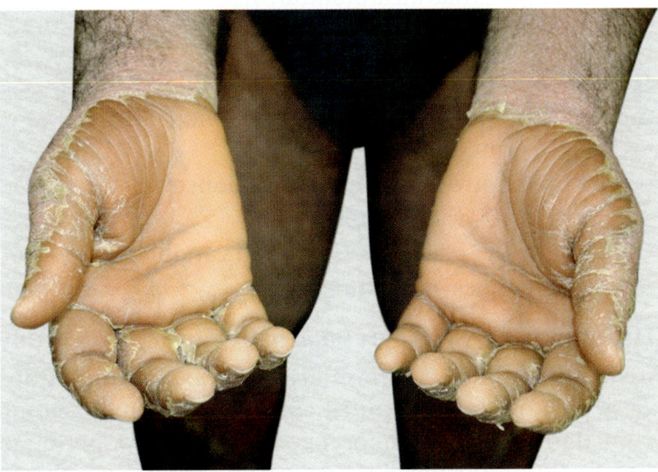

Fig. 3: Thickening of skin of palms

Q1. What is the most probable clinical diagnosis?

a. Erythroderma
b. Psoriasis
c. Pityriasis rubra pilaris
d. Papulo-erythroderma of Ofuji

Ans: c. Pityriasis rubra pilaris (PRP). Erythema and scaling over the body with islands of sparing, cephalocaudal progression of lesions and palmoplantar involvement favor diagnosis of PRP.

Q2. What are the clinical characteristics of pityriasis rubra pilaris?

Ans: Circumscribed follicular keratoses, branny scales, orange-red erythema and waxy diffuse palmoplantar keratoderma (PRP sandal).

Q3. How do you classify PRP?

Ans: Classification scheme as per Griffiths and Gonzales – Lopez classifies PRP into 6 subtypes:

Type	*Nomenclature*	*%*	*Clinical characteristics*	*Course*
I	Classical adult type	>50	Generalised involvement, cephalo-caudal progression, erythroderma with islands of normal skin, follicular hyperkeratosis, PRP sandal	Usually resolves within 3 yrs
II	Atypical adult type	5	Follicular hyperkeratosis at some sites, lamellar ichthyosis on legs. Less tendency to become erythrodermic	Prolonged (>20 yrs)
III	Classical juvenile type	10	Age of onset—1–2 yrs of life Similar to type I	Usually resolves within 2 yrs
IV	Circumscribed juvenile	25	Prepubertal, well-demarcated plaques of follicular plugging on knees and elbows	Uncertain course
V	Atypical juvenile	5	Early onset, overlaps with ichthyosis and erythrokeratoderma. Follicular plugging with scleroderma-like change of digits. Most familial PRP cases are of this type	Chronic course
VI	HIV associated	-	HIV associated follicular syndrome, classical PRP or filiform pattern of keratosis	Responds to anti-retroviral therapy

Q4. What are the histopathological features of PRP?

Ans: Varies with stage of disease and site involved

- Hyperkeratosis
- Acanthosis with broad short rete ridges
- Foci of parakeratosis
- Follicular plugging
- Dilated dermal capillaries
- Lymphohistiocytic dermal infiltrate.

Q5. What are the clinical features that help in differentiating between PRP and psoriasis?

Ans:

Feature	*Pityriasis rubra pilaris*	*Psoriasis*
Age at onset	Bimodal	Second decade
Scalp scaling	Furfuraceous	Adherent
Islands of pale skin	Constant	Less common
Keratoderma	Constant	Less common
Nail changes	No salmon patches	Present
Nail growth rate	Moderate increase	Marked increase
Epidermal kinetics	Moderate increase	Marked increase
Seronegative arthropathy	Rare	Common
Response to UVB, corticosteroids	Poor	Good
Response to methotrexate	Variable	Good

Q6. Which of the following nail changes are not seen in PRP?

a. Distal discoloration
b. Splinter hemorrhages
c. Dystrophy of nail plate
d. Pitting

Ans: c. Dystrophy of nail plate. Unlike psoriasis, dystrophy of nail plate is never seen in psoriasis. Pitting, although minimal can be seen in PRP.

Q7. What are the histopathology features that help in differentiating PRP and psoriasis?

Ans:

Feature	*Pityriasis rubra pilaris*	*Psoriasis*
Follicular plugging	Present	Absent
Granular layer	Increased	Decreased
Munro-micro abscess	Absent	Present
Suprapapillary thinning	Absent	Present
Dermal capillaries	Dilated	Dilated and tortuous

Q8. What differential diagnoses would you like to consider?

Ans: The differential diagnosis are as follows:

- Psoriasis
- Seborrheic dermatitis
- Follicular eczema
- Lichen planus
- Ichthyosis
- Pityriasis lichenoides chronica
- Dermatophytosis
- Secondary syphilis
- Erythrokeratoderma
- Cutaneous T-cell lymphoma
- Subacute lupus erythematosus.

Q9. What changes can one see on laboratory investigations?

Ans: There are no specific diagnostic tests for PRP. Serum vitamin A levels may be normal. There are reports of reduction in the levels of the serum retinol binding protein. An elevation in the cellular retinol and retinoic acid binding protein level has been found.

Q10. Which of the following topical agents is least effective in PRP?

a. Emollients
b. Calcipotriol
c. Topical steroids
d. Tazarotene

Ans: c. Topical steroids. Topical steroids provide little long-term therapeutic effect in PRP. Topical therapy includes emollient application, vitamin D analogues and keratolytics like salicylic acid and urea. Vitamin A analogues like tazarotene are reserved as second-line agents.

Q11. What are the systemic agents used in PRP?

Ans:

- Retinoids—Acitretin, Isotretinoin—First line of treatment
- Methotrexate—Variable response
- PUVA—variable response
- HAART—for HIV associated variant
- Biologics—Infliximab.

Q12. Describe the progression of PRP to erythroderma.

Ans: As pityriasis rubra pilaris evolves, erythematous perifollicular papules coalesce to form a scaling dermatitis with an orange red hue over a period of 2–3 months developing into erythroderma. Islands of normal skin (nappes claires) are diagnostic.

A waxy yellow palmoplantar keratoderma also develops along with nail and mucous membrane changes. Prolonged erythema may give rise to peripheral edema and high-output cardiac failure in the elderly. Progression to erythroderma is commonly seen in the classic adult, classic juvenile and HIV-associated forms. The atypical adult type has lesser tendency of becoming erythrodermic. The juvenile circumscribed variant does not progress to a widespread involvement.

Q13. What is the prognosis for this condition?

Ans: In the classical adult form, spontaneous resolution may occur in 1–3 years but recurrences have been recognised. Spontaneous clearance in 1–2 years has been reported in the juvenile classical variant. The prognosis is uncertain in the juvenile circumscribed form, with a few reports of clearance in the late teens. Juvenile atypical form has a chronic course and may not resolve spontaneously. HIV associated PRP is usually severe and can occasionally be fatal.

CHAPTER 64

Darier's Disease

Anuradha Babu

Case study Darier's Disease

Presenting Complaints

Doctor, these dirty lesions have been developing in my underarms and groin for the last 5 years. I have noticed some changes in my nails for the last 2 years.

Setting

Dermatology outpatient department

History of Present Illness

A 20-year-old man presented to the dermatology outpatient department with complaints of dirty skin lesions on scalp, face, neck, chest and back for the last 5 years. He also complained of malodorous growths in the underarms and groin for the last 2 years. There was aggravation of lesions during summer. He has also developed some nail changes and skin-colored lesions on the back of hands and feet.

General Physical Examination and Systemic Examination

No abnormality detected.

Dermatological Examination

- Hyperpigmented papules on margins of scalp, face, neck, back and chest (Fig. 1)
- Maceration and warty plaques in axillae and groin
- Flat-topped skin-colored papules on dorsa of hands and feet (Fig. 2)
- Pits on palms and soles
- Nails—Longitudinal red and white lines and V-shaped notches on distal ends (Fig. 3).

Q1. What is the most likely diagnosis?

a. Seborrheic dermatitis

b. Grover's disease

c. Darier's disease

d. Hailey-Hailey disease

Ans: c. Darier's disease. Presence of warty papules in seborrheic areas, maceration and vegetating masses in axillae and groin, skin-colored warty papules on dorsa of hands and feet, palmoplantar pits and nail changes are suggestive of Darier's disease.

Q2. What is the etiology of Darier's disease?

Ans: The etiology is as follows:

- Darier's disease is due to mutations in the *ATP2A2* gene at chromosome 12q24.1, which encodes the

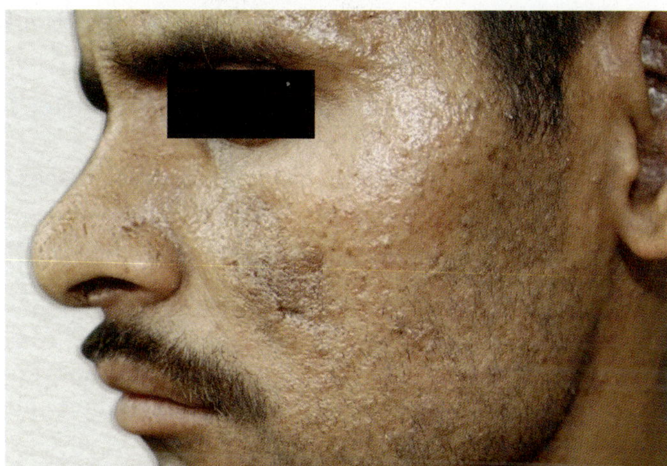
Fig. 1: Dirty papules on face

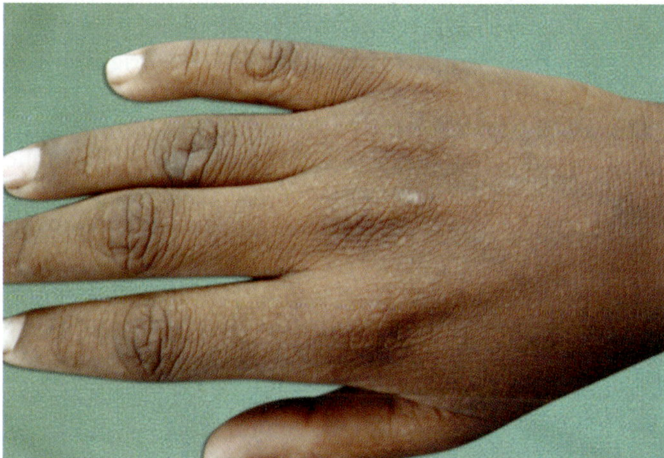
Fig. 2: Flat topped papules on dorsum of hands

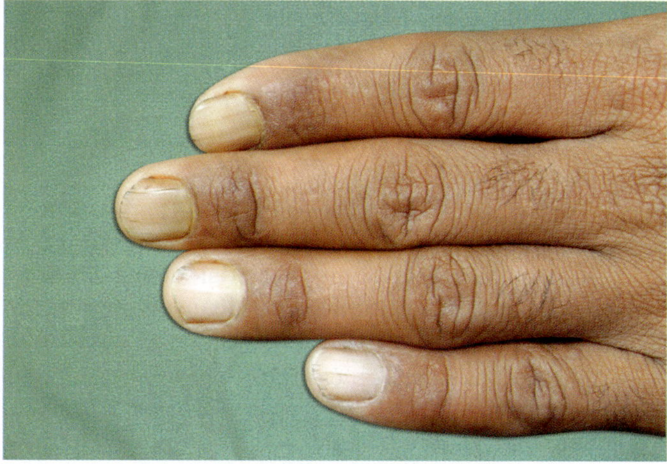
Fig. 3: V shaped notching of nails

sarco/endoplasmic reticulum calcium ATPase type 2 (SERCA2)

- One hypothesis proposes a failure in compensatory mechanisms when the endoplasmic reticulum is stressed. The consequent reduced calcium concentrations leads to folding of secreted or membrane proteins and therefore transport is disrupted. In Darier's disease, keratinocytes exhibit reduced trafficking of desmosomal proteins to the cell membrane, resulting in failure of adhesion
- An impaired stress response may also predispose to apoptosis, which could explain the dyskeratotic cells.

Q3. What are the clinical features of Darier's disease?

Ans: Clinical features:

- The disease usually begins between the ages of 6 and 20 years, with a peak onset during puberty
- The rash is typically exacerbated by heat and light
- The primary lesions are keratotic red to brown papules, which develop in a "seborrheic" distribution involving the trunk, scalp margins, face and neck (Fig. 1)
- The lesions tend to become confluent and may form papillomatous masses which may become vegetating and malodorous especially in flexures
- Flat and freckle-like lesions may appear as pale macules (Guttate leukoderma) in pigmented skin
- On the dorsa of hands and feet, discrete papules are clinically indistinguishable from acrokeratosis verruciformis of Hopf (Fig. 2)
- The characteristic nail changes include red and white longitudinal bands, longitudinal ridging and fissuring,wedge-shaped subungual hyperkeratosis, brittle nails leading to V-shaped notches distally (Fig. 3)
- Palms and soles show minute pits or, punctuate or filiform keratoses
- White umbilicate or cobblestone papules may be seen on the palate
- Patients have an increased susceptibility to herpes simplex. Kaposi's varicelliform eruption and chronic pyogenic infections are common
- Salivary duct narrowing can cause recurrent salivary gland swelling
- Various neuropsychiatric conditions, such as epilepsy, intellectual impairment and mood disorders have been reported in association with Darier's disease

- Ocular complications like corneal ulcerations and staphylococcal endophthalmitis may occur rarely
- Pulmonary involvement
- Bone cysts.

Q4. What are the morphological variants of Darier's disease?

Ans: Morphological variants:
- Acral hemorrhagic
- Segmental
- Vesiculobullous
- Flexural erosive disease
- Hyperkeratotic lesions
- Acantholytic dyskeratotic epidermal nevi (Blaschkoid)
- Comedones and cysts with Darier's disease.

Q5. What are the differential diagnoses of Darier's disease?

Ans: Differential diagnosis:
- Seborrheic dermatitis—The involvement of seborrheic areas is seen in both seborrheic dermatitis and Darier's disease. Darier's disease is distinguishable by the presence of warty papules, involvement of acral skin, nails and oral mucosa. Histological findings will aid in differentiation of both conditions
- Grover's disease (transient and persistent acantholytic dermatosis)—The pruritic crusted papules are not confluent and they typically appear after occlusion or sweating. Histology may mimic Darier's disease
- Hailey-Hailey disease (familial benign pemphigus)—Flexural Darier's disease may clinically and histologically overlap with this. However, a predominantly vesicular eruption is rare in Darier's disease. The presence of palmoplantar pits, longitudinal erythronychia, distal notching of nails and mucosal lesions serve as clues to the diagnosis of Darier's disease. Histologically, acantholysis in Darier's disease occurs primarily in discrete foci whereas the loss of intercellular bridges in Hailey-Hailey disease is generally more widespread within the epidermis giving rise to the "dilapidated brick wall" appearance
- Acrokeratosis verruciformis of Hopf—An autosomal dominant disorder with flat-topped, wart-like papules on the dorsal aspects of the extremities which is indistinguishable from similar lesions in Darier's disease. Both have traditionally been separated on the basis of their histological features, with acrokeratosis verruciformis of Hopf lacking acantholysis and dyskeratosis.

Q6. How do you confirm the diagnosis of Darier's disease?

Ans: In a patient with clinical features of Darier's disease a skin biopsy will help to confirm the diagnosis.

There are two prominent histologic features in Darier's disease, acantholysis and dyskeratosis. Acantholysis is due to a disturbance in cell adhesion that leads to suprabasilar cleft formation. Dyskeratosis is due to apoptosis of keratinocytes and is characterized by nuclear condensation and perinuclear keratin clumping.

Two types of dyskeratotic cells are seen in Darier's disease.

1. "Corps ronds"—Acantholytic enlarged keratinocytes in the malphigian layer with darkly staining and partially fragmented nuclei surrounded by a clear cytoplasm and encircled by a bright ring of collapsed keratin bundles.
2. "Grains"—Small, oval cells in the stratum corneum characterized by an intensely eosinophilic cytoplasm composed of collapsed keratin bundles containing shrunken parakeratotic nuclear bundles.

The epidermis overlying acantholytic and dyskeratotic foci is thickened and shows papillomatosis and hyperkeratosis. There is mild-to-moderate perivascular inflammatory infiltrate in the superficial dermis.

Q7. Acantholytic dyskeratosis is seen in all except?

a. Darier's disease
b. Grover's disease
c. Hailey-Hailey disease
d. Pemphigus foliaceus

Ans: d. Pemphigus foliaceus

Q8. What are the treatment options for Darier's disease?

Ans: *General measures:* Lightweight clothes and sunscreen help prevent exacerbation due to heat, sweating and sun exposure. Malodorous bacterial colonization may be prevented by antimicrobial cleansers. Keratolytic emollients will help to reduce scaling and irritation.

Topical therapy: Topical tretinoin, adapalene and tazarotene have been reported to be effective. However, retinoid-associated irritation is common and can be reduced by liberal use of emollients and combination therapy with mid-potency topical corticosteroids. Intermittent use of topical antibiotics and antifungal agents is helpful in treating malodor due to microbial colonization and mild secondary infections.

Systemic therapy: Isotretinoin and acitretin are very effective treatments for Darier's disease, with significant improvement and control of disease. There are case reports of cyclosporine being used to control severe Darier's disease, and it may be helpful for patients who cannot tolerate or do not respond to oral retinoids.

Surgical therapy: Surgical therapy may be an effective alternative for focal recalcitrant lesions, particularly in the flexural and gluteal areas. Excision followed by split-thickness grafting, dermabrasion or laser (CO_2 or erbium:YAG) may yield a long-term remission.

CHAPTER 65

Follicular Keratotic Disorders

Anupam Das

Case study Follicular Keratotic Disorders

Presenting Complaints

Doctor, I have developed these small, dark raised bumps over my outer arms and thighs for the last 3 years.

Setting

Outpatient department of dermatology

History of Present Illness

A 18-year-old girl presented with dark goose bump like rough lesions distributed over the upper part of both arms and thighs, present for the preceding 3 years. To start with, there were very few lesions over the arms but gradually, they increased in number to involve the entire arm and the thighs as well. The patient complains of occasional itching and burning over the lesions.

General Physical Examination and Systemic Examination

No significant abnormality detected.

Dermatological Examination

- Inspection shows numerous small (1–2 mm) folliculocentric erythematous keratotic papules distributed over the outer arms and thighs, bilaterally (Fig. 1). Small coiled hair could be seen arising out of the papules
- Palpation gave the feeling of fine sandpaper-like texture. Whitish material could be expressed from the keratotic papules.

Q1. What is the most likely diagnosis?

a. Lichen scrofulosorum

b. Lichen spinulosus

c. Keratosis pilaris

d. Pityriasis rubra pilaris

Ans: c. Keratosis pilaris. The typical morphology (folliculocentric keratotic papules) of the lesions distributed over the classical site (outer arms and thighs) confirms the diagnosis.

Q2. What are the common sites of involvement in keratosis pilaris?

Ans: Common sites of involvement

- Postero-lateral aspect of upper arms (92%)
- Anterior aspect of thighs (59%)

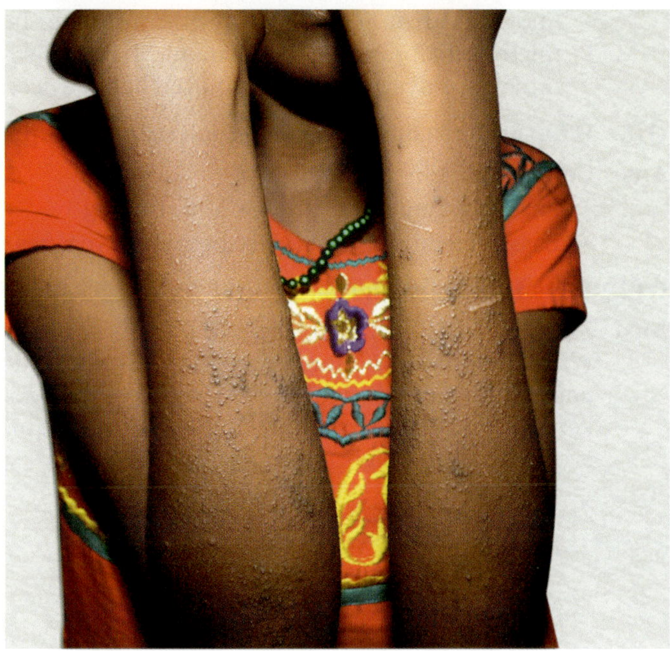

Fig. 1: Keratotic papules on extensor aspect bilaterally
Courtesy: Dr MS Sadeep

- Buttocks (30%)
- Cheeks.

Q3. What are the differential diagnoses to be considered in a case of keratosis pilaris?

Ans: Differential diagnosis includes:
- Lichen spinulosus
- Phrynoderma
- Follicular atopic eczema
- Follicular lichen planus
- Pityriasis rubra pilaris
- Lichen scrofulosorum
- Lichen nitidus
- Perforating disorders
- Eruptive vellus hair cysts
- Eruptive xanthoma
- Erythromelanosis follicularis faciei et colli.

Q4. What is the basic pathomechanism behind this entity?

Ans: Defective keratinization of the follicular epithelium resulting in the development of a keratotic infundibular plug.

Q5. What is the mode of inheritance of keratosis pilaris?

a. Autosomal dominant
b. Autosomal recessive
c. X-linked dominant
d. X-linked recessive

Ans: a. Autosomal dominant

Q6. What are the histological findings in keratosis pilaris?

Ans: It is characterised by a triad of hyperkeratosis, hypergranulosis and follicular plugging.

Q7. What are the causes of follicular plugging?

Ans: Causes of follicular plugging include:
- Discoid lupus erythematosus
- Acne vulgaris
- Keratosis pilaris
- Follicular lichen planus
- Pityriasis rubra pilaris
- Darier's disease
- Lichen sclerosus et atrophicus
- Demodicidosis
- Trichostasis spinulosa
- Eruptive vellus hair cysts
- Perforating disorders.

Q8. What are the associations of keratosis pilaris?

Ans: Associations of keratosis pilaris include:
- Atopic dermatitis
- Ichthyosis vulgaris
- Scarring alopecia
- KID syndrome
- Obesity
- Cardio-facio-cutaneous syndrome
- Down's syndrome
- Ectodermal dysplasia
- Prolidase deficiency
- Atrichia with papular lesions.

Q9. What are the dermoscopic features of keratosis pilaris?

Ans: Dermoscopic features:
- Follicular plugging may or may not be present
- Coiled hair shaft emerging from the infundibulum of the hair follicle
- Hair shaft may take the shape of a semicircle or a loop.

Q10. What is keratosis pilaris atrophicans faciei?

Ans: It is a rare variant of keratosis pilaris characterised by the presence of erythematous horny papules over the eyebrows and cheeks. It is also known as ulerythema ophryogenes as there is loss of eyebrows.

Q11. Is there any grave cosmetic concern in case of ulerythema ophryogenes?

Ans: Yes, it can lead to complete loss of eyebrows, causing a serious cosmetic concern for the patient.

Q12. What are the treatment options?

Ans: Treatment options include:
- Use of mild cleansers
- Proper lubrication with moisturising lotions
- Topical retinoids
- Topical mid-potent steroids (if inflammation present)
- Hydroquinone 4%, azelaic acid 10% and kojic acid for pigmentation
- Surgical procedures: Glycolic acid peels, microdermabrasion, photodynamic therapy, 595-nm pulsed dye laser, intense pulsed light devices.

Q13. What are the complications which may develop?

Ans: Complications:
- Postinflammatory pigmentation, scarring
- Loss of lateral eyebrows (ulerythema ophryogenes).

Q14. What is antenna sign?

Ans: Antenna sign is characteristic of keratosis pilaris. When light is shone tangentially on the keratotic papule, the individual follicles show a long strand of keratin which appears popped up and shining. This is called antenna sign.

CHAPTER 66

Erythroderma

Ankan Gupta

Case study Erythroderma

Presenting Complaint

Doctor, I have severe itching all over body and extensive flaking of skin since last 2 weeks.

Setting

Emergency department

History of Present Illness

A 43-year-old man presented with history of redness and scaling initially involving the upper extremities which gradually progressed to involve the trunk, face and lower extremities since 2 weeks. He gives no history of any skin complaints prior to this episode.

General Physical Examination

- The patient is well oriented to time, place and person
- The patient is conscious and cooperative
- Pulse rate: 90 beats/min
- BP: 100/60 mm Hg
- She is afebrile, has pallor and pitting pedal edema around the ankle joint.

Systemic Examination

No abnormality detected.

Dermatological Examination

- Diffuse erythema and scaling is present over the trunk and limbs with sparing of palms and soles (Figs 1 and 2)
- BSA (body surface area) involved >90%
- Diffuse thick scaling noted on the scalp with fissuring in the retroauricular areas (Fig. 3)
- Face has erythema and scaling with prominent bilateral ectropion
- Mucosae and nails are normal.

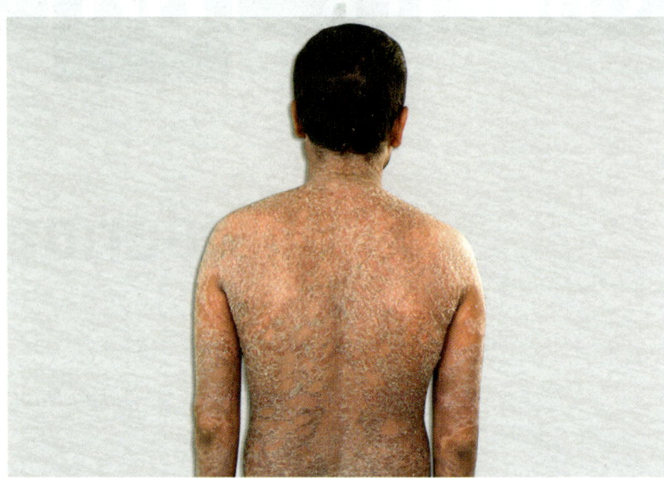

Fig. 1: Diffuse erythema and scaling is present over the trunk

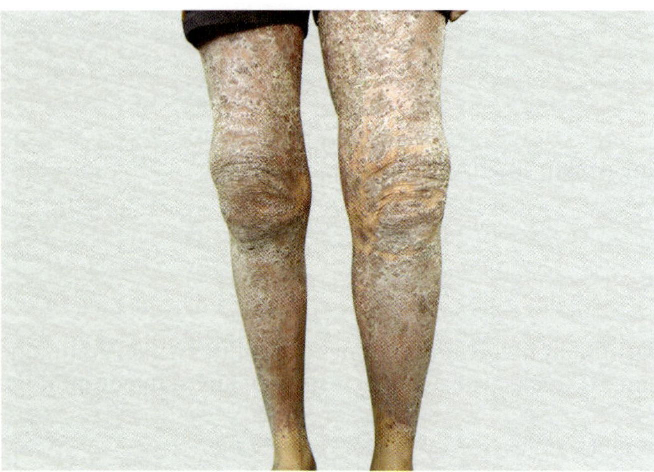

Fig. 2: Similar lesions on the lower limbs

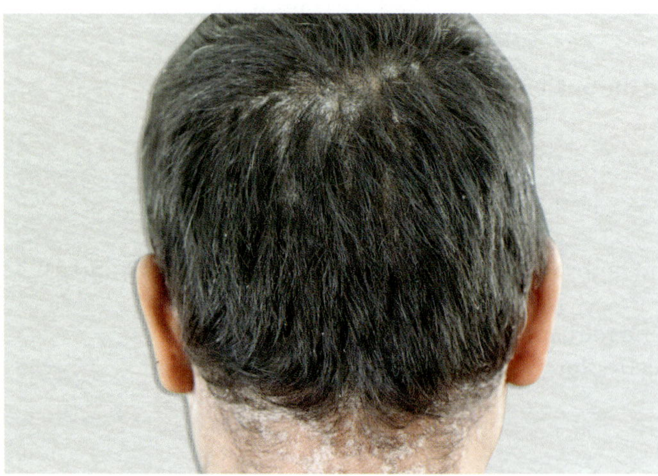

Fig. 3: Diffuse thick scaling noted on the scalp

Q1. What is the first step in the management of this patient?

a. Performing a skin biopsy
b. Administration of intravenous antibiotics
c. Administration of corticosteroids
d. Managing the patient conservatively and waiting for investigation results

Ans: d. Managing the patient conservatively and waiting for investigation results.

Q2. What clinical differential would be foremost in this case?

a. Drug hypersensitivity syndrome
b. Erythroderma
c. Psoriasis
d. Seborrheic dermatitis

Ans: b. Erythroderma. Extensive scaling and erythema over the body involving more than 90% BSA points toward the diagnosis of erythroderma.

Q3. Enumerate various causes of erythroderma?

Ans: The causes of erythroderma are as follows:

- *Eczema of various types*: Atopic dermatitis, seborrheic dermatitis, allergic contact dermatitis, irritant contact dermatitis, stasis dermatitis
- *Papulosquamous disorders*: Psoriasis, lichen planus, pityriasis rubra pilaris, reactive arthritis
- *Malignancy related*: Lymphomas, leukemias, graft-versus-host disease
- *Drug induced*: Antiepileptics, gold, lithium salts and allopurinol. Antibiotics, such as penicillins, sulphonamides and antitubercular drugs
- *Bullous diseases*: Pemphigus foliaceus, bullous pemphigoid
- *Connective tissue disorders*: Systemic lupus erythematosus, dermatomyositis
- Hereditary disorders: Ichthyosiform erythroderma
- *Others*: Dermatophytosis, Norwegian scabies, HIV (human immunodeficiency virus)
- Idiopathic/Unknown.

Q4. What are the key features in history that point toward the cause of erythroderma?

Ans: Key features in etiology are as follows:

- Acute onset of erythroderma suggests drug-induced cause or lymphoma
- Excessive pruritus is a feature of atopic eczema or lymphoma leading to erythroderma
- A positive family history is seen in atopics

- Preexisting scaly skin lesions on extensor aspects with seasonal variation points toward psoriasis
- A cephalocaudal spread is suggestive of pityriasis rubra pilaris
- Photoexacerbation/photosensitivity/radiation exposure (if therapeutic—indication, no. of sessions, adjuvant chemotherapy) might exacerbate preexisting dermatosis/systemic lupus erythematosus (SLE)/chronic actinic dermatitis/radiation dermatitis eventually leading to erythroderma
- Preexisting medical illness and treatment history is relevant in association with erythroderma or its management viz. recent change in antiepileptics, initiation of antiretroviral therapy (ART), antituberculosis treatment (ATT), antibiotics (sulfonamides, fluoroquinolones), chemotherapy drugs, and adverse drug reactions secondary to primary drug initiated or cross-reaction between drugs that affect pharmacokinetics of each other
- In many cases, treatment with topical ayurvedic or herbal medications can precipitate erythroderma
- Presence of constitutional symptoms (weight loss, pyrexia of unknown origin, malaise) with generalized lymphadenopathy and hepatosplenomegaly on clinical examination suggests malignancy
- Immune status of individuals with HIV, hemophiliacs on routine transfusions, and post organ transplantation being compromised is more susceptible to an exacerbated tissue response secondary to infections and infestations (scabies, tuberculosis, dermatophytosis) that readily precipitates erythroderma.

Q5. What clues in physical examination could help ascertain the most likely cause of erythroderma?

Ans: It is important to assess the hue of the erythema, type of scaling, areas of sparing, involvement of palms and soles which could all point toward an underlying etiology.

Areas of Sparing

- Face is spared in psoriasis mostly.
- Nose sparing (Pavithran's sign) is nonspecific.

Erythematous Hue

- Deep purple-red hue in cutaneous T-cell lymphoma (CTCL)
- Orange in platelet-rich plasma (PRP).

Palms and Sole Involvement

- Suggests PRP and psoriasis
- Fissured keratoderma suggests CTCL.

Nature of Scales

- Most prominent with psoriasis
- Fine scales with atopic dermatitis/dermatophyte infection
- Bran-like scales with seborrheic dermatitis
- Posterythema desquamation is common with drug reactions or bacterial infections
- Coarse scales seen in early erythroderma while fine scales noted in late/recovery phase.

Additional Mucocutaneous Findings

- Blisters and crusting—suggestive of secondary infection, autoimmune blistering disorders (bullous pemphigoid, pemphigus foliaceus)
- Nail changes (subungual hyperkeratosis, nail pitting suggests psoriasis, shore line nails in drug-induced erythroderma, periungual telangiectasia in dermatomyositis)
- Oral ulcers suggest systemic lupus erythematosus (SLE)
- Alopecia suggests CTCL.

Systemic Findings

- Organomegaly (hepatomegaly suggests drug-induced erythroderma, splenomegaly may be associated with lymphoma)
- Lymphadenopathy may be associated with lymphoma
- *Musculoskeletal features*: Arthritis in SLE, psoriasis, muscle weakness in dermatomyositis.

Q6. What investigations should be performed to ascertain the cause of erythroderma?

Ans: Investigations:

Baseline Investigations

Skin Biopsy

- A biopsy should be taken from multiple skin sites, and it should be repeated when the nonspecific clinical signs improve
- *Histopathologically*: Psoriasiform, spongiotic or ichthyosiform pattern, epidermotropism, and keratinocyte apoptosis may give a clue to the possible underlying etiology. It may be repeated on a 6 monthly basis to look for CTCL

Complete Hemogram along with Peripheral Smear

- Low hemoglobin and variations in red blood cell (RBC) indices may indicate anemia of chronic disease, increased loss of blood from the skin, or malabsorption in the gut
- A high white blood cell (WBC) total count could indicate infection, or isolated WBC cell variations in differential counts especially atypical

lymphocytosis and abnormal cells can indicate a leukemic condition

- Eosinophilia may be associated with allergic contact dermatitis, bullous pemphigoid, drug reactions, idiopathic hypereosinophilic syndrome (HES), parasitic infestations
- Pancytopenia suggests collagen vascular disorders, hematopoietic malignancies.

Other Routine Investigations

Erythrocyte sedimentation rate (ESR), serum blood urea nitrogen, sodium, potassium, and chloride along with an albumin level, liver function tests (LFT), renal function test (RFT), chest X-ray, and urinalysis.

Additional Tests—Investigations Which May Be Performed Depending on Clinical Suspicion

- *Scales*: KOH, Gram stain, culture and sensitivity
- Nail fold capillaroscopy
- Antinuclear antibodies (ANA)
- Absolute eosinophil counts and serum immunoglobulin E (IgE)
- Lymph nodes: FNAC (fine-needle aspiration cytology), biopsy
- Lactate dehydrogenase (LDH)
- Pap smear, CA-125, prostate-specific antigen (PSA)
- Patch test (2 weeks after discharge)
- Serum calcium, angiotensin converting enzyme (ACE) levels
- Direct immunofluorescence
- Immunophenotyping of skin and blood.

Q7. What are the principal management modalities in erythroderma?

Ans: The principal elements include nursing care, monitoring hemodynamic changes, fluid and electrolyte balance, nutrition, prevention of complications, topical therapy, and treatment of underlying cause.

- The patient should be admitted and nursed in a warm room
- Strict monitoring of urine input-output and vitals charting is needed
- Optimum hydration and electrolyte balance should be maintained, along with supplementation of proteins, zinc, iron and folic acid
- Pedal edema can be managed with bandages and in severe cases with furosemide
- Topically, bland emollients or petrolatum or a low-potency topical steroid (e.g. 1% hydrocortisone) or simply lukewarm compresses with oatmeal baths could help reduce the inflammation and scaling
- Parenteral antibiotics.

Q8. In addition to the conservative management, what are the cause-specific treatment modalities in the case of erythroderma?

Ans: Specific treatment modalities:

- Psoriatic erythroderma is best managed with methotrexate, cyclosporine A, acitretin, and tumor necrosis factor (TNF) alpha inhibitors
- In spongiotic dermatitis, secondary to allergic contact dermatitis, and photodermatitis leading to erythroderma—steroids (0.5 mg/kg/day and tapering by 5 mg every 5 days) could be used, and in uncontrolled/severe cases, steroid sparing agents, such as cyclosporine, azathioprine, and methotrexate could be used
- In cases of erythroderma due to lymphoma/leukemia—phototherapy, potent topical steroids, IV denileukin diftitox, bexarotene, vorinostat or romidepsin have all been found effective
- In case of drug reactions, it is essential to discontinue all drugs and manage the patient conservatively. Oral corticosteroids can be used in severe cases.

SECTION 14

Eczemas

Anju George

Irritant Contact Dermatitis

Blistering Beetle Dermatitis

CHAPTER 67

Seborrheic Dermatitis

Saloni Katoch

Case study — Seborrheic Dermatitis

Presenting Complaints

Doctor, I have persistent dandruff on my scalp since 2 years. I have also noticed these red rashes with white flakes along my hairline, behind my ears and sides of nose since 2 weeks.

Setting

Dermatology outpatient department.

History of Presenting Illness

A 28-year-old male patient presented with complaints of excessive dandruff over his scalp since 2 years. He gives history of associated itching and aggravation during the colder months of the year. The patient also noticed red rashes with white flakes along his hairline, behind ears and sides of nose since 2 weeks.

General Examination and Systemic Examination

No abnormality detected.

Dermatological Examination

- Diffuse white bran-like scales present over the scalp
- Bilateral, symmetrical, and multiple erythematous patches with occasional greasy yellowish scales and mostly white scales present over the anterior hairline, medial eyebrows, nasal alar creases, nasolabial folds, retroauricular and presternal regions.

Q1. What is the most likely diagnosis?

a. Seborrheic dermatitis
b. Psoriasis
c. Rosacea
d. Darier's disease

Ans: a (Seborrheic dermatitis)

The characteristic history with examination findings, absence of telangiectases, thick plaques with silvery scales, nail involvement, palmar pits, and greasy scaly papules favor the diagnosis of seborrheic dermatitis.

Q2. How do you diagnose seborrheic dermatitis?

Ans: The diagnosis is usually made on clinical grounds. It is a chronic recurrent inflammatory skin condition characterized by sharply marginated areas of erythema with yellow bran-like and sometimes greasy scales primarily affecting sebum-rich areas like the scalp, face, upper chest, back, and flexures. The noninflammatory variant is dandruff (pityriasis capitis) presenting with visible desquamation from the scalp. Possibility of HIV (human immunodeficiency virus) infection to be considered in patients with severe seborrheic dermatitis.

The histopathology is not diagnostic, the changes seen in various stages include:

- *Acute*: Orthokeratosis and focal parakeratosis, mild focal spongiosis, sparse superficial perivascular lymphocytic, and histiocytic infiltrates
- *Subacute*: Mild psoriasiform hyperplasia, numerous yeasts in stratum corneum
- *Chronic*: Psoriasiform hyperplasia, folliculocentric scales, superficial dilation of capillaries and venules, minimal spongiosis.

Q3. How would you manage a patient of seborrheic dermatitis?

Ans: The main goal of therapy is to clear visible signs of the disease and to ameliorate the associated symptoms. Patients should be counseled regarding the relapsing nature of the condition and the need for preventive regimens

- Scalp
  - *Mild to moderate*: Ketoconazole (1–2% shampoo, creams, lotions or foams) or ciclopirox (1% shampoo, cream or gel) twice weekly for 4 weeks
  - *Severe*: Topical corticosteroids in solution, foam or spray once daily for the first 1–2 weeks along with antifungal preparations
  - *Frequent relapses*: Continue topical antifungals for long term, once or twice a week
  - *Others*: Shampoos containing zinc pyrithione, selenium sulphide (1–2.5%), salicylic acid (shampoos and creams) and coal tar (creams and shampoos).
- Face and other sites
  - *Antifungals*: Ketoconazole 2% cream, ciclopirox 1% cream, miconazole 2% cream, terbinafine 1% cream
  - *Topical corticosteroids*: Low to low-mid potency. Lead to rapid clearance in 1–4 weeks. Long-term use is discouraged
  - *Topical calcineurin inhibitors*: Pimecrolimus 1% cream, tacrolimus 0.03% and 0.1% cream and ointment
  - Metronidazole 0.75 and 1% gel, azelaic acid 15% gel, sulphur, benzoyl peroxide wash 5–10%, 5% lithium succinate ointment
  - *Mild-to-moderate*: Twice daily application of antifungal creams or topical calcineurin inhibitors (1–4 weeks)
  - *Moderate-to-severe*: Topical corticosteroids, once or twice daily for 1–2 weeks with long-term topical antifungals/nonsteroidal preparations to prevent relapse.
- Severe inflammatory disease
  - Short course of systemic glucocorticoids (prednisolone 0.5 mg/kg/day) when patients fail to respond to topical therapy.
- Severe refractory cases
  - *Oral antifungals*: Itraconazole (100 mg daily for up to 21 days), terbinafine
  - Oral isotretinoin in low doses (0.1–0.3 mg/kg/day) over 3–5 months
  - NBUVB (narrowband ultraviolet B) and PUVA (photochemotherapy) can also be used in refractory cases.

Q4. What are the key points in its etiopathogenesis?

Ans: The key points in etiopathogenesis are as follows:

- *Increased activity of sebaceous glands*: At birth (under the influence of maternal androgens), and peaks between 18 years and 40 years of age
- *Increased skin colonization with yeast of the genus Malassezia:* Due to altered cell-mediated immune responses to the organism
- Inflammation of the skin results due to metabolic products produced and activation of complement pathways
- Mild abnormalities in surface lipids could result from ineffective keratinization
- Epidermal hyperproliferation or dyskeratinization may result due to increased activity of calmodulin
- Low humidity and cold temperature aggravate the disease
- Is found to be more common in myocardial ischemia, malabsorption, epilepsy, obesity and alcoholism.

Q5. Which neurological disorders are associated with seborrheic dermatitis?

Ans: Excessive pooling of sebum on immobile skin has been reported in patients suffering from neurological disorders. Depression and emotional stress are found to trigger and aggravate the dermatitis. Disorders such as Parkinson's, Alzheimer's, syringomyelia, epilepsy, cerebrovascular infarcts, post-encephalitis, mental retardation, poliomyelitis, quadriplegia, trigeminal and facial nerve palsies can be associated with seborrheic dermatitis.

Q6. Which drugs can cause a seborrheic dermatitis like eruption?

Ans: Griseofulvin, cimetidine, lithium, methyldopa, arsenic, gold, buspirone, chlorpromazine, haloperidol, ethionamide, interferon alpha, stanozolol, psoralen, methoxsalen and trioxsalen.

Q7. What are the clinical patterns of adult seborrheic dermatitis?

Ans: It is chronic, recurrent, marked by periods of exacerbation during emotional stress, fatigue, dry and cold climate, systemic infections and use of certain medications. Itching occurs when scalp is involved.

Morphological variants:

- Scalp
  - *Dandruff*: Mild dry desquamation
  - *Inflammatory*: Perifollicular erythema and scaling, sharply marginated patches sometimes extending beyond anterior hairline
  - "Corona seborrheica", also onto the occiput and neck
  - Reversible hair loss in chronic cases.
- Face
  - Involve medial eyebrows, forehead, nasolabial folds and lateral nares
  - *Eyes*: Blepharitis (Fig. 1), conjunctivitis
  - *Ears*: Retroauricular region, external auditory canal, auricle and conchal bowl.
- Trunk
  - *Petaloid*: Petal shaped, seen on the front of chest and interscapular region
  - *Pityriasiform*: Generalized erythemato-squamous eruption, similar to pityriasis rosea, involves neck up to the hair margin, resolves spontaneously
  - *Flexural*: Axillae, groin, anogenital and submammary regions can be involved, presents as intertrigo; crusted fissures, secondary infection and weeping dermatitis may develop
  - Eczematous plaques
  - Follicular.
- *Generalized*: May result in erythroderma.

Q8. What is pityriasis amiantacea?

Ans: Pityriasis amiantacea describes an inflammatory reaction pattern of the scalp characterized by thick, adherent asbestos like scales attached in layers to the scalp and hair shaft. Also known as asbestos scalp, tinea asbestina, keratosis follicularis amiantacea and porrigo amiantacea. Primarily affects young adults and is more common in females. Most commonly seen with psoriasis, seborrheic dermatitis and atopic dermatitis. Less commonly associated with tinea capitis, lichen planus and Darier's disease. Can lead to temporary or scarring alopecia especially when associated with secondary infection with Streptococcus or Staphylococcus. Therapy should be directed at the underlying dermatoses.

Q9. How does the clinical presentation and prognosis differ in infantile seborrheic dermatitis?

Ans: The infantile form occurs during the first few weeks to 3 months of life. Is self-limiting with good prognosis in contrast to the adult form, usually clearing by about 12 months of age. Clinical patterns include:

- *Cradle cap*: Greasy yellow brown adherent scales over the vertex of scalp (Fig. 2)
- Greasy scaly lesions elsewhere on scalp
- *Trunk*: Flexures and napkin area can be involved.
- *Erythroderma desquamativum (Leiner's disease)*: Widespread erythrodermic form, could be familial or nonfamilial.

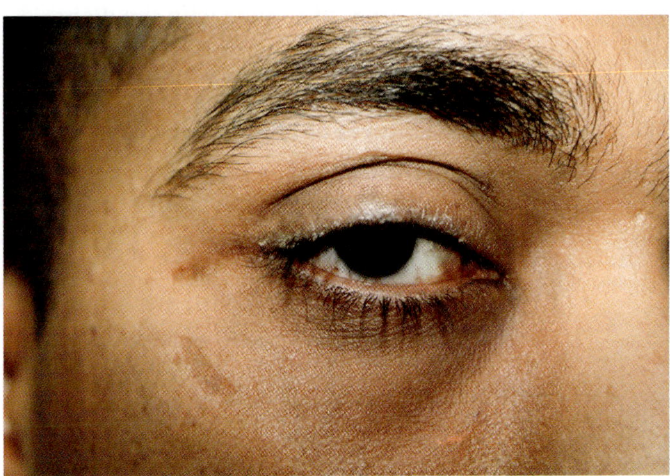

Fig. 1: Blepharitis due to seborrheic dermatitis

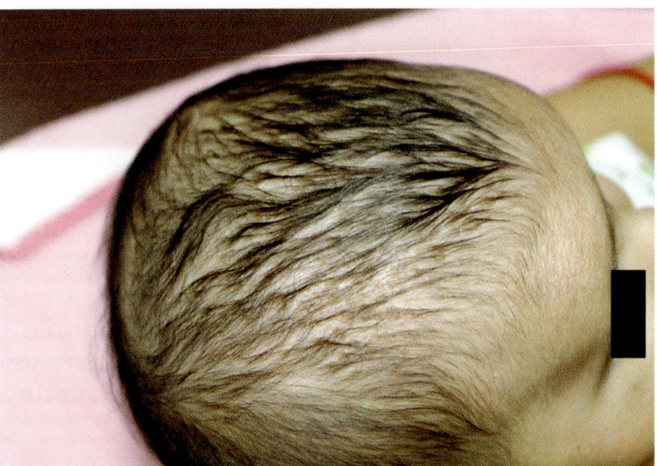

Fig. 2: Infantile seborrheic dermatitis

Management: Responds readily to shampoos, emollients and mild topical steroids. Low potency topical corticosteroids (hydrocortisone 1% cream or lotion) and topical imidazoles (2% ketoconazole cream or 1% shampoo) can be used for areas with prolonged inflammation. Mild baby shampoo with or without 3% salicylic acid can be used to gently remove thick adherent scales on the scalp.

Q10. Describe features of seborrheic dermatitis associated with HIV?

Ans: Seborrheic dermatitis in HIV patients is severe and extensive.

- Attributed to enhanced growth of yeasts secondary to immunosuppression
- Possible marker of early HIV infection, occurring with CD4 counts between 200 cells/cumm and 500 cells/cumm
- Histopathology shows more follicular involvement, parakeratosis, necrosis, lymphocytes, plasma cells, focal leucocytosis and prominence of Malassezia yeasts
- May be refractory to standard therapy, treatment with oral antifungals may be necessary.

Q11. What are the differential diagnoses of seborrheic dermatitis?

Ans: The site-specific differential diagnoses are as follows:

- *Scalp*: Psoriasis, atopic dermatitis, impetigo, tinea capitis
- *Face*: Psoriasis, rosacea, contact dermatitis, impetigo, discoid lupus erythematosus, drug-induced photosensitivity
- *External auditory canal*: Psoriasis, contact dermatitis
- *Eyelids*: Atopic dermatitis, psoriasis
- Trunk: Pityriasis rosea, pityriasis versicolor, subacute cutaneous lupus erythematosus, psoriasis
- *Buttock and groin*: Intertrigo, extramammary Paget's disease, zinc deficiency
- *Intertriginous*: Inverse psoriasis, candidiasis, erythrasma, intertrigo, langerhan cell histiocytosis
- *Generalized*: Scabies, secondary syphilis, pemphigus foliaceous and erythematosus, drug eruption
- *Erythrodermic (should be biopsied)*: Psoriasis, pityriasis rubra pilaris, drug eruption, mycosis fungoides, lichen planus, chronic actinic dermatitis, HIV, Hodgkin's disease, paraneoplastic syndrome, leukemia cutis.

Q12. Which of the following can be considered as differential diagnosis for infantile seborrheic dermatitis?

a. Atopic dermatitis
b. Scabies
c. Psoriasis
d. All of the above

Ans: d (All of the above)

The differential diagnoses for infantile seborrheic dermatitis are as follows:

- Scalp
  - *Tinea capitis*: Noninflammatory type, scaly areas with broken hair, KOH mount will help differentiate from seborrheic dermatitis
  - Psoriasis.
- Body
  - *Atopic dermatitis*: Family history of atopy may be present, pruritic, involvement of shin and forearms with sparing of axilla has a relapsing course
  - *Scabies*: Family history of similar complaints, extensive lesions with involvement of palms and soles, pruritic, demonstration of mite will confirm diagnosis
  - Psoriasis
  - *Langerhans cell histiocytosis*: Moist erythematous plaques and petechial lesions in intertriginous areas and scalp, associated hepatosplenomegaly and lymphadenopathy, biopsy will confirm diagnosis.
- Diaper area
  - *Diaper dermatitis*: Spares the deeper folds, present in areas of contact with the diaper
  - *Candidiasis*: Presence of satellite pustules, culture will confirm the diagnosis.

Q13. Describe the features of Leiner's disease.

Ans: Leiner described a disease of young babies characterized by extensive dermatitis, failure to thrive and diarrhea. Also known as erythroderma desquamativum.

- Familial and nonfamilial forms have been reported, the hereditary form is associated with deficiency of complement C3, C5 and phagocyte malfunction

- May be present at birth but more commonly presents within the first few months of life.
- Clinical features include severe, widespread and erythrodermic form of infantile seborrheic dermatitis, fever, anemia, diarrhea, vomiting, weight loss and sometimes death
- Prone to recurrent skin and internal infections, complications such as pneumonia, meningitis and septicemia may arise.
- Management includes maintaining fluid balance, temperature regulation and antibiotics if there is secondary bacterial infection.
- Fresh frozen plasma and whole blood may be required to supplement complement deficiencies.
- Administration of biotin appears to be useful.

CHAPTER 68

Atopic Dermatitis

Tarang Goyal, Samipa S Mukherjee

Case study Atopic Dermatitis

Presenting Complaints

Doctor, our child is having a reddish rash all over her body with mild oozing from few lesions, for the last 15 days. She has severe itching and sneezes very frequently.

Setting

Dermatology outpatient department.

History of Present Illness

A 12-year-old girl child presented with complaints of itchy red rash all over the body since last 15 days. She has been having these episodes on and off since early infancy with a seasonal variation. The lesions show worsening in winter months. She also has a tendency for running nose and frequent sneezing. All her vaccinations are updated. Family history revealed asthma in maternal grandmother. Overall the itching is severe so as to disrupt the normal sleeping pattern of the child.

General Examination and Systemic Examination

A well-oriented child, with no lymphadenopathy, hepatosplenomegaly. Mild pallor was present.

Dermatological Examination

Edematous, erythematous, excoriated oozing ill-defined plaques predominantly present over face, periorbital area, neck, trunk, antecubital fossae, popliteal fossae and ankles (Figs 1 to 3). Scalp shows redness and fine scaling. Palms and soles show hyperlinearity. Nails, mucosae normal.

Q1. What is the clinical diagnosis?

a. Seborrheic dermatitis
b. Atopic dermatitis
c. Erythroderma
d. Nummular eczema

Ans: b (Atopic dermatitis)

Q2. What is atopic dermatitis (AD)?

Ans: Atopy is derived from the greek word "*atopos*" which means out of place or strange and refers to the predisposition to develop Allergic rhinitis, bronchial asthma, or AD with resultant surfaces where the body contacts the allergen, being "overreactive". Atopic dermatitis is a chronic, pruritic inflammatory skin disease that occurs most frequently in children.

Q3. What is the incidence of AD globally?

Ans: Atopic dermatitis affects up to 20% of children and up to 3% of adults; recent data show that its prevalence is still increasing, especially in low-income countries. It is very common in infancy and early childhood.

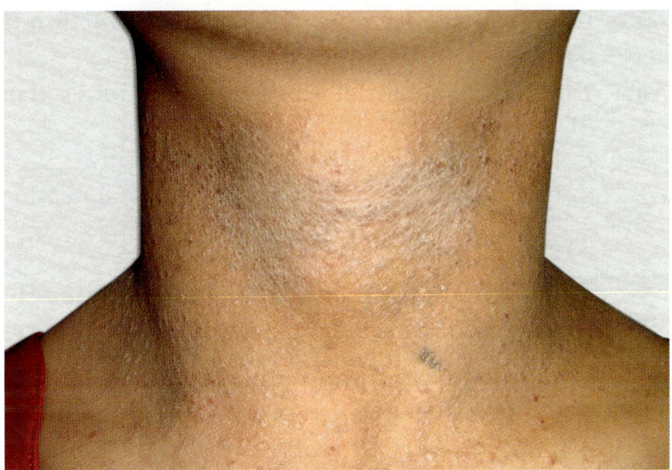

Fig. 1: Erythematous, excoriated ill-defined plaques predominantly present over neck

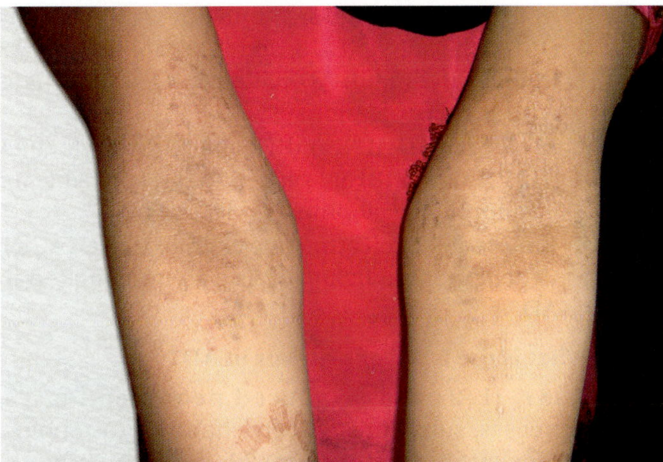

Fig. 2: Similar lesions on flexural aspect of elbows

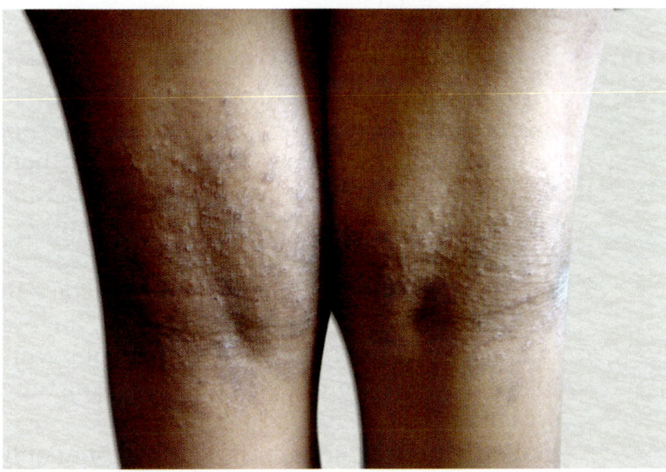

Fig. 3: Similar lesions on flexural aspect of knees

Q4. What is "atopic diathesis"?

Ans: Allergic rhinitis, bronchial asthma, or atopic dermatitis occurrence in patients.

Q5. What is atopic march?

Ans: The term "Allergic March" (also called "Atopic March") refers to the natural history of atopic manifestations, which is characterized by a typical sequence of immunoglobulin E (IgE) antibody responses and clinical symptoms which may appear early in life, persist over years or decades, and often remit spontaneously with age.

Q6. What are the diagnostic features of AD?

Ans: The Hanifin and Rajka criteria

- Major features:
  - Pruritus
  - Typical morphology and distribution
  - Chronically relapsing dermatitis
  - Personal or family history of atopy.
- Minor features (three or more):
  - Xerosis
  - Ichthyosis, palmar hyperlinearity, or keratosis pilaris
  - Immediate (type 1) skin-test reactivity
  - Raised serum IgE
  - Early age of onset
  - Tendency toward cutaneous infections (especially *Staphylococcus aureus* and herpes simplex) or impaired cell-mediated immunity
  - Tendency toward nonspecific hand or foot dermatitis
  - Nipple eczema
  - Cheilitis
  - Recurrent conjunctivitis
  - Dennie-Morgan infraorbital fold
  - Keratoconus
  - Anterior subcapsular cataracts
  - Orbital darkening
  - Facial pallor or facial erythema
  - Pityriasis alba
  - Anterior neck folds
  - Itch when sweating
  - Intolerance to wool and lipid solvents
  - Perifollicular accentuation
  - Food intolerance
  - Course influenced by environmental or emotional factors
  - White dermographism or delayed blanch.

Q7. What are etiopathological factors in development of AD?

Ans: The following are the etiopathological factors in development of AD:

- Decreased skin barrier function
- Immune responses (T helper-2 in acute AD and T helper-1 like in chronic AD)
- Genetic predisposition
- Altered skin barrier function
- Environmental factors and infectious agents.

Q8. What are the scoring systems used in AD?

Ans: The Diepgen score, EASI (eczema area scoring index), SCORAD (SCORing Atopic Dermatitis) and POEM (Patient-Oriented Eczema Measure) are used as scoring systems in AD.

Q9. What are the potential risk factors associated with rise in AD?

Ans: The following are the potential risk factors associated with rise in AD:

- Small family size
- Increased income and education
- Rural to urban migration
- Increased use of antibiotics.

Q10. What is "hygiene hypothesis" in AD?

Ans: Allergic diseases may be prevented by avoiding them acquiring "infections" from older siblings in early childhood. Reduced exposure to bacterial and parasitic infections in childhood leads to an abnormal development of the immune system, which later tends to overreact to innocuous antigens.

Q11. What are extrinsic and intrinsic types of AD?

Ans: Atopic dermatitis can be classified into two types based on the presence or absence of elevated IgE and specific IgE sensitization. (1) "Extrinsic type" of AD, also known as "allergic type", is associated with elevated IgE (45–80%). (2) In "intrinsic type", also known as "atopiform" dermatitis or "nonallergic" type, the IgE levels are normal (20–40%). Extrinsic type is more common in adult onset AD unlike intrinsic AD.

Q12. What is the role of decreased barrier function in AD?

Ans: The decreased barrier function leads to increased allergen absorption into skin and microbial colonization. The epicutaneous sensitization to allergen results in higher allergic immune responses in children.

Q13. In what ways the epidermal barrier function is compromised in AD?

Ans: The epidermal barrier function is compromised in AD in many ways:

- Downregulation of filaggrin and loricrin
- Decreased ceramide and antimicrobial peptide levels
- Increased levels of proteolytic enzymes
- Colonization by *S. aureus* and house dust mites
- Increased transepidermal water loss.

Q14. What are the strong and consistent risk factors in development of AD?

Ans: A family history of atopy and loss-of-function mutations in the filaggrin gene, which codes for filaggrin.

Q15. What cytokines are responsible for AD?

Ans:

- *In acute AD*: T helper-2 cytokines; interleukins (IL) such as IL-4, IL-13, and IL-31 are seen. IL-13 induces itching in AD patients. IL-31 correlates with severity of lesions
- *In chronic AD*: IL-5 and T helper-1 like cytokines (IL-12 and IL-18) are seen. IL-5 is responsible for eosinophil development and survival
- Cutaneous T cell attracting chemokine (CTACK); CC chemokine ligand 27 is also upregulated in AD.

Q16. What is the basis of pruritus in AD?

Ans: IL-31, IL-2, stress-induced neuropeptidases, proteases, substance P, acetylcholine, prostanoids, and calcitonin are responsible for itching in AD patients. Thereby the itching in AD is not controlled with antihistaminics; they have only a sedative role which is beneficial.

Q17. What are the patterns of AD presentation by age?

Ans:

- *Infantile (2 months–2 years)*: Symmetric involvement of cheeks, forehead, ears, scalp, extensor surfaces of extremities, and trunk. There is intense pruritis. Erythema, oozing, crusting, papules, and vesicles are commonly present.
- *Childhood (2 years to puberty)*: Wrists, ankles, neck, posterior thighs, buttocks, antecubital and popliteal fossae are commonly involved. Intense itching with poorly defined erythematous scaly plaques with secondary crusting, oozing, and erosions.
- Adults: Face, neck, arms, back, flexures commonly involved. Intense itching with thick lichenified plaques.

Q18. What infections are usually seen in AD?

Ans: The following infections have been shown to be commonly associated with AD:

- *Viral infections*: Herpes simplex (Kaposi varicelliform eruption or eczema herpeticum), small pox vaccination-induced eczema vaccinatum
- *Superficial fungal infections*: *Trichophyton rubrum, Malassezia sympodialis*
- *Bacterial infections*: *S. aureus* [particularly MRSA (methicillin-resistant *S. aureus*)].

Q19. What causes facial predominant AD?

Ans: Facial predominant atopy has a high colonization of the yeast *Pityrosporum sympodialis*.

Q20. What are the poor prognostic factors in AD?

Ans: The following are the poor prognostic factors in AD:

- Widespread AD
- Early onset AD
- Associated allergic rhinitis or bronchial asthma
- Family history of AD in parents or siblings
- Only child
- Very high serum IgE levels.

Q21. What physical findings are associated with AD?

Ans: The following physical findings are associated with AD:

- Xerosis
- Keratosis pilaris
- Pityriasis alba
- Hyperlinear palms and soles
- Hertoghe's sign
- Dennie-Morgan folds
- Dermatographism
- *Ocular complications*: Chronic blepharitis, atopic keratoconjunctivitis, vernal conjunctivitis, keratoconus, cataract (particularly anterior subcapsular cataract).

Q22. What is Hertoghe's sign?

Ans: Thinning or absence of hair on the lateral aspect of eyebrows.

Q23. What are the differential diagnoses of AD?

Ans:

- Allergic contact dermatitis
- Immunodeficiency
- Irritant contact dermatitis
- Lichen simplex chronicus
- Nummular dermatitis
- Scabies with eczematization
- Psoriasis
- Seborrheic dermatitis
- Extensive tinea corporis.

Q24. Are investigations necessary in AD?

Ans: Investigations are not needed in all cases of AD. Investigations may be done only in cases of suspected syndrome or as a pretreatment work up with systemic medications. IgE levels, skin prick test, radioallergosorbent testing (RAST), food-specific IgE levels, immunocap to know whether the child has outgrown the allergy may be done.

Q25. What are the common trigger factors of AD?

Ans: Certain foods especially cow's milk, milk products, soy, nuts, egg white can sometimes worsen AD. Aeroallergens such as animal dander, pollen, molds, and house dust mites should be avoided. Woolen clothes, carpets, furry toys, and pets are other common triggers. Psychological triggers such as stress of examination, anxiety, social pressure also play a role.

Q26. What are the general treatment plans for AD patients?

Ans: The following are the general treatment plans for AD patients:

- Avoid trigger factors
- Continue breastfeeding and delay exposure to solid foods (though not proven)
- Adequate moisturization of skin by an emollient which is customized according to patient
- Avoid long and very warm water baths, use bleach baths
- Use a mild soap or syndet
- Wear cotton clothes
- Keep humidity to 35-40%
- Avoid kissing the child
- Counseling and good psychological support remains the cornerstone.

Q27. What is "wet-wrap" therapy?

Ans: It is also known as "two-pajama", "two-caps", "two-gloves", "two-shirts", etc. treatment therapy according to the site involved. Immediately after bathing, put a mild-to-mid potency corticosteroid to skin. Soak one pajama in warm water and wear it wrung-out. Then wear a dry one on top of it and sleep.

After waking up in morning, remove both and apply moisturizer.

Q28. What are the topical treatments available for AD?

Ans: The following topical treatments are available for AD:
- Moisturizers and emollients
- Topical antiinflammatory therapies (topical glucocorticoids, topical calcineurin inhibitors)
- Topical antibiotics.

Q29. What is the role of probiotics in treatment of AD?

Ans: A Cochrane review done recently had concluded that probiotics are not an effective treatment for eczema in children and this could even lead to risk of few adverse effects.

Q30. What are the syndromes associated with AD?

Ans: Syndromes:
- Job's syndrome
- Hyper IgE syndrome
- Netherton's syndrome
- Wiskott-Aldrich syndrome.

Q31. What is the drug of choice for atopic erythroderma?

Ans: Cyclosporine is the drug of choice for atopic erythroderma due to its rapid onset of action, excellent control, and lesser side effects.

Q32. What are the other treatment options for AD?

Ans:
- Oral corticosteroids
- Cyclosporine
- Methotrexate
- Azathioprine
- Antihistaminics
- *Phototherapy*: Preferably narrowband ultraviolet B.

Q33. Which is the latest biological treatment that is undergoing phase 3 trial for AD?

Ans: Dupilumab: It is a monoclonal antibody against IL-4.

CHAPTER 69

Hand Eczema

Boby Krishna

Case study Hand Eczema

Presenting Complaints

Doctor, I have itchy raised lesions over both hands since the last 5 years with an acute exacerbation for 2 weeks.

Setting

Dermatology outpatient department.

History of Present Illness

A 29-year-old construction worker presented with history of recurrent episodes of numerous itchy raised lesions on the palms for the last 5 years. He consulted a local hospital and was treated with topical steroid creams and antihistamines, following which the lesions improved but to reappear later. He has noticed exacerbation of the skin lesions at work place. Presently since 2 weeks he has developed fresh lesions on hands with oozing, crusting and severe itching.

General Examination and Systemic Examination

No abnormality detected.

Dermatological Examination

Hyperkeratotic plaques on the palmar aspect of both hands along with oozy crusted lesions on the dorsum of both hands (Fig. 1). Excoriation marks were present. Edema of hands present.

Patch Test

Positivity to potassium dichromate.

Q1. What is the most likely diagnosis?

a. Psoriasis of the hands
b. Allergic contact dermatitis leading to chronic hand eczema
c. Dermatophytic infection of the hands
d. Irritant contact dermatitis leading to chronic hand eczema

Ans: b (Allergic contact dermatitis leading to chronic hand eczema)

Chronic relapsing course especially exacerbating at work place and patch test positivity to potassium dichromate (ingredient in cement) all favors allergic contact dermatitis to cement.

Q2. What is hand eczema?

Ans: Dermatitis largely confined to hands with or without minor involvement of other areas. It accounts for 20–35% of all dermatitis. The disease can be acute,

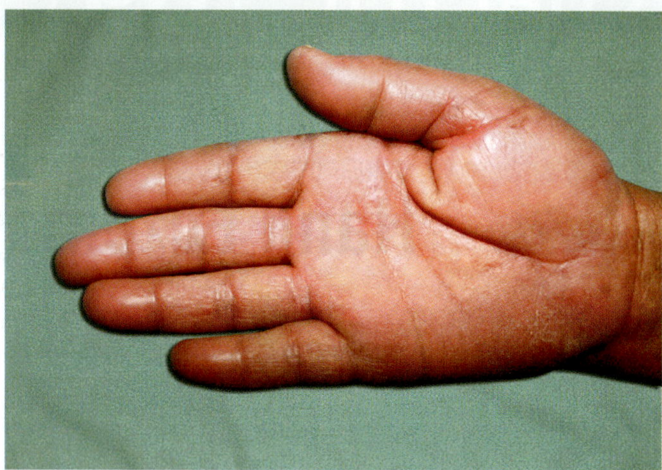

Fig. 1: Hyperkeratotic scaly lesions on palm with edema

lasting less than 3 months, or chronic or appear as recurrent flares in between periods with normal skin.

Q3. How do you classify hand eczema?

Ans: Classification of hand eczema:

Etiological

- Endogenous
  - *Immunological*: Atopy
  - *Psychosomatic*: Stress (e.g.: repeated picking, rubbing)
  - *Dyshidrosis*: Increased sweating
  - *Idiopathic*: Hyperkeratotic hand eczema
- Exogenous
  - Irritant contact dermatitis
    - *Chemical*: Detergents, soaps, etc.
    - *Physical*: Friction trauma, cold dry air, sweat
  - Allergic contact dermatitis
    - *Type I hypersensitivity reaction*: Contact urticaria to vesiculation
    - *Type IV hypersensitivity reaction*: Dermatitis to rubber, nickel, chromium, etc.
  - Ingested allergens
    - Food or drugs containing nickel chromium, etc.
  - Infection
    - Secondary to bacterial, fungal or viral infection.

Morphological

- Apron eczema
- Chronic acral dermatitis
- Discoid eczema (nummular eczema)
- Fingertip eczema
- Gut eczema
- Hyperkeratotic palmar eczema
- Pompholyx
- Recurrent focal palmar peeling
- Ring eczema
- Wear and tear dermatitis
- Others (patchy, vesiculosquamous).

Q4. What is the differential diagnosis of hand eczema?

Ans:
- *Psoriasis*: Well demarcated, erythematous, scaly plaques with nail changes
- *Palmoplantar pustulosis*: Persistent pustulosis usually on an erythematous base affecting central palm and instep of foot
- *Tinea manuum*: Unilateral patch, with scaly or pustular edge with positive mycology
- *Keratolysis exfoliativa*: Recurrent focal peeling on fingers, palms and soles
- *Bowen's disease*: Persistent red scaly patch resembling chronic dermatitis.

Q5. What are the risk factors for hand eczema?

Ans: Risk factors for hand eczema are listed in Table 1.

Table 1: Risk factors for hand eczema

Extrinsic factors
• *Wet work*: Ongoing exposure to liquids, frequent hand washing or occlusion with gloves • *Smoking*: Association between smoking and hand eczema • *Stress*: Exacerbates • *Site*: Back of hands more permeable than skin on palms therefore more vulnerable to irritants • Fat soluble chemicals enters skin even through undamaged horny layer • *Temperature*: High temperature—decreased barrier function, increased penetration of irritants and allergens • *Air flow*: Cold dry air—chapping of skin increased sensitivity of skin • *Low humidity*: Decreased water content and plasticity of stratum corneum—chapping and cracking • *Occlusion*: Promotes percutaneous absorption (gloves, wrist watch, straps, rings, shoes, boots, etc.). • *Occupation*: Healthcare workers, food service workers, beauticians, construction workers, homemakers, machinists and warehouse workers • *Medications*: Opiates—enhances allergic and irritant contact dermatitis • *Socioeconomic*: Exposure to cheap metals such as nickel and tattooing—dyes allergy.
Intrinsic factors
• *Age*: As age increases, barrier function deteriorates. • *Atopy*: Principal endogenous factor • *Dry skin*: more sensitive to irritants • *Ethnicity*: Whites more prone • *Sex*: Females more affected • *Genetic*: TNF α (tumor necrosis factor alpha) gene polymorphism • Coincidental diseases, e.g. cancer, HIV (decreased T lymphocyte function). • *Hormones*: Premenstrual flare up, e.g. nickel allergy.

Q6. How to differentiate irritant contact hand eczema and allergic contact hand eczema?

Ans: Both cannot be reliably distinguished based on clinical features alone (Table 2). Most often ICD (irritant contact dermatitis) precedes ACD (allergic contact dermatitis).

Q7. What are the features of vesicular hand dermatitis?

Ans: Popularly known as pompholyx or dyshidrotic eczema. There is no sweat gland dysfunction in dyshidrotic eczema, so it is a misnomer. Long-lasting, pruritic, vesicular and primarily involves the palmar surface of hand. Vesicles surmount on an erythematous base. Does not involve wrist and spares the dorsal surfaces of hands completely or limited to dorsal fingertips. Soles usually affected. Difficult to treat condition.

- Sudden onset of large bullae on palms can occur.
- They usually resolve in 2–3 weeks and recur at varying intervals.

Q8. Which among the following is not a synonym for housewives' dermatitis?

a. Wear and tear dermatitis
b. Apron eczema
c. Dermatitis palmaris sicca
d. Asteatotic eczema

Ans: b (Apron eczema)

Unlike housewives' dermatitis, apron eczema is an endogenous eczema which involves proximal palmar aspect of two or adjacent fingers and contiguous palmar skin over the metacarpophalangeal joints resembling an apron. Housewives' dermatitis occurs due to a combination of asteatosis, irritant exposure (soaps and detergents) and mild trauma. In this eczema, palmar skin feels dry and criss-crossed with superficial cracks along with chapping of the skin over the dorsa of knuckle joints.

Table 2: Difference between irritant contact hand dermatitis and allergic contact hand dermatitis

Irritant contact hand eczema	*Allergic contact hand eczema*
Finger web space involvement with extension to dorsal or ventral surfaces of hand	Fingertip, nail fold and dorsal hand involvement
Localization on palms and ball of thumb. Nonvesicular pattern	Frequently with vesiculation. Palms rarely primarily affected
Often begins around 3 months after exposure, usually wet work	Local reaction after 5–25 days
Upon re-exposure, quickly recurs	Re-exposure, reaction within 24–48 hours
Upon removal, the reaction improves—decrescendo pattern	Reaction often crescendo over 1–3 weeks before improving
Direct cell injury	Type IV hypersensitivity reaction. Patch testing helps to identify the antigen

Q9. How to diagnose hand eczema?

Ans:

- A thorough history including medical, occupational and social history is important.
- Physical examination
  - Hands
    - dorsal and palmar involvement
    - any vesicles or pustules
    - finger-tip and finger web involvement
    - wrist involvement
    - nail pitting
  - Any other area involved
- Patch testing
  - Considered in chronic hand dermatitis
  - Gold standard for diagnosing ACD
- Potassium hydroxide examination and fungal culture
- Biopsy to rule out other noneczematous skin diseases: Psoriasis, keratoderma, dermatomyositis, vesicular bullous pemphigoid, CTCL (cutaneous T-cell lymphoma)
- Radio allergosorbent testing (RAST) or prick testing for contact urticaria to foods, latex and other allergens.

Q10. What are the treatment modalities in hand eczema?

Ans: *Behavioral Changes*

- Elimination of known irritants and allergens
- Creating physical barriers with gloves
  - Vinyl gloves—for wet works and irritants
  - Rubber gloves/plastic—only with cotton lining especially if used for more than 10 minutes.
- Emollient barrier creams and ointments applied before work and reapplied after washing and whenever skin dries out
- Changing occupations
- Educating atopic patients to avoid irritants and wet work in home and at work is critical.
- Avoid excessive sweating and dry conditions which triggers hand eczema
- Minimize frequent hand washing with soap
- Stress avoidance

Topical Therapy

- *Topical corticosteroids*: Ultra potent creams/ointments for 2–4 weeks, then pulsed at weekends. Ointments are more effective than creams because of greater penetration and less potentially sensitizing preservatives than creams. Preservatives such as formaldehyde releasers, parabens, MCI/MI in topical steroid creams are responsible for ACD.

- *Topical immunomodulators*: Topical pimecrolimus and tacrolimus inhibit inflammatory cytokine production by T-lymphocytes and mast cells. Twice daily application, with or without occlusion overnight. Transient skin burning and warmth are adverse effects. Pimecrolimus safer for long-term and widespread use due to lipophilicity and lower potential for systemic immunosuppression.
- *Intradermal injection of triamcinolone* (10 mg/mL): In recalcitrant localized patches.
- Nontraditional agents for topical use
  - Vitamin D_3 analogs
    - Calcitriol
    - Calcipotriol
    - Tacalcitol especially in hyperkeratotic palmar eczema
  - Tazarotene: Hyperkeratotic hand dermatitis
  - Tar and salicylic acid preparation: Hyperkeratotic hand dermatitis.

Wet dressings for early vesicular phase of pompholyx using 3% acetic acid or potassium permanganate compresses and the use of steroid-antiseptic or antibiotic preparation may help to lessen the risk of infection and improve the response.

Radiation and Light Therapy

- Grenz Rays
- PUVA (photochemotherapy), NBUVB (narrow-band ultraviolet B)

Systemic Therapy

In severe and recurrent cases of hand eczema.

- Systemic steroids: Start with 20–40 mg of prednisolone single daily dose in the morning for 3–7 days to a maximum of 10–14 days. This is repeated if necessary.
- Cyclosporin: 3 mg/kg per day for 6 weeks for resistant cases
- Mycophenolate mofetil: 2–3 g/day
- Methotrexate: 12.5–22.5 mg/week
- Azathioprine: 50–150 mg/day
- Oral antibiotics
- Retinoids: Acitretin proven effective. Alitretinoin, a new oral retinoid once daily treatment with 10, 20 or 40 mg/day. It can be used for severe, never go away completely or recurrent hand eczema.
- Biologicals: Etanercept in recalcitrant pompholyx and alefacept and ustekinumab in hyperkeratotic hand eczema
- Other therapies.

Iontophoresis

- *Botulinum toxin A injection*: Both are effective therapies for hyperhidrosis thereby, decreases sweat-induced irritation that occurs in occupational and atopic dermatitis.
- *Vitamin E, oral iron and oral zinc*: All showed benefits in hand eczema due to metal allergy.

CHAPTER 70

Discoid Eczema

Preema Sinha

Case study **Discoid Eczema**

Presenting Complaints

Doctor, I am getting recurrent itchy red raised round lesions over both legs since last 1 year.

Setting

Dermatology outpatient department.

History of Present Illness

A 52-year-old male presented with complaints of recurrent red raised itchy round lesions over both legs since last 1 year. Onset was insidious with a progressive course. He also gave history of few lesions developing aggregated fluid-filled lesions over surface with mild oozing of clear nonfoul smelling discharge. There is no history of known allergies.

General Physical Examination and Systemic Examination

No abnormality detected.

Dermatological Examination

- Few coin-shaped erythematous plaques with a sharp border, distributed over both legs (Fig. 1). Vesiculation seen over few of the lesions
- Few of the plaques show yellowish crusts on the surface.

Q1. What is the most likely diagnosis?

a. Discoid eczema
b. Psoriasis vulgaris
c. Asteatotic eczema
d. Tinea corporis

Ans: a [Discoid eczema (nummular dermatitis)].

Presence of small sharply bordered erythematous plaques with vesiculation and yellowish crusts over the legs, along with pruritus point toward the diagnosis.

Q2. How do you clinically diagnose discoid eczema?

Ans: Discoid eczema has clinical features which sets it apart.

- It is a disease commonly occurring in the middle-aged and elderly with a winter exacerbation. Male predominance is noted
- Each patch begins as a small group of red spots and tiny blisters, which enlarge rapidly into a red swollen moist round patch

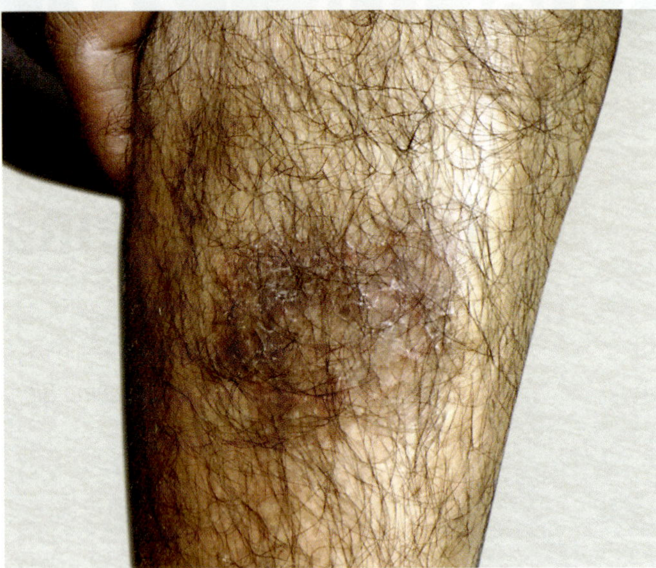

Fig. 1: Discoid eczema (nummular dermatitis)

- They may become edematous and have a few vesicles
- As the acute inflammation leads to rupture of the vesicles, the larger expanding lesions tend to have yellow crust and scale. Pruritus is present and is generally very severe
- Typical lesions are generally 1–3 cm or more in diameter and are usually round. Most patients have two or three lesions but some may develop a symmetric generalized eruption
- Typical locations include the legs and the back of the hand. Other frequently affected areas include extensor aspects of forearms, lower legs, flanks and hips
- Hyperpigmentation is common in Indian skin in cases of chronic relapsing discoid dermatitis.

Q3. What is the etiology and pathogenesis of the disease?

Ans: Etiopathogenesis:

- The exact cause is not known. It was earlier thought to be mediated by an allergy to bacterial antigens, hence called as "microbial dermatitis"
- Frequently seen in patients with xerotic skin, denoting a relationship with asteatotic eczema. Patients with atopic dermatitis often have such nummular lesions
- Substance P and calcitonin gene-related peptide positive nerve fibers were found in one study, to be more in lesional papillary dermis
- Allergic contact dermatitis is commonly seen in persistent discoid eczema with up to 50% patients being patch test positive. Common allergens include rubber chemicals, formaldehyde, neomycin, chromium, cobalt and nickel
- Severe forms of nummular dermatitis also found in patients with hepatitis, treated with pegylated interferon and ribavirin.

Q4. Which of the following has been associated with the development of nummular dermatitis?

a. TNF-alpha blockers
b. IL-1 antagonists
c. PDE-IV inhibitors
d. All of the above

Ans: a [TNF-alpha (tumor necrosis factor alpha) blockers]
TNF-alpha (tumor necrosis factor alpha) blockers have been reported to cause nummular dermatitis, in patients of rheumatoid arthritis.

Q5. How will you confirm the diagnosis?

Ans: Confirmation of diagnosis:

- Diagnosis is made on clinical grounds
- Allergy contact patch tests done to look for allergic contact eczema
- Examination of skin scales for a fungal infection
- Swabs may be taken to check for a bacterial infection
- Skin biopsy shows histopathological features that are not unique:
  - The acanthotic epidermis shows spongiosis, blisters and serous crust
  - Dermis shows a perivascular lymphocytic infiltrate
  - In few severe cases the epidermal reaction pattern maybe psoriasiform with absent microabscesses.

Q6. What is the differential diagnosis?

Ans: Differential diagnosis:

- Tinea corporis
- Plaque psoriasis
- Pityriasis rosea (Herald patch)
- Asteatotic eczema
- Lichen simplex chronicus
- Fixed drug eruption
- Cutaneous T cell lymphoma.

Q7. Which is the course and prognosis of this disease?

Ans:
- The course is chronic and frequently recurrent.

- Since the etiology is unknown, it is hard to do much more than treat the lesions as they arise.

Q8. How do you manage this chronic disease?

Ans: Management:

- Nummular eczema is relatively corticosteroid responsive. Start with high potency corticosteroid cream or lotion in the exudative phase and switch to a weaker corticosteroid in a firmer vehicle once the lesions improve
- Stubborn, nonexudative thick lesions: corticosteroids under occlusion
- Role of emollients is important: Applied after bath
- For bacterial secondary infection: Topical antibiotics
- If doubt of systemic infection is there, then culture-directed oral therapy; generally antistaphylococcal antibiotics
- Antipruritic sedative antihistaminics
- In severe cases, short course of oral corticosteroids can be given
- Sometimes in chronic cases narrowband ultraviolet B has proven to be very useful.

Q9. What is nummular neurodermatitis?

Ans: The lesions of nummular eczema itch and scratching often becomes habitual. In such cases the term nummular neurodermatitis has been used.

Q10. What is oid-oid disease?

Ans:

- Also known as Savill's syndrome/Sulzberger-Garbe syndrome.
- It is a syndrome of chronic exudative discoid and lichenoid dermatitis with severe nocturnal pruritus.

CHAPTER 71

Airborne Contact Dermatitis

Rajesh Kumar Mandal

Case study Airborne Contact Dermatitis

Presenting Complaints

Doctor, I am having severe itching along with red-colored dry rashes over my face, neck, chest, and hands for last 1-week or so. The itching increases on going outside my house. Last year also I had similar rashes during the same season.

Setting

Dermatology outpatient department.

History of Present Illness

A 37-year-old farmer presented with complaints of severe itching along with red, dry rash over his face, neck, upper chest, forearms, and hands of 1-week duration. The rash started on face with redness and itching while working in the wheat fields and slowly increased to present situation. The itching increases on going outdoors. He had a similar episode last year also. There is no history of associated systemic illness and any medication prior to the eruption. There is no personal and family history of asthma and rhinitis.

General Physical Examination and Systemic Examination

No abnormality detected.

Dermatological Examination

Diffuse erythematous, non-oozing, scaly plaques were present over photoexposed areas like face, "V" area of neck along with chest, forearms, and feet. On careful examination non- photoexposed parts of face like both the eyelids, nasolabial folds, under surface of chin, back of ears, under surface of collar over neck, flexors of elbow and legs were also involved (Fig. 1). Slight lichenification was also noticed over under collar area of neck and elbow flexors. Trunk was relatively spared. There was no involvement of mucosa, hair and nails.

Q1. What is the most likely diagnosis?

a. Photo dermatitis
b. Atopic dermatitis (AD)
c. Airborne contact dermatitis (ABCD)
d. Seborrheic dermatitis

Ans: c. ABCD.

There is presence of erythematous, non-oozy scaly, eczematous plaques over photoexposed and non-photoexposed parts. Especially involvement of the non-photoexposed areas like eyelids, nasolabial folds, under surface of the chin, back of ears, elbow flexors, and legs in a farmer with history of recurrence suggests the diagnosis of ABCD. Other clues favoring

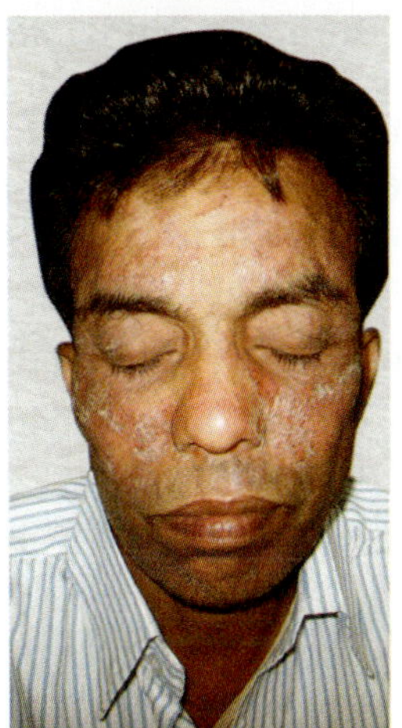

Fig. 1: Involvement of non-photoexposed parts of face like eyelids and nasolabial folds

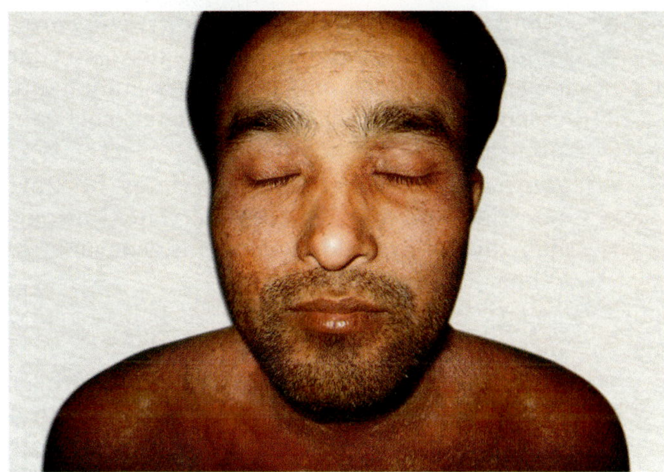

Fig. 2: Characteristic involvement in airborne contact dermatitis

diagnosis of ABCD are late-age of onset, no personal and family history of atopy.

Q2. How will you differentiate photo dermatitis from airborne-contact dermatitis?

Ans: Quite often photodermatitis may resemble ABCD and clinically it becomes very difficult to distinguish the two. Usually photodermatitis involves only the photoexposed areas. There is sparing of both the eyelids, under surface of the chin, back of ear, elbow flexors and legs. This sparing of the non-photoexposed area is very important sign to differentiate photo dermatitis from ABCD where these areas are also involved. ABCD starts over photoexposed areas but with due course it may extend to non-photoexposed parts also (Fig. 2). Photopatch test is positive in photodermatitis.

Q3. How will you differentiate it from atopic dermatitis?

Ans: In majority of cases the age of onset of AD is during infancy or childhood. There is personal or family history of atopy present. Clinically there is typical flexural involvement. In difficult cases patch test may help which is negative in AD cases.

Q4. How will you confirm your diagnosis?

Ans: Airborne contact dermatitis is a morphological diagnosis and is usually done on clinical grounds based on history, morphology, and distribution of lesions. In difficult cases patch test and prick test can be done which are positive in ABCD. Photopatch test can be performed to differentiate ABCD from photo dermatitis. In ABCD photopatch test is usually negative.

Q5. How will you classify airborne contact dermatitis?

Ans: Classification of ABCD

- *Epidemiologically*
  - Occupational and nonoccupational ABCD.
- *According to pathogenesis*
  - Airborne allergic contact dermatitis, airborne irritant-contact dermatitis, airborne photoallergic reactions, airborne phototoxic reactions, and airborne contact urticaria.
- *According to causative agent*
  - Plant origin and non-plant origin.

Q6. What is the most common cause of airborne-contact dermatitis in India?

Ans: In India a plant-antigen derived from *Parthenium hysterophorus* is considered to be the most common cause of ABCD. It is a wind-pollinated plant and produces huge amount of pollen.

Q7. What is the chemical compound or allergen in Parthenium plant?

Ans: Parthenin, a sesquiterpene lactone (SL) is the major allergen in Parthenium plant. Sesquiterpene lactones are the class of chemical compound or allergens causing sensitization of an individual leading to ABCD. They contain a lactone ring, hence the name and are found in many plants including Parthenium. SLs are lipophilic and are present in oleoresin fraction of plant.

Q8. What are the other common allergens causing and precipitating airborne contact dermatitis?

Ans: Common allergens causing and precipitating ABCD are:

- *Plants source allergen*: *Parthenium hysterophorus, Ambrosia deltoidea, Acacia melanoxylon*, cedar pollen, citrus fruits, cinnamon, chrysanthemum, essential oils, garlic, sunflower, latex, soybean, tropical and domestic wood
- *Plastic, rubbers and glues*: Acrylates, benzoyl peroxide, epoxy resin, epoxy acrylates, formaldehyde and formaldehyde resins, isocyanates, rubber additives
- *Metals:* Arsenic salts, chromates, cobalt, mercury, nickel, silver, and gold
- *Industrial and pharmaceutical chemicals:* Formaldehyde, gluteraldehyde, isoflurane, methyl chloroform, paraphenyldiamine, phosphorus sesquisulphide, para-aminobenzoic acid (PABA), potassium metabisulphite, azathioprine, azithromycin, budesonide, famotidine, methotrexate, meropenem, pantoprazole
- *Pesticides*: Carbamates, pyrethrum, dyrene, ethoxyquin
- *Miscellaneous:* Agricultural dusts, cigarettes, disperse dyes.

Q9. What is the most common area of involvement in airborne-contact dermatitis?

Ans: In classical ABCD the exposed areas of face, "V" area of neck, forearms, hands, and the Wilkinson's triangle, nasolabial folds, eyelids, and under surface of chin are the most common areas of involvement.

Q10. What is Wilkinson's triangle? What is its importance?

Ans: Wilkinson's triangle refers to small triangular area behind the ear lobes. Involvement of Wilkinson's triangle and other non-photoexposed areas like back of ear and flexors clinically helps to differentiate ABCD and other photo-related dermatitis where it is spared. During an epidemic of photosensitive reaction to salicylinides containing soaps during 1970s Wilkinson noticed sparing of a small area behind lobe of ears in photosensitive individuals with eczematous rash over face. This area is known as Wilkinson's triangle.

Q11. How will you treat airborne contact dermatitis?

Ans: Treatment is difficult and individualized according to severity. Treatment measures include:
- Exposure to the contact has to be minimized
- Barrier creams and emollients
- Photo-protection (sunscreens, full sleeve shirts, hats, etc.)
- Topical steroids in limited disease
- Immunosuppressives in widespread, recalcitrant disease
- Hyposensitization.

Q12. What is the immunosuppressive of choice to treat airborne contact dermatitis?

a. Cyclosporine
b. Mycophenolate mofetil
c. Azathioprine
d. Systemic steroids

Ans: c. Azathioprine.

Azathioprine is preferred due to its steroid sparing effect with well-established long-term safety profile with minimum adverse effects. There are studies which showed excellent control of dermatitis within few months of starting azathioprine.

Q13. What is Hyposensitization?

Ans: It refers to challenging the body with an antigen in a low dose and from a route different from the natural one to induce an immunological response without producing clinical manifestation of the disease.

CHAPTER 72

Blistering Beetle Dermatitis

Ishad Aggarwal, Anju George

Case study Blistering Beetle Dermatitis

Presentation

Doctor, since early morning I am having a burning sensation with itching on my right shoulder and chest. Soon after waking up, I noticed few reddish-raised lesions and now there are some fluid-filled lesions at the same site.

Setting

Dermatology outpatient department.

History of Presenting Complaints

A 35-year-old male presented with complaints of pruritic erythematous rash on the right shoulder which developed a few hours ago. The patient woke up the same day early morning with a burning sensation on his right shoulder and noticed few reddish-raised lesions, extending to the right chest. The lesions were pruritic and slightly painful. Gradually few of the erythematous lesions started developing blisters atop them. He was apparently asymptomatic till previous night. No history of fever, drug intake or any topical application. No history of similar episodes in the past.

General Examination and Systemic Examination

No significant abnormality detected.

Dermatological Examination

Multiple discrete and confluent, erythematous, and edematous papules on the right shoulder and chest in a linear and bizarre pattern. Multiple vesicles containing clear fluid are present in the center of the small papules (Fig. 1). Mild edema present in the same region.

Q1. What is the most likely diagnosis?

a. Herpes zoster
b. Phytophotodermatitis
c. Blister beetle dermatitis
d. Irritant-contact dermatitis

Ans: c. Blistering beetle dermatitis. The characteristic symptoms especially noticed towards early morning and the linear configuration of lesions, adds strength to the diagnosis of blister beetle dermatitis.

Q2. What is blister beetle dermatitis?

Ans: Blister beetle dermatitis is an acute irritant-contact dermatitis provoked by insects belonging to the families *Meloidae and Staphylinidae*. It is clinically characterized by erythematous and bullous lesions of sudden onset on exposed areas of the body. The beetle does not bite or sting, rather accidental brushing against or crushing the beetle over the skin, provokes the release of its coelomic fluid, which contains a potent vesicant.

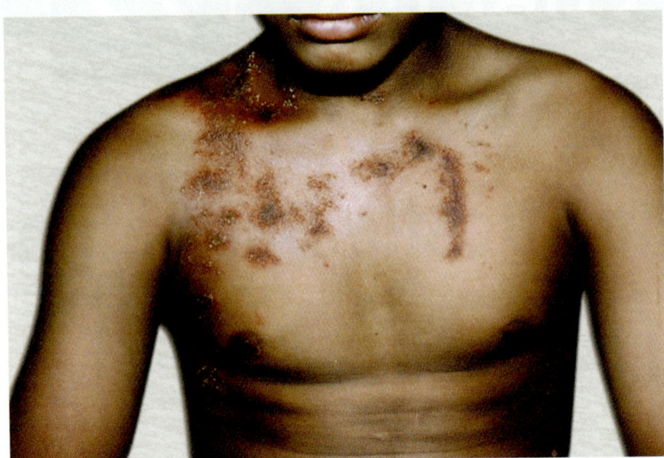

Fig. 1: Linearly arranged vesicles and papules on right shoulder and chest

Q3. What are the synonyms?

Ans: Blister beetle dermatitis is often referred to as "Paederus dermatitis" or "dermatitis linearis". Although blister beetle dermatitis and Paederus dermatitis are synonymously used, they are slightly different.

Q4. Briefly explain the etiology of blister beetle dermatitis.

Ans: The beetles that irritate humans belong to two families: *Meloidae (oil beetles and blister beetles) and Staphylindae (rove beetles).* The family Meloidae contains blister beetles namely *Lytta vesicatoria*, commonly known as the Spanish fly, and *Epicauta solani*. The family Staphylindae contains the rove beetles, which belong to the genus Paedurus.

Q5. Explain the pathogenesis of the condition.

Ans: Blister beetles, usually the Spanish fly, release a defensive compound called *cantharidin*, which is a bicyclic terpenoid. These beetles get crushed on the skin at night, emitting their vesicating fluid but some may exude the toxin without being crushed. Contact with the skin produces an irritant dermatitis.

Rove beetles release *pederin*, an amide which is a more potent vesicant and chemically-distinct from cantharidin.

Q6. What are the other properties or uses of cantharidin?

Ans: Cantharidin was used previously in the treatment of warts and molluscum contagiosum. It has been used in blistering plasters and hair restorers. Cantharidin is also an aphrodisiac.

Q7. What is the epidemiology of blister beetle dermatitis?

Ans: The dermatosis shows a seasonal variation depending on the habits of the insect. In South India it is common after the onset of monsoons, in June and July months. The beetles occupy moist habitats and are beneficial to agriculture because they feed largely on crop pests.

Though the beetles fly, they usually prefer to run. Adults are attracted to incandescent and fluorescent lights at night, and as a result, inadvertently come into contact with humans, especially if windows or doors are left open. The dermatitis can affect all age groups without any gender predisposition as it is solely dependent on the insect's habitats and the patient activities.

Q8. What are the common clinical patterns seen?

a. Kissing lesions
b. Whiplash dermatitis
c. Herpetiform pattern
d. All the above

Ans: d. All the above.

The classical lesion starts as a wheal which blisters in 12 hours, surrounded by erythema and edema. Occasionally they may turn necrotic. "Kissing" lesions occur when the irritant comes in contact with adjacent skin. Occasionally, a drip mark may occur when the toxin has run down the skin, producing the pattern called as linear or "whiplash" dermatitis. Other patterns include herpetiform, zosteriform, patchy or bizarre patterns. The response varies depending on the concentration of toxin, duration of exposure, and individual characteristics. Mild cases manifest only erythema lasting for a few days. In severe cases, the erythema evolves into vesicles and bullae over a few days, which might take over a week to subside. Postinflammatory hyper- or hypopigmented patches are common. Scarring usually does not occur.

Q9. What are the usual sites and symptoms?

Ans: Exposed sites like face, neck, and trunk are usually involved. Eyes may also be involved. The symptoms include pruritus, burning sensation, pain, and occasionally swelling of the affected site.

Q10. What are the complications?

Ans: Postinflammatory hyperpigmentation, secondary infections, and rarely ulceration may occur. In East Africa the species Paederus sabaeus can cause conjunctivitis along with dermatitis, known as "Nairobi Eye".

Q11. How will you diagnose the condition?

Ans: Often the patient would not have noticed a bite but the diagnosis can be made based on the symptoms and clinical patterns. Histopathological examination shows spongiosis and necrosis of superficial epidermal cells with a variable density of focal round cell infiltration in upper dermis.

Q12. What are the differential diagnoses?

Ans: These include herpes zoster, phytophotodermatitis, liquid burns, acute allergic or irritant-contact dermatitis, millipede dermatitis.

Q13. What is the treatment?

Ans: The first step is washing the affected area with soap and water to remove the irritant. This should be followed by cool wet-soaks and further application of a strong topical steroid. Systemic antibiotics and a short course of oral steroids in tapering doses may be added, depending on the severity of the condition.

Q14. Are preventive measures useful?

Ans: Yes, preventive measures should be considered in moist habitats. These include:

- Use of insect screens, light-proof curtains and yellow light (which do not attract insects).
- Doors and windows to be preferably kept closed.
- Sleeping under a bed net can minimize the chances of a beetle falling on the skin during the night.
- Maintaining a light trap—an external floodlight is placed over a container filled with soapy water so as to drown the insects. This keeps the insects away from buildings.
- Clearing decaying animal and vegetable matter from the close premises of residence.
- Patients should be advised to avoid crushing the beetle on the skin (if visualized), manipulating primary lesions or rubbing the eyes following primary involvement.

In a suspicious scenario, immediately wash the affected area with soap and water.

SECTION 15

Skin Tumors

Indrashis Podder

CHAPTER 73

Bowen's Disease

Navya Handa

Case study — Bowen's Disease

Presenting Complaints

Doctor, I have a red scaly lesion on my right foot since 10 months which sometimes itches and has slowly increased in size.

Setting

Dermatology outpatient department

History of Present Illness

A 64-year-old woman presented with a single red-raised lesion on right foot for 10 months. The lesion initially started as an asymptomatic elevated lesion following a minor blunt injury at the site. The lesion gradually enlarged to the present size associated with moderate pruritus and occasional clear oozing. She had been previously treated with topical steroid antibiotic combinations for few weeks without any improvement.

General Physical Examination and Systemic Examination

No abnormality detected

Dermatological Examination

Single 3 × 2 cm round to oval well-defined erythematous irregular, scaly plaque on dorsum of the right foot covered with thick semi-adherent yellow-crust, removal of which showed a nonindurated erythematous mildly oozy base without frank bleeding (Fig. 1).

Q1. What is the most likely diagnosis?

a. Seborrheic keratosis

b. Actinic keratosis

c. Basal cell carcinoma (BCC)

d. Bowen's disease

Ans: d. Bowen's disease: It is a form of squamous cell carcinoma (SCC) in situ that may occur both in skin and mucous membranes. Lesions are erythematous, scaly patches or plaques with a sharply demarcated, irregular border that may become hyperkeratotic, crusted, fissured, or ulcerated. If it presents as an erythematous, moist, velvety or smooth plaque on the glans penis, it is referred to as erythroplasia of Queyrat.

Q2. What are the differential diagnoses for Bowen's disease?

Ans: Differential diagnosis for Bowen's disease has been described as:

- *Actinic keratosis***:** Begin as small, rough spots on sun exposed areas that are easier felt than seen

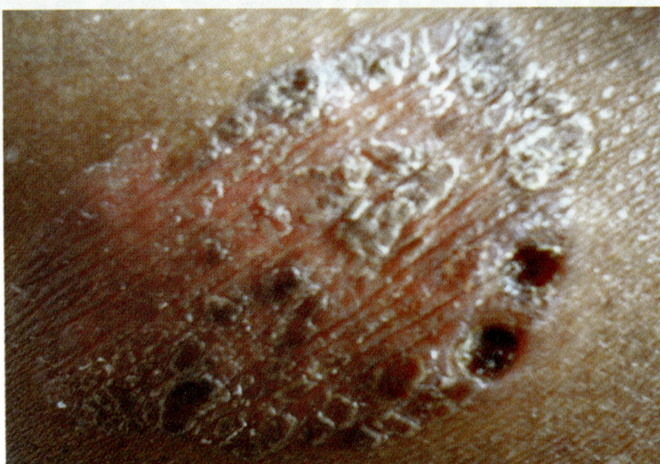

Fig. 1: Solitary plaque with crusts and mild scaling over dorsum of foot

with a sandpaper-like texture and a dry rough adherent and often yellow- or brown-colored scale which can be picked to reveal a hyperemic base with punctate bleeding points. The edge is usually sharply demarcated and the reddening is usually closely confined to the area immediately below the area of abnormal scaling

- *Seborrheic keratosis:* Usually larger, darker and multiple with raised "greasy" warty surface with a stuck on appearance
- *Basal cell carcinoma:* Superficial variant may mimic Bowen disease but is usually less hyperkeratotic and usually they have a pearly whipcord edge
- *Squamous cell carcinoma:* Early invasive SCC may present as a diagnostic challenge but generally patients give a history of change and the plaque may have evolved to form a small nodule and induration is seen
- *Discoid dermatitis:* Often large multiple pruritic plaques
- *Psoriasis:* Thickened plaque with marked scaling. Often multiple and also seen on other sites like extensors, scalp, nail.

Q3. What are the predisposing factors for Bowen's disease?

Ans: Predisposing factors are:

- Sun exposure
- Arsenic ingestion
- Ionizing radiation
- Human papillomavirus (HPV) infection: HPV16 and HPV18, both are common in anogenital Bowen's disease and HPV16 has also been implicated in 60% of palmoplantar and periungual lesions
- Immunosuppression following solid-organ transplant, hematological malignancies, in particular chronic lymphocytic leukemia or human immune deficiency virus (HIV)
- Skin injury or chronic inflammation, such as lupus vulgaris and chronic lupus erythematosus.

Q4. What are the common sites for Bowen's disease?

Ans: Common sites for Bowen's disease are:

- Lower legs of elderly women.
- Head and neck
- Perianal skin
- Subungual region
- Palms and soles
- Oral and genital mucosa (anal intraepithelial neoplasia, penile intraepithelial neoplasia, and vulval intraepithelial neoplasia).

Q5. What are the clinical variants for Bowen's disease?

Ans: Clinical variants-

- Subungual, periungual: Affects younger women and is associated with high-risk HPV16. Associated with higher risk of invasion and recurrence
- Pigmented Bowen's disease: Usually found in the flexures, perianal, or subungual sites
- Verrucous Bowen's disease: May raise the suspicion of invasive carcinoma.

Q6. How will you confirm the diagnosis?

Ans: Diagnosis is often made clinically. Laboratory evaluation is required mainly to diagnose cases with atypical presentations, to assess severity of disease and systemic involvement.

- *Dermatoscopy*
  - Glomerular vessels and a scaly surface
  - Pigmented Bowen's disease: Small brown globules regularly packed in a patchy distribution and structureless gray to brown pigmentation.
- *Biopsy*
  - Full-thickness epidermal dysplasia and keratinocyte disorganization. However, the basement membrane remains intact.
  - Epidermis is often acanthotic, with varying amounts of parakeratosis or hyperkeratosis. Within the entire epidermis, pleomorphic keratinocytes show loss of polarity, atypia and mitosis, producing a "windblown" appearance.
  - The basal layer is more uniform and looks like eyeliner (i.e. "eyeliner sign")

- Chronic inflammatory infiltrate composed of lymphocytes, plasma cells and histiocytes is commonly found in the upper dermis
- Other histologic variants: Psoriasiform, atrophic, verrucous, acantholytic and pigmented
- Stain for high-molecular weight cytokeratin.

Q7. How do you treat Bowen's disease?

Ans: Treatment**:**

- *General Measures:*
  - Sun protection
    - Stay indoors
    - Barrier clothing
    - Apply SPF50+, broad-spectrum sunscreens generously to exposed skin
    - Avoid indoor tanning
- *Specific Measures*
  - Simple excision (Recurrence rates of 5%)
  - Mohs micrographic surgery: Area where there is an increased incidence of recurrence (perianal and subungual) or when tissue sparing is a priority (e.g. face, genitals)
  - Cryosurgery, 5% 5-*Fluorouracil* (FU), and imiquimod have been reported with conventional excision
  - The superficial, large, and sometimes multifocal lesions of Bowen's disease may be considered an ideal indication for photodynamic therapy.
- *Others*
  - Diclofenac gel
  - Topical retinoids
  - Chemical Peel
  - Radiotherapy
  - Electron beam therapy
  - Carbon dioxide laser ablation
  - Erbium: Yttrium-aluminum garnet (YAG) laser ablation.

Q8. What is the course and prognosis for Bowen's disease?

Ans: Prognosis:

- Invasive SCC arises in about 5% of lesions.
- Where there is malignant transformation, it results in an invasive SCC, which may metastasize if left untreated.

CHAPTER 74

Squamous Cell Carcinoma

Indrashis Podder

Case study Squamous Cell Carcinoma

Presenting Complaints

Doctor, I have developed these ulcers over my burn scar on right leg during the last 4 months. These ulcers have gradually increased in size, with associated pain. Recently, I have developed some swellings over my right groin.

Setting

Dermatology outpatient department of a tertiary medical center.

History of Present Illness

A 68-year-old man presented with complaints of development of ulcers over his burn scar, situated on the distal part of his right lower limb. The burn scar has been present for the last 12 years. Recently, he noticed the development of some hard swellings along the margin of his scar which gradually increased in size and later ruptured to form multiple raw areas in quick succession over the last 4 months. These raw areas coalesced over time, to form a large ulcer. There is associated pain and occasional bloody discharge. There is no history of preceding trauma. Lately the patient has noticed the development of some hard swellings over his right groin.

General Examination and Systemic Examination

No abnormality detected

Dermatological Examination

- Large crateriform ulcers over the burn scar, measuring approximately 6 cm in diameter
- Pigmented, irregular borders (no eversion seen)
- Necrotic floor with punched-out edges; indurated base
- Hyperkeratotic gray-brown indurated nodules present in the vicinity
- Hard, swollen, painless discreet right inguinal lymph nodes
- Hair, nail, mucosa have been spared.

Q1. What is the most probable diagnosis?

a. Basal cell carcinoma

b. Squamous cell carcinoma (SCC)

c. Melanoma

d. Infected postburn keloid

Ans: b. SCC

SCC developing in an old scar as in this patient is called Marjolin's ulcer.

Q2. What are the points in favor of your diagnosis from history?

Ans: The points in favor of diagnosis from history are as follows:

- Rapid development of indurated nodules and ulcerations only over 4 months
- Preexisting burn scar
- Old age, male sex
- Asymptomatic lesions
- Development of hard, discreet right inguinal lymphadenopathy

Q3. How will you confirm your diagnosis?

Ans: Although, clinical presentation and other predisposing factors (preexisting burn scar, old age, rapid development, etc.) suggest the diagnosis, a histopathological examination (HPE) is necessary to confirm the diagnosis. The HPE should be done from the edge of ulcerative lesion.

Q4. Describe briefly the histopathological features of squamous cell carcinoma.

Ans: The characteristic histological features of SCC are briefly discussed below:

- *Epidermis:* Presence of dysplastic keratinocytes (large cells, hyperchromatic nucleus, loss of polarity, abnormal mitoses ±) involving the entire breadth of epidermis and showing downward proliferation with dermal infiltration. Based on the degree of differentiation, SCC can be of two types:
  1. *Well-differentiated*: Intercellular bridges preserved, increased keratinization leading to the formation of keratin pearls (concentric pearls of squamous cells with increased keratinization towards the center), horn cysts, etc. (better prognosis)
  2. *Poorly differentiated*: Intercellular bridges lost, absence of keratin pearls (poor prognosis).

  Note:
  - When dysplastic keratinocytes are restricted to the epidermis without any dermal infiltration.
  - SCC in situ (e.g. Bowen's disease) (a premalignant condition).
- *Dermis:* Presence of atypical and dysplastic keratinocytes, often infiltrating the vascular and lymphatic structures (invasive SCC).

Q5. Mention briefly the different histopathological variants of squamous cell carcinoma.

Ans: Some of the important histological variants are briefly discussed below:

- *Keratoacanthoma like:* Central keratin-filled crater with surrounding overhanging epidermis (lip or buttress pattern); severe dysplasia.
- *Spindle cell type:* Whorls of spindle-shaped cells, occasional giant cells (D/d fibroxanthoma)
- *Acantholytic or adenoid or pseudoglandular:* acantholysis of keratinocytes along hair follicles, well-circumscribed; resembling glands
- *Mucinous:* Large, pale cells containing mucinous material
- *Papillary:* Presence of finger-like or papillomatous projections.
- *Pseudovascular:* Cords of cells forming pseudolumina
- *Verrucous:* Epidermis shows hyperkeratosis, acanthosis and papillomatosis with downward proliferation of keratinocytes in the dermis leading to compression of collagen fibers (bulldozing phenomenon). There is absence of cellular atypia, keratin pearls, and lymphatic or vascular infiltration. Dermis shows edema and lymphohistiocytic infiltrate
- *Uncommon histological variants:* Signet ring, clear cell, basaloid, pigmented, desmoplastic, and rhabdoid.

Q6. How will you investigate such a patient?

Ans: We would perform the following investigations in such patients:

- Investigations to confirm our diagnosis
- Investigations to assess the spread of tumor and its staging

Investigations to confirm our diagnosis

- Biopsy from the lesion and HPE (findings discussed above)
- Immunohistochemistry (IHC) may be done: positive for high-molecular weight cytokeratin markers (AE 2/3); negative for low-molecular weight cytokeratin markers (AE 1, CAM 5.2)

Investigations to assess the spread of tumor and its staging

- Computed tomography (CT) scan, magnetic resonance imaging (MRI) to assess the spread of tumor
- *Fine needle aspiration cytology* (FNAC) from enlarged lymph nodes may be done.

Q7. Briefly mention the tumor, nodes and metastasis staging of squamous cell carcinoma.

Ans: SCC is staged according to the tumor, lymph nodes and metastasis (TNM) system of staging:

- T (tumoral status)
  - T_x: Primary tumor cannot be assessed
  - T_0: No primary tumor
  - T_1: Maximum diameter of the tumor less than 2 cm or equal to 2 cm
  - T_2: Maximum diameter of tumor greater than 2 cm
  - T_3: Involvement of maxilla, mandible, orbital, or temporal bone
  - T_4: Involvement of axial or appendageal skeleton, perineural invasion
- N (status of lymph nodes)
  - N_x: Lymph node cannot be assessed
  - N_0: No palpable lymph node
  - N_1: Single ipsilateral lymph node; less than or equal to 3 cm
  - N_{2a}: Single ipsilateral lymph node; size greater than 3 cm but less than 6 cm
  - N_{2b}: Multiple ipsilateral lymph nodes; size 3–6 cm
  - N_3: Any lymph node sized greater than 6 cm
- M (status of distant metastasis)
  - M_0: No distant metastasis
  - M_1: Presence of distant metastasis.

Q8. How will you treat such a patient?

Ans: Several treatment modalities are available for treatment of SCC which are briefly discussed below:

- *Medical therapy:* Topical (5% Imiquimod or resiquimod, 3% diclofenac gel, 5-Fluorouracil); Intralesional (methotrexate, bleomycin); Systemic chemotherapeutic agents (cisplatin or carboplatin, taxanes, epidermal growth factor receptor (EGFR) inhibitors, etc.).
- *Surgical therapy:* It is the mainstay of therapy. Consists of several modalities:
  - Electrodessication (ED) with curettage: Small lesions (<10 mm diameter); superficial lesion on trunk, chest, forehead; postradiation SCC
  - Excision with wide margin (2 cm healthy skin around tumor): large lesions (> 3 cm diameter); involvement of high-risk areas like scalp, forehead, eyelid, lip; SCC over preexisting scar (Marjolin's ulcer), bone and cartilage infiltration
  - Moh's micrographic surgery: tissue preservation needed, high risk cases, recurrent cases
- *Radiation therapy:* Inoperable cases, greater than 1 cm diameter, lesion over nasolabial fold, preauricular area (*Contraindicated for verrucous carcinoma*)
- *Other therapeutic modalities:* Cryotherapy, Photodynamic therapy (PDT), Laser ablation (CO_2 laser, Er-YAG laser).

Q9. What are the poor prognostic factors of squamous cell carcinoma?

Ans: Some of the important poor prognostic factors of SCC are given below:

- Involvement of certain body sites viz lip, ear, genitalia, forehead, scalp, temple, dorsum of hands, etc. (high risk of metastasis)
- Poorly differentiated tumor
- Perineural spread
- Invasion of adnexal structures, viz sweat glands
- Certain histological variants, viz acantholytic and mucinous variants
- SCC developing over irradiated areas, scars (Marjolin's ulcer), tar keratosis, etc.
- Thickness of tumor greater than 5 mm; diameter greater than 2 cm—increased risk of metastasis.

Q10. Which type of SCC shows the highest risk of metastasis?

a. SCC developing over irradiated areas
b. SCC developing over tar keratosis
c. Marjolin's ulcer (SCC developing over scar m/c post burn scar)
d. Lip SCC

Ans: c. Marjolin's ulcer (scar SCC) shows the highest risk of metastasis.

Q11. What is the most common route of metastasis in squamous cell carcinoma?

Ans: The most common route of metastasis is the lymphatic route for SCCs. In late stage, hematogenous dissemination may also take place.

Q12. What are the different clinical variants of squamous cell carcinoma?

Ans: Some of the important clinical types of SCC are given below:

- *Keratotic invasive:* Usually presents with a raised firm papule or plaque, with a smooth or verrucous or papillomatous surface, associated with induration, infiltration, ulceration and hemorrhage.
- *Nodular:* Firm to hard well-circumscribed elevated and indurated swellings (Figs 1 and 2).
- *Arsenic-induced SCC:* Develops over arsenical keratoses primarily involving the palms, soles and trunk; painful, non-hemorrhagic, non-healing ulcers.

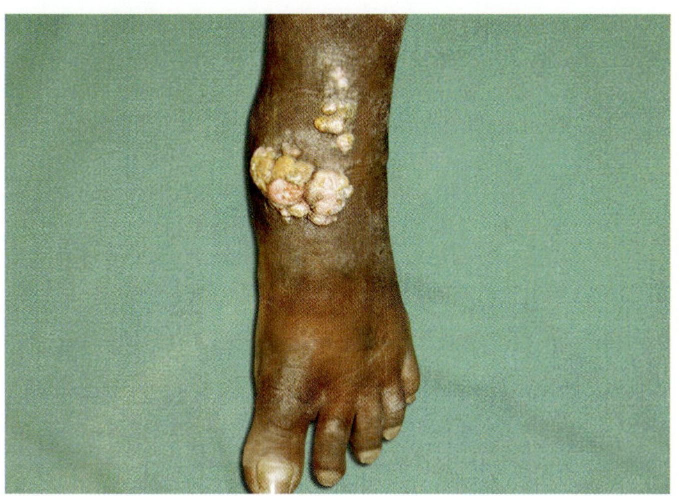
Fig. 1: Nodular– firm to hard well-circumscribed elevated and indurated swellings on the leg

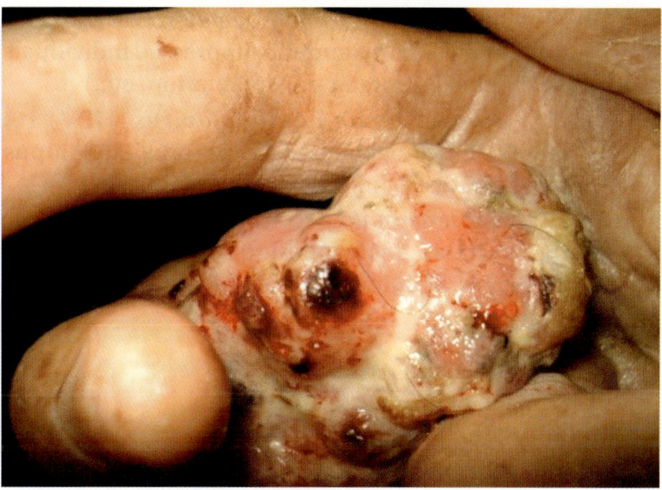
Fig. 2: Similar lesions on the hand

- *Thermal SCC:* May develop over the lesions of erythema ab igne.
- *Radiation-induced SCC:* Develops over a background of chronic radiation-induced skin damage (telangiectasis, hyperpigmentation, or fibrosis, etc.)
- SCC developing over long standing scar (Marjolin's ulcer)
- *Oral SCC:* The most common sites are the lower lips, commissures, lateral tongue, floor of the mouth, soft palate; history of chronic tobacco abuse, betel-nut use, etc. usually presents as noduloulcerative lesions, fissuring, atrophic areas, crusting, etc. Preexisting actinic cheilitis is an important risk factor
- *Genital SCC:* Most common is glans penis (lack of circumcision, poor hygiene, phimosis, presence of premalignant lesions like Lichen sclerosis et atrophicus (LSA), erythroleukoplakia, Erythroplasia of Queyrat, etc. are notable risk factors); usually presents as a fungating mass with destruction of surrounding tissues
- *Periungal SCC:* Hyperkeratotic mass beneath the nails; often confused with subungal verruca
- *Acantholytic SCC:* Usually develops over the sun exposed areas like face, ears, lower lip; central ulceration with induration
- Verrucous carcinoma.

Q13. What is a verrucous carcinoma?

Ans: It is a low-grade SCC which is locally invasive (invades soft tissue and bone) but distant metastasis is extremely rare. It presents as a slow growing mass with a verrucous or cauliflower-like surface. Radiotherapy is contraindicated in verrucous carcinoma as it increases the chance of metastasis. There are 4 varieties of verrucous carcinoma:

1. Oral florid papillomatosis or Ackerman's tumor: accounts for approximately 2–12% of all oral cancers; occurs in the oral cavity (retromolar area, gingiva, floor of mouth, tongue, etc.) in patients (elderly females) with poor oral hygiene, ill-fitting dentures, tobacco abuse.
2. Epithelioma cuniculatum: occurs on the soles; increased fissuring (rabbit burrow-appearance)
3. Buschke-Lowenstein tumor: occurs in the anogenital area, mimics giant condyloma acuminata; mainly involves the glans penis, prepuce, coronal sulcus, vulva and vagina.
4. Papillomatous cutis carcinoides: papillomatous lesions occur over the trunk, buttocks, extremities, chronic ulcer, scar, etc.

Q14. Discuss briefly the etiopathogenesis and predisposing factors for development of squamous cell carcinoma.

Ans: The following factors play important roles in the etiopathogenesis of SCC:

- *Genetic factors:* Loss-of-function mutation of tumor suppressor genes (*p53, Bcl 2, RAS*, etc.), altered signal transduction pathways [EGFR, cyclooxygenase (COX)]
- *Environmental factors:* ↑ exposure to ultraviolet rays → DNA damage →↑ chance of SCC

- *Immunosuppression:* More aggressive SCC, higher recurrence rate in immunosuppressed individuals (HIV-positive, organ transplantation, etc.)
- *Infections: Human papillomavirus* (HPV) 16, 18, 31, 33 (anogenital, cervical, oral, etc.), lupus vulgaris, dissecting cellulitis of scalp, etc.
- *Preexisting dermatoses*: Xeroderma pigmentosum, ataxia-telangiectasia, Bloom syndrome, porokeratosis, actinic keratoses, discoid lupus erythematosus (DLE), *lichen planus* hypertrophic (LPH), etc.
- *Chronic scar or ulcer:* Burn scar, thermal injury, venous ulcer, radiation dermatitis, ulcerative LP, etc.
- *Chronic arsenic exposure:* Environmental or therapeutic
- *Chemicals and toxins:* Polyaromatic hydrocarbons, poly vinyl alcohols, etc.

CHAPTER 75

Basal Cell Carcinoma

Tarang Goyal

Case study Basal Cell Carcinoma

Presenting Complaints

Doctor, I have a nonhealing slowly enlarging dark-raised painless lesion on nose since last 3 years. It often bleeds on trivial trauma.

Setting

Outpatient department of dermatology

History of Present Illness

A 65-year-old lady presented with chief complaint of a nonhealing lesion on the tip of the nose. The lesion increased in size and depth gradually over time and at present some blood stained oozing is present over the lesion. She also complained of lesional bleeding resulting from trivial trauma.

General Physical Examination and Systemic Examination

No abnormality detected

Dermatological Examination

A well-defined plaque sized approximately 2.5 × 2.0 cm is present over the tip of nose with involvement of both alae nasi as well as columellar regions (Fig. 1). The margins are elevated, rolled, and pigmented. The lesion shows yellowish crust deposition with some serosanguineous discharge. Hair, nails, and mucosae are spared.

Q1. What do you think is the most probable diagnosis?

a. Bowen's disease
b. Actinic keratosis
c. Basal cell carcinoma (BCC)
d. Melanoma

Ans: c. BCC

Q2. How is the diagnosis established in these cases?

Ans: Clinical and histopathological approach is sufficient in most of the cases of BCC. Dermoscopy and reflectance confocal microscopy are becoming useful as noninvasive methods for the same.

Q3. What are the dermoscopic findings in basal cell carcinoma?

Ans: The dermoscopic hallmark of BCC is well-focused arborizing vessels with foci of microulcerations. Large blue-gray ovoid nests, blue-gray globules, leaf-like structures, spoke wheel areas have also been seen.

Q4. Describe the pathology of superficial basal cell carcinoma.

Ans: Superficial BCC shows proliferation of atypical basaloid cells that form an axis parallel to the epidermal surface and demonstrate slit-like retraction

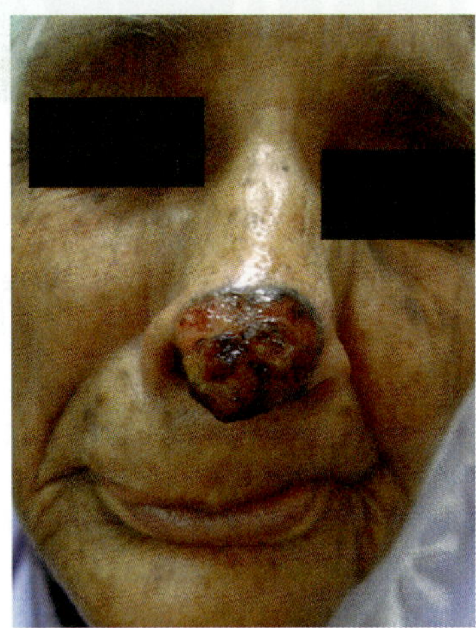

Fig. 1: Solitary well-defined crusted plaque on nose

of the palisaded basal cells from the subjacent stroma. The cleft-like spaces often contain alcian blue-positive mesenchymal mucoid material, a presumed product of the stromal cells. Also, sometimes heavy band-like infiltrate may be present.

Q5. What is its incidence?

Ans: BCC, first described by Jacob in 1827, is the most common cancer in humans. It arises from basal cells (small, round cells) found in the lower layer of epidermis. It accounts for 75% of all nonmelanoma cancers and 25% of all cancers.

Q6. What are the risk factors associated with basal cell carcinoma?

Ans: The following are risk factors associated with BCC:

- Old age (although now incidence in young females is rising)
- Light or red hair color and eye color (Blue eyes)
- Northern European ancestry
- Inability to tan
- Exposure to arsenic, coal tar derivatives and irradiation; although by far ultraviolet (UV) light is the most important factor in lesion development and progression.
- BCC may also arise from scars, draining sinuses, ulcers, burn sites and foci of chronic inflammation just like squamous cell carcinoma

Q7. What genetic mutation is associated with basal cell carcinoma?

Ans: The phenotypic expression of BCC is linked to spontaneous mutation involving the patched-1 (PTCH) gene at the 9q22.3 chromosomal locus.

Q8. Which lineages of cells give rise to basal cell carcinoma?

Ans: Traditionally, it has been agreed upon that BCC have originated from the folliculosebaceous-apocrine germ, also known as trichoblast.

Q9. What are the macroscopic types of basal cell carcinoma?

Ans: Following are the major macroscopic types of BCC:

- Localized: Nodular, nodulocystic, pigmented, cystic and nevoid
- Generalized superficial and infiltrative: Generalized superficial is multifocal and spreading type ("field-fire" type of lesion), whereas infiltrative types are morpheaform, cicatrizing and ice-pick types.

Q10. What are the major clinic-pathologic types of basal cell carcinoma?

Ans: There are four major clinicopathologic types of BCC:

1. Nodular
2. Superficial
3. Morpheaform
4. Fibroepithelial (Fibroepithelioma of Pinkus).

Q11. Which of the following is not regarded as an aggressive variety of basal cell carcinoma?

a. Morpheaform BCC
b. Infiltrative BCC
c. Fibroepithelioma of Pinkus
d. Basosquamous BCC

Ans: c. Fibroepithelioma of Pinkus is not an aggressive variety of BCC.

Q12. What is meant by "Giant" basal cell carcinoma?

Ans: As defined by the American Joint Committee on Cancer (AJCC), giant BCC (GBCC) is a tumor 5.0 cm or more in maximum dimension. Thus, it is classified as T3 tumor as per tumor, nodes and metastasis (TNM) classification.

Q13. What is rodent ulcer?

Ans: In the ulcerative type of BCC, the lesions are nonhealing and simulate a rodent has "gnawed" upon the tissue, so the name "rodent ulcer". It is also called as "Jacob's ulcer".

Q14. Why it is called a "field-fire" type of cancer?

Ans: Lesions of the superficial variety are frequently multifocal and are thus termed as the so-called "field fire" BCC due to their rapid peripheral spread.

Q15. What is meant by "tear drop" morphologic type of basal cell carcinoma?

Ans: Due to frequent involvement of nasolabial area by BCC, the morphologic distribution is similar to dropping area of tears; it is called as "tear-drop" morphology.

Q16. Describe the pathology of nodular type of basal cell carcinoma?

Ans: The nodular form of BCC is characterized by discrete large or small nests of basaloid cells in either the papillary or reticular dermis accompanied by slit-like retraction from a stroma.

Q17. What are the treatment modalities available for basal cell carcinoma?

Ans: The following are the treatment modalities available for BCC:

- Surgical approach: Mohs micrographic surgery, standard excision
- Curettage and desiccation, cryosurgery and CO_2 laser (tried in some very superficial BCCs)
- Topical treatment: Imiquimod, 5- Fluouracil, intralesional-α-2b
- Others: Photodynamic therapy, radiation therapy.

Q18. What is the novel Hedgehog pathway inhibitor being used now in basal cell carcinoma?

Ans: Vismodegib is the novel Hedgehog pathway inhibitor being used now in BCC. It is used orally in a dose of 150 mg daily. The common side effects are muscle spasms, alopecia, weight loss, fatigue, nausea, vomiting diarrhea, constipation, and arthralgia. Its use is contraindicated in pregnancy.

Vismodegib was approved by the US Food and Drug Administration (USFDA) in 2012 for treatment of adults with locally advanced BCC that has recurred following surgery, metastatic BCC, patients who are not candidates for surgery or radiation.

Q19. What are the rates of metastases in various organs?

Ans: The most common sites of distant metastasis are lymph nodes (40–83%), followed by lung (35–53%), bone (20–28%), skin (10–17%), and liver (9%). The rate of metastasis for BCC ranges from 0.003% to 0.55%, but it goes up to 1.9% for tumor size more than 3.0 cm.

Q20. What is "Halo Basal cell carcinoma"?

Ans: The presence of a surrounding hypo- or hyper-pigmented flare has been designated as "halo" BCC.

Q21. Enumerate the syndromes associated with predisposition for basal cell carcinoma?

Ans: Inherited familial cancer syndromes that involve a predisposition to BCC are:

- Gorlin-Goltz Syndrome
- Bazex–Dupré–Christol Syndrome
- Rombo syndrome.

Q22. Syndromes that are associated with a predisposition to nonmelanoma skin cancer are?

Ans: Syndromes with predisposition to nonmelanoma skin cancer (NMSC):

- Xeroderma pigmentosum
- Albinism
- Epidermodysplasia verruciformis.

Q23. What are the main features of Gorlin-Goltz syndrome?

Ans: The three main features of this syndrome are (1) multiple BCCs, (2) odontogenic jaw cysts and (3) palmar pits.

CHAPTER 76

Melanoma

Indrashis Podder

Case study Melanoma

Presenting Complaints

Doctor, I have developed an irregular area of blackish discoloration on the lateral aspect of my right great toe near the nail. It was initially small in size, which is growing rapidly. Often there is bleeding even on minor trauma. Recently, I have developed some swellings over my right groin and lost weight.

Setting

Dermatology outpatient department (OPD)

History of Present Illness

A 67-year-old man presented with scaly, brown-black lesion around his right great toe on the lateral aspect. History revealed he had a mole at that site since birth, which grew bigger in size and became more darkly pigmented over the last 4 months. He also complained of bleeding from the lesion even on trivial trauma. Recently, he reported the development of dark-colored bands over his toenail. There is no history of trauma. Lately the patient has developed few swellings over his right groin and also complaints of profound weakness and weight loss (around 5 kg).

General Examination

Alert, conscious, co-operative.
Vitals: Stable, pallor present; right-sided inguinal lymphadenopathy (discreet, hard, painless). Height: 158 cm, Weight: 41 kg, BMI:16.46

Systemic Examination

No abnormality detected.

Dermatological Examination

- Asymmetric brownish black plaque with irregular borders, sized approximately 4.5 cm in diameter on the lateral aspect of right great toe
- Irregular borders
- *Surface*: Variegated appearance, scaling
- *Palpation*: Induration present, bleeding on trivial manipulation (trauma)
- *Nails*: Brown longitudinal band on right great toe, width 3.5 mm.

Laboratory Investigations (Routine Blood Biochemistry)

All parameters are within normal limits except for Hb 7.5 mg/dL (anemia).

Q1. What is the most probable diagnosis?

a. Squamous cell carcinoma
b. Melanoma
c. Traumatic hematoma
d. Dysplastic nevus

Ans: b. Melanoma.

Q2. What are the points in favor of your diagnosis?

Ans: Important points in favor of my diagnosis are given below:

- Rapid progressive development of asymmetric, brownish-black raised lesion with irregular borders and variegated surface
- History of pre-existing nevus/mole at the site of affection
- History of bleeding on trivial trauma
- Discreet, hard painless lymph nodes in groin
- Generalized malaise, weakness, weight loss in recent period.

Q3. How will you confirm your diagnosis?

Ans: The best way to confirm such a diagnosis is skin biopsy and histopathological examination.

Q4. Which biopsy technique is suitable for malignant melanoma?

Ans: Preferred biopsy technique is narrow excisional biopsy that encompasses entire breadth of lesion with clinically negative margins to a depth sufficient to ensure that lesion is not transected. This may be accomplished by elliptical or punch excision with suturing, or shave removal to depth below anticipated plane of lesion. Partial sampling (incisional biopsy) can be done for facial or acral location, low clinical suspicion or uncertainty of diagnosis, or very large lesion. Repeat biopsy is recommended if initial biopsy specimen is inadequate for diagnosis or microstaging of primary lesion.

Q5. Describe briefly the histopathological features of melanoma.

Ans: Histopathological features of melanoma are:

- Hallmark feature is the presence of atypical melanocytes (larger hyperchromatic nuclei, larger cell size, anisocytosis, nuclear atypia, presence of mitotic figures and necrosis).
- Atypical melanocytes, initially are intraepidermal (confined to epidermis-dysplastic nevus), later invade dermis and form sheets/nests.
- In late stage, they may invade the follicular epithelium, nerves and/or blood vessels both singly and in small nests.
- Presence of neoplastic melanocytes (pagetoid, spindled, small and large rounded, polygonal and multinucleate cytomorphological features) seen.

Q6. What are types of primary cutaneous melanoma?

Ans: There are four major subtypes of primary cutaneous melanoma according to the growth pattern as described in Table 1.

Q7. What is the most common type of melanoma seen on darker skin?

a. Superficial spreading melanoma
b. Nodular melanoma

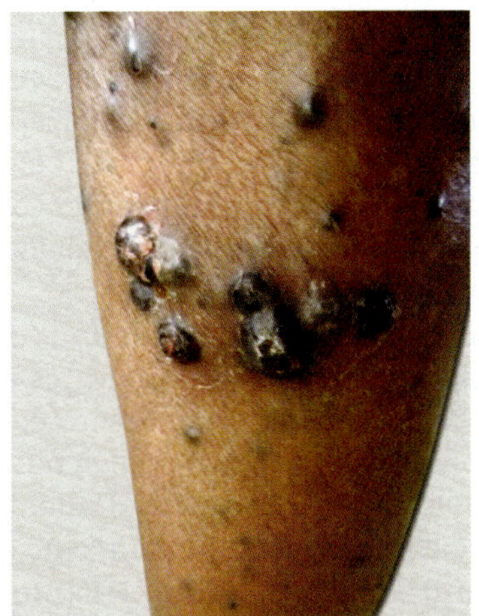

Fig. 1: Nodular melanoma on the leg

Table 1: Types of primary cutaneous melanoma

Subtype of melanoma	*Preferred site*	*Characteristic feature(s)*	*Overall incidence*	*Radial growth*
Superficial spreading	Any site; lower extremities >trunk	Pagetoid melanocytes, less relation to sun-damage	60–70% (most common)	Present
Nodular melanoma (Fig. 1)	Any site, esp. trunk, head and neck	Nodular lesion with more vertical growth	15–30%	Absent
Lentigo maligna melanoma	Face esp. nose and cheeks	Occurs over sun-damaged skin, slow growth	5–15%	Present
Acral lentiginous melanoma	Palms, soles, nail	Occurs in the acral parts, may involve the nail unit	5–10	Present

c. Lentigomaligna melanoma
d. Acral lentiginous melanoma

Ans: a. Acral lentiginous melanoma. Although acral lentiginous melanoma has the least incidence overall globally, the rarity of other types of melanoma in the darker skin makes it the most common type of melanoma affecting the dark skin.

Q8. What are the melanoma variants?

Ans: Apart from these four major subtypes, there are some other rare and unusual varieties which are called the melanoma variants. Some of the important melanoma variants are given below:

- *Amelanotic melanomas*: Any subtype lacking the characteristic hyperpigmentation.
- *Nevoid melanomas*: These melanomas resemble either a spitz nevus or acquired/congenital melanocytic nevus. Presence of atypical melanocytes in the dermis confirms the diagnosis.
- *Malignant blue nevus*: Rare intradermal melanocytic tumor most commonly affecting scalp and face. It appears as a blue-black nodule, usually more than 1 cm on diameter; histologically characterized by the presence of spindle-shaped atypical melanocytes. This variant shows high rate of recurrence and metastasis.
- *Desmoplastic/spindled/neurotropic melanoma*: Histological variant characterized by presence of fibrous stroma (desmoplastic) and/or spindle-shaped atypical melanocytes. Clinically, it is indistinguishable from lentigo maligna melanoma occurring on sun-exposed sites.
- *Clear cell sarcoma (melanoma of soft parts)*: Occurs on the distal extremities of young and adolescents. Clinically, it resembles a soft tissue tumor or sarcoma having a high rate of metastasis or recurrence. Histopathological presence of atypical melanocytes confirms the diagnosis.
- *Animal-type melanoma*: Histological variety characterized by the presence of nodules and fascicles of epithelioid melanocytes with pleomorphic nuclei, striking hyperpigmentation, abundant melanophages and a scarce lymphocytic infiltration. It is named so because of its histopathological resemblance to melanocytic neoplasms seen in white/gray horses.
- *Ocular melanoma*: Extremely rare, broadly of two types—conjunctival and uveal/choroidal. Increased risk of ocular melanoma has been reported in dysplastic nevus syndrome and nevus of Ota.
- *Mucosal melanoma*: Extremely rare variant which may affect oral, nasopharyngeal, laryngeal, vaginal and anal mucosa. Usually starting near the mucocutaneous junctions, these melanomas have a very poor prognosis.

Q9. What is the ABCDE of melanoma?

Ans: For quick clinical diagnosis even by nondermatologists, the ABCDE criteria have been highlighted in public awareness programs, which stands for:

A → Asymmetric appearance
B → Border irregularity
C → Color becoming darker or variegated
D → Diameter > 5 mm
E → Evolution of the above changes over a short span of time (in months).

Q10. How will you investigate a case of melanoma?

Ans: Following clinical examination, we have to confirm our diagnosis by performing histopathological examination. Other investigations like CT scan, MRI and PET scan using 18F-fluorodeoxyglucose (FDG) need to be done to assess the extent of spread. USG or CT-guided lymph node biopsy may be done in cases of lymph node involvement. Immunohistochemistry (IHC) may be done to detect the presence of melanocytic markers like Melan A, Mart 1, S-100, etc. to aid in diagnosis.

Q11. What are the dermoscopic findings of melanoma? How can we differentiate it from a benign melanocytic lesion?

Ans: Dermoscopy is a relatively newer noninvasive investigation which may help us to differentiate benign and melanocytic lesions based on the findings given in Table 2.

Q12. Mention briefly the staging of melanomas and the parameters on which the staging is dependent.

Ans: The staging of melanoma is dependent on several parameters as given below:

Table 2: Difference between benign melanocytic lesion and malignant melanoma

Benign melanocytic lesion	*Malignant melanoma*
Pigment network (network of brownish lines over a tan background) Typical network (brown-colored regular meshwork, narrow-spaced) Regular dots and globules Regular black-brown blotches Comma-like vessels	Atypical network (irregular meshwork and thick brown-black lines) Irregular dots and globules Streaks (irregular, linear lines) Blue-whitish veil (irregular, confluent blue-white diffuse pigmentation) Irregular black-brown blotches Dotted or irregular vessels

- Tumor thickness is graded as less than or equal to 1 mm, 1–2 mm, 2–4 mm and more than 4 mm (Breslow depth).
- The T1 stage is further classified based on Clark level of invasion.
- Presence of microscopic ulceration is considered a grave prognostic factor.
- Local recurrence, presence of satellite lesions and local invasion are all considered to be stage III melanoma.
- Recently the number of involved lymph nodes is being considered for staging instead of the size of affected lymph nodes.
- Elevated serum lactate dehydrogenase (LDH) level is considered a bad prognostic factor
- The site of distant metastasis is important for prognosis.

Staging of melanoma: Recently the revised AJCC staging (American Joint Committee on Cancer) system is in vogue for staging of melanoma:

- Stage I → tumors with Breslow depth less than or equal to 1 mm (low risk)
- Stage II → tumors with Breslow depth more than 2 mm (high risk)
- Stage III → involvement of regional lymph nodes
- Stage IV → distant metastases.

Q13. Breslow thickness is measured from which layer of epidermis?

a. Stratum corneum
b. Stratum granulosum
c. Stratum basale
d. Stratum spinosum

Ans: b. Stratum granulosum. It is measured from the granular layer of the overlying epidermis or base of a superficial ulceration to the deepest malignant cells invading dermis to the nearest 0.1 mm, not including deeper adventitial extension and microsatellitosis.

Q14. What are microsatellitosis and its significance?

Ans: Nest(s) of tumor cells (0.05 mm in diameter) located in reticular dermis, subcutis, or vessels, separated from invasive component of tumor by more than or equal to 0.3 mm of normal tissue. Its presence upstages the tumor to N2c (Stage IIIB) TNM staging.

Q15. Briefly mention the treatment of melanoma.

Ans: Although there are several guidelines for the treatment of melanoma, an acceptable treatment protocol is given below according to the stage of disease. The mainstay of treatment is surgical excision (Table 3).

Table 3: Treatment of melanoma

Stage of melanoma	*Treatment modality*
Stage I and II	Wide local excision of the primary tumor (0.5 cm margin for in-situ melanoma, 1 cm margin if Breslow depth < 2 mm, 2 cm margin if depth = 2 mm, 2–3 cm margin if depth more than 4 mm
Stage III (regional lymph node metastasis)	At first sentinel lymph node biopsy is to be done (SLNB) à if metastasis found in the sentinel lymph node à complete regional lymph node dissection Recent AJCC guidelines recommend SLNB for all primary melanomas > 1 mm thickness
Stage IV (distant metastasis)	Palliative measures, systemic chemotherapy (dacarbazine, cisplatin, taxols, etc.), immunotherapy [IL-2, antibodies against melanoma-associated antigen (MAA)], vaccine therapy (BCG, M-VAX, etc.). Whole brain radiotherapy may be employed in cerebral metastasis. Extremely poor prognosis with survival rates ~6% and median survival period (7.5 months)

Newer modalities of therapy:

- *Biochemotherapy*: This modality encompasses the combination of biological response modifiers and chemotherapy. The most promising combinations have been that of interferon alpha (IFN-α) or interleukin 2 (IL-2) with cisplatin-based chemotherapy regimens.
- *Molecular targeted therapy*: This is an experimental therapy targeting the genes, their products and the genetic pathways playing a role in the progression of melanoma. Most of the studies are centered on two genes *BRAF* (Raf kinase inhibitors) and *VEGF* (thalidomide, bevacizumab, etc.).

Q16. What are the common sites of systemic metastasis of melanoma?

Ans: Skin, brain, gastrointestinal (GI) tract, lung and bone.

Q17. How is the prognosis affected by the site of metastasis?

Ans: The prognosis worsens in the following order: GI > lung > brain/bone.

CHAPTER 77

Cutaneous Lymphoma

Tanumay Raychaudhury, Navya Handa

Case study Cutaneous lymphoma

Presenting Complaints

Doctor, I am having multiple elevated lesions on my chest, buttocks and upper thigh for the past 2 months.

Setting

Dermatology outpatient department

History of Present Illness

A 60-year-old male patient developed erythematous raised lesions on his trunk with associated pruritus for the past 2 months. He has applied topical steroids on and off without any significant improvement. Since the last one month, he has developed large raised lesions on his buttocks and both upper thighs.

General Physical Examination

No abnormality detected except for the presence of discrete, mobile, nontender cervical, axillary and inguinal lymphadenopathy.

Systemic Examination

No splenomegaly or hepatomegaly noted.

Dermatological Examination

- Multiple, well-defined, annular, hypopigmented scaly plaques with irregular borders and central clearing on the trunk with size ranging from 3 × 4 cm to 6 × 8 cm.
- Multiple, nontender skin colored nodules,1–3 cm in size on buttocks and upper thighs, mobile over underlying structures but attached to the overlying skin (Fig. 1).
- There is no peripheral nerve thickening or history of extramarital sexual contact.

Laboratory Investigations

The venereal disease research laboratory (VDRL) and enzyme-linked immunosorbent assay (ELISA) for HIV are negative. Slit skin smear for acid-fast bacilli (AFB) (L) is negative. Histopathology from the lesions reveals atypical lymphocytes in the epidermis with no granulomas.

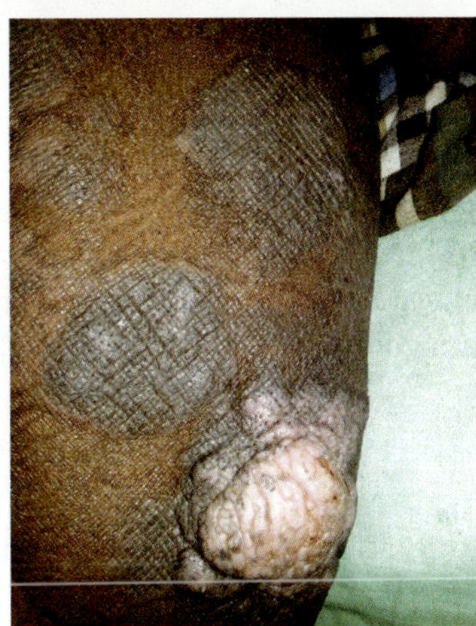

Fig. 1: Multiple hyperpigmented plaques on the thigh with a solitary nodular lesion

Q1. What is the most likely diagnosis?

a. Secondary syphilis
b. Lepromatous leprosy
c. Mycosis fungoides
d. Cutaneous B cell lymphoma

Ans: c. Mycosis fungoides (MF). MF is the most common cutaneous T cell lymphoma subtype.

Q2. Describe a typical case of mycosis fungoides.

Ans: Mycosis fungoides has a predilection for older males (>50 years). Classical Alibert-Bazin type of MF presents with mild erythematous scaly annular or arcuate patches which classically involve sun-shielded areas ("bathing suit distribution"). Though the early patches have predilection over unexposed areas, later they may become eczematous, hypopigmented or hyperpigmented. In a few patients, erythroderma may arise *de novo* or from progression of patch/plaque MF. Patients who develop erythroderma and do not meet hematologic criteria for Sezary syndrome (SS) are considered as "erythrodermic MF".

Q3. What are the different variants of mycosis fungoides?

Ans: Subtypes and variants of MF include folliculotropic MF, pagetoid reticulosis and granulomatous slack skin. Other atypical variants including syringotropic, bullous/vesicular, hyperpigmented, hypopigmented, unilesional, palmoplantar, hyperkeratotic/verrucous, vegetating/papillomatous, ichthyosiform, pigmented purpura-like and pustular variants have been reported in literature. Few atypical variants including hypopigmented, pityriasis lichenoides-like, and ichthyosiform mycosis fungoides are more prevalent in Asians compared to the West.

Q4. What are the histopathological changes seen in mycosis fungoides?

Ans: Diagnosis of MF is supported by the following histopathologic findings:

- Superficial lymphoid infiltrate
- Epidermotropism without spongiosis
- Atypical lymphoid infiltrate (cells with enlarged, hyperchromatic nuclei and irregular or cerebriform nuclear contours). Presence of such atypical lymphocytes in the epidermis is 100% sensitive and 92% specific for the diagnosis of MF.
- Although considered classical, well-formed Pautrier microabscesses are seen in only a minority of patients.

Q5. Discuss briefly the immunohistochemistry of mycosis fungoides.

Ans: Expression of CD4, which is a marker of mature helper T-cells, is a hallmark finding of MF. Immunophenotypical markers which are commonly observed in MF include CD2+, CD3+, CD4+, CD5+, CD45RO+, CLA+ (cutaneous lymphoid antigen), CD8- (cytotoxic T-cell marker) and CD30-. Low levels of CD7 expression (<10%) has a sensitivity of 40% and specificity of 80–100% which helps to distinguish early MF from benign mimics.

Q6. What is the staging of mycosis fungoides?

Ans: Staging is based on morphology of skin lesions, extent of involvement, nodal involvement, extracutaneous dissemination and blood involvement.

The International Society for Cutaneous Lymphomas (ISCL)/European Organization of Research and Treatment of Cancer (EORTC) revised clinical staging and classification of mycosis fungoides and Sezary's syndrome (Table 1)

Tumor stage (skin)

- T1: Limited patches, papules, and/or plaques covering less than 10% of skin surface (T1a: patch only and T1b: plaque with or without patch)
- T2: Patches, papules, or plaques covering 10% or more of skin surface (T1a: patch only and T1b: plaque with or without patch)
- T3: One or more tumors equal to or greater than 1 cm diameter
- T4: Confluence of erythema, covering 80% or more of body surface area.

Table 1: The International Society for Cutaneous Lymphomas (ISCL)/European Organization of Research and Treatment of Cancer (EORTC) revision to the staging of mycosis fungoides and Sezary's syndrome

Stage	*T*	*N*	*M*	*B*
IA	1	0	0	0,1
IB	2	0	0	0,1
II	1,2	1,2	0	0,1
IIB	3	0-2	0	0,1
III	4	0-2	0	0,1
IIIA	4	0-2	0	0
IIIB	4	0-2	0	1
IVA1	1-4	0-2	0	2
IVA2	1-4	3	0	0-2
IVB	1-4	0-3	1	0-2

Nodal stage

- N0: No clinically abnormal peripheral lymph nodes; biopsy not required
- N1: Clinically abnormal peripheral lymph nodes; histopathological involvement, no atypical lymphocytes (N1a: clone-negative and N1b: clone-positive)
- N2: Clinically abnormal peripheral lymph nodes; histopathological involvement, aggregates of atypical lymphocytes (N1a: clone-negative and N1b: clone-positive)
- N3: Clinically abnormal peripheral lymph nodes; histopathological involvement, partial or complete effacement of nodal architecture by atypical lymphocytes or neoplastic cells; clone-positive or negative
- N_x: Clinically abnormal peripheral lymph nodes; no confirmed histological involvement.

Metastatic stage (visceral)

- M0: No visceral disease
- M1: Visceral disease.

Blood stage

- B0: No hematological involvement; less than 5% atypical or Sezary's cells in peripheral blood (B0a: clone-negative and B0b: clone-positive)
- B1: Sezary's count 5% or more of peripheral blood lymphocytes, but does not meet criteria of B2 (B0a: clone-negative and B0b: clone-positive)
- B2: 1000/μL or more Sezary's cells; clone-positive.

Q7. What are the poor prognostic markers for mycosis fungoides?

Ans: Some of the important poor prognostic factors of MF are given below:

- Clinical parameters like male sex and increasing age
- Hematological parameters like elevated lactate dehydrogenase (LDH) level in the blood
- Histological features such as folliculotropism
- Certain genetic mutations like NAV3/TNFRSF1B, PIK3, etc.

Q8. How do you classify cutaneous lymphomas?

Ans: The World Health Organization (WHO)-EORTC classification of cutaneous lymphomas is tabulated below (Box 1).

Clinically, primary cutaneous lymphomas refer to those cutaneous T-cell lymphomas (CTCL) and

Box 1

World Health Organization (WHO)/European Organization of Research and Treatment of Cancer (EORTC) classification of cutaneous lymphomas

Cutaneous T-cell and NK-cell lymphomas
Mycosis fungoides (MF)
Subtypes of MF
- Pagetoid reticulosis
- Granulomatous slack skin
- Folliculotropic MF
- Sezary syndrome
- Adult T-cell leukemia/lymphoma

Primary cutaneous CD30+ lymphoproliferative disorders (CD30+ LPD)
- Lymphomatoid papulosis
- Primary cutaneous anaplastic large cell lymphoma

Subcutaneous panniculitis-like T-cell lymphoma (SPTL)*
Extranodal NK/T-cell lymphoma, nasal type (Extranodal NKTL)
Primary cutaneous peripheral T-cell lymphoma, unspecified (PTCL, NOS)
- Primary cutaneous aggressive epidermotropic CD8+ T-cell lymphoma (provisional)
- Cutaneous δ/γ T-cell lymphoma (provisional)
- Primary cutaneous CD4+ small/medium-sized pleomorphic T-cell lymphoma(provisional)

Cutaneous B-cell lymphomas (CBCL)
Primary cutaneous marginal zone B-cell lymphoma (PCMZL)
- Primary cutaneous immunocytoma
- Primary cutaneous plasmacytoma
- Follicular hyperplasia with monotypic plasma cells

Primary cutaneous follicle center lymphoma (PCFCL)
- Growth patterns: follicular, follicular and diffuse, diffuse

Primary cutaneous diffuse large B-cell lymphoma, leg type (DLBCL)
Primary cutaneous diffuse large B-cell lymphoma, other
Intravascular large B-cell lymphoma (IVLBCL)
Precursor hematological neoplasm
- CD4+/CD56+ hematodermic neoplasm (formerly blastic NK cell lymphoma)

* By definition, phenotype is T-cell receptor α/β chain positive

cutaneous B-cell lymphomas (CBCL) without any extracutaneous disease at the time of diagnosis. Secondary CL represents infiltrates of a disseminated nodal or extranodal lymphoma into the skin.

Q9. What is Sezary syndrome (SS)?

Ans: Sezary syndrome (SS) is a triad of erythroderma, generalized lymphadenopathy, and the presence of neoplastic T cells (Sezary cells) in skin, lymph nodes and peripheral blood. It has a poor prognosis. SS usually occurs in a short time period de novo and progresses rapidly. Though it was considered separate from MF, rarely SS may follow classic MF. Patients with SS usually present with generalized exfoliative erythroderma with keratoderma and fissures on the palms and soles which may be associated with electrolyte imbalance, hypothermia, hair loss and eyelid changes/ectropion.

Q10. What are the diagnostic criteria for Sezary syndrome?

Ans: International Society for Cutaneous Lymphomas (ISCL) recommended criteria for diagnosis of SS include one or more of the following:

- Absolute Sezary cell count of 1,000 cells/mm^3 or more
- Specific immunophenotypical abnormalities (CD4/CD8 ratio more than 10, loss of any or all of the T-cell antigens CD2, CD3, CD4, and CD5, or both)
- Demonstration of a T-cell clone in the peripheral blood by molecular or cytogenetic methods.

Q11. What are the histopathological features of Sezary syndrome?

Ans: Classical histopathological features including epidermotropism, Pautrier microabscesses are variable and less prominent in SS. Traditional determination of Sezary cells quantification was largely replaced by flow cytometry analysis which identifies neoplastic T cells, which are characterized as CD4+ CD7- and/or CD4+ CD26-.

Q12. What are the prognostic factors of Sezary syndrome?

Ans: Sezary syndrome is an aggressive disease with a median survival of 2–4 years and an overall survival rate at 5 years of between 11% and 20%. Transformation into a large-cell lymphoma may also occur in the course of SS as in classical MF.

Q13. What are primary cutaneous CD30+ lymphoproliferative disorders (CD30+ LPD)?

Ans: The primary cutaneous CD30+ LPDs are the second most common form of CTCL contributing around 25% of all CTCLs. Lymphomatoid papulosis (LyP) and cutaneous anaplastic large cell lymphoma (C-ALCL) form a spectrum of CD30+ LPDs which is usually differentiated by clinical appearance, course and histological criteria.

Q14. What is lymphomatoid papulosis (LyP)?

Ans: LyP generally occurs in adults with male predominance but may occur in children as well. Clinically, LyP is usually characterized by a chronic course of self-healing skin eruption of erythematous papules and nodules that may become hemorrhagic, necrotic, and/or ulcerative lesions each of which undergoes spontaneous regression after weeks or months.

Q15. What is subcutaneous panniculitis-like T-cell lymphoma (SPTL)?

Ans: Subcutaneous panniculitis-like T-cell lymphoma (SPTL) which accounts for 1% of all CL's is defined based on the new WHO/EORTC classification as a cytotoxic T-cell lymphoma showing an α/β+, CD3+, CD4-, CD8+ phenotype which is primarily limited to subcutaneous infiltrates with an indolent clinical course.

Q16. What are cutaneous B-cell lymphomas (CBCL)?

Ans: Cutaneous B-cell lymphomas always remain a great challenge for the clinicians and pathologists in terms of definitive diagnosis and treatment. The different types of cutaneous B-cell lymphomas include primary cutaneous marginal zone B-cell lymphoma (PCMZL), primary cutaneous follicle center lymphoma (PCFCL), primary cutaneous diffuse large B cell lymphoma leg type (PCDLBCL–LT), primary cutaneous diffuse large B-cell lymphoma, other and intravascular large B-cell lymphoma. Primary cutaneous follicle center lymphomas constitute the most common type of CBCL.

SECTION 16

Skin and Systemic Disease

Shilpa K

- Neurofibromatosis
- Tuberous Sclerosis
- Systemic Amyloidosis
- Lipoid Proteinosis
- Xanthomatosis
- Endogenous Ochronosis
- Calcinosis Cutis
- Mastocytosis

CHAPTER 78

Neurofibromatosis

Lakshmi DV

Case study Neurofibromatosis

Presenting Complaints

Doctor, I have these pigmented skin lesions since birth and multiple swellings over my trunk since 9 months and my father also had similar lesions.

Setting

Dermatology outpatient department.

History of Present Illness

A 24-year-old male, presented with complaints of pigmented patches over the trunk, back and lower extremities since birth. He has noticed multiple smooth, soft, painless, compressible swellings over the trunk and back since 9 months. There is no history of any impairment of vision, seizures, or learning disabilities. The pedigree of the family members is as shown in Figure 1. Father and maternal uncle had similar lesions.

General Physical Examination

- Well oriented to time, place and person
- BMI: 17 kg/m^2, Pulse: 80 bpm, BP: 124/86 mm Hg

Systemic Examination

- *Ocular examination*: Lisch nodules seen in both iris on slit lamp microscopy.
- *Musculoskeletal system:* Scoliosis present
- No other systemic abnormality detected.

Dermatological Examination

Multiple smooth, soft, nontender, compressible swellings with the largest measuring around 2 × 3 cm, seen over the trunk and back (Fig. 2). Swelling invaginates easily into the underlying structures (*Buttonhole sign*—Fig. 3). Freckling is seen in axillae, groins and inframammary area (*Crowe's sign*) and freckling also seen in palms (*Patrick Yesudian sign*). Well-defined hyperpigmented patches with smooth borders present (7 patches present over trunk, back and thighs, largest measuring 15 × 10 cm, smallest 5 × 3 cm).

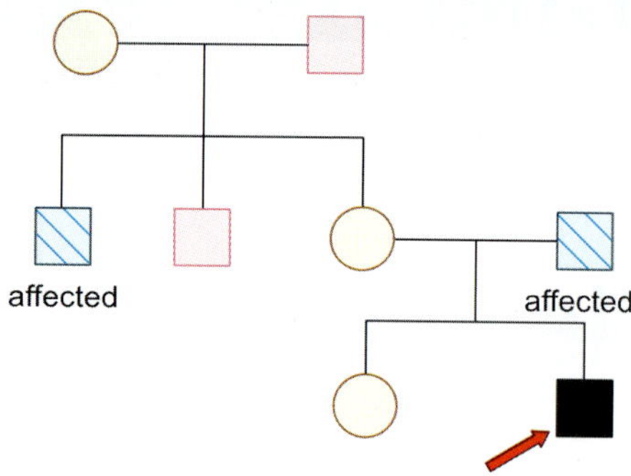

Fig. 1: Family pedigree showing the proband and affected family members

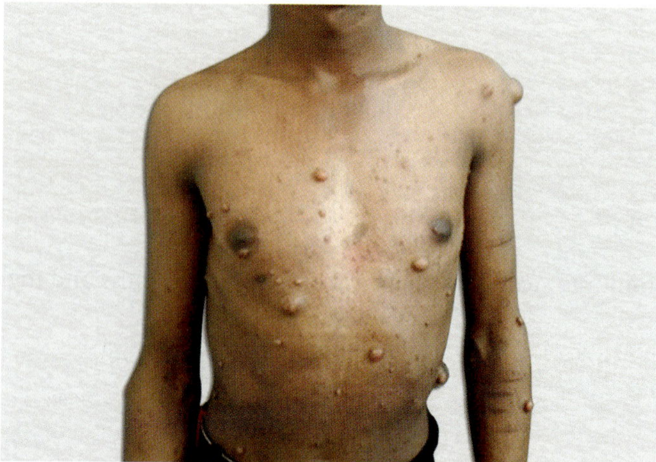

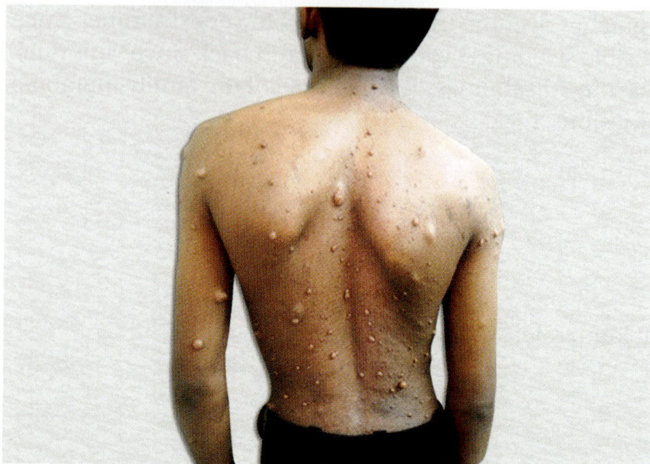

Fig. 2: Multiple neurofibromas, café-au-lait macules (CALMS) and scoliosis

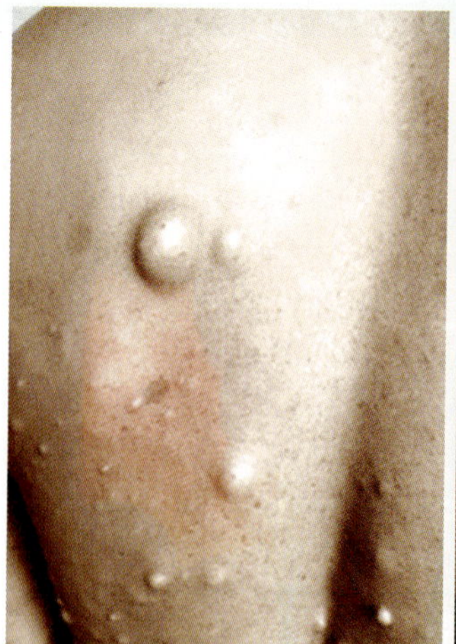

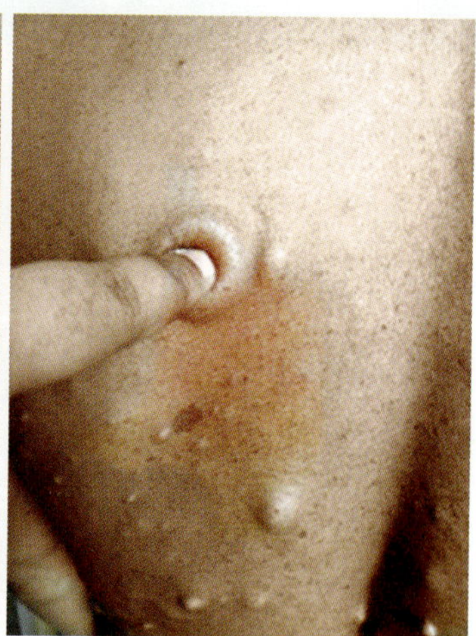

Fig. 3: Buttonhole sign

Table 1: Diagnostic criteria for neurofibromatosis 1 (NF1) (National Institute of Health Consensus Development Conference, 1988)

1	Six or more café-au-lait macules (CALMs) >5 mm in greatest diameter at prepubertal age and >15 mm in greatest diameter in adults	Presence of two or more of the following criteria are needed for diagnosis
2	Two or more neurofibroma of any type or one plexiform neurofibroma	
3	Axillary or inguinal freckling	
4	Optic glioma	
5	Two or more Lisch nodules	
6	A distinctive osseous lesion, e.g. sphenoid dysplasia/thinning of cortex of long bones with or without pseudarthrosis	
7	First-degree relative (parent, sibling, offspring) with NF1 by the above criteria.	

Q1. What is the most likely diagnosis?

a. Tuberous sclerosis
b. Schwannomatosis
c. Neurofibromatosis 1 (NF1)
d. Klippel–Trenaunay–Weber syndrome

Ans: c. Neurofibromatosis 1.

Q2. How do you diagnose and how will you confirm it?

Ans: A thorough clinical examination of the patient and other family members is a must as diagnosis is mainly clinical. A diagnostic criterion is proposed for NF1. The above patient fulfilled required criteria for NF1 (Table 1).

Q3. What is the pattern of inheritance and chance of inheritance in each offspring?

Ans: It has an autosomal dominant pattern of inheritance. So, if one parent is affected then each child born will have 50% chance of having neurofibromatosis. If both the parents are normal, then incidence of the child to get affected is as that of incidence in general population 1 in 3,000 for NF1 (1 in 40,000 for NF2) which is due to sporadic mutation.

Q4. Enumerate Riccardi's classification for neurofibromatosis 1.

Ans: Riccardi's classification of neurofibromatosis -1 has been described in Table 2.

Q5. Enumerate the major cutaneous and systemic manifestations of neurofibromatosis 1 (NF1).

Ans: Major cutaneous and systemic manifestations of NF1 have been discussed in Table 3.

Table 2: Riccardi's classification of neurofibromatosis-1

NF1	von Recklinghausen (Syn: NF 1/peripheral neurofibromatosis)
NF2	Acoustic schwannoma (Syn: NF 2/central neurofibromatosis)
NF3	Mixed (multiple brain and spinal tumors with café-au-lait macules (CALM) and neurofibroma; CALMs are large, pale, and fewer than in NF1)
NF4	Variant (both neurofibroma and CALM are present but further categorization is not possible; CALMs may spontaneously disappear)
NF5	Segmental CALM or neurofibromas or both in one or more dermatomes (Syn: Mosaic localized NF 1)
NF6	CALM only
NF7	Late onset (manifestations after 20 years of age; CALMs may be absent)
NF8	Not otherwise specified (definite NF, but not characteristic of any other category; CALMs may be absent)

Table 3: Major cutaneous and systemic manifestations of neurofibromatosis-1 (NF-1)

System involved	*Manifestations and frequency*	*Age of onset in major clinical features*
Cutaneous	• Café-au-lait macules (CALMs) (>99%) • Cutaneous neurofibroma • Plexiform neurofibroma • Axillary freckling	• *CALMs:* Birth—12 years • *Cutaneous NF:* >7 years (late adolescence) • *Plexiform NF:* Birth–18 years • *Axillary freckling:* 3 years—adolescence
Ocular	• Lisch nodule (90%) • Hypertelorism (25%) • Glaucoma	• *Lisch nodule:* > 3 years of age
Skeletal	• Cranial: Macrocephaly (20–50%), sphenoid wing dysplasia (<5%) • Spinal: Scoliosis (5–10%), spina bifida • Limbs: Dysplasia of long bones—tibia (14%) • Pseudarthrosis (2%), thinning of long bone cortex, long bony overgrowth, absent patella	• *Sphenoid wing dysplasia:* Congenital • *Scoliosis:* Birth—18 years • *Pseudarthrosis of tibia:* Birth—13 years
Tumors	• Optic glioma (10–15%) • Malignant peripheral nerve sheath tumors (3–15%) • Central nervous system (CNS) tumors • Cerebral glioma • Pheochromocytoma (1%) • Juvenile myelomonocytic leukemia • Rhabdomyosarcoma • Retinoblastoma • Duodenal carcinoid • Somatostatinoma • Parathyroid adenoma	• *Peripheral nerve sheath tumors:* 5–75 years • *Cerebral glioma:* Lifelong • *Pheochromocytoma:* >10 years
Neurologic	• Unidentified bright objects on Magnetic resonance imaging (MRI) (50–75%) • Learning difficulties (30–50%) • Seizures (5%) • Mental retardation (<5%) • Aqueductal stenosis (2%) • Hydrocephalus	• *Learning difficulties:* Birth • *Seizures:* Lifelong • *Mental retardation:* Intelligence quotient (IQ) < 70—Birth • *Aqueductal stenosis:* Lifelong
Cardiovascular	• Hypertension (30%) • Pulmonic stenosis • Renal artery stenosis	
Renal	• Renal artery stenosis	*Renal artery stenosis:* Lifelong
Endocrinal	• Precocious puberty • Gynecomastia • Acromegaly • Addison's disease • Hyperparathyroidism • Pheochromocytoma	

Q6. What are the different types of neurofibromas?

Ans: Types of neurofibroma:

- *Cutaneous neurofibroma*: These are asymptomatic, skin-colored to pink, tan or brown, polypoid or pedunculated nodules, soft in texture that invaginates easily into the underlying tissue. Cutaneous neurofibromas (CNFs) can appear as early as 4–5 years of age but more typically develop around puberty with occasional acceleration during pregnancy.
- *Subcutaneous neurofibromas*: They occur deeper in the dermis, less well circumscribed and more firm than CNFs. Nearly one-fifth of NF1 patients have at least one subcutaneous neurofibroma (SNF) and one-quarter of these develop local complications from the tumor.
- *Plexiform neurofibromas*: These track along nerves to create tender, firm nodules or masses in the subcutaneous tissue *(palpation—bag of worms consistency)*, or they can infiltrate diffusely to involve all layers of the skin, fascia, muscle or even internal structures. Approximately 25% of NF1 patients have plexiform neurofibromas (PNFs), and often these lesions lead to such soft tissue and bony hypertrophy that massive distortion of the head, neck or extremities may result. Impingement upon nerves may lead to neurologic deficits.

Q7. What are the histopathological features of a neurofibroma?

Ans: Well circumscribed encapsulated, spindle cell proliferations with a mucinous background and many masts cells. Proliferation of Schwann cells, perineurial cells, endoneurial cells, mast cells and blood vessels.

Q8. What are the radiological features of central nervous system (CNS) seen in neurofibromatosis-1 (NF1)?

Ans: Brain MRI of children demonstrates regions of increased signal intensity on T2-weighted images referred as UBOs (Unidentified Bright Objects) seen commonly in internal capsule, basal ganglia, cortex, cerebellar hemispheres, optic tract and brainstem.

Target sign refers to radiological finding seen on MRI of neurofibroma in CNS, wherein plexiform neurofibroma demonstrates a targetoid appearance showing bright peripheral and dark central signals. Neurofibroma arising from dorsal root ganglion, when grows through neural foramina, compresses the spinal cord and causes dumbbell appearance.

Q9. What are the close differentials corresponding with the cutaneous manifestations?

Ans: The close differentials corresponding with the cutaneous manifestations have been described in Table 4.

Q10. Which condition is an allelic variant of neurofibromatosis-1 (NF 1)?

a. LEOPARD syndrome
b. Watson syndrome
c. Legius syndrome
d. McCune-Albright syndrome

Ans: a. Watson syndrome.

It is an autosomal dominant condition characterized by Lisch nodules, axillary freckling, pulmonary valvular stenosis, short stature and neurofibroma and defect attributed to NF1 gene on chromosome 17q.

Q11. What are the investigations that should be done to evaluate them and for periodic assessment?

Ans: Investigations of neurofibromatosis that should be done for periodic assessment have been discussed in Table 5.

Table 4: The close differentials corresponding with the cutaneous manifestations

Neurofibromas	***Multiple café-au-lait macules (CALMs)***
Other forms of neurofibromatosis: Segmental/mosaic NF1 Watson syndrome Autosomal dominant multiple café-au-lait patches alone (some allelic with NF1) Neurofibromatosis 2 *Tumors confused with neurofibromas:* Lipomatosis Bannayan-Riley-Ruvalcaba syndrome Fibromatoses Multiple endocrine neoplasia type 2B	NF 1 NF 2 LEOPARD syndrome McCune-Albright syndrome Tuberous sclerosis Fanconi anemia Multiple endocrinal neoplasia Bannayan-Riley-Ruvalcaba syndrome Bloom syndrome Ataxia telangiectasia Familial café-au-lait spots
Plexiform neurofibromas	Pigmented macules/lentiginosis
Localized overgrowth syndromes Klippel-Trenaunay-Weber syndrome Proteus syndrome	LEOPARD syndrome Neurocutaneous melanosis Peutz–Jeghers syndrome Piebaldism

Note: In NF, CALMs are round or oval, flat lesions of light brown pigmentation, present since birth, having smooth borders (Coast of California) unlike seen in McCune-Albright syndrome which has ragged borders (Coast of Maine).

Table 5: Parameters to be assessed periodically

• Development and progress at school	• Optic pathway glioma, glaucoma
• Visual symptoms, visual acuity and fundoscopy until age 7 years	• Rapid increase might indicate tumor or hydrocephalus
• Head circumference	• Abnormal pubertal development
• Height and Weight	• Delayed/precocious puberty due to pituitary/hypothalamic lesion
• Pubertal development	
• Blood pressure	• Consider renal artery stenosis, pheochromocytoma
• Cardiovascular examination	• Congenital heart disease, especially pulmonary stenosis
• Evaluation of spine	• Scoliosis and underlying plexiform neurofibromas
• Evaluation of the skin	• Cutaneous, subcutaneous and plexiform neurofibromas
• System examination if specific symptoms	

Baseline investigations:
- An ophthalmological evaluation (especially slit lamp examination, assessment of color vision and visual fields), skeletal survey and neurological screening (CT scan and magnetic resonance imaging (MRI) are to be advised.
- Awareness about unusual symptoms, particularly the clinical features of malignant peripheral nerve sheath tumors and of spinal cord compression are minimum requirements for an asymptomatic adult to seek medical consultation.

Q12. How do you manage a case of neurofibromatosis?

Ans: *Management*:
- The mainstay of management is age-specific monitoring of disease manifestations and patient education. Monitoring during adolescence and adulthood depends on patient preference and disease severity.
- *Café-au-lait macules (CALMs)*: Camouflage and Lasers (QS Ruby 694 nm, Copper vapor 511 nm, Er:YAG 2740 nm)
- *Neurofibromas*: Large and disfiguring—excision or CO_2 laser
- *Pruritus*: Antihistamines (Mast cell stabilizers preferred)
- *Pirfenidone*: Antifibrotic agent and it inhibits collagen matrix synthesis, fibroblast proliferation and farnesyl transferase inhibitor which downregulates RAS proto-oncogene
- Tipifarnib, a farnesyl transferase inhibitor that targets RAS
- *Imatinib*: It is a mast cell C-kit inhibitor showed promising results in unresectable plexiform neurofibroma
- Interferon α-2b and a combination of methotrexate and vinblastine also tried.
- *Newer drugs*: Cediranib [inhibitor of vascular endothelial growth factor (VEGF) receptor tyrosine kinase], Sirolimus [Mammalian target of rapamycin (mTOR) pathway inhibitor], pegylated interferon (PEG INF)α2b
- Photodynamic therapy.

Q13. What is the prognosis of neurofibromatosis 1 (NF1)?

Ans: As the onset of various manifestations is unpredictable, the prognosis depends on manifestations and time of occurrence. Early onset, rapid progression before puberty and extensive involvement have poor prognosis. Malignant transformation, sarcomatous changes, psychological morbidity due to extensive lesion further worsen the quality of life.

Q14. Is prenatal diagnosis useful in neurofibromatosis (NF)?

Ans: Yes. Multiplex polymerase chain reaction (PCR) for microsatellite markers linked to the *NF1* gene has been reported, helpful in preimplantation genetic diagnosis and prenatal diagnosis.

Q15. What are the characteristic features of neurofibromatosis 2 (NF2)?

Ans: Autosomal dominant in inheritance. Caused due to mutation in gene on chromosome 22q11, encodes for Merlin (also known as Neurofibromin 2/Schwannomin). Characterized by bilateral acoustic schwannomas, meningeal and glial tumors, neurofibromas, juvenile posterior subcapsular cataract and fewer CALMs, unlike NF1. No Lisch nodules and learning disability.

Q16. Outline the diagnostic criteria of neurofibromatosis 2.

Ans: Diagnostic criteria of neurofibromatosis 2 have been discussed in Box 1.

Box 1

Manchester clinical diagnostic criteria for neurofibromatosis-2 (NF2)

Bilateral vestibular schwannomas seen by magnetic resonance imaging (MRI) scan

Or

A first-degree relative with NF2 and unilateral vestibular schwannoma

Or

Two of the following criteria: Meningioma, glioma, schwannoma, juvenile posterior subcapsular cataract

Or

Unilateral vestibular schwannoma

Or

Two of the following criteria: Meningioma, glioma, schwannoma, juvenile posterior subcapsular cataract

Or

Multiple meningiomas (two or more) and unilateral vestibular schwannoma and any two of the following: Schwannoma, glioma, neurofibroma, cataract

CHAPTER 79

Tuberous Sclerosis

Kirti S Jangid

Case study Tuberous Sclerosis

Presenting Complaints

A 12-year-old girl presented with asymptomatic skin lesions over the face since childhood and history of recurrent seizures since the last 7 years.

Setting

Dermatology outpatient department.

History of Present Illness

A 12-year-old girl presented with history of asymptomatic reddish to skin colored elevated lesions over the face which progressively increased in size and number. She subsequently developed asymptomatic elevated skin colored lesions over the lower back. She had a history of recurrent seizures since the age of 5 years. She was born to nonconsanguineous parents. There was no history of similar skin findings or associated symptoms in siblings or parents. Family history was not relevant.

General Physical Examination

- Well oriented to time, place and person
- BMI–19 kg/m^2, Pulse–80 bpm, BP–110/60 mm Hg

Systemic Examination

No abnormality detected. Central nervous system (CNS) examination was normal.

Dermatological Examination

On examination, she was found to have skin colored to erythematous, asymptomatic, sessile and pedunculated lesions over face, hypopigmented plaques over lower back and gluteal region hypopigmented. She also had ivory-white macules ranging in size between 5 mm to 10 mm, four in number, well defined with irregular margins distributed over the trunk, coarse pits on the teeth, longitudinal grooves over toenails of both feet and a few periungual tumors. The mucous membrane of the oral cavity was normal. Ophthalmological evaluation was normal. Neurological examination too was normal.

Q1. What is the diagnosis?

a. Neurofibromatosis 1
b. Neurofibromatosis 2
c. Tuberous sclerosis
d. SLE

Ans: c. Tuberous sclerosis (TS). The characteristic skin lesions, epilepsy and an early onset point toward the diagnosis of tuberous sclerosis. Onset before the age of 5 years with cutaneous changes or with epilepsy is usual, although the disease may remain latent until adolescence or adult.

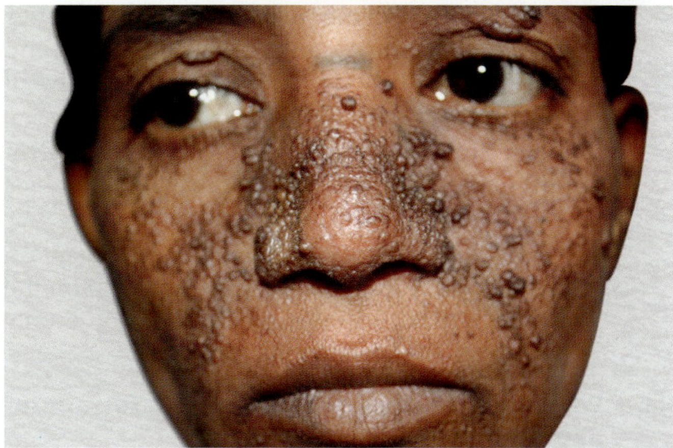

Fig. 1: Facial angiofibromas

Q2. What are the clinical features of tuberous sclerosis?

Ans: Tuberous sclerosis is clinically characterized by the triad; refractory epilepsy, mental retardation (sometimes severe) and angiofibromas of the face (typical for 70–90% of the patients, along with other types of cutaneous lesions). In the brain, there are hamartomas and calcified tubers and nodules (cortical brain stones), which determine refractory epilepsy and hydrocephalus. Angiofibromas (formerly misnamed adenoma sebaceum) consist of hyperplastic blood vessels and sebaceous glands of immature hair follicles. Other lesions include angioleiomyomas of the kidneys, liver, adrenal gland, rhabdomyomas of the heart and retinal glial nodules.

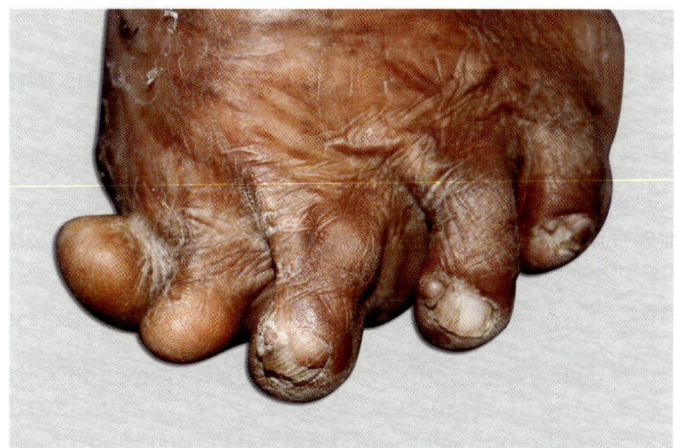

Fig. 2: Periungual fibromas

Q3. What are the cutaneous features of tuberous sclerosis?

Ans: Skin lesions are found in 60–70% of cases. Lesions of four types are pathognomonic which include angiofibromas, periungual fibromas (Koenen's tumors), shagreen patch, and white ovoid or ash-leaf-shaped macules.

- Angiofibromas usually appear between the age of 3 years and 10 years and sometimes later. Firm, discrete, red-brown, telangiectatic papules, 1–10 mm in diameter, extend from the nasolabial furrows to the cheeks and chin (Fig. 1).
- Periungual fibromas (Koenen's tumors) appear at or after puberty as smooth, firm, flesh-colored excrescences emerging from the nail folds (Fig. 2).
- The shagreen patch is an irregularly thickened, slightly elevated, soft, skin-colored plaque, usually in the lumbosacral region (Fig. 3).
- White ovoid or ash-leaf-shaped macules 1–3 cm in length, detectable by examination under Wood's light, may be found at birth or in early infancy, and may suggest the correct diagnosis in infants with convulsions.

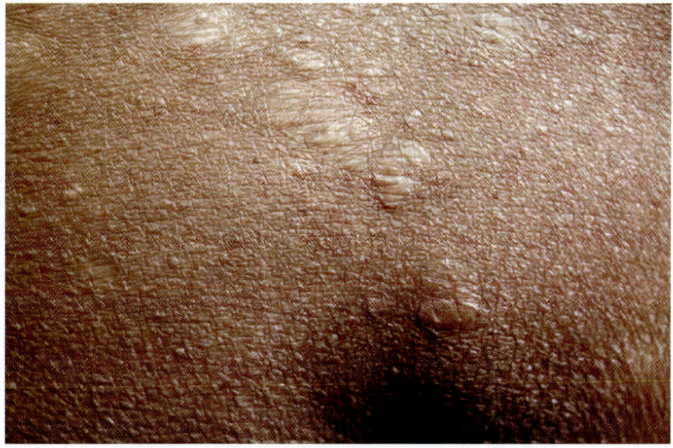

Fig. 3: Shagreen patch on the lower back

- Hypopigmented macules are seen in 2–3 per 1,000 of apparently normal newborn babies and therefore alone their presence is not indicative of tuberous sclerosis complex (TSC).
- Other cutaneous manifestations include firm fibromatous plaques, soft pedunculated fibromas around the neck and axillae and poliosis.
- Fibromatous tumors are occasionally present on the gums and palate and rarely are found on the tongue, larynx and pharynx. Small pits commonly occur in the tooth enamel.

Q4. What is the differential diagnosis for angiofibromas?

Ans: Acne vulgaris, rosacea, fibrous papules, multiple endocrine neoplasia 1, angiofibromas, Birt–Hogg–Dube syndrome, trichoepitheliomas, fibrofolliculomas, trichilemmomas, syringomas, dermal melanocytic nevi.

Q5. In which other conditions do you get ash-leaf macules?

Ans: Nevus depigmentosus, piebaldism, vitiligo, MEN 1 hypomelanotic macules, nevus anemicus.

Q6. What are the differential diagnoses for shagreen patch?

Ans: Shagreen patches are nothing but collagenomas. Differential diagnoses include familial cutaneous collagenoma, eruptive collagenomas, dermatofibrosis lenticularis disseminata (in Buschke-Ollendorff syndrome), sclerotic fibromas (Cowden syndrome), isolated connective tissue nevus, juvenile elastoma and nevus elasticus.

Q7. Give other names for tuberous sclerosis.

Ans: EPILOIA (epilepsy, low intelligence, adenoma sebaceum), Bourneville's disease, Pringle disease.

Q8. What is the inheritance pattern of tuberous sclerosis?

Ans: Tuberous sclerosis is inherited in an autosomal dominant fashion, though approximately 60–70% cases of tuberous sclerosis are attributed to new mutations. Molecular studies have identified pathogenic mutations in *TSC1* or *TSC2* genes in 75–90% of patients. However, 10–25% of patients do not show any genetic mutation with currently available testing. The *TSC2* gene that encodes tuberin is present on chromosome 16q13 and *TSC1* gene which encodes for hamartin and is present on chromosome 9q34. Loss of tuberin activity is thought to lead to activation of Rap1 in tumors of patients with TSC. Hamartin and tuberin act synergistically to regulate cellular growth and differentiation. Disturbance in this balance leads to interference in organogenesis resulting in hamartoma formation.

Q9. Enumerate the criteria for diagnosis of tuberous sclerosis.

Ans: International TSC Consensus Conference Revised Diagnostic criteria for TSC laid out in 2012:

- *Genetic diagnostic criteria:* The identification of either a TSC1 or TSC2 pathogenic mutation in DNA from normal tissue is sufficient to make a definite diagnosis of TSC. (Note that 10–25% of TSC patients have no mutation identified by conventional genetic testing, and a normal result does not exclude TSC, or have any effect on the use of clinical diagnostic criteria to diagnose TSC).
- *Clinical diagnostic criteria*
  - ***Major features***
    - Hypomelanotic macules (≥3, at least 5 mm diameter)
    - Angiofibromas (≥3) or fibrous cephalic plaque
    - Ungual fibromas (≥2)
    - Shagreen patch
    - Multiple retinal hamartomas
    - Cortical dysplasias
    - Subependymal nodules
    - Subependymal giant cell astrocytoma
    - Cardiac rhabdomyoma
    - Lymphangioleiomyomatosis (LAM)
    - Angiomyolipomas (≥2)
  - ***Minor features***
    - "Confetti" skin lesions
    - Dental enamel pits (>3)
    - Intraoral fibromas (≥2)
    - Retinal achromic patch
    - Multiple renal cysts
    - Nonrenal hamartomas.

Definite diagnosis: Two major features or one major feature with more than or equal to two minor features.

Possible diagnosis: Either one major feature or more than or equal to two minor features.

Q10. What are the systemic features of tuberous sclerosis?

Ans: *Learning difficulties* is present in 60–70% of cases.

Epilepsy is seen in almost all mentally retarded patients and in some 70% of those with average intelligence. It usually begins in infancy or early childhood.

Brain: Periventricular (subependymal) nodules, parenchymal hamartomas (cortical tubers), ventriculomegaly and rarely subependymal giant cell astrocytomas.

Ocular signs occur in 50%. Retinal phacomas, pigmentary and other retinal abnormalities, hypopigmented spots in the iris.

Cardiac and renal tumors: Cardiac rhabdomyomas detected by echocardiography occur in over 50% of infants. Renal involvement includes angiomyolipoma and renal cysts.

Pulmonary changes: Lymphangioleiomyomatosis is occasionally seen. Death can occur from tension pneumothorax or cor pulmonale.

Gastrointestinal tumor: Hamartomatous colonic polyps. Colonoscopy should be considered in the investigation of patients with TSC.

Endocrine and other metabolic disturbances: Pituitary–adrenal dysfunction, thyroid disorders and premature puberty.

Hands and feet: Cyst-like lesions of the phalanges and irregular thickening of the cortex of metatarsals and metacarpals.

Q11. Enlist the types of adenoma sebaceum.

Ans: Types of adenoma sebaceum are:

- *Balzer type:* There are only slight changes in the sebaceous glands.
- *Pringle type:* There is enormous hyperplasia of the sebaceous glands.
- *Hallopeau-Leredde type*: There is a predominance of the fibrous tissue with a verrucous surface.
- *Mixed type*: Mixed appearance where one lesion shows great hyperplasia of the sebaceous gland and neighboring lesion shows no sebaceous change.
- Epithelioma adenoides cysticum (misnomer, as they are actually trichoepitheliomas).

Q12. What investigations will you perform in a case of tuberous sclerosis?

Ans: Investigations:

- Routine evaluation in the form of complete blood count, liver and renal function tests
- Complete ophthalmological evaluation
- Baseline electrocardiogram (ECG) is recommended for all patients newly diagnosed with TSC
- The electroencephalograph (EEG), computed tomography (CT) or magnetic resonance imaging (MRI) scans of the brain to identify the extent and number of cortical tubers, renal ultrasounds for angiomyolipoma or cysts
- Echocardiograms for cardiac rhabdomyomas
- Molecular genetic testing where available
- Complete examination and further evaluation, where indicated of first-degree relatives.

Q13. What are the treatment modalities in such cases?

Ans: Multidisciplinary approach is used when systemic involvement presents. The cosmetic appearance may be improved by treating angiofibromas with the pulsed dye vascular laser (wavelength 585 nm), which reduces redness. The more papular/nodular lesions are best treated with carbon dioxide (CO_2) or erbium:YAG laser surgery, dermabrasion and surgical removal. Neurosurgery should be considered when epilepsy is uncontrolled by drugs and there is a fixed, circumscribed and electroencephalographic focus.

Q14. Which is the latest medication which has been devised for treating tuberous sclerosis?

a. Sirolimus
b. Tacrolimus
c. Rapamycin
d. Ruxolitinib

Ans: c. Rapamycin

Q15. What is the role of rapamycin in tuberous sclerosis complex?

Ans: Rapamycin is an immunosuppressant which forms an inhibitory complex with immunophilin FKBP12, and binds to and inhibits mammalian target of rapamycin (mTOR). It prevents activation of T and B cells by inhibiting their response to interleukin 2. It also has antineoplastic effects exerted through the downregulation of angiogenesis and the correction of aberrant growth signals. It has been found to reduce associated tumors in the brain, skin and kidneys. It is available in the market in two formulations: oral solution (60 mg per 60 mL) and tablets of 1 and 2 mg. Rapamycin for systemic manifestations is usually initiated at 0.2 mg/kg/day (1 mg/day) and titrated with adverse effects to as high as 5 mg/day. Everolimus, a derivative and prodrug for rapamycin has been approved for subependymal giant cell astrocytoma not amenable to surgery. It is also proposed as an antiepileptic medication in cases of epileptogenic cortical dysplasia and has been shown to reduce seizures and cognitive defects.

Rapamycin also has a role in reducing skin lesions, especially facial angiofibromas. Inhibition of mTOR pathway by topical rapamycin decreases the output of vascular endothelial growth factor (VEGF). Presently, rapamycin is only available as pharmacy made preparations of 0.1% in white soft paraffin ointment for facial angiofibromas. Rapamycin tablet crushed into 30 mL of 1% ointment or oral solution of rapamycin (1 mg/mL) is the usual methods employed for topical use.

CHAPTER 80

Systemic Amyloidosis

Anuradha Babu

Case study Systemic Amyloidosis

Presenting Complaints

Doctor, I have been developing bruises around my eyes for past 1 year. I have also noticed enlargement of my tongue for past 6 months. I have been suffering from tingling and numbness of fingers for past 3 months which has now become unbearable.

Setting

Dermatology outpatient department.

History of Present Illness

A 55-year-old woman presented with complaints of ecchymotic patches around her eyes for past 1 year. She also noticed progressive enlargement of her tongue over the past 6 months. She has been suffering from nocturnal pain that radiates from wrist to fingers, tingling and numbness of thumbs, index and middle fingers for past 3 months and now it has become very severe.

General Physical Examination

- Well-built and nourished
- Well oriented to time, place and person
- Pulse—80 beats per minute; Respiratory rate—20 breaths per minute
- Blood pressure—130/80 mm Hg
- Bilateral pitting pedal edema present
- No pallor/icterus/clubbing/lymphadenopathy.

Systemic Examination

Nervous system: Tinel's sign—positive. Tinel's sign is elicited by tapping over the median nerve as it passes through the carpal tunnel in the wrist. A sensation of tingling in the distribution of the median nerve over the hand denotes a positive response.

Dermatological Examination

- Macroglossia with dental impressions on the tongue
- Periorbital purpura
- Skin colored waxy papules and plaques in the periorbital area (Fig. 1).

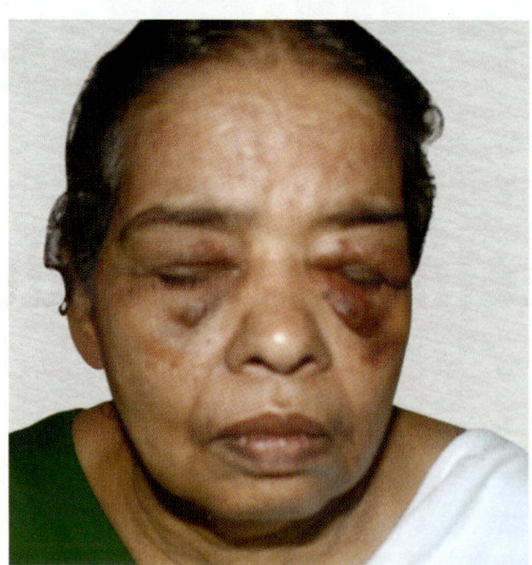

Fig. 1: Waxy purpuric nodules around the eyelids

Q1. What is the most probable diagnosis?

a. Lipoid proteinosis
b. Myxedema
c. Primary systemic amyloidosis
d. Sarcoidosis

Ans: c. Primary systemic amyloidosis. Cutaneous lesions like periorbital purpura, waxy papules and plaques along with macroglossia and carpal tunnel syndrome form the classical triad of primary systemic amyloidosis.

Q2. How do you classify systemic amyloidosis?

Ans: Classification:

- *Primary systemic amyloidosis (AL>AH amyloid protein)*
  - Plasma cell dyscrasias (more common)
  - Multiple myeloma-associated
- *Secondary systemic amyloidosis (reactive; AA amyloid protein)*
  - Chronic inflammation (e.g. Rheumatoid arthritis)
  - Chronic infection (e.g. Tuberculosis)
- *Hemodialysis-associated amyloidosis*
- *Genetic (inherited) forms of amyloidosis*
  - Familial amyloid polyneuropathy
  - Muckle-Wells syndrome and other cryopyrin-associated periodic syndrome
  - Familial Mediterranean fever
  - Tumor necrosis factor (TNF) receptor-associated periodic syndrome (TRAPS)
  - Familial amyloidosis, Finnish type.

Q3. Explain the pathogenesis of systemic amyloidosis.

Ans: The major component of amyloid is the fibril protein and the minor components are amyloid P component, glycosaminoglycans and apoE lipoprotein. Approximately 18 distinct forms of amyloid fibril proteins and their precursors have been identified, including AL (amyloid light chains), containing immunoglobulin light chains and AA (amyloid associated), a protein synthesized by the liver.

Each condition is associated with a specific precursor protein. The precursor proteins are initially soluble proteins. Then they undergo changes leading to aggregation, polymerization, fibril formation, and, finally, extracellular deposition in tissues as insoluble amyloid. This transformation process is multifactorial. In primary systemic amyloidosis, substitution of amino acids in specific positions in the variable region of the immunoglobulin light chain potentially destabilizes the light chains and increases their likelihood of being converted to amyloid fibrils. The accumulation of these relatively inert amyloid fibrils within the vital organs leads to pressure atrophy and eventually interferes with the normal functioning of the organ.

Q4. What are the systemic features of primary systemic amyloidosis?

Ans: Primary systemic amyloidosis is associated with a wide spectrum of organ involvement. The presenting symptoms are often varied and nonspecific, such as fatigue, weight loss, paresthesia, dyspnea or syncopal attacks. Other findings include:

- The tongue may be uniformly enlarged and firm or it may have hemorrhagic papules, plaques and blisters on its surface
- Renal involvement manifests as proteinuria and hypoalbuminemia
- Cardiac involvement may eventually lead to restrictive cardiomyopathy and congestive cardiac failure resulting in dyspnea, hepatomegaly and pedal edema
- Autonomic involvement can result in postural hypotension, impotence and gastroparesis
- Sensory neuropathies are also common
- Muscle weakness may be caused by neuropathy, or by amyloid infiltration of muscle or its vascular supply
- Amyloid deposits in joints may mimic rheumatoid arthritis, and deposition around shoulders may cause extensive soft tissue enlargement (the shoulder-pad sign)
- Hepatomegaly occurs in about 50%, splenomegaly in 10%, nephrotic syndrome in 30% and congestive cardiac failure in 30% of patients

- The carpal tunnel syndrome has been reported in up to 25% of patients with primary systemic amyloidosis.

Q5. What are the cutaneous features seen in primary systemic amyloidosis?

Ans: Cutaneous features:
- Following minor trauma, petechiae, purpura and ecchymoses are often observed, especially on the eyelids, neck, axillae and anogenital region due to infiltration of blood vessels by amyloid deposits
- Characteristically, periorbital purpura (the "raccoon eyes" sign) may be precipitated by coughing, the Valsalva maneuver, or proctoscopy as well as after pinching or rubbing the skin (pinch purpura)
- About 25% of individuals with primary systemic amyloidosis show clinically evident skin involvement. Skin infiltration by amyloid presents as waxy, translucent or purpuric papules, nodules and plaques
- Less often, sclerodermoid appearance, bullous lesions, nail dystrophy, acquired acral cutis laxa and cutis verticis gyrata with diffuse alopecia may be seen.

Q6. What are the histopathological findings and special staining characteristics for amyloid?

Ans: Histopathological features and special stains:
- Homogeneous, hyaline, eosinophilic deposits in H&E-stained sections
- Crystal violet metachromasia
- Positive staining with alkaline Congo red
- Apple-green birefringence under polarized light after Congo red staining; also dichroic
- Fibrillar structure on electron microscopy
- Stains brightly by ultraviolet fluorescence microscopy after thioflavin T staining
- Staining with antibodies to amyloid P component
- Staining with antibodies directed against specific precursors (e.g. Keratin).

Q7. What is the percentage of patients with primary systemic amyloidosis in whom amyloid deposits can be demonstrated in random rectal biopsies or in abdominal subcutaneous fat aspirates?

a. 50–60%
b. 60–70%
c. 70–80%
d. 80–90%

Ans: d. 80–90%

Q8. What are the treatment options for primary systemic amyloidosis?

Ans: Treatment options for primary systemic amyloidosis:
- Without therapy the prognosis for primary systemic amyloidosis is poor; median survival is about 13 months, especially if there is cardiac involvement
- The treatment of choice for younger patients with minimal cardiac involvement is high-dose melphalan followed by autologous peripheral blood stem cell transplantation
- For older patients with or those with cardiac involvement, newer targeted agents (e.g. lenalidomide, bortezomib) are used alone or in combination with systemic corticosteroids and melphalan
- Supportive measures are administered according to the organs affected and the consequent manifestations.

Q9. What are the causes for secondary systemic amyloidosis?

Ans: Causes of secondary systemic amyloidosis:
- Secondary systemic amyloidosis occurs as a complication of severe chronic inflammatory diseases of an infectious or noninfectious nature, such as tuberculosis, lepromatous leprosy, rheumatoid arthritis and ankylosing spondylitis. It has also been observed in patients with hidradenitis suppurativa, dystrophic epidermolysis bullosa, generalized psoriasis, scleroderma, systemic lupus erythematosus and dermatomyositis
- Secondary systemic amyloidosis is characterized by the deposition of a distinctive nonimmunoglobulin protein designated AA (amyloid A protein)
- AA amyloidosis usually affects kidneys, liver, spleen, adrenals and heart. Cutaneous lesions of amyloidosis are rare in this type of amyloidosis
- Successful treatment of underlying infectious or inflammatory disease may halt the progression of reactive amyloidosis.

Q10. How do you evaluate a patient with suspected primary amyloidosis?

Ans: Investigations:
- Routine evaluation in the form of complete blood count, liver and renal function tests
- Conventional urine heat testing and electrophoresis of serum and urine samples may fail to demonstrate small quantities of monoclonal paraprotein or Bence-Jones protein

- Immunoelectrophoresis of serum and concentrated urine samples is essential
- Echocardiography is valuable in the evaluation of amyloid heart disease. It usually reveals a concentrically thickened left ventricle and often a thickened right ventricle, with a normal-to-small cavity
- Doppler studies are useful and may show abnormal relaxation early in the course of the disease. Advanced involvement is characterized by restrictive hemodynamics
- 18F-Fluorodeoxyglucose positron-emission tomography has been used in primary systemic amyloidosis evaluation
- Biopsy of a cutaneous lesion, if present, has the advantage of safety and a high diagnostic yield. Biopsy results in clinically normal skin may be positive in as many as 50% of cases of primary systemic amyloidosis
- Findings from abdominal fat aspiration are positive in almost 80% of patients
- Rectal biopsy reveals positive findings in about 80% of patients
- If specimens from the biopsy sites are negative for amyloid, tissue should be obtained from an organ or area with suspected involvement, such as the kidney, liver, heart, or sural nerve.

CHAPTER 81

Lipoid Proteinosis

Tanumay Raychaudhury, Navya Handa

Case study Lipoid Proteinosis

Presenting Complaints

Doctor, my 7-year-old boy has started to develop scars over the face and dorsum of hands, and multiple raised lesions around eyes, knees and elbows since 1 year. His voice also is totally different from the others since infancy.

Setting

Dermatology outpatient department.

History of Present Illness

7-year-old male patient, born to consanguineous parents, was normal at birth, but after 6 months of life developed weak cry and a different muffled voice. At 6 years of age, he started to develop multiple skin colored raised lesions on the back of the hands, knees, elbows, face and eyelid margins. Some of the lesions have healed with brown depressed scars. He has no history of frontal headache, seizures or visual disturbance and his intelligence is normal.

General Physical and Systemic Examination

No abnormality detected.

Dermatological Examination

- Beaded papules along the margins of the eyelids
- Multiple small atrophic varioliform scars over the face
- Thick tongue which cannot be protruded
- Verrucous nodules present over the knees and elbows.

Q1. What is the most likely diagnosis?

a. Lipoid proteinosis
b. Hydroa vacciniforme
c. Erythropoietic protoporphyria
d. Amyloidosis

Ans: a. Lipoid proteinosis (LP or Urbach-Wiethe disease). The presence of hoarseness of voice since birth with atrophic varioliform scars, beaded papules along eyelid (moniliform blepharosis) suggests the diagnosis of LP. Absence of photosensitivity rules out hydroa vacciniforme and erythropoietic protoporphyria.

Q2. How do you confirm the diagnosis of lipoid proteinosis?

Ans: Confirmation of diagnosis:

- Lipoid proteinosis can be diagnosed based on clinical feature. It can be confirmed by histology: Disruption and/or duplication of the basement membrane along with deposition of periodic acid-Schiff (PAS) positive, diastase-resistant hyaline material at the dermo-epidermal junction, papillary dermis, surrounding capillaries, and around adnexal epithelia with appearance of sweat coils

- *Immunofluorescence*: Labeling with anti-collagen antibody shows type IV and V collagen accumulation and reduction of type I and III collagen around blood vessels
- *Gene analysis*: Demonstration of pathogenic *ECM1* gene mutation in LP now provides a definite means of diagnosis
- Computed tomography scan brain: Calcification.

Q3. What is the genetics behind lipoid proteinosis?

Ans: The cause of LP (hyalinosis cutis et mucosae) has been identified as loss-of-function mutations in the gene encoding extracellular matrix protein 1 on chromosome 1q21. The function of the protein ECM1 is still unclear, although an important role in skin physiology and homeostasis has been hypothesized.

Q4. What is the etiopathogenesis of lipoid proteinosis?

Ans: The etiopathogenesis of the LP is not still completely understood, but it seems to be related to an alteration in the synthesis and metabolism of the collagen, leading to an increase in the synthesis of types IV and V collagen by the endothelial cells of the blood vessels, a glycoprotein substance by the fibroblasts, and a decrease in the production of collagen types I and II.

Q5. What are the characteristic cutaneous changes in lipoid proteinosis?

Ans: Characteristic features:

Cutaneous findings: The skin of children with LP is highly susceptible to damage, being reflected in the appearance of chicken pox-like scars and yellowish papules (Fig. 1). Early lesions include collection of recurrent blood or pus-filled vesicles, bullae, macules, papules, and skin-colored nodules, which are often pruritic and may coalesce resulting in diffuse thickening of the skin and mucous membrane. Beaded papules along the eye margin is characteristic (Fig. 2).

Oral cavity: Infiltration of the oral mucosa may lead to xerostomia, dysphagia, limited tongue movements and speech difficulties. Papules on the tongue, frenulum, and lips may coalesce to give cobblestone appearance. Tongue may be thickened, firmed, and enlarged crenated which may interfere with mastication (Fig. 3). Other findings include hyperkeratosis on the labial, buccal, and palatal mucosa, hyperplasia or aplasia of the teeth, as well as recurrent inflammation of the parotid and submandibular glands.

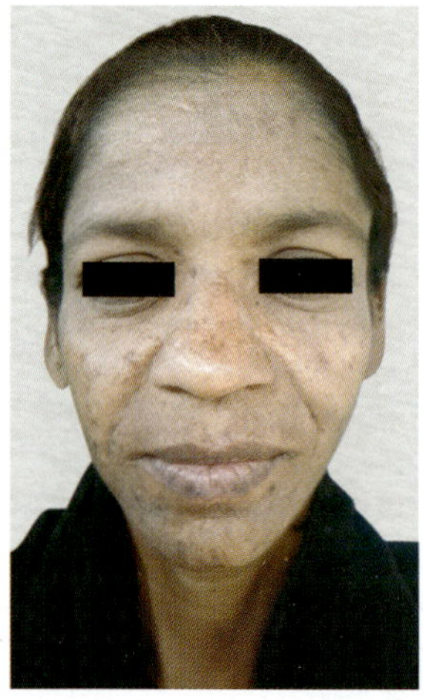

Fig. 1: Yellow papules over face and mild scarring

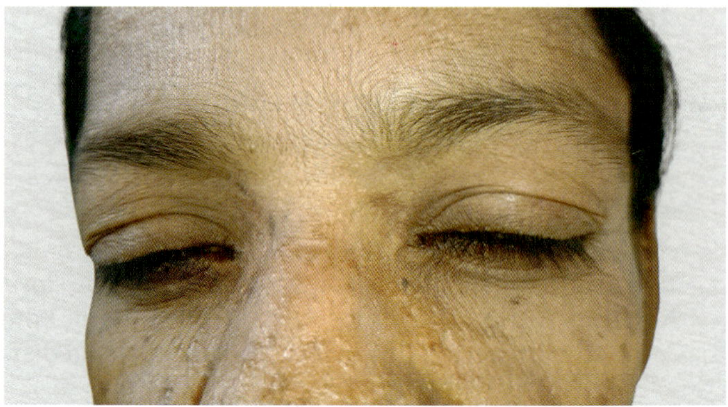

Fig. 2: Close up showing the yellow papules and also beaded papules on eyelids

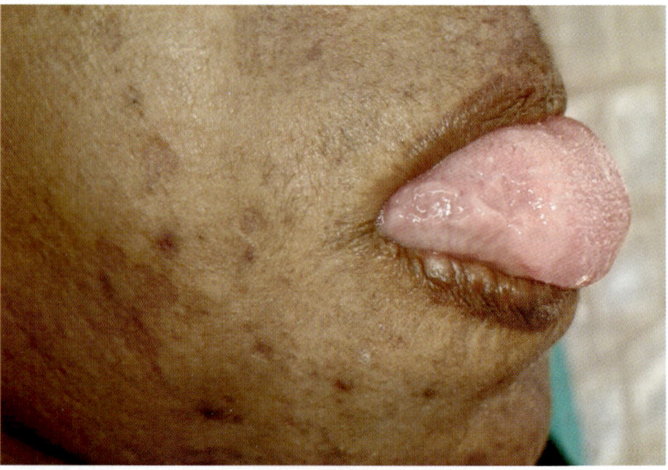

Fig. 3: Large protruding tongue with impressions of teeth laterally

Hair and nail: Infiltration of the scalp often gives patchy or diffuse alopecia. Nail dystrophy with hemorrhagic blisters on the wrists, fingers, and nail bed is a common finding.

Q6. Enumerate the systemic involvement and what are the investigations that should be done to evaluate them.

Ans: Although autopsy studies have shown LP to be a generalized disorder with microscopic deposits of hyaline material in practically every organ, symptoms related to these deposits are minimal or absent. The respiratory system, upper gastrointestinal tract, central nervous system, blood vessels, and lymph nodes may be involved.

Ocular manifestation: Hyaline deposits have been described in the conjunctiva, cornea, trabeculum, and retina leading to corneal opacities or secondary glaucoma.

Investigations: Slit lamp examination, tonometry.

Gastrointestinal involvement: The characteristic yellowish nodules have been found in esophagus, stomach, duodenum, and colon. Deposition of hyaline material in the small bowel may lead to intestinal bleeding.

Investigations: Endoscopy and colonoscopy can demonstrate gastrointestinal deposits. Biopsy shows the typical deposition of eosinophilic PAS-positive hyaline material, similar to the findings in the skin biopsies. Small bowel follow through shows multiple well-defined, round, small filling defects all over the jejunum.

Central nervous system involvement: Epilepsy, memory loss, schizophrenic behavior, mental retardation, emotional changes, and other neuropsychiatric abnormalities may be seen in some patients.

Investigations: Computed tomography shows calcification in the temporal lobes or hippocampus.

Respiratory tract involvement: Involvement of epiglottis and vocal cords results in hoarseness of voice.

Investigations: Laryngoscopy reveals beaded deposits.

Q7. How will you treat a case of lipoid proteinosis?

Ans: There is no effective and precise treatment regimen for LP. This disease compromises the quality of life due to its disfiguring scars and multisystem involvement. The disease is not life-threatening except for the respiratory obstruction in severe cases. If the lesions start at an early age, it is found to be self-limiting.

- However, for esthetic consideration, dermabrasion and chemical skin peeling can be done.
- Treatment with dimethyl sulfoxide, D-penicillamine, etretinate, intralesional heparin has also been tried. None of them have given a promising result.
- Laser microlaryngoscopy, mucosal stripping, or dissection of the vocal cords and excision of deposits may be performed to preserve or improve the quality of voice.
- In very severe cases, if there is diffuse infiltration of the pharynx and larynx causing respiratory distress, tracheostomy is required.

Q8. Calcification in lipoid proteinosis is seen in:

a. Hippocampus
b. Falx cerebri
c. Dura
d. Cerebellum

Ans: a. Hippocampus.

Q9. What is the prognosis of lipoid proteinosis?

Ans: Lipoid proteinosis has a stable or slowly progressive course. The presence of this disease is compatible with a normal life span unless altered by airway obstruction or fatal seizure activity. Mortality rates in infants and adults are slightly increased because of laryngeal obstruction. Patients with significant airway compromise may require permanent tracheostomy.

CHAPTER 82

Xanthomatosis

Nagendra Beniwal

Case study Xanthomatosis

Presenting Complaints

Doctor, I have developed painless, yellowish- to skin-colored swellings involving both lower eyelids for last 3 years.

Setting

Dermatology outpatient department.

History of Present Illness

A 47-year-old lady presented with complaints of asymptomatic yellowish linear lesions involving both lower eyelids for last 3 years which was insidious in onset and gradually progressive. There is no history of photosensitivity, oral ulcers or joint pains. She has regular menstrual cycles and two healthy children.

General Physical Examination and Systemic Examination

No abnormality detected.

Dermatological Examination

Fairly well-circumscribed yellowish plaques measuring approximately 0.5 cm involving medial aspect of both the lower eyelids symmetrically. There is also a large 2.5 cm linear lesion on the left lower eyelid extending from the medial lesion (Fig. 1).
Soft in consistency.
No eye involvement.

Q1. What is the most likely diagnosis?

a. Xanthelasma
b. Sebaceous hyperplasia
c. Sarcoidosis
d. Lipoma

Ans: a. Xanthelasma.

Asymptomatic yellowish plaques involving medial aspect of both the lower eyelids suggests diagnosis of xanthelasma (xanthelasma palpebrarum).

Q2. How do you diagnose xanthelasma?

Ans: Diagnosis of xanthelasma is based on clinical presentation.

Q3. How will you confirm the diagnosis?

Ans: Diagnosis is made on clinical grounds; however, excisional biopsy or punch biopsy can be done for histopathological correlation in case of atypical presentation or for research purpose.

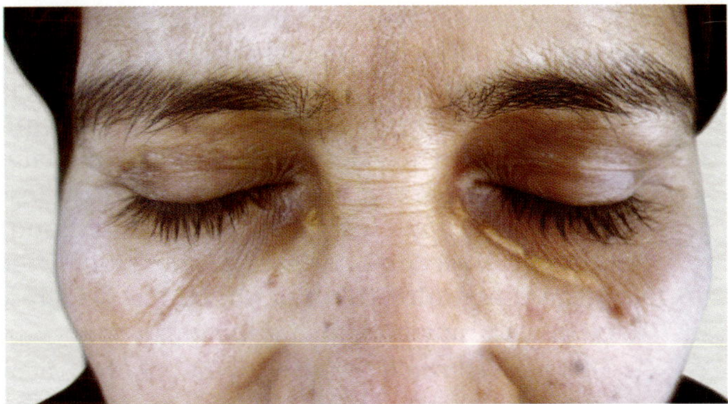

Fig. 1: Well-circumscribed yellowish plaques involving medial aspect of both lower eyelids. Large 2.5 cm linear lesion on the left lower eyelid extending from the medial lesion

Evaluation of other laboratory parameter is required mainly to diagnose associated metabolic disturbances.

Q4. What is xanthelasma?

Ans: Xanthelasma [Greek word: xanthos (yellow), elasma (beaten metal plate)]. Xanthelasma palpebrarum being the most common form of xanthomas may be associated with familial hypercholesterolemia and familial hypercholesterolemia. However, 50% of them may have normal lipid levels.

Q5. What are the other xanthomas you know of?

Ans: Other xanthomas:

- Eruptive xanthomas
- Tuberous xanthomas
- Tendinous xanthomas
- Planar xanthomas
  - Palmar xanthoma
  - Intertriginous xanthomas
  - Diffuse xanthoma
- Corneal arcus
- Tonsillar xanthoma.

Q6. What are the typical presentations and associations of various xanthomas?

Ans: Typical presentation and associations of various xanthomas are listed in Table 1:

Other common associations:

- Obesity
- Cholestasis
- Diabetes
- Hypothyroidism.

Q7. What all investigations will you advise?

Ans: Investigations:

- Lipid profile
- Blood sugar

Table 1: Typical presentations and associations of various xanthomas

Type	*Presentation*	*Association*
Xanthelasma palpebrarum	• Most common type • Subtype of plane xanthoma • Consultation is mainly for esthetic reasons • Yellowish-orange, soft papules-plaque involving eyelids particularly medial canthus and upper eyelids	• 50% of patients have lipid disorders • Familial hypercholesterolemia • Familial dysbetalipoproteinemia
Eruptive xanthomas	• Sudden onset, in crops • Multiple reddish-yellow papules involving extensor surface of extremities and buttocks • Often transient course	• Familial hypertriglyceridemia with chylomicronemia (fasting level > 1,000 mg/dL) • Familial lipoprotein lipase deficiency • Medications: Protease inhibitors, estrogen therapy, retinoids
Tuberous xanthomas	• Yellowish, indurated, firm nodules involving extensor aspect of elbows, knees, knuckles and buttocks	• Familial hypercholesterolemia • Familial dysbetalipoproteinemia
Tendinous xanthomas	• Firm subcutaneous nodule attached to Achilles tendon, extensor tendons of hands, knees and elbows	• Familial hypercholesterolemia • Familial dysbetalipoproteinemia • Cerebrotendinous xanthomatosis
Planar xanthomas • Generalized • Palmar • Intertriginous	Yellowish macules, papules or plaques over face, neck, chest	Monoclonal gammopathies
Corneal arcus	White ring in front of the periphery of the iris	• Familial hypercholesterolemia

- Thyroid profile
- Complete blood count
- Ultrasonography
- Biopsy.

Q8. What are its histopathological features?

Ans: Histopathological examination (HPE) is not must for establishing diagnosis since it is based predominantly on clinical presentation. HPE shows characteristic foamy macrophages which are vacuolated macrophages filled with lipid droplets.

Foamy histiocytes generally have one nucleus, but Touton giant cells which are multinucleated histiocytes can also be present.

Along with foam cells:

- Eruptive xanthomas have lymphoid cells, neutrophils and free lipid in dermis.

Tuberous and tendinous xanthomas have cholesterol clefts.

Xanthelasma have superficial location of foam cells.

Q9. What are common differential diagnoses of various xanthomas?

Ans: Common differential diagnoses of various xanthomas are discussed in Table 2.

Q10. Which type of xanthoma is associated with neurological disease?

a. Eruptive xanthomas
b. Xanthelasma palpebrarum
c. Cerebrotendinous xanthoma
d. Corneal arcus

Ans: c. Cerebrotendinous xanthoma.

It is a rare genetic metabolic disorder of cholesterol and bile acid metabolism. There is defect in the *CYP27A1* gene that codes for sterol 27-hydoxylase leading to subsequent overproduction and accumulation of cholestanol (a physiological sterol) in multiple tissues of the body. These patients cannot convert cholesterol to chenodeoxycholate, which is an important bile acid. Patients manifest with cataract in adolescence or early childhood, xanthomas in second or third decade along with significant neurological impairment like seizures, dementia, extrapyramidal dysfunctions.

Diagnosis can be ascertained by finding of elevated plasma cholesterol levels as measured with gas chromatography.

Treatment: Chenodeoxycholate 250 mg TDS which arrests progression of neurological symptoms as well as xanthomas.

Table 2: Common differential diagnoses of various xanthomas

Eruptive xanthomas	Xanthoma disseminatum Sarcoid Juvenile xanthogranuloma
Plane xanthomas	Amyloidosis Sarcoidosis Pseudoxanthoma elasticum
Xanthelasma	Syringoma Sebaceous hyperplasia Adnexal neoplasm
Tuberous or tendinous xanthomas	Lipoma Cyst Neurofibroma

Q11. What is the rate-limiting enzyme in lipid metabolism and which lipid-lowering medicine group is based on that?

Ans: HMG-CoA reductase enzyme (3-hydroxy-3-methylglutaryl coenzyme A reductase) is the rate-limiting enzyme in cholesterol synthesis. Statins cause competitive inhibition of HMG-CoA enzyme.

Q12. What are common drugs associated with hyperlipidemia?

Ans: Common drugs associated with hyperlipidemia are:

- Glucocorticoids
- Anabolic steroids
- Estrogens
- Antihypertensive medications
- Retinoids
- Calcineurin inhibitors: cyclosporine
- Cimetidine
- Antiepileptic drugs.

Q13. How will you treat this case? What all other modalities you can think of for better aesthetic outcome?

Ans: Treatment:

- Chemical Cautery
  - Trichloroacetic acid
  - Bichloroacetic acid
- Laser
  - Ultrapulse CO_2 laser
  - 1450-nm diode laser
  - 1064-nm Q-switched Nd:YAG Laser
  - Er:YAG laser
- Radiofrequency
- Excision with blepharoplasty.

Q14. What medication or advice will you offer to a patient who turns out to have associated hyperlipidemia?

Ans: Management:

- *Lifestyle modification:*
  - Increased physical activity
  - Weight control
  - Dietary management:
    - Restriction of dietary saturated fat and trans fat
    - Replacing animal fat with vegetable oils (Polyunsaturated fatty acids)
    - Restriction of high fat/high sugar desserts
- Drug therapy:
  - Statins
  - Ezetimibe resins
  - Fibrates
  - Niacin.

CHAPTER 83

Endogenous Ochronosis

Nikita Lodha

Case study Endogenous Ochronosis

Presenting Complaints

Doctor, my eyes, face and back of hands have a black discoloration since 12 years. Now, I have difficulty in walking since the past 2 weeks.

Setting

Dermatology outpatient department.

History of Present Illness

A 42-year-old lady presented with complaints of darkening of face since the last 12 years. The pigmentation appeared over her ears, nose and cheeks, and gradually progressed to involve the forehead. On enquiry, she revealed dark staining of underwear since childhood. There was no history of photoexacerbation or systemic complaints. No history of exposure to topical or systemic medications, including heavy metals, in the past. She has now developed severe pain in her hips and is finding it difficult to walk without support since the last 2 weeks. She was born of a nonconsanguineous marriage. The family history was not contributory.

General Physical Examination

Well-oriented to time, place and person
Body mass index: 25 kg/m^2
Vitals: Stable

Systemic Examination

Muskuloskeletal: Tenderness of bilateral hip joints with severe restriction of movements.

Dermatological Examination

- Blue-gray diffuse macular pigmentation over nose tip, cheeks and forehead
- Thickening and blue-gray tinge over ear cartilage
- Brown pigmentation over sclera, between limbus and lateral canthi
- Mucosa, teeth and nails were normal.

Q1. What is the most likely diagnosis?

a. Endogenous ochronosis
b. Exogenous ochronosis
c. Argyria
d. Chrysiasis

Ans: a. Endogenous ochronosis (EO or Alkaptonuria)
Cutaneous and scleral pigmentation (ochronosis), thickened and pigmented ear cartilage and dark staining of the underwear (due to staining by urine) suggests diagnosis of EO. No history of exposure to topical phenolic compounds rules out exogenous ochronosis. No history of gold or silver therapy rules out argyria and chrysiasis. No mucosal pigmentation also is a point against argyria.

Q2. What is endogenous ochronosis?

Ans: Endogenous ochronosis, also called as alkaptonuria, is a rare (1:2,50,000) autosomal recessive metabolic disorder caused due to homogentisic acid oxidase (HGO) deficiency. HGO is essential for the metabolism of homogentisic acid (HGA), an intermediate byproduct of phenylalanine and tyrosine metabolism. Excessive HGA accumulates in the connective tissues, including the dermis (ochronosis) and is excreted in the urine, which often turns dark. The nomenclature 'alkaptonuria' is based on the affinity of HGA to alkalize (alkapton) and its excretion in the urine (uria). Alkaptonuria has the distinction of being the first disease in which a Mendelian recessive inheritance pattern was proposed.

Q3. What is the cause of blue-gray pigmentation?

Ans: Endogenous ochronosis is characterized by the deposition of oxidized and polymerized forms of HGA, i.e. benzoquinone acetic acid in connective tissues (including skin, bone, tendon, cartilage, sclera). However, the affected tissues appear bluish-gray because of the Tyndall effect.

Q4. What are the clinical manifestations of endogenous ochronosis?

Ans: Dark urine, cutaneous pigmentation, and arthropathy are the hallmarks of this disorder.

- Dark urine (Homogentisic aciduria)
  - Earliest and probably the only symptom in pediatric patients. Parents may complain of 'spotting or staining' of the diapers after cleansing in soap (alkaline). Urine turns black on exposure to air for many hours.
- Cutaneous pigmentation (Ochronosis)
  - Becomes obvious by 2nd or 3rd decade. Pigmentation is more pronounced in sun-exposed sites, cartilaginous areas and areas with sweat glands (forehead, cheeks, axilla, genitalia, palms and soles). Sweat can stain clothes brown.
  - Thickened and blue-gray pigmentation of the ear cartilage. Pigment also appears in earwax. Calcification of the ear cartilage may occur.
  - Blue-brown pigmentation of the sclera is observed midway between the limbus and the outer and inner canthi at the insertion of the recti muscles (Osler's sign). Pigment deposit may also be seen in the conjunctiva and cornea. However, vision is unaffected.
  - Blue-black discoloration may be seen on the skin of the hands, corresponding to the underlying tendons, or in the web between the thumb and index finger.
  - Brown staining of the nails may be seen.
  - Buccal mucosa and larynx may be pigmented.
- Ochronotic arthritis and arthropathy
  - Starts around the 4th decade. It causes progressive degenerative arthropathy, mainly affecting the axial and weight-bearing joints like intervertebral joints in the spine and the knees. It begins in the lumbar region, and may progress to involve the thoracic spine leading to respiratory dysfunction due to restricted chest expansion.
- Other visceral manifestations
  - Aortic or mitral valvulitis and calcification
  - Atherosclerosis
  - Urolithiasis, ochronotic prostate stones
  - Pigment deposits may occur in the respiratory tract (larynx, trachea and bronchi), nervous system, teeth and endocrine organs.

Q5. How will you confirm the diagnosis of endogenous ochronosis?

Ans:

- Identification and quantification of HGA in urine using gas-liquid chromatography and mass spectrophotometer in blood is the best choice of a confirmatory test
- Polymerase chain reaction (PCR): Screening for mutations in *HGD* gene on Chromosome 3, the gene encoding HGO.

Q6. What investigations would you like to do to support your diagnosis?

Ans:
- Biochemical tests on urine sample and their results
  - Urine turns black on exposure to air for many hours
  - Addition of 10% alkali: Positive (dark black color)
  - Benedict's test: Positive (black color)
  - Ferric chloride test: Positive (transient green color)
  - Addition of equal volume of ammoniacal silver nitrate ($AgNO_3$): Black precipitate of reduced silver
  - Thin layer chromatography followed by staining with ammoniacal $AgNO_3$: Black color spot comparable to pure standard of benzoquinone
  - Radiographs of the spine showing flattened and calcified intervertebral disks are pathognomonic. Calcification of the pinna may be seen.

Q7. How to investigate the patient following the initial diagnosis of endogenous ochronosis?

Ans: To establish the extent of disease, the following evaluations are recommended:
- Complete physical examination with particular attention to range of motion in the spine and large joints
- Ophthalmologic evaluation
- Electrocardiogram and echocardiogram in individuals older than 40 years of age
- Ultrasound or abdominal CT examination to evaluate for the presence of renal calculi
- Medical genetics consultation.

Q8. What is the treatment of endogenous ochronosis?

Ans: Treatment:
- No effective therapy is available
- Dietary restrictions of proteins (predominantly phenylalanine and tyrosine) play a limited role in halting the progression of the disease
- Vitamin C (ascorbic acid) in the dose of 500 mg twice daily, inhibits the polymerization of HGA, but its efficacy has not been proven
- Nitisinone, a triketone herbicide, inhibits the enzyme 4-hydroxyphenylpyruvate dioxygenase (HPPD) that is responsible for the synthesis of HGA. Clinical trials show promising results in arthropathy.

Q9. What should you look out for in follow-ups?

Ans: Active surveillance for arthropathy, cardiac, renal, and prostatic complications should be done after the 4th decade.

Q10. How to evaluate relatives at risk?

Ans: Presence of elevated urinary HGA in siblings of affected individuals allows early diagnosis and intervention to prevent secondary complications. However, biochemical testing cannot detect the carrier state.

Q11. What is the role of genetic counseling in endogenous ochronosis?

Ans: Endogenous ochronosis is an autosomal recessive disease. At conception, each sibling of an affected individual has a 25% chance of being affected, a 50% chance of being an asymptomatic carrier, and a 25% chance of being unaffected and not a carrier. Once an at-risk sibling is known to be unaffected, the chance of his/her being a carrier is 2/3. Carrier testing for at-risk family members is possible by PCR, if the disease-causing mutations in the family are known.

Prenatal diagnosis and preimplantation genetic diagnosis for at-risk pregnancies require prior identification of the disease-causing mutations in the family.

Q12. What is the prognosis of endogenous ochronosis?

Ans: Life expectancy is normal although they are at an increased risk for cardiac problems and may require surgical intervention for arthropathy.

Q13. Enumerate the other types of ochronosis.

Ans: *Exogenous ochronosis:* It is an acquired condition and lack of any systemic involvement is the key differentiating feature from alkaptonuria. It most commonly results from the use of topical hydroquinones (usually used as bleaching creams) but has also been associated with the use of phenol, quinine injection, resorcinol, picric acid, mercury, and oral antimalarials.

Idiopathic ochronosis: It is characterized by the absence of the use of any drug and features of alkaptonuria. Features of ochronosis per se are present. Laboratory tests of blood and urine are negative.

Q14. How to classify exogenous ochronosis?

Ans: Dogliotti classified exogenous ochronosis into three clinical stages:

a. Erythema and mild hyperpigmentation
b. Hyperpigmentation, pigmented colloid milium (Caviar-like lesions) and scanty atrophy
c. Papulonodular lesions.

Q15. Describe the histopathological features of ochronosis?

Ans: Histopathological features:

- Banana-shaped fibers or ocher bodies in the dermis. The ochre or yellow-brown pigment is present within collagen bundles which tend to fracture transversely resulting in pointed ends
- Fine pigment granules are also seen in the endothelium, macrophages and basement membrane of sweat glands. Collagen degeneration or granuloma formation may be occasionally seen.

Q16. Which are the special stains for the ocher pigment?

a. Methylene blue
b. Crystal violet
c. Van Gieson
d. Pearl's stain
e. Masson-Fontana

Ans: Both a and b.

Methylene blue and crystal violet. Ochronotic pigment stains black with methylene blue or crystal violet.

CHAPTER 84

Calcinosis Cutis

Nikita Lodha

Case study Calcinosis Cutis

Presenting Complaints

Doctor, I have developed painless swellings over my elbows and right knee since the past 2 years.

Setting

Dermatology outpatient department.

History of Present Illness

An 18-year-old girl presented with complaints of multiple, painless, slowly-progressing hard swellings over both the elbows and around the right knee joint since the last 2 years. The lesions over the right elbow had formed an open wound and was discharging chalky white material intermittently.

There was no history of muscle weakness, joint pains, photosensitivity, difficulty in swallowing or Raynaud's phenomenon. She denied excessive milk or antacid intake. There was no history of any inciting trauma. The family history was unremarkable.

General Physical Examination and Systemic Examination

No abnormality detected.

Dermatological Examination

- Multiple, firm-to-hard, nontender, skin-colored to whitish, irregular, tumorous nodules over the lateral aspect of the right knee measuring 12 × 8 cm, and over both elbows measuring about 6 × 4 cm. The nodule over the right elbow had eroded forming an ulcer and was extruding white discharge. Skin overlying the nodules showed few atrophic scars
- There was no restriction of movements at the joints.

Q1. What is the most likely diagnosis?

a. Calcinosis cutis
b. Gouty tophi
c. Rheumatoid nodules
d. Osteosarcoma
e. Mycetoma

Ans: a. Calcinosis cutis

Hard nodules discharging chalky white material around major joints in an otherwise healthy individual suggests calcinosis cutis (Tumoral variant).

Q2. What is calcinosis cutis?

Ans: Calcinosis cutis is a term used to describe a group of disorders in which aberrant calcium deposits form in the skin. Virchow initially described calcinosis cutis in 1855.

Q3. What are the types of calcinosis cutis?

Ans: Calcinosis cutis can be divided into four main groups:

1. *Dystrophic:* associated with local tissue injury such as alterations in collagen, elastin, or subcutaneous fat. Calcium and phosphate metabolism and serum levels are normal, e.g. connective tissue disorders like scleroderma (Fig. 1), dermatomyositis, lupus erythematosus.
   Hereditary: Pseudoxanthoma elasticum, Ehlers-Danlos syndrome
   Metabolic: Porphyria cutanea tarda, calciphylaxis
   Tumors: Pilomatricoma, pilar cyst, nevi, basal cell carcinoma, hemangioma, scrotal sebaceous cysts (Fig. 2), etc.
   Infections: Onchocerciasis, cysticercosis.
2. *Metastatic:* Associated with abnormal calcium and phosphate metabolism with calcium precipitates in normal tissue (skin, vessels, fat, muscles, organs). It is associated with hyperparathyroidism, milk alkali syndrome (excessive intake of foods or antacids containing calcium), and hypervitaminosis D. Ectopic calcification can occur in the setting of hypercalcemia and/or hyperphosphatemia when the calcium-phosphate product exceeds 70 mg^2/dL^2, without preceding tissue damage.
3. *Idiopathic:* Not associated with any tissue damage or metabolic disorder. It comprises tumoral calcinosis, subepidermal calcified nodules, and scrotal calcinosis
4. *Iatrogenic:* Calcinosis cutis arises secondary to a treatment or a procedure, e.g. intravenous calcium or para-aminosalicylic acid, use of saturated calcium chloride electrode paste in electroencephalography.
   Other rare types described include calcinosis cutis circumscripta, calcinosis cutis universalis, tumoral calcinosis, and transplant-associated calcinosis cutis.

Q4. What is calciphylaxis?

Ans: Calciphylaxis (or calcific uremic arteriolopathy): Small-vessel calcification mainly affecting blood vessels of the dermis or subcutaneous fat. The vasculopathy causes ischemia and frank tissue infarction. It may involve visceral organs and skeletal muscles.

Disturbances in calcium and phosphate metabolism and hyperparathyroidism are associated. This potentially fatal syndrome predominantly occurs in patients with end-stage renal disease undergoing long-term renal dialysis.

Q5. How will you investigate a case of calcinosis cutis?

Ans:
- Complete blood count
- Renal function tests
- Autoantibody screen, rheumatoid factor
- Serum calcium and phosphate levels
- Alkaline phosphatase levels
- Hormonal assays (vitamin D, parathormone)
- Fine-needle aspiration cytology (FNAC) reveals amorphous chalky granular material

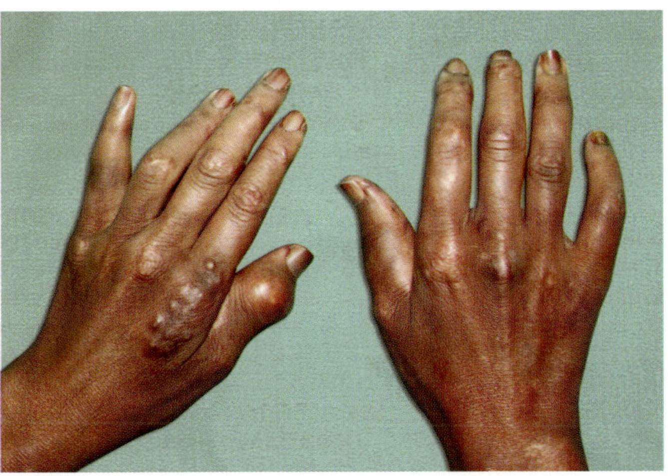

Fig. 1: Calcinosis cutis in scleroderma

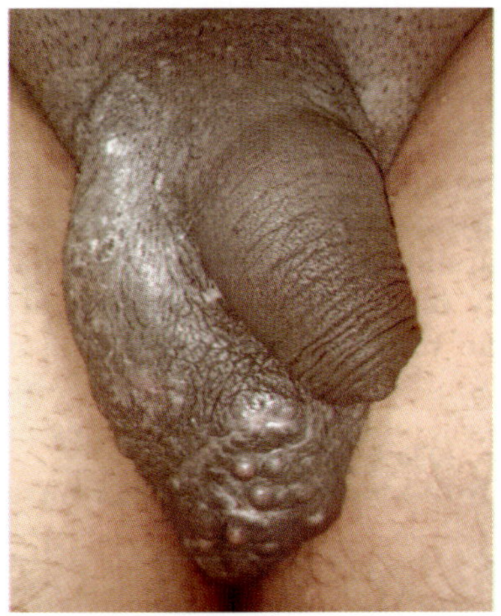

Fig. 2: Calcification in scrotal cysts

- Radiology: X-ray, bone scintigraphy, ultrasound, computed tomography scan, magnetic resonance imaging
- Skin biopsy: Shows deeply basophilic amorphous granular material of varying size surrounded by foreign body reaction.

Q6. What is the special stain for calcium?

a. Von-Kossa
b. Periodic acid-Schiff
c. Gentian violet
d. Methylene blue

Ans: a. Von-Kossa stains calcium deposits black.

Q7. What is the treatment of calcinosis cutis?

Ans: Treatment of calcinosis cutis is challenging with lack of controlled clinical trials. There are no standard treatment guidelines, and therapy depends upon the type of calcification and the underlying disease.

- Small calcified deposits have been successfully treated with warfarin, surgical excision, carbon dioxide laser, ceftriaxone, and intravenous immunoglobulin
- Larger calcified lesions may benefit from curettage, surgical excision, probenecid, diltiazem (2–4 mg/kg/d), aluminum hydroxide, and bisphosphonates (etidronate and alendronate)
- Minocycline has been reported to decrease inflammation surrounding calcified deposits. A slight reduction in size has also been observed
- Extracorporeal shock wave lithotripsy has been used for pain control
- There is a single report of successful use of topical sodium metabisulfite in four cases of calcinosis cutis
- Diet low in calcium and phosphate may prove beneficial.

Q8. What is tumoral calcinosis cutis?

Ans: Tumoral calcinosis cutis (TCC) is a morphological diagnosis characterized by calcium deposits in skin over large joints resembling neoplasm. Patients usually present with asymptomatic, single or multiple, unilateral or bilateral, firm swellings over hip, shoulder, elbow, and knee joints. It mainly appears in otherwise healthy adolescents.

Q9. What is the pathogenesis of tumoral calcinosis cutis?

Ans: Tumoral calcinosis cutis is considered a variant of idiopathic calcinosis. However, it has been reported with diseases like chronic renal failure, primary hyperparathyroidism, hypervitaminosis D, milk-alkali syndrome, and massive osteolysis, leading to the hypothesis that tumoral calcification is a form of metastatic calcification. Again, the occurrence of nodules over joints, which are often subject to local tissue injury, suggests it is a form of dystrophic calcification. A hyperphosphatemic familial tumoral calcinosis, an autosomal recessive condition has also been described.

However, many cases of TCC are not associated with any detectable biochemical abnormality.

Q10. What are the complications of tumoral calcinosis cutis?

Ans: Complications include pain due to nerve compression, ulceration, bacterial infection, cosmetic disfigurement, and restricted joint mobility. Severe complications are uncommon.

Q11. How to treat tumoral calcinosis cutis?

Ans: Complete surgical removal is the treatment of choice. When this cannot be undertaken, the use of partial surgical resection and concomitant dietary therapy with oral aluminum hydroxide, low calcium, low phosphate diet may be effective.

Calcium channel blocker diltiazem and bisphosphonates have been useful in idiopathic sporadic tumoral calcinosis.

Antacids, sevelamer (phosphate-binders) and acetazolamide are found useful in hyperphosphatemic cases.

Q12. What is calcinosis universalis?

Ans: Calcinosis universalis is a rare condition characterized by extensive deposits of calcium salts in skin, subcutaneous tissue, tendons and muscles. Most cases become apparent during the first decade of life. Patient may present with arthralgia to movement limitation, with calcification of soft tissues.

They should be evaluated for autoimmune diseases, though no underlying disease may be demonstrable in a number of cases.

Differential diagnosis should exclude fibrodysplasia ossificans progressive, progressive osseous heterodysplasia, myositis ossificans and dermatopolymyositis.

Q13. What is the difference between calcification and ossification?

Ans: Calcification is the deposition of insoluble calcium salts in an unorganized manner, e.g. calcinosis cutis.

Ossification is the formation of organized bony tissue by the deposition of calcium and phosphorus in a proteinaceous matrix as hydroxyapatite crystals, e.g. Albright hereditary osteodystrophy.

Q14. What is miliary osteoma cutis or osteomatosis of the face?

Ans: Post-acne osteoma cutis has been reported in patients with acne vulgaris. It is known as miliary osteoma cutis or osteomatosis of the face. They represent metaplastic bone formation in the mid- or reticular dermis. They present as multiple, small firm nodules on the face. Treatment consists of topical retinoids or surgical excision.

CHAPTER 85

Mastocytosis

Debdeep Mitra, Ajay Chopra

Case study Mastocytosis

Presenting Complaints

Doctor, my 4-year-old son has been developing recurrent fluid-filled lesions over different parts of his body for the last 2½ years. These eruptions are associated with severe itching which is exacerbated on sun exposure.

Setting

Dermatology outpatient department of a tertiary care hospital.

History of Present Illness

A 4-year-old boy, product of second-degree consanguineous marriage, presented with a history of recurrent fluid-filled eruptions since the age of 1½ years. Eruptions occurred every 2–3 months and were associated with severe pruritus at their onset. The lesions were ruptured forcibly, and they healed with scarring and hyperpigmentation.

General Physical Examination and Systemic Examination

No abnormality detected.

Dermatological Examination

- Multiple tense bullae over the chest, abdomen, and proximal extremities with few erosions over the trunk
- The bullae were present on a non-urticated base and contained clear fluid
- Bulla spread sign and Nikolsky's sign: Negative
- Darier's sign was positive
- Hair, nail and mucosa have been spared.

Laboratory Investigations

No abnormality detected apart from the presence of higher serum tryptase level.

Q1. What is the most probable diagnosis?

a. Bullous mastocytosis
b. Epidermolysis bullosa
c. Incontinentia pigmenti
d. Chronic bullous disease of childhood

Ans: a. Bullous mastocytosis

Q2. What are the points in favor of your diagnosis?

Ans:
- Early age of onset (1.5 years)
- Recurrent eruption of tense bullous lesions, on and off
- Lesions associated with severe pruritus which was aggravated on photoexposure

- The lesions healed by themselves with residual hyperpigmentation
- Negative Nikolsky's sign and bulla spread sign (rules out immunobullous and mechanobullous disorders)
- Positive Darier's sign.

Q3. How will you further evaluate this patient?

Ans: Further tests are needed to confirm the diagnosis. Some useful modalities are given below:

- *Tzanck smear:* This is a bedside test. Fluid collected from the blister is stained with Giemsa stain and viewed under a microscope. It will reveal a large number of mast cells but no acantholytic cells
- *Skin biopsy:* Must be done from an intact bulla to confirm the diagnosis. Skin biopsy and histological examination show subepidermal bulla and an upper dermal inflammatory infiltrate comprising mainly mast cells, which are more abundant around blood vessels and appendages. Toluidine blue staining confirms the infiltration by mast cells
- Recently, detection of monoclonal antibodies against tryptase and CD117 (KIT) is also being done and is regarded as a very sensitive test for the diagnosis of mastocytosis
- Chest X-ray, abdominal ultrasound, bone marrow aspiration, and X-ray of long bones to rule out systemic mastocytosis
- Serum and urinary histamine levels are increased in systemic mastocytosis. Serum tryptase level is elevated in all types of mastocytosis (mast cells produce the enzyme tryptase).

Q4. What is mastocytosis?

Ans: Mastocytosis is a rare disease characterized by abnormal expansion and accumulation of tissue mast cells with an altered immunophenotype in one or multiple organs. It usually presents in the skin, but may affect other tissues, especially the bone marrow and gastrointestinal tract.

Q5. What is the clinical classification of mastocytosis?

Ans: Metcalfe has proposed a clinical classification including the dermatological and hematological presentations of mastocytosis as given below:

- Cutaneous
  - Urticaria pigmentosa
  - Mastocytoma
  - Telangiectasia macularis eruptiva perstans
  - Diffuse cutaneous mastocytosis
- Systemic (extracutaneous mast cells in at least one organ)
  - Indolent systemic mastocytosis
    - Isolated bone marrow mastocytosis
    - Smouldering systemic mastocytosis
  - Mastocytosis with an associated hematological disorder (AHNMD)
    - Myeloproliferative disorders
    - Myelodysplastic disorders
  - Aggressive systemic mastocytosis
  - Mast cell leukemia
  - Mast cell sarcoma
  - Extracutaneous mastocytoma.

Q6. What is the prevalence of mastocytosis?

Ans: Mastocytosis is a rare disease included in the National Organization of Rare Diseases. The prevalence is less than 1 per 300,000 with no sexual predilection. Cutaneous mastocytosis is more common than systemic mastocytosis; amongst which urticaria pigmentosa is the most common type (34%), followed by mastocytoma (<1%) and diffuse mastocytosis. Mastocytosis has a bimodal age distribution often presenting in children from birth to 2 years of age and in those between the ages of 20 and 40.

Q7. What is the clinical presentation of commonest cutaneous variant urticaria pigmentosa?

Ans: Numerous reddish-brown or pale monomorphic maculopapules, plaques or nodules appear in a symmetrical distribution anywhere on the body except the face, head, palms and soles, with the highest concentration usually being on the trunk. They show a positive Darier's sign. Flushing, alcohol intolerance, pruritus, heat or cold intolerance, recurrent diarrhea and headache are few of the other associated systemic findings.

Q8. What is Darier's sign?

Ans: It is the development of urticarial wheals within minutes of gentle rubbing of normal skin which disappears after about 1 hour. It is not 100% specific for mastocytosis, since it has also been described rarely in juvenile xanthogranuloma and acute lymphoblastic leukemia of neonates.

Q9. What is the World Health Organization's criteria for diagnosis of systemic mastocytosis?

Ans: *Major criteria*

- Multifocal dense aggregates of mast cells (≥15) in bone marrow or other tissues (not skin).

Minor criteria

- On biopsy of bone marrow or other extracutaneous tissue more than or equal to 25% of mast cells in the infiltrate are spindle-shaped or have atypical morphology OR more than or equal to 25% of mast cells on bone marrow aspirate are immature or atypical

- Detection of a KIT point mutation at codon 816 in bone marrow, blood or other organs (not skin)
- Mast cells in bone marrow, blood or other extracutaneous organs that coexpress CD117 with CD2 and/or CD25
- Total blood tryptase persistently more than or equal to 20 ng/mL (unless there is an associated clonal myeloid disorder in which case this parameter is not valid)

Diagnosis of systemic mastocytosis may be made if one major and one minor criteria or three minor criteria are fulfilled.

Q10. What is the histopathological finding in mastocytosis?

Ans: The histopathology of mastocytosis shows the following features:

Epidermis

Epidermis is normal apart from the presence of increased basal layer melanization.

Dermis

The dermis shows increased numbers of mast cells in all types of mastocytosis. The mast cells are usually oval or spindle-shaped and have granules that stain metachromatically with toluidine blue. They are also well-demonstrated by Giemsa or chloroacetate esterase stains in formalin-fixed biopsies. Mast cell infiltrates are predominantly found around blood vessels and skin appendages in the papillary dermis.

Q11. What are the potential mast cell degranulating stimuli?

Ans: Some important stimuli which may promote the degranulation of mast cells are given below:

- Physical triggers (especially rubbing)
- Alcohol
- Nonsteroidal anti-inflammatory drugs (including aspirin, diclofenac)
- Allergens (confirmed IgE-mediated reactions, e.g. latex allergy)
- Insect and snake venoms (allergic and/or toxic effects)
- Radiocontrast media (especially if iodinated)
- Plasma expanders (especially dextran)
- Opiates (including codeine and morphine)
- General anesthetic agents
  - Nondepolarizing muscle relaxants (especially benzylisoquinolinium group, e.g. atracurium, gallamine)
  - Anticholinergic drugs (e.g. hyoscine)
- Immunoglobulin E.

Q12. How to approach an adult with mastocytosis?

Ans: *Baseline assessment*

Presenting complaints and enquire about allergic reactions, bowel symptoms and bone pain.

- Investigations:
  - Skin biopsy
  - Blood counts, biochemistry and serum tryptase level estimation
- Optional investigations
  - If eosinophilia or serum tryptase more than 20 ng/mL, bone marrow examination with KIT mutational analysis may be done
  - Bone densitometry, abdominal ultrasound if systemic mastocytosis suspected
  - Gastroscopy if peptic ulceration suspected.

Follow-up assessment

Annual blood counts and biochemistry and serum tryptase

- 3-yearly bone densitometry
- Other investigations as guided by disease progression.

Q13. What is the management protocol for a case of mastocytosis?

Ans: Management:

- Prophylactic prevention of mast cell degranulation triggers
- Antihistamines
- Mast cell stabilizing and anti-inflammatory drugs
- Photochemotherapy and phototherapy (PUVA and NBUVB)
- Corticosteroids
- Interferon alpha-2a and alpha-2b
- Chemotherapy.

SECTION 17

Infections-1 (Bacterial, Mycobacterial and Fungal)

Lakshmi DV

CHAPTER 86

Pyoderma (Folliculitis)

Ananta Khurana

Case study Pyoderma (Folliculitis)

Presenting Complaints

Doctor, I have pus-filled bumps on my face and thighs since past 1 week.

Setting

Dermatology outpatient department

History of Present Illness

A 35-year-old man presented with pus-filled lesions over the face and thighs for a week. He complained of developing such lesions frequently over these sites for the past 6 months. All lesions respond well to antibiotics each time. He denies history of diabetes mellitus, any other systemic disease, drug intake/application or frequent oiling.

General Physical Examination and Systemic Examination

No abnormality detected

Dermatological Examination

- Follicular pustules over the beard region and thighs
- Central hair shaft noted in many
- No evidence of scarring or vesicular lesions on face
- Scars over sites of healed lesions over thighs

Q1. How would you proceed in investigating this case?

Ans: Investigations which should be carried out:

- Gram stain of the pus can help in confirming the diagnosis of bacterial etiology.
- KOH scraping to look for a fungal etiology. Tzanck smear for herpetic folliculitis.
- Culture examination of the pus to identify the causative organism and its drug sensitivity pattern is optional.
- *Gram stain from the pus in the lesion revealed pathogenic gram-positive cocci.*

Q2. What is the most likely diagnosis now?

a. Superficial folliculitis (Bockhart's impetigo)
b. Eosinophilic pustular folliculitis
c. Lupoid sycosis
d. Actinic folliculitis

Ans: A. Superficial folliculitis (Bockhart's impetigo).

Q3. What is folliculitis?

Ans: Folliculitis is an inflammation of the hair follicles. It can affect any hair bearing part of the skin.

Q4. How do you classify folliculitis?

Ans: Classification of folliculitis has been given in Table 1.

Q5. How would you treat such a case?

Ans: Treatment

General measures:

- Good hygiene practices especially hand hygiene
- Avoiding oil application and tight clothing
- Shaving in one direction in recurrent cases of beard folliculitis

Specific measures:

Mild folliculitis: Topical antibiotics (mupirocin, fusidic acid, retapamulin) and antiseptics; Retapamulin is a newer antibiotic available as 1% ointment, and shows good activity against *Staphylococcus* including methicillin-resistant *Staphylococcus aureus* (MRSA) and *Streptococci*.

Severe and extensive folliculitis: Systemic antibiotics—amoxicillin, penicillinase resistant penicillin group molecules (cloxacillin, dicloxacillin, flucloxacillin) and the first (cefadroxil, cephalexin) and second generation (cefuroxime) cephalosporins. Macrolides (azithromycin, erythromycin, clarithromycin) can be used in those sensitive to β-lactams. The antibiotics are given for 5-7 days or till the lesions clear.

Q6. What is the significance of methicillin-resistant *Staphylococcus aureus* (MRSA)?

Ans: MRSA is an organism resistant to methicillin by means of the *mecA* gene which encodes for a variant penicillin-binding protein (PBP2a), leading to low affinity to beta-lactams antibiotics (flucloxacillin, oxacillin, cephalosporins and carbapenems). Macrolides, tetracyclines, fluoroquinolones, and sulfonamides can also present with these resistance patterns. MRSA occurs as healthcare associated-MRSA and community acquired-MRSA. The majority of the infections present as abscesses or folliculitis. MRSA infections are associated with a higher rate of adverse outcome and treatment failure as well as higher economic costs of care compared to methicillin-sensitive *S. aureus* and other organisms.

Q7. What are the antibiotics effective against methicillin-resistant *Staphylococcus aureus* (MRSA)?

Ans: Oral antibiotics active against MRSA include cotrimoxazole, clindamycin, doxycycline, minocycline and linezolid. For hospitalized patients options for empirical therapy of MRSA are—intravenous (I/V) vancomycin, oral or I/V linezolid, I/V daptomycin, I/V telavancin, and IV or oral clindamycin.

Q8. What is the importance of *Staphylococcus aureus* carriage?

Ans: *S. aureus* nasal carriage has been variably reported to occur in 10–40% of healthy population in different

Table 1: Classification of folliculitis

Classification		
1. Depth of invasion	a. Superficial (Involvement limited to follicular infundibulum)	*Folliculitis, furunculosis*
	b. Deep: Involvement deeper than the follicular ostia)	*Carbuncle, sycosis barbae* *Lupoid sycosis*
2. Etiology	a. Infective	i. Bacterial: *Staphylococcus, Pseudomonas, gram-negative organisms* (Fig. 1), *Streptococcus, Proteus, coliform organisms* ii. Fungal: *Dermatophytes, Pityrosporum, candida* iii. Viral: *Herpes simplex, Molluscum contagiosum* iv. Parasitic: *Demodicidosis*
	b. Noninfective	Physical and chemical agents like occlusive dressings, adhesive tapes, after use of mineral oil, coal tar preparations
	c. Unknown etiology	*Sycosis barbae* *Acne keloidalis* *Actinic folliculitis* *Eosinophilic pustular folliculitis* *Folliculitis decalvans* *Hidradenitis suppurativa* *Dissecting cellulitis*

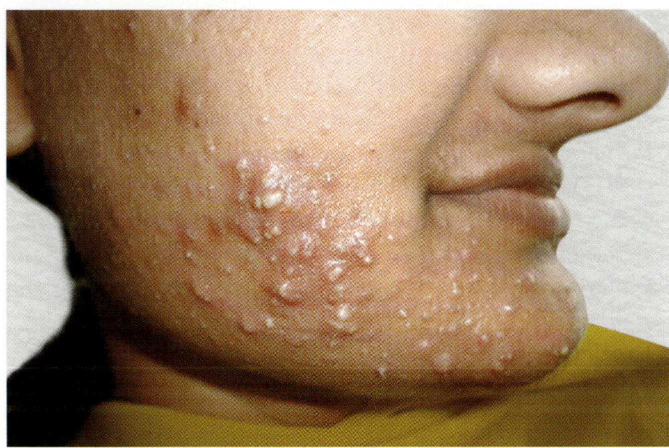

Fig. 1: Gram-negative organisms causing folliculitis

studies from India and other countries. In addition, other important sites of *S. aureus* carriage are perineum (20%), axillae (5–10%) and toe-webs (5–10%).

Nasal carriers act as reservoirs of the organism for themselves and their contacts. Nasal carriage of *S. aureus* has been identified as a major risk factor for the subsequent development of community-acquired and nosocomial infections. At present, two categories of nasal carriers are distinguished, namely persistent and nonpersistent carries. Persistent carriers carry higher bacterial load and can lead to more extensive dispersal.

Q9. When is treatment of carrier state indicated?

Ans: Elimination of carrier state is indicated in those having recurrent staphylococcal infections (and their household contacts) and healthcare workers, especially those working in sensitive sites like neonatal units and operation theatres.

Q10. How is *S. aureus* carriage state treated?

Ans: Intranasal application of a 2% mupirocin for 5 days eliminates *S. aureus* nasal carriage in 70% of healthy individuals for up to 3 months. A 5-day course of nasal mupirocin ointment every month for 1 year reduces positive nasal cultures in a majority. Application to other colonized sites (axilla, perineum) is desirable.

Rifampicin (600 mg orally daily for 10 days) eradicates *S. aureus* from most nasal carriers for up to 3 months. However, selection of rifampicin-resistant strains can occur rapidly with such therapy. The addition of a second drug (dicloxacillin for methicillin susceptible *S. aureus*; trimethoprim-sulfamethoxazole, ciprofloxacin, or minocycline for MRSA) has been used to reduce the emergence of rifampicin resistance.

Clindamycin in the dose of 150 mg daily for 3 months is another alternative.

Q11. What are the other common skin infections caused by gram-positive bacteria?

Ans: Common skin infections caused by gram-positive bacteria have been described in Table 2.

Q12. What are the drugs effective in corynebacterial infections?

Ans: The following drugs have been useful in treatment of the abovementioned corynebacterial infections:

- *Topical antimicrobials*: Clindamycin, erythromycin, fusidic acid
- *Topical imidazoles*: Clotrimazole, miconazole
- *Benzoyl peroxide*: In the form of washes and 5% gel
- *Oral antimicrobials (for extensive erythrasma)*: Erythromycin 250 mg QID, clarithromycin 1 g single dose, tetracyclines.

Q13. What is the clinical presentation and etiology of impetigo?

Ans: Impetigo is superficial infection of the nonhair bearing skin and can present in nonbullous or bullous forms (Table 3).

Q14. What is botryomycosis?

Ans: Botryomycosis is an uncommon chronic suppurative granulomatous bacterial infection (hence a misnomer) that can affect the skin and viscera.

- *Causative organism*: *Staphylococcus aureus* and *Pseudomonas aeruginosa*, occasionally *E. coli*, *Proteus* spp, *Bacillus* spp, *Prevotella melaninogenica* and *Actinobacillus*.
- *Predisposing factors*: Immunosuppression, alcoholism and diabetes mellitus
- *Pathogenesis*: Unknown. Interplay of host immune status (T cell defects and impaired neutrophil, monocyte and/or macrophage function) and microbial infectivity implicated
- Clinically presents as small tender nodules which breakdown to form discharging sinuses commonly over extremities
- Histopathology shows bacterial colonies are arranged in a distinctive "bunch of grapes" pattern with surrounding eosinophilia, known as the Splendore-Hoeppli phenomenon.
- *Treatment*: Prolonged antibiotic therapy depending on the organism cultured and its sensitivity profile.

Table 2: Common skin infections caused by gram-positive bacteria

Organism	***Infection***	
a. *Staphylococcus sp.*		
Staphylococcus aureus	Direct infection	Nonfollicular—impetigo (Fig. 2), ecthyma, erysipelas, cellulitis. Follicular—folliculitis, furunculosis, carbuncle, sycosis
	Secondary infection	Occurs over pre-existing skin conditions (eczema, scabies) (Fig. 3)
	Toxin-mediated diseases	Staphylococcal scalded skin syndrome, Toxic shock syndrome, Staphylococcal scarlatina, recurrent toxin-mediated perineal erythema
Staphylococcus epidermidis (Coagulase negative)	Secondary infections of wounds and implanted devices, occasionally minor skin infections like folliculitis, internal infections including endocarditis and septicemia (especially in patients with immune deficiencies)	
b. *Streptococcus sp.*		
Streptococcus pyogenes	Direct infection	Impetigo, ecthyma, erysipelas, cellulitis, vulvovaginitis, perianal infection, streptococcal ulcers, blistering distal dactylitis, necrotizing fasciitis
	Secondary infection	Occurs over pre-existing skin conditions (Eczema, scabies, ulcers)
	Toxin-mediated diseases	Scarlet fever, toxic-shock-like syndrome, recurrent toxin-mediated perineal erythema
Group C streptococci (colonize diseased skin)	Impetigo, erysipelas and cellulitis	
Group G streptococci (colonize pharynx, intestine, vagina or skin)	Cellulitis or erysipelas in patients with vascular disease or those who have undergone cardiac surgery and venous ligation	
Group B streptococci (colonize the anorectum and vagina)	Severe infections in neonates; cause invasive disease in adults, particularly in patients with chronic disease; causal role in bacterial intertrigo; rarely cause erysipelas, cellulitis, necrotizing fasciitis and blistering distal dactylitis	
Group F streptococci	Secondary pathogens in suppurative hidradenitis	
Group D streptococci (enterococci)	Occasionally cellulitis and necrotizing fasciitis	
c. *Coryneform bacteria*		
Corynebacterium minutissimum	Erythrasma	
Corynebacterium tenuis	Trichomycosis (Trichobacteriosis) axillaris	
Corynebacterium sp	Pitted keratolysis	Micrococcus sedentarius, (a gram-positive staphylococcus-related bacteria), dermatophilus congolensis also implicated

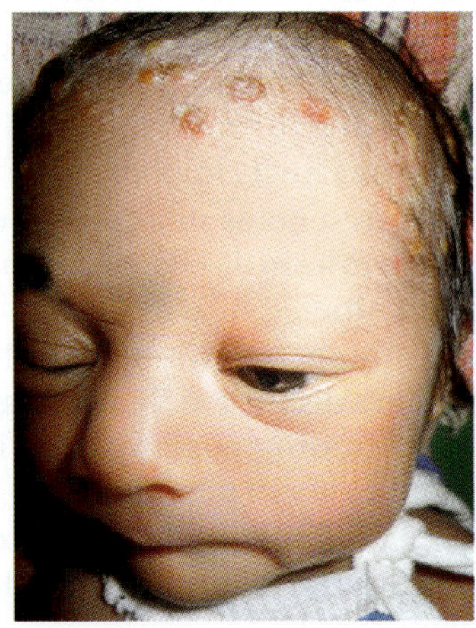

Fig. 2: Impetigo contagiosa on scalp of infant

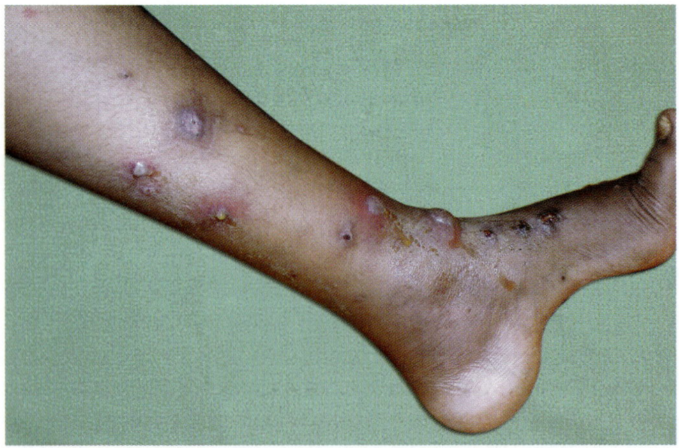

Fig. 3: Secondary infection of eczema

Table 3: Clinical presentation and etiology of impetigo

	Bullous impetigo	***Nonbullous impetigo***
Age	Infancy, any age	Preschool, children
Causative organism	*S. aureus* phage group II esp. stains 77 and 55 (Toxin mediated-A and B exfoliative toxin)	*Staphylococcus aureus*, Streptococcus
Site	Face, perioral, nares, diaper area	Nose, mouth, face, extremities
Bulla	Flaccid, thin walled bullae ruptures forms varnish like crusts at center	Begins as small 1–2 mm red papule/pustule/thin-roofed vesicle/bullae, honey-colored crusts. Stuck on appearance
Base	Little or no erythema	Surrounded by erythema
Erythema	Extends peripherally with central clearing	Extends peripherally with central clearing with satellite lesions
Clinical patterns	Annular, circinate, polycyclic	Annular, gyrate
Regional adenitis	Rare, seen in later course of disease	Common and early
Complications	Sepsis, osteomyelitis, septic arthritis, lymphadenopathy, pneumonia	Cellulitis, erythema multiforme, urticaria, poststreptococcal glomerulonephritis, scarlet fever

CHAPTER 87

Erythrasma

Meenaz Khoja

Case study Erythrasma

Presenting Complaints

Doctor, I have these dark-colored patches in my underarms and groin folds for 6 months. They look ugly and itch occasionally. I also have this foul smelling thick deposition between my toes for 6 months.

Setting

Dermatology outpatient department

History of Present Illness

A 45-year-old obese, diabetic male came with occasionally pruritic dark brown patches over bilateral axillae, inframammary area and groins for 6 months. The patches were erythematous initially and then became dark brown. He also gives history of a foul smelling maceration in the fourth toe web space.

General Physical Examination and Systemic Examination

No abnormality detected.

Dermatological Examination

- Dark brown, well-demarcated, wrinkled thin patches with minimal scaling present over bilateral axillae, groins and inframammary folds (Fig. 1)
- No maceration was noted
- Scratch sign (rubbing the lesion or scratching it with a blunt object so as to enhance the scaling) was negative
- Wood's lamp examination revealed coral red fluorescence over the lesions. The fourth toe web space showed hyperkeratotic macerated plaques and had a foul odor.

Q1. What is the most likely diagnosis?

a. Pityriasis versicolor
b. Erythrasma
c. Intertrigo
d. Flexural psoriasis

Ans: B. Erythrasma

Presence of tan brown, well-demarcated, wrinkled plaques characteristically located over intertriginious areas with minimal scaling and giving coral red fluorescence on Wood's lamp is suggestive of erythrasma.

Negative scratch sign and a coral red fluorescence under Wood's lamp rule out pityriasis versicolor. Psoriasis and intertrigo do not show any fluorescence under Wood's light.

Q2. What causes erythrasma?

Ans: Erythrasma is a common, chronic, cutaneous infection caused by the gram positive, aerobic,

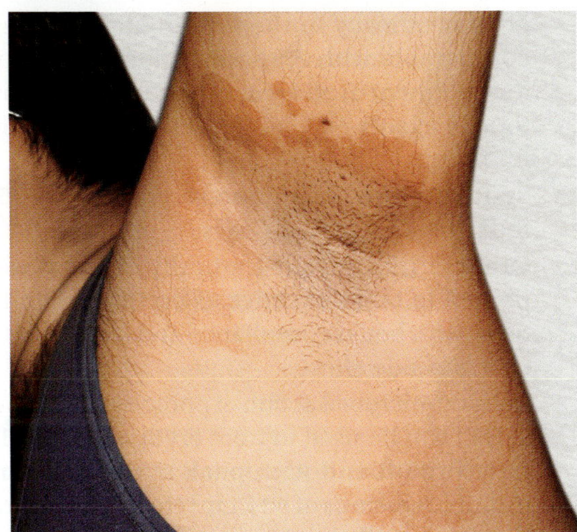

Fig. 1: Classical hyperpigmented plaques over axillae, showing wrinkled appearance and mild scaling
Courtesy: Dr Sanjay Khare, Madhya Pradesh, India

nonsporing bacilli—*Corynebacterium minutissimum*. These bacilli are filamentous, nonspore forming and lipophilic. These corynebacteria are part of the normal flora of the skin and have been isolated from genital regions in 4–20%, and interdigital regions of the feet in 69% in some populations *Corynebacterium aurimucosum* and *Microbacterium oxydans* may rarely cause erythrasma.

Q3. Which is the commonest area involved in erythrasma?

a. Axillae
b. Groin folds
c. Inter web spaces of toes
d. Infra-mammary areas

Ans: C. Inter web spaces of toes.

Q4. What are the manifestations and characteristic skin changes in erythrasma?

Ans: Erythrasma shows well-demarcated, irregularly shaped (usually oval) erythematous plaques (early) or dark brown to tan plaques (late lesions) with mild scaling and wrinkled appearance mainly over intertriginous areas such as interspaces of the toes axillae, groins, inframammary folds, genitocrural and intergluteal folds. In toe web spaces, erythrasma presents as yellowish (due to hyperkeratosis) plaques with maceration. Rarely, toe web lesions have a vesiculobullous appearance. It may appear macerated with concomitant infection with yeasts and dermatophytes; usually asymptomatic and occasionally pruritic condition. When nails are affected, they appear thickened and yellow and show hyperkeratosis of the nail bed and onycholysis.

Q5. What are the systemic associations of erythrasma?

Ans: Erythrasma may be the presenting feature in diabetes. It is commonly associated with obesity and seen in adults from institutions. It may rarely be associated with systemic disease like recurrent abscesses or endocarditis.

Q6. How do you diagnose erythrasma?

Ans: It is mainly a clinical diagnosis which is substantiated by Wood's lamp examination.

Q7. How will you confirm the diagnosis?

Ans: Confirmation of diagnosis:

- *Wood's lamp examination*: *Corynebacterium minutissimum* secretes coproporphyrin III which exhibits the coral red fluorescence under the Wood's lamp. Sometimes, due to bathing, the coproporphyrins may be washed away and the Wood's lamp may not show fluorescence.
- *Skin swab test*: Done for Gram, periodic acid–Schiff (PAS), Grocott, Giemsa or methylene blue stains which show bacilli arranged in characteristic V-shaped or Chinese letter pattern.
- *Skin biopsy*: The biopsy is unremarkable on hematoxylin and eosin staining (H&E) except for mild hypergranulosis and superficial perivascular lymphocytic infiltrate. The biopsy of erythrasma is considered as one of the "invisible dermatosis". Erythrasma may be missed on routine H&E staining as the *Corynebacterium minutissimum* is a tiny coccobacilli and they do not incite much inflammatory reaction. The organisms can be made more prominent by using special stains such as Gram stain, periodic acid-Schiff or methenamine silver stains.
- Potassium hydroxide mount and culture on Sabouraud's Dextrose agar (SDA) —subjecting skin scraping to 10% potassium hydroxide and for culture on SDA may be done to rule out dermatophyte or yeast infection. These may be positive in cases of concomitant dermatophytosis and candidiasis.
- Skin swab test for bacterial culture on blood agar and Colombia agar grows cream-colored colonies after 24 hours at 37°C. These colonies are urease positive, can hydrolyze esculin and produce acid from glucose, maltose and saccharose but not lactose. The corynebacterium colonies also exhibit coral red fluorescence on Wood's lamp examination.

Q8. What are the differential diagnoses of erythrasma?

Ans: Differential diagnoses of erythrasma:

- Pityriasis versicolor—individual lesions are smaller, hypopigmented or hyperpigmented plaques with scaling
- Tinea cruris—lesions over thighs, genitocrural folds mimic tinea but in erythrasma there is absence of vesiculation, inflammatory edges and satellite lesions
- Tinea pedis and candidiasis—difficult to differentiate clinically cases of toe space erythrasma from candidiasis and dermatophytosis, they also usually coexist
- Flexural psoriasis—shiny appearance
- Seborrhoeic dermatitis.

Q9. What are the treatment options of erythrasma?

Ans: Various topical and systemic modalities are available for the treatment of erythrasma:

- Topical treatments include sodium fusidate ointment, imidazoles, clindamycin. Whitfield's ointment, which has equal efficacy to systemic erythromycin in the axillae and groin, shows greater efficacy in the interdigital areas and is comparable with 2% sodium fusidate ointment for treatment of all areas. Antibacterial soaps and topical agents may be needed for treatment and for prophylaxis.
- Systemic drugs include oral erythromycin 250 mg four times a day for 14 days.
- Oral clarithromycin 1 g orally single dose was proven to be as effective as erythromycin for 14 days, with better compliance and lesser treatment cost and side effects.
- The antimicrobial action of photodynamic therapy (PDT) can be used to treat erythrasma. PDT (red light broadband with peak at 635 nm) one or multiple sessions of 80 J/cm^2 clear the erythrasma due to photodynamic reaction causing activation of the porphyrins, no external photosensitizers are needed.

Q10. Which are the other skin conditions caused by corynebacteria?

Ans: Cutaneous diseases caused by corynebacteria species include trichomycosis axillaris (*C. tenuis*) and pitted keratolysis.

CHAPTER 88

Pitted Keratolysis

Sujala S Aradhya, Sacchidanand S

Case study Pitted keratolysis

Presenting Complaints

Doctor, my soles have developed multiple pits since 4 weeks and they also smell badly.

Setting

Dermatology outpatient department

History of Present Illness

A 35-year-old male, farmer by profession presented with complaints of multiple pits over both his feet for 4 weeks and associated malodor with no itching or burning sensation.

General Physical Examination and Systemic Examination

No abnormality detected

Dermatological Examination

- Multiple crateriform pits are seen over both plantar regions (Fig. 1)
- Pits are shallow, circular, discrete that coalesce at places to form large irregular erosions (Fig. 2)
- Some areas show maceration
- No associated scaling, excoriations or discharge but malodor is noted
- Mucosa (buccal, genital, ocular)/hair/nails: normal.

Q1. What is the most likely diagnosis?

a. Plantar warts
b. Pitted keratolysis
c. Punctate keratoderma
d. Punctate porokeratosis

Ans: b. Pitted keratolysis (Multiple, discrete to coalescing, circular, shallow pits).

Q2. What is pitted keratolysis?

Ans: Pitted keratolysis is an acquired, chronic, usually asymptomatic, noninflammatory, superficial bacterial infection of the skin, confined to the stratum corneum of the soles, characterized clinically by multifocal, discrete, superficial crateriform pits and superficial erosions. It can rarely occur on the palms.

Q3. What are the synonyms of pitted keratolysis?

Ans: Keratoma plantare sulcatum (currently not used), keratolysis plantare sulcatum, keratolysis sulcata, ringed keratolysis.

Q4. What are the points that aid in the diagnosis of pitted keratolysis?

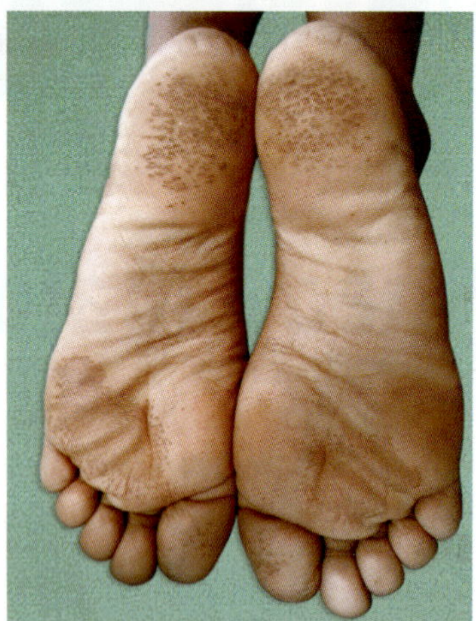

Fig. 1: Pitted lesions on both the feet

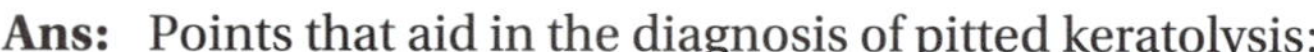

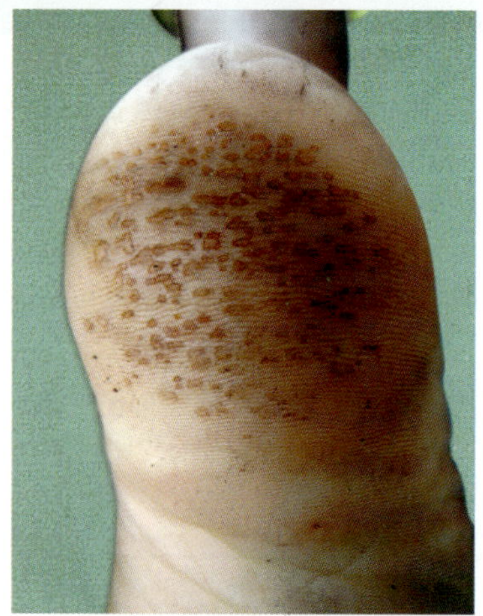

Fig. 2: Close-up image of the pits

Ans: Points that aid in the diagnosis of pitted keratolysis:
- Multiple, conspicuous, discrete, shallow circular lesions with punched-out appearance that coalesce in places to form superficial irregular erosions
- Usually associated with malodor and hyperhidrosis, may be surrounded by maceration and associated stickiness.
- Commonly seen over soles and rarely on palms, and more frequently involve the pressure bearing and friction prone areas.
- Patient may give a history of frequent immersion of hands and feet in water.
- Soaking the feet in water for 15 minutes causes swelling of the horny layer and accentuates the lesions.
- More common among barefooted people living in tropical regions, especially during summers and rainy seasons.
- Also commonly reported in barefooted laborers/farmers, marine workers, soldiers and industrial workers wearing occluded shoes for prolonged periods.
- Interdigital intertrigo and paronychia may coexist but does not influence the onset or course of the disease.

Q5. What are the differential diagnoses for pitted keratolysis?

Ans: Differential diagnosis:
- Plantar warts
- Keratosis punctata
- Keratolysis exfoliativa
- Punctate keratoderma
- Darier's disease
- Punctate porokeratosis
- Pits of basal cell nevus syndrome
- Arsenic poisoning
- Acropigmentation of Kitamura
- Tungiasis
- Yaws.

Q6. Which organisms cause this condition?

Ans: Pitted keratolysis is caused by a cutaneous infection with either *Kytococcus sedentarius* (earlier known as *Micrococcus sedentarius*), *Dermatophilus congolensis*, Corynebacterium species (*Corynebacterium minutissimum*) and some species of *Streptomyces*.

Q7. How does the infection occur?

Ans: Under appropriate conditions (i.e. prolonged occlusion, hyperhidrosis, increased skin surface pH or contact with wet surfaces) these bacteria proliferate and produce proteinases that destroy the stratum corneum, creating pits. *Kytococcus sedentarius* has been found to produce two keratin-degrading enzymes, protease P1 (30 kd) and P2 (50 kd) respectively. The malodor associated with pitted keratolysis is presumed to be due to the production of sulfur-compound byproducts, such as thiols, sulfides and thioesters.

A variant of markedly enlarged lesions, called crateriform pitted keratolysis, also has been described. In addition to pits, erythematous to violaceous macules to plaque-like lesions may be present.

Q8. What could be the complications of pitted keratolysis?

Ans: Complications:

- Usually asymptomatic but may have a chronic course
- Associated malodor and sliminess (hyperhidrosis)
- Occasionally soreness, itching and pain while walking.

Q9. What are the histopathological features of pitted keratolysis?

Ans: Presence of crater with coccoid and filamentous microorganisms seen at the base and margin of the crater (in the most superficial parts of stratum corneum) are the characteristic features. These organisms may extend downward between keratinocytes with associated lysis of keratin. To highlight these organisms, special stains like Gram stain, periodic acid–Schiff (PAS) stain and methenamine silver can be used. The mid-dermis may contain a spotty infiltrate of round cells.

Two types of pitted keratolysis can be distinguished histologically:

a. Superficial or minor type—there is only a small depression due to focal lysis and coccoid bacteria are distributed in groups or chains.
b. Classical or major type—organisms exhibit dimorphism with septate hyphae as well as coccoid forms, which extend into the stratum corneum forming more definitive pits.

Q10. How to confirm the diagnosis?

Ans: The diagnosis can be confirmed by:

- Skin biopsies are not routinely performed since diagnosis is easy due to the unique clinical presentation and characteristic odor.
- Wood's ultraviolet light examination is not consistently helpful, but the affected areas may display a characteristic coral red fluorescence.
- The organisms obtained from the pitted lesions are more easily detected in Gram-stained scrapings.
- Culture on brain–heart infusion agar, incubated at 37 °C in a mixture of pure nitrogen containing 5–10% carbon dioxide, gives minute irregular colorless colonies within 3–5 days. However, given the existing confusion over the identity of the bacteria, culture is not a useful diagnostic process.

Q11. What is the treatment of pitted keratolysis?

Ans: Pitted keratolysis has an excellent prognosis; effective treatment clears both the lesion and the odor in 3–4 weeks.

- Topical therapy with twice daily application of antibiotics like erythromycin solution or gel, 1% clindamycin hydrochloride solution, fusidic acid cream, 2% sodium fusidate and mupirocin cream to the entire plantar surfaces of the feet.
- Various other medications, like 0.1% triamcinolone acetonide, iodochlorhydroxyquin-hydrocortisone cream, flexible collodion, benzoic and salicylic acid ointment, Castellani's paint, gentamicin sulfate cream, 1% clotrimazole cream, 2% miconazole nitrate cream, benzoyl peroxide wash or gel and Whitfield's ointment have been used with limited success. Successful treatment with topical antiseptics, such as 2% buffered glutaraldehyde, formaldehyde, and 5% formalin solution have been advocated. Oral erythromycin is another option, especially for resistant cases.
- Treatment of hyperhidrosis slowly brings the condition under control including potassium permanganate soaks, 20% aluminium chloride solution, iontophoresis and botulinum toxin.
- Avoiding use of occlusive footwear, reduction of foot friction with properly fitting footwear, using absorbent cotton socks, wearing open toed sandals whenever possible, washing feet with soap or antibacterial cleanser twice a day and avoiding sharing of footwear or towels.

CHAPTER 89

Actinomycosis

Piyush Kumar

Case study Actinomycosis

Presenting Complaints

Doctor, I have a swelling in left neck region for last 6 months. Recently, it has developed 2–3 openings and pus along with yellowish grain-like material is coming out through them.

Setting

Dermatology outpatient department

History of Present Illness

A 40-year-old male presented with the complaints of a firm swelling on the left jaw that softened and broke down to form multiple openings discharging pus containing yellowish granules (Fig. 1). He has undergone root canal treatment of two left lower molar teeth prior to onset of neck swelling.

General Physical Examination and Systemic Examination

Nothing abnormally detected

Dermatological Examination

- Firm nodule with multiple discharging sinuses—left submandibular region
- Pus and yellowish granules were expressed on pressure.
- No cervical lymphadenopathy.

Q1. What is the most likely diagnosis?

a. Actinomycosis
b. Scrofuloderma
c. Hidradenitis suppurativa
d. Squamous cell carcinoma

Ans: a. Actinomycosis—presence of multiple draining sinuses and discharging yellowish granules suggest the diagnosis of actinomycosis.

Q2. What are the causative organisms of actinomycosis?

Ans: Causative organisms:

- *Actinomyces israelii*
- *A. gerencseriae*
- *A. viscosus*
- *A. naeslundii*
- *A. odontolyticus*
- *A. meyeri*

Actinomyces spp. are anaerobic or microaerophilic, gram positive, nonacid-fast filaments which fragment into bacillary and coccoid forms without any spores. They colonize the oropharynx, gastrointestinal tract and urogenital tract. *Propionibacterium propionicum*

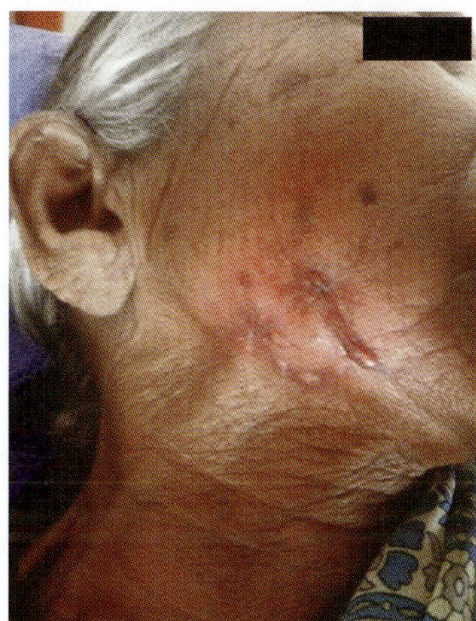

Fig. 1: Multiple nodules and sinuses on right jaw

(formerly known as *Arachnia propionica*) has been reported to cause actinomycosis-like infection.

Q3. What are the types of actinomycosis?

Ans: Types of actinomycosis:

- Cervicofacial actinomycosis
- Thoracic actinomycosis
- Abdominal actinomycosis
- Pelvic actinomycosis
- Actinomycosis involving other sites.

Q4. What are the common presentations of actinomycosis?

Ans: The signs and symptoms depend on the site of involvement.

Cervicofacial actinomycosis: It is the most common actinomycosis and is seen in association with odontogenic infection. The common predisposing conditions include poor oral hygiene (dental caries, gingivitis) and oral mucosa trauma (dental extraction, gingival trauma), male sex, diabetes mellitus, immunosuppression, alcoholism and malnutrition.

It usually starts as a firm painful swelling along the alveolar ridge that softens and breaks down to form multiple sinuses discharging a typical thick yellow exudate with characteristic sulfur granules. Infection here is commonly known as "lumpy jaw". Regional adenopathy is rare. The underlying bone may be involved with periostitis or osteomyelitis. It can lead to distant organ dissemination, including brain, lungs and digestive tract.

Thoracic (respiratory tract) actinomycosis: It includes pulmonary, bronchial, and laryngeal actinomycosis. It results from direct extension of the disease from the neck or abdomen or as a primary infection from aspiration of organism from the mouth. Extrapulmonary spread may involve pleura, mediastinum, and chest wall, resulting in fistula and multiple draining sinuses.

Abdominal (digestive tract) actinomycosis: Appendix, cecum, and colon are the most common abdominal sites of actinomycosis, which follow gastrointestinal mucosa disruption and surgery for appendicitis or colonic diverticulitis with perforation. Signs and symptoms of patients with digestive tract actinomycosis depend on the anatomical location of the disease. Patients with ulcerative involvement of the esophagus mainly have dysphagia. Patients with appendix, cecum, or colon actinomycosis frequently have abdominal pain with a palpable mass; abdominal wall involvement results in fistula and draining sinuses.

Pelvic (genitourinary) actinomycosis: Genitourinary tract actinomycosis is the second most frequent clinical form of actinomycosis. The most common presentation of genitourinary tract actinomycosis is pelvic actinomycosis in women using an intrauterine device (IUD). It presents with pain and an enlarging mass in the ovary or fallopian tube, abdomen or surrounding areas.

Other actinomycosis

- *Central nervous system actinomycosis: Actinomyces* spp. are mainly involved in brain abscess, but meningitis, meningoencephalitis, epidural abscess and subdural empyema have also been described. The central nervous system involvement occurs hematogenously from the lung or contiguously from a cervicofacial actinomycosis or following a penetrating head injury.
- *Primary cutaneous actinomycosis:* Primary skin and soft-tissue actinomycosis results from skin disruption followed by invasion of *Actinomyces* spp and presents with progressive skin and soft-tissue inflammation, which can become an abscess or cold mass, or nodular lesions with fistulas.
- *Extrafacial bone and joint actinomycosis:* Extrafacial bone and joint infection may result from hematogenous spread of localized actinomycosis; contiguous spread of pulmonary actinomycosis to the spine; and polymicrobial bone and joint infection following bone exposure.

Q5. What is the differential diagnosis of actinomycosis?

Ans: In general, actinomycosis mimics malignancy, tuberculosis and nocardiosis. Other differentials diagnoses include:

- Cervicofacial actinomycosis—tuberculosis (scrofuloderma, tubercular lymphadenitis), chronic osteomyelitis, hidradenitis suppurativa, glanders, gumma, tularemia.
- Thoracic actinomycosis—lung abscess, bronchiectasis, psoas abscess, chronic osteomyelitis
- Abdominal actinomycosis—appendicitis
- Pelvic actinomycosis—lymphogranuloma venereum.

Q6. How will you confirm the diagnosis?

Ans: Isolation of Actinomyces from a sterile site confirms the diagnosis of actinomycosis. The most appropriate clinical specimens are tissue from surgical biopsy or pus; swabs must be avoided (FNAC from the sinuses may be tried, reference available). However, the identification of Actinomyces in mucosa, where these bacteria are normal inhabitants, is of little significance in the absence of sulfur granules or a typical clinical picture.

Gram stain: Actinomyces spp are seen as nonspore-forming gram-positive rods. All species, except *A. meyeri*, are branching filamentous rods.

Culture: Strict anaerobic processing (rapid transport to the laboratory and/or transport in an anaerobic transport medium) and anaerobic growth conditions are necessary for primary isolation. Growth of Actinomyces is slow; it may take up to 15–20 days. Actinomyces spp can be cultured on chocolate blood agar media or brain heart infusion broth at 37 °C. Semiselective media (such as phenylethyl alcohol or mupirocin-metronidazole blood agar) may be used to increase isolation rates.

Histopathology: Chronic suppurative granulomatous reaction with sulfur granules (organized aggregates of bacterial filaments). Sulfur granules (called so because of their yellow color) are composed of delicate, branched, gram-positive filaments, about 1 micrometer in diameter, haphazardly arranged in an amorphous matrix. Eosinophilic clubs composed of immunoglobulin are seen at the periphery of the granule (*Splendore-Hoeppli phenomenon*). These sulfur granules are not specific for actinomycosis and may be seen in nocardiosis and chronic cervicofacial fungal infections. Immunofluorescence techniques can help identify Actinomyces spp.

16s rRNA Polymerase chain reaction can also be used for direct detection of Actinomyces in tissue samples. Antibody tests are available too.

Q7. How to manage actinomycosis?

Ans: Check for immunosuppression and diabetes.

- *Medical:* Actinomyces spp. are usually extremely susceptible to beta-lactams, and penicillin G or amoxicillin is considered drugs of choice for the treatment of actinomycosis. As Actinomyces spp. do not produce beta-lactamases, it is not useful to combine amoxicillin with beta-lactam inhibitors such as clavulanic acid, except if copathogens are involved in the disease. Penicillin is used in a dose of 10–20 million units of penicillin G intravenously for 4–6 weeks followed by penicillin V 250–500 mg, 4–6 times a day for 12–18 months. Other effective drugs include macrolides, doxycycline and clindamycin, tetracycline, ceftriaxone, imipenem and aztreonam.
- *Surgical* incision and drainage, debridement (Just debulks and always an add-on therapy and needs antibiotics concurrently).

CHAPTER 90

Lupus Vulgaris

Soumya Jagadeesan

Case study Lupus vulgaris

Presenting Complaints

Doctor, I have slowly enlarging asymptomatic reddish raised lesions on the right leg of 11 months duration.

Setting

Dermatology outpatient department

History of Presenting Illness

A 45-year-old housewife presented with reddish raised lesions on the right leg since 11 months. Initially, the lesions were small and later, they slowly increased in size with peripheral extension of the lesions and central clearing. No history of preceding trauma or any significant systemic illness was present.

General Physical and Systemic Examination

No abnormality detected

Dermatological Examination

Clinical examination revealed three well-demarcated erythematous to hyperpigmented annular plaques on the right leg with raised borders and central atrophy (Fig. 1). Sensations were intact. No nodules/papules were seen in the surrounding skin. No peripheral nerve thickening present.

Investigations

- Routine biochemical analysis, complete blood count and urine microscopy were normal. Chest radiograph and computed tomography findings were normal. Mantoux test showed increased reactivity with a 15 mm induration after 48 hours.
- Histopathologic examination revealed multiple noncaseating granulomas in the upper dermis with no acid fast bacilli. No suppuration or sclerotic bodies were found. No atypical cells were seen.

Q1. What is the most likely diagnosis?

a. Sarcoidosis
b. Hansen's disease
c. Chromoblastomycosis
d. Lupus vulgaris

Ans: D. Lupus vulgaris

Lupus vulgaris is a form of cutaneous tuberculosis, usually paucibacillary, where the patient is a previously sensitized individual with a high degree of immunity to tuberculin. It is one of the most common presentations of cutaneous tuberculosis and can present in myriad ways.

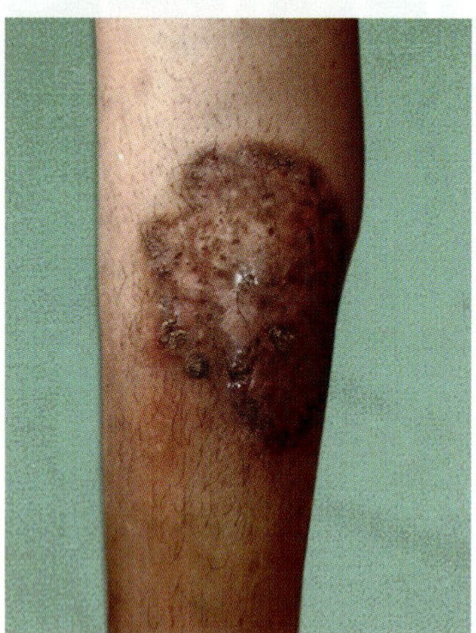

Fig. 1: Annular plaque with raised borders and central atrophy

Q2. How is lupus vulgaris transmitted?

a. Exogenous
b. Hematogenous dissemination
c. Lymphatic spread
d. All of the above.

Ans: D. All the above

Lupus vulgaris most commonly occurs due to hematogenous spread. However, it may occur after exogenous inoculation or as a complication of Bacille Calmette-Guerin (BCG) vaccination. It commonly arises from an underlying focus of tuberculosis, in a bone, joint or lymph node, by either contiguous extension or hematogenous or lymphatic spread. Sometimes the underlying focus is not clinically apparent; in such cases, reactivation of a latent cutaneous focus is suspected.

Q3. How do we classify cutaneous tuberculosis?

Ans: Cutaneous tuberculosis is classified depending upon the host's cell-mediated immunity and also the route of transmission (Table 1).

Q4. What are the clinical features of lupus vulgaris?

Ans: The classical presentation of lupus vulgaris is with slowly enlarging lesions which expand peripherally, showing a central clearing and a peripheral raised border. The lesions may be covered with scales or there may be central scarring. In some cases, reddish brown soft papules or nodules may be evident, which on diascopy exhibits the characteristic "apple jelly" consistency.

The clinical variants of lupus vulgaris include: 1) classic plaque; 2) hypertrophic; 3) ulcerative; 4) vegetating and 5) papular and nodular forms. The common sites affected, especially in children are the face and extremities following scratches, lacerations, boils, pin-pricks, etc. Lupus vulgaris may also occur at the BCG vaccination site.

Q5. What are the main differential diagnoses of lupus vulgaris?

Ans: Deep mycoses, especially chromoblastomycosis may resemble the vegetating and crusted type of lupus vulgaris. Cultures and histopathology will help to differentiate the two. Lupoid leishmaniasis may also pose diagnostic difficulty clinically. But, the histopathologic appearance, cultures and serological investigations will be of help. Sarcoidosis and leprosy are the other main differentials. The nodules of sarcoidosis resemble "grains of sand" rather than "apple jelly". The nodules in leprosy are firmer and there are other associated signs including sensory loss, nerve thickening, nerve palsies, etc. Syphilis, lupus erythematosus, psoriasis, etc. are the other differentials.

Q6. What are the histopathological features of lupus vulgaris?

Ans: There are tuberculoid granulomas with a tendency to become confluent throughout the dermis. Lymphocytes are usually prominent. Langerhans cells are present in moderate numbers in the granulomas. Central caseation may be scanty or absent. The bacilli

Table 1: Classification of cutaneous tuberculosis

Host immunity	*Method of inoculation*	*Disease*
Multibacillary forms		
Näive host	Direct inoculation	Tuberculous chancre (primary inoculation)
Low	Contiguous spread	Scrofuloderma
Low	Autoinoculation	Orificial tuberculosis
Low	Hematogenous spread	Acute miliary cutaneous
Low	Hematogenous spread	Tuberculous gumma (abscess)
Paucibacillary forms		
High	Direct inoculation	Warty tuberculosis
High	Direct inoculation	Lupus vulgaris (some)
High	Hematogenous spread	Lupus vulgaris
High	Hematogenous spread	Tuberculids Lichen scrofulosorum Papulonecrotic tuberculid Erythema induratum (Bazin)

are hard to demonstrate, occasionally numerous bacilli may be seen. The overlying epidermis may be atrophic or hyperplastic.

Q7. How do we diagnose lupus vulgaris? What are the investigations that help in the diagnosis?

Ans: The diagnosis of lupus vulgaris is based on clinical features, demonstration of acid-fast bacilli on smear, tissue culture, skin biopsy, and in recent years, polymerase chain reaction (PCR). Tissue culture is the gold standard for diagnosis, but lupus vulgaris being a paucibacillary form of tuberculous infection, culture is often negative. The Mantoux test is often positive, but it does not allow for precise diagnosis, only indicates that the patient has had previous contact with *Mycobacterium tuberculosis*. PCR is a useful, rapid method that has become available in recent years, but its sensitivity is reduced when used with smear-negative specimens or paucibacillary samples. Interferon-gamma releasing assays may also be helpful in some cases. However, in certain cases, where the diagnosis cannot be established conclusively, a therapeutic trial with standard antituberculosis therapy regimen might be helpful. Failure to respond within 4–6 weeks may suggest an alternate diagnosis.

Q8. What are the complications of lupus vulgaris?

Ans: Squamous cell carcinoma is the most important serious complication of long-standing lupus vulgaris; incidence varies between 0.5% and 10%. Other malignancies like basal cell carcinomas, melanomas and lymphomas have also been reported. Scarring, contractures and ulceration are the other major complications. Some scars may also develop keloids. If the lesions are on cosmetically important areas like the face (especially the nose), the impact can be quite disfiguring.

Q9. Discuss the management of lupus vulgaris.

Ans: A careful search for an underlying focus of disease and coexistent infections including HIV is essential before starting antituberculosis chemotherapy. It is also vital to confirm the diagnosis bacteriologically whenever possible and to obtain drug susceptibilities, in view of the increasing rates of drug-resistant tuberculosis.

The standard recommended antituberculosis regimen consists of four drugs: a combination of rifampicin, isoniazid, ethambutol and pyrazinamide for 2 months, followed by a 4 months continuation phase of rifampicin and isoniazid.

- Isoniazid (300 mg daily) for the full 6 months
- Rifampicin (450 mg daily for those weighing less than 50 kg; 600 mg daily for those above this weight) for the full 6 months.
- Pyrazinamide for the first 2 months (1.5 g daily for those weighing less than 50 kg; 2.0 g daily for those above this weight).
- Ethambutol for the first 2 months (15 mg/kg body weight daily).

All the drugs are taken on an empty stomach, once daily.

With appropriate treatment, a clinical response is seen as early as 5 weeks into treatment and usually marked improvement by 10 weeks. Second-line drugs may be considered, if there is a suspicion of resistance or if the patient develops serious adverse effects. Surgical excision of early lesions of lupus vulgaris may also be effective in some cases.

CHAPTER 91

Tinea Corporis

Lakshmi DV

Case study Tinea Corporis

Presenting Complaints

Doctor, I have noticed itchy circular patch over the forearm and upper back since 20 days. It has been increasing and spreading since then.

Setting

Dermatology outpatient department

History of Present Illness

A 30-year-old female presented with circular, itchy patch over the upper back since 20 days. The lesion has been increasing with partial clearance in central area. A similar patch has occurred over left forearm. She is not a known diabetic. No history of similar complaints in family members. No history of any topical cream application.

General Physical Examination and Systemic Examination

No abnormality detected

Dermatological Examination

An annular scaly plaque with central clearing measuring around 5 × 5 cm is seen over the left upper back (Fig. 1). A larger scaly plaque with marginal accentuation is present over the distal end of the forearm involving both flexor and extensor aspect of forearm around 10 × 7 cm (Fig. 2).
Potassium hydroxide (KOH) examination showed branching filamentous hyphae (Fig. 3).

Q1. What is your diagnosis?

a. Tinea circinata
b. Tinea imbricata
c. Tinea corporis
d. Tinea manuum

Ans: c. Tinea corporis.

It is defined as dermatophytosis of the glabrous skin with the exclusion of the palms (tinea manuum), soles (tinea pedis), and groins (tinea cruris).

Q2. What are the predisposing factors and routes of transmission of tinea corporis?

Ans: Predisposing factors are poor personal hygiene, poor nutrition, geographic locations (hot humid climates), and debilitating systemic diseases like diabetes, leukemia, and other endocrine disorders (Cushing's syndrome).

Direct contact with infected persons or animals, infection from other sites in the same patient, e.g.

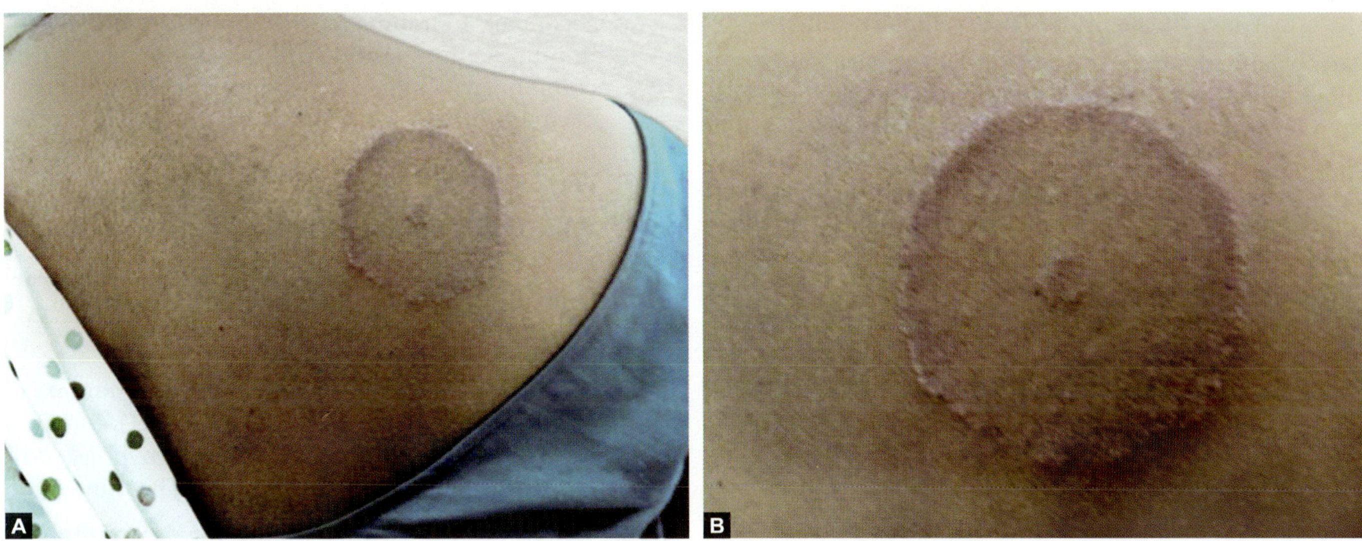

Figs 1A and B: Annular scaly plaque with central clearing over the left upper back

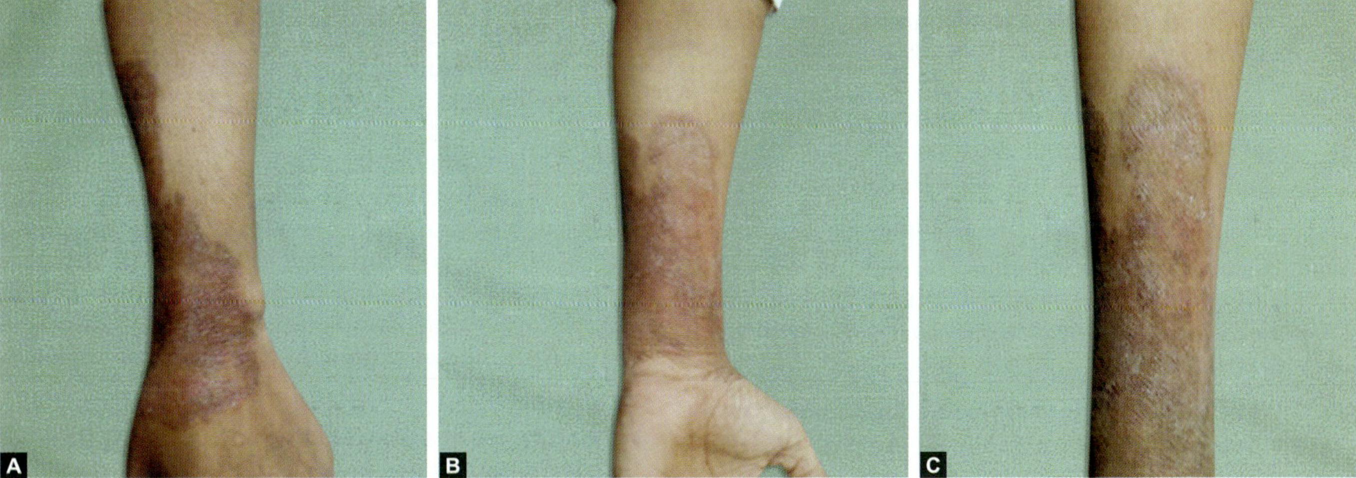

Figs 2A to C: Large scaly plaque with marginal accentuation over the distal end of the forearm involving both flexor and extensor aspect

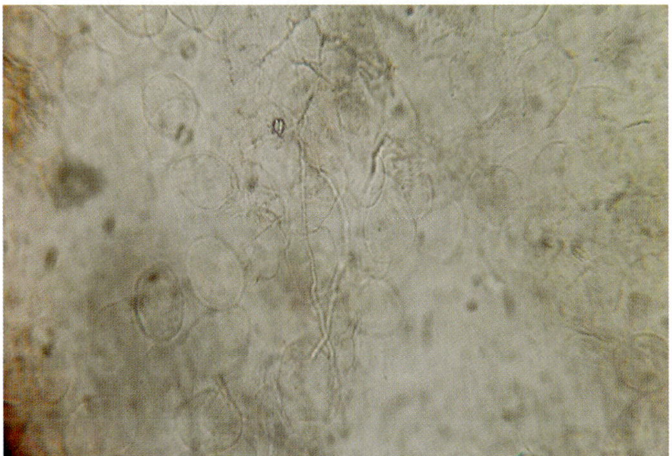

Fig. 3: KOH examination showed branching filamentous hyphae and mosaic pattern of outline of keratinocytes

reservoir of infection on the feet or scalp, and fomites are the common routes of transmission.

Q3. Which are the most common causative organisms of tinea corporis?

Ans: The three most common causative organisms are (1) *Trichphyton rubrum,* (2) *Trichophyton mentagrophytes* and (3) *Microsporum canis.*

Q4. Why is tinea corporis less inflammatory than other dermatophytosis?

Ans: The degree of inflammation varies depending on the species of the fungus, the immune status of the host and the extent of follicular invasion. Thus, tinea corporis is generally less inflammatory than other dermatophytosis.

Q5. Why are the characteristic lesions annular?

Ans: The dermatophyte invades the uppermost, keratinized layer, the stratum corneum, produces exoenzyme keratinase and induces inflammatory reaction at the site of infection. Inflammation causes increase in epidermopoiesis, and the pathogen to move away from the site of infection and take residence at a new site with central clearance. This movement of the organism away from the infection site produces the classical ringed lesion. The central skin shows normal or postinflammatory hyperpigmentation, a change of texture or residual erythematous dermal nodules.

Q6. List the morphological variants of tinea corporis.

Ans: Annular type, eczematous annular type, crusted type, herpetiform type, and plaque type

Q7. What is tinea profunda and tinea imbricata?

Ans: Tinea profunda is a clinical variant of tinea corporis characterized by excessive inflammatory response to a dermatophyte analogous to a kerion on the scalp whereas tinea imbricata is a another variant caused by the anthropophilic dermatophyte *T. concentricum* clinically characterized by overlapping scaly annular plaques that form a concentric lamellar lesion.

Q8. What is Tinea pseudo imbricata?

Ans: Tinea imbricat like lesions occurring in patients who have used topical steroids. Usually *Trichophyton* mentagrophytes is isolated instead of Trichophyton concentricum.

Q9. What are the differentials to be considered in a case of tinea corporis?

Ans: Differential diagnosis:

- When lesions are annular and noninflammatory, pityriasis rosea, impetigo circinata, nummular eczema, erythema annulare centrifugum, and granuloma annulare.
- If inflammatory concurrent bacterial, candidal, or deep fungal infections to be considered.
- If the lesion is more papulosquamous, then psoriasis, seborrheic dermatitis, pityriasis rosea, lichen planus, polymorphous light eruption, or secondary syphilis to be ruled out.

Q10. What is granuloma trichophyticum?

Ans: Granuloma trichophyticum is synonymous with Majocchi's granuloma, also known as granuloma tricofitico, and nodular granulomatous perifolliculitis commonly caused by *Trichophyton rubrum*.

It is a granulomatous dermal response caused by dermal penetration of fungi, by follicular invasion secondary to trauma or break in epidermis seen in immunocompetant individuals (follicular-variant common in young girls). Subcutaneous nodular type occurs solitary or as multiple well-circumscribed oval patches or as indistinct scaly ones and evolve into perifollicular papulopustules and nodules.

Q11. What is sandwich sign?

Ans: It is the histopathological appearance of the fungal hyphae trapped in the layers of stratum corneum.

Q12. What is mosaic fungus?

Ans: It is microscopic artifact caused by the borders of the keratinocytes on wet-mount (KOH), partially lysed simulating fungal hyphae. True hyphae show branching and crosses the borders of keratinocytes.

Q13. Which are the culture media for dermatophyte isolation?

Ans: Sabouraud's dextrose agar (SDA, 4% peptone, 1% glucose, agar, water) is the most commonly used isolation media for dermatophytosis and development of colony takes 7–14 days. Modified SDA, with addition of gentamicin, chloramphenicol, and cycloheximide is more selective media for dermatophytes as chroramphenicol inhibits the growth of saprophytic fungus. Dermatophyte test medium is an alternative to isolation media that contains pH indicator phenol red. Dermatophytes utilize the protein resulting in excess ammonium ion and alkaline environment which turn the medium from yellow to bright red.

Q14. What are the newer diagnostic modalities of dermatophyte detection?

Ans: The newer methods include:

- Uniplex polymerase chain reactiom (PCR) and multiplex PCR. Multiplex PCR tests enable simultaneous amplification of 21 dermatomycotic pathogens with subsequent DNA detection by means of agarose gel electrophoresis.
- Matrix-assisted laser desorption ionization time-of-flight mass spectrometry: It is based on the detection of biochemical characteristics, proteolytic degradation product which is a result of the activity of mycological infections. The peptide patterns of affected samples are then identified by comparison with known peptide spectra from skin disorders.
- Reflectance confocal microscopy provides *in vivo* imaging of the epidermis and superficial dermis at cellular level resolution and can be used to detect cutaneous fungi and parasitic infestations.

Q15. What is Trichophyton rubrum syndrome?

Ans: It refers to chronic dermatophytosis with episodes of relapse and remissions caused by *Trichophyton rubrum*. It is characterized by involvement of atleast four body sites such as feet (plantar), hands (palmar), nails, as well as one other site with exclusion of inguinal area along with identification of *Trichophyton rubrum* in microscopy and culture.

Q16. What is trichophytin test?

Ans: It is an intradermal test performed to detect allergic hypersensitivity towards dermatophytes. Trichophytin antigen is a glycopeptide obtained (using acetone-ethylene glycol extraction method) from the spores and mycelia of dermatophytes, especially *Trichophyton mentagrophytes.* Trichophytin in the concentration of either 10 µg, 1 µg, or 0.1 µg in 0.1 mL of normal saline is injected intradermally into the flexor forearm. The test is read after 20 minutes for an immediate reaction and after 24 or 72 hours for a delayed response. A wheal larger than 10 mm in diameter at 20 minutes and induration more than 5 mm at 72 hours is considered a positive response.

Q17. Enumerate the line of management in a case of tinea corporis.

Ans: *General measures:* Good personal hygiene, avoid tight fitting clothing or use of moist clothing.

Specific measures:

- *Topical therapy:* Miconazole, clotrimazole, ketoconazole, econazole or terbinafine cream twice daily for 2–4 weeks
- *Systemic therapy:*
  - Itraconazole: 200–400 mg OD for 2 weeks
  - Fluconazole: 150–300 mg weekly for 4–6 weeks
  - Terbinafine: 250 mg OD for 14 days.

Presently longer duration of therapy upto 4-6 weeks is being considered in view of large amount of resistant cases

CHAPTER 92

Tinea Pedis

Rahul Arora

Case study Tinea Pedis

Presenting Complaints

Doctor I have white itchy lesions in between my toes.

Setting

Dermatology outpatient department

History of Present Illness

A 38-year-old factory worker presented with complaints of itchy white-colored thick lesion in the interdigital area of fourth and fifth toe of left leg of 2-weeks duration. Patient further gave history of prolonged wearing of tight fitting rubber boots as a protective wear for long hours.

General and Systemic Examination

No abnormality detected

Dermatological Examination

There was erythema, maceration, fissuring, and scaling, present between the fourth and fifth left toes. The dorsal surface of the foot was clear, but some extension onto the plantar surface of the foot was seen. There was presence of distal leukonychia and subungual hyperkeratosis in the left great toe. The right foot and finger nails were absolutely normal.

Q1. What is your diagnosis?

a. Tinea pedis
b. Contact allergic dermatitis to boots
c. Psoriasis
d. Dyshidrotic eczema

Ans: a. Tinea pedis

Q2. What is Tinea pedis?

Ans: Tinea pedis or athlete's foot is the term used for a dermatophyte infection of the plantar aspect of the feet and the interdigital spaces.

Q3. What are the causative organisms of tinea pedis?

Ans: *Trichophyton rubrum* is the most common cause of tinea pedis worldwide although *Trichophyton mentagrophytes,* and *Epidermophyton floccosum* also cause tinea pedis. Nondermatophyte moulds causing tinea pedis include *Scytalidium dimidiatum, Scytalidium hyalinum,* and rarely, *Candida* species.

Q4. What is the pathophysiology of tinea pedis infection?

Ans: Pathophysiology:

- *Agent factors:* Dermatophyte fungi release keratinases and invade the superficial keratin of the skin. Dermatophyte cell walls also contain mannans, which can inhibit the body's immune response and reduce keratinocyte proliferation, resulting in a decreased rate of sloughing and a chronic state of infection.

- *Host factors:* Breaks in the skin and maceration of the skin may aid in dermatophyte invasion. The cutaneous presentation of tinea pedis is also dependent on the host's immune system and the infecting dermatophyte.
- *Environmental factors:* Temperature and serum factors, such as beta globulins and ferritin, appear to have a growth-inhibitory effect on dermatophytes; however, this pathophysiology is not completely understood. Sebum also is inhibitory, thus partly explaining the propensity for dermatophyte infection of the feet, which have no sebaceous glands.

Q5. What are the clinical variants of tenia pedis?

Ans: Various clinical variants include:

- *Interdigital tinea pedis*: The interdigital variant is characterized by erythema, maceration, fissuring, and scaling, most often seen between the fourth and fifth toes. A secondary bacterial infection following a fungal infection is not uncommon and is known as the dermatophytosis complex. Interdigital variety is usually caused by *Trichophyton rubrum*. Other possible causative organisms in tinea pedis include *Trichophyton mentagrophytes* var *interdigitale* and *Epidermophyton floccosum*.
- *Chronic hyperkeratotic tinea pedis*: A distinctive pattern of lesion, manifesting as scaling and thickening of the soles, which often extends beyond the plantar surface in a moccasin distribution commonly caused by *Trichophyton rubrum* (Fig. 1). It may be asymptomatic and both feet are usually affected. Other possible causative organisms include *Trichophyton mentagrophytes* var *interdigitale*, *Epidermophyton floccosum*, and the nondermatophyte molds *Scytalidium hyalinum* and *Scytalidium dimidiatum*.
- *Inflammatory or vesicular tinea pedis*: It is a rare form characterized by painful, pruritic vesicles or bullae mimicking pompholyx, most often on the instep or anterior plantar surface which may contain either clear or purulent fluid and on rupturing leave behind persistant erythema (Fig. 2). It may be associated with complications like cellulitis, lymphangitis, adenopathy, and id-reaction.
- *Ulcerative tinea pedis*: It is characterized by rapidly spreading vesiculopustular lesions, ulcers, and erosions, typically in the web spaces, and is often accompanied by a secondary bacterial infection. Cellulitis, lymphangitis, pyrexia, and malaise can occur. This type is commonly seen in immunocompromised and diabetic patients. Both inflammatory and ulcerative varieties are rare and are caused by the zoophilic fungus *Trichophyton mentagrophytes* var *mentagrophytes*.

Q6. What is 2-feet—1-hand syndrome?

Ans: Tinea manuum is often unilateral and associated with moccasin-type tinea pedis. The scratching habits of the infected individual can cause the spread of the dermatophytes from the feet to the hand.

Q7. What are the predisposing factors which must be asked in the history?

Ans: Predisposing factors include:

- Age: Adult more than children
- Sex: Males more than females
- Hot, humid, tropical environment
- Occlusive footwear and bare foot walking
- Hyperhidrosis
- Immunodeficiency states, e.g. medication such as azathioprine, or infection with human immunodeficiency virus
- Compromised peripheral circulation, e.g. due to lymphoedema.

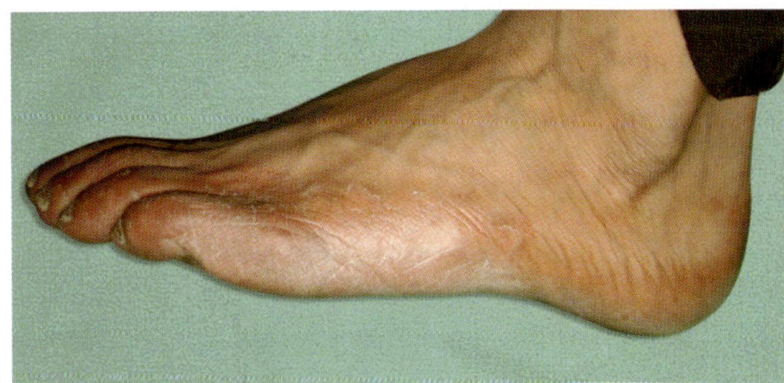

Fig. 1: Chronic hyperkeratotic moccasin leather type Tinea pedis

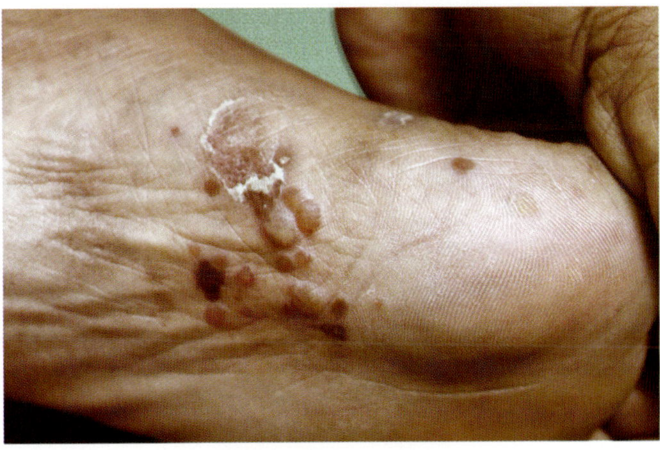

Fig. 2: Bullous tinea pedis

Q8. What are the relevant differential diagnosis?

Ans: Differential diagnosis:
- Allergic-contact dermatitis
- Cutaneous candidiasis
- Dyshidrotic eczema
- Erythema multiforme
- Erythrasma
- Friction blisters
- Syphilis
- Pityriasis rubra pilaris
- Plaque psoriasis
- Pustular psoriasis
- Reactive arthritis.

Q9. What is the treatment of tinea pedis?

Ans: Treatment principles:
- Usually treated by topical antifungal cream as for tinea corporis
- Chronic infections require oral antifungal therapy which is similar to treatment of tinea corporis.
- Secondary bacterial infections may occur and require oral antibiotics
- Using antifungal powders on feet and shoes can help prevent reinfection
- Wearing open shoes can help with healing.

Q10. What are the preventive measures that should be advised to the patient?

- Keep feet clean and dry
  - Dry thoroughly and between the toes after bathing, showering, or swimming
  - Do not put on socks and shoes when feet are wet
- Wash with soap and/or shampoo after sports or exercise
- Change socks at least once a day. Cotton socks will absorb sweat
- Wear shoes that are roomy and allow some air to circulate
  - Shoes that are made of breathable materials, such as leather, are best
  - Shoes made of materials such as vinyl, cause the feet to remain moist and thus provide a good place for fungi to grow
- Wear flip-flops or other footwear in gym shower or locker room to prevent contact
- Avoid sharing nail tools, such as clippers and scissors
- Avoid sharing sports gear, shoes, and towels with others.
- Use antifungal foot powders, both on the feet (between the toes) and in the shoes
- When washing clothing, use hot water and bleach to increase the chance of killing fungi.

Q11. What are the causes of treatment failure?

Ans: Main causes of treatment failure include:
- Untreated or persistent infection, e.g. of the nails (onychomycosis)
- Reinfection from close contacts.

Q12. What are the common concurrent problems?

- Secondary bacterial infection especially gram-negative bacteria
- Erythrasma due to *Cornyebacterium minutissimum*
- Complications: cellulitis, erysipelas, id reactions.

Q13. Which are the most common oral antifungals that are used in the treatment?

Ans: Oral antifungals in adults:
- Terbinafine: 250 mg OD for 2–6 weeks
- Fluconazole: 150–300 mg weekly for 4–6 weeks
- Itraconazole: 100 mg BD for 4 weeks
- Griseofulvin: 500 mg BD for 4–8 weeks.

CHAPTER 93

Onychomycosis

Aarti Sarda, Abhishek De, Lakshmi DV

Case study Onychomycosis

Presenting Complaints

Doctor, I have noticed yellowish discoloration of my finger nails since 1 month.

Setting

Dermatology outpatient department

History of Present Illness

A 35-year-old male presented with discoloration of his left fourth and little finger nails since 1-month. He is a gardener by occupation. There was history of similar nail involvement in the past which improved with some oral medication. He is not a known diabetic. No history of similar complaints in family members.

General Physical Examination and Systemic Examination

No abnormality detected

Dermatological Examination

Diffuse yellowish dyschromia over the left little finger nail plate with a white-patch overlapping the yellow discoloration (Fig. 1). There was relative sparing of the lateral and proximal periungual region. Similar changes more localized to distal half of nail plate were present in the fourth finger nail. Rest of the finger nails spared. Toe nails uninvolved. Palmar aspect, lateral borders of palms and interdigital spaces appear normal. Potassium hydroxide (KOH) examination revealed long, septate, branching hyphae in the nail specimen (Fig. 2).

Q1. What is your diagnosis?

a. Onychomycosis
b. Lichen planus of nail
c. Psoriatic nail
d. Trachyonychia

Ans: a. Onychomycosis (mixed pattern onychomycosis). Here there is a combination of clinical pattern: Distal subungual onychomycosis with superficial onychomycosis.

Q2. What are the risk factors in onychomycosis?

Ans: The risk factors include:

- Nail trauma
- Diabetes mellitus
- Psoriasis
- Advanced age, family history
- Environmental factors: hot, humid regions, barefoot walking, occlusive footwear
- Immunocompromised states

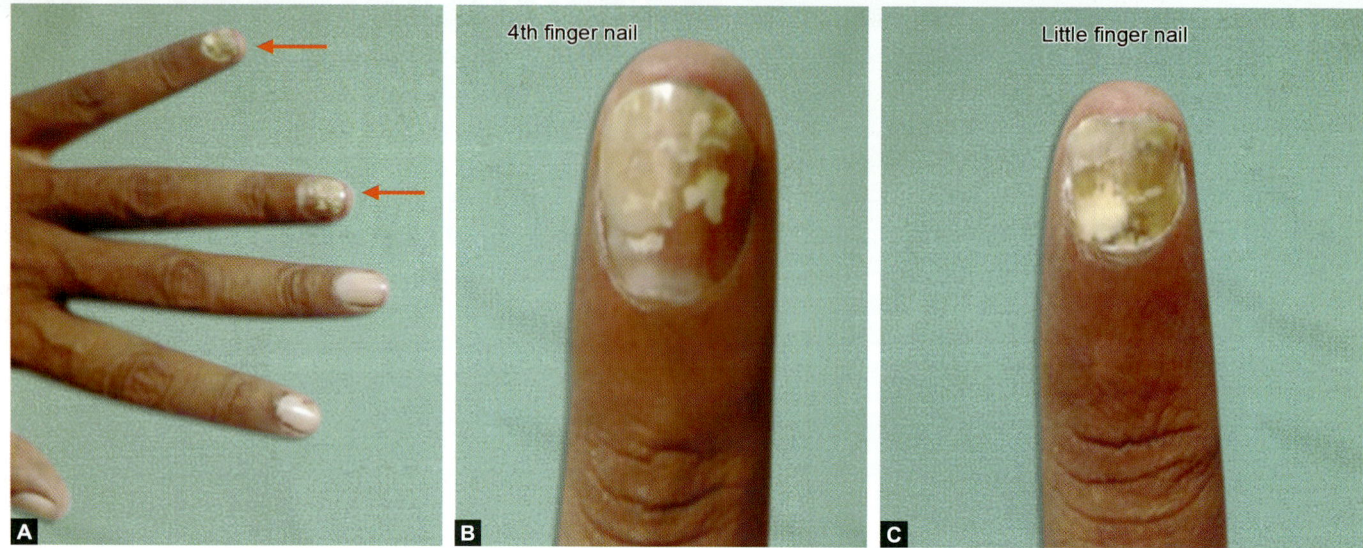

Figs 1A to C: Diffuse yellowish dyschromia over the left little finger nail plate with a white-patch overlapping the yellow discoloration

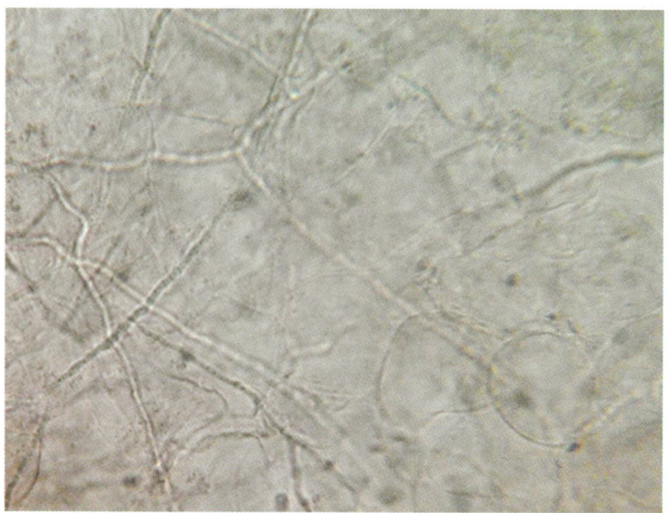

Fig. 2: KOH examination revealed long, septate, branching hyphae in the nail specimen

Table 1: Fungi responsible for causing onychomycosis

1	Dermatophytes	• *Trichophyton rubrum* • *Trichophyton mentagrophytes* • *Epidermophyton floccosum*
2	Nondermatophytes	• *Acremonium species* • *Alternaria species* • *Aspergillus* • *Scytalidium dimidiatum* • *Scytalidium hyalinum* • *Scopulariopsis brevicalis* • *Geotrichum candidum* • *Botryodiplodia theobromae* • *Fusarium species* • *Onycochola Canadensis* • *Cladosporium carrionii*
3	Yeast	• *Candida albicans*

- Peripheral vascular diseases.

Note: Interdigital and moccasin type of tinea pedis increases risk for nail infection.

Q3. What are the fungi responsible in causation of onychomycosis?

Ans: The fungi responsible in causation of onychomycosis has been described in Table 1.

Q4. What are the clinical types of onychomycosis?

Ans: The clinical types of onychomycosis are:

1. *Distal subungual onychomycosis* (DLSO): Invasion through distal nail bed, most common type
2. *Proximal subungual onychomycosis* (PSO): Invasion through newly formed proximal nail plate seen as white to beige opacity which eventually affects the entire nail, and causes subungual hyperkeratosis, leukonychia, proximal onycholysis.
3. White superficial onychomycosis (WSO): Invasion of the superficial layers of nail plate resulting in white to dull-yellow sharply bordered-patches anywhere on the surface of the toe nail.
4. *Total dystrophic onychomycosis* (TDO): Entire nail plate and bed involved.
5. Mixed pattern onychomycosis: combination of different clinical patterns in the same nail or in different nails. DLSO plus WSO, SWO plus PSO, DLSO plus PSO

Q5. What is endonyx onychomycosis?

Ans: Endonyx onychomycosis is an unusual variant of onychomycosis which involves the inner surface of nail plate without inflammation of the nail bed, onycholysis or subungual hyperkeratosis. The classic nail lesion shows milky-white discoloration in the nail plate without nail surface change. It is caused by *Trichophyton soudanense* and *Trichophyton violaceum*.

Q6. What are the salient features of candidal onychomycosis and its subtypes?

Ans: It is caused by mostly *C. albicans*, and also *C. parapsilosis*, *C. tropicalis* and *C. krusei*. Both toe and finger nails can be involved.

It has three subtypes:

1. Candidal paronychia: The most common type marked by swelling and erythema of proximal and lateral nail folds.
2. Candidal granuloma: Characterized by direct invasion and thickening of nail plate and associated paronychia seen in immunocompromised individuals. In advanced cases, entire nail is involved with swelling of proximal and lateral nail folds till digits causing pseudoclubbing giving "chicken drumstick" appearance.
3. Candidal onycholysis: Resembles DLSO, seen as yellowish-gray mass lifts off nail plate from bed. Hence, the name onycholysis.

Q7. Enumerate the differentials in a case of onychomycosis.

Ans: Differentials include nail conditions due to:

- Psoriasis
- Lichen planus
- Alopecia areata
- Paronychia
- Bacterial infections
- Yellow nail syndrome
- Twenty-nail dystrophy
- Nail changes secondary to systemic diseases
- Contact dermatitis or atopic dermatitis or nail changes due to nail cosmetics
- Nail bed tumors.

Q8. How should you obtain a nail clipping for microscopic evaluation and culture?

Ans: The patient should be off both topical and systemic drugs for 2–4 weeks prior to sample collection. Sample collected to be divided into two parts (one for direct microscopy, other for culture).

- Cleanse affected nails with alcohol or soap or water and allow it to dry.
- A curette is preferable than blade as it minimizes bleeding.
- For a subungual sample, clip nails to the most proximal point possible (without causing discomfort), trim back the nail to access the underside of nail plate, moist debris that lies behind the dry, flaky material at the end of distal nail.
- In PSO, normal surface of nail plate is paired with no. 15 surgical blade at lunula and white debris is collected with curette from deeper portion of the plate and the proximal nail bed.
- In WSO, white spots on nails scraped, outermost surface discarded, debris directly underneath collected.
- In TDO, any part of affected nail plate or bed can be used.

Q9. Which are the diagnostic modalities useful in onychomycosis?

Ans: *Conventional microscopy:* KOH, special stains, fungal culture, histopathological examination (HPE), nail dermoscopy.

Other modalities: Immunohistochemistry, dual-flow cytometry, DNA-based methods: polymerase chain reaction-restriction fragment length polymorphism (PCR-RFLP) assay, double-round PCR, real-time PCR, PCR-direct sequencing, optical coherence tomography, matrix-assisted laser desorption, phase contrast hard X-ray microscopy.

Q10. Should nail biopsy be advocated routinely and why?

Ans: No. HPE does not help to differentiate between viable or nonviable organisms nor does it help to identify the particular pathogen as both dermatophytes and moulds produce hyphae and large, thick-walled arthrospores. It may be done if KOH and culture are repeatedly negative with high clinical suspicion of onychomycosis.

Histopathology reveals hyphae between the nail laminae parallel to the surface, with often on ventral nail and nail bed stratum corneum. The epidermis may show spongiosis and focal parakeratosis, with minimal dermal inflammatory response. In SWO, the organisms are present superficially on the dorsal nail and display unique "perforating organs" and "eroding fronds". In candidal onychomycosis, pseudohyphae invades the entire nail plate, adjacent cuticle, granular layer and stratum spinosum of the nail bed, and the hyponychial stratum corneum.

Q11. Which special stains accentuate the fungal hyphae when added to KOH preparation?

Ans: Parker blue-black ink, Calcofluor-white and Chlorazol black E.

Q12. List the culture media useful in onychomycosis.

Ans: Culture media:

- *Primary medium*: Containing cycloheximide that inhibits the growth of nondermatophytic moulds and bacteria, e.g. Dermatophyte medium, Sabouraud peptone-glucose agar (Emmon's modification), Mycosel (BBL) and Mycobiotic (DIFCO).
- *Secondary media*: Free of cycloheximide and allow isolation of non-dermatophytic moulds, e.g. Sabouraud dextrose agar (SDA), Littman Oxgall medium, and potato dextrose agar (PDA) that are antibiotics like chloramphenicol and gentamicin may be added to SDA or PDA to eliminate bacterial contamination from non-sterile sites. Specimens should be incubated at 25–30°C.
- Growth on both types of media is indicative of a dermatophyte while growth only on cycloheximid-free media is suggestive of nondermatophytic mould.

Q13. If a culture yields a nondermatophyte, when is it significantly considered as primary causative pathogen?

Ans: Nondermatophytes can be obtained as contaminants. So in case of culture of a mold or yeast, it should be considered a pathogen only if hyphae, spores, or yeast cells are seen on microscopic examination. Finally, confirmation of an infection by a nondermatophyte requires isolation of the organism on at least 5 out of 20 inocula without concurrent isolation of a dermatophyte.

Q14. Define a lacquer and how does it help in onychomycosis.

Ans: Lacquers are specialized transungual drug delivery systems that produce a nonwater-soluble film after application and following evaporation of solvent, active ingredient remains in contact with the nail for long periods and the concentration of the active ingredient in the remaining film reservoir increases manifold, thus providing the high concentration gradient essential for maximal penetration. Lacquer also acts as occlusive agent, transungual water loss is further reduced, enhancing the mass transport of the drug into and through the nail plate.

Q15. Enumerate the topical antifungal available for onychomycosis.

Ans: The topical antifungals available for onychomycosis has been described in Table 2.

Method of application: The lacquer is painted evenly on affected nail plates using applicatory brush daily for 48 weeks. Also apply under the tip of each affected nail. Application to be done preferably at night time for better compliance. Lacquer to be removed once weekly with a alcohol wipe. Do not use nail polish during treatment period. Amorolfine is applied 1–2 times/week.

Q16. How do you manage a case of onychomycosis?

Ans: Treatment:

- *General measures*: To wear loose shoes, keep nails short, avoid nail polish and bare foot walking.
- *Specific measures:*
  - Topical therapy
    - Antifungal nail lacquers (discussed above).
    - Chemical avulsion of the nail: 30% salicylic acid, 50% potassium iodide or 40% urea under occlusion. Etching of nail plate with 20% tartaric acid and 10% phosphoric acid increases surface area and adhesion of active compound resulting in formation of profuse microporosities that enhance topical antifungal delivery.

Table 2: Topical antifungals and its mechanism of action

S.No.	*Drugs*	*Mechanism of action*
1	Ciclopirox olamine 8%	Inhibits metal-dependent enzymes responsible for the degradation of peroxides within the fungal cell as well as upregulation of fungicidal reactive oxygen formation within the fungal cytoplasm. Used for dermatophytics and nondermatophytic molds
2	Amorolfine 5%	It affects membrane fluidity by inhibiting two important enzymes viz 14-α-reductase and δ-7,8 isomerase involved in ergosterol biosynthesis
3	Efinaconazole 10%	Formulation has low surface tension, causes wicking action thereby draws the drug around the nail
4	Tavaborole 10%	It is boron-based therapy, due to low molecular weight, highly reactive molecules, targets protein synthesis (inhibition of the enzyme leucine aminoacyl-transfer ribonucleic acid synthetase)

- Physical techniques like manual or electric nail abrasion, microporation, application of low frequency ultrasound and electric currents. These techniques enhance the action of topical antifungal.
- *Systemic therapy*: Oral antifungals are given when more than 75% of the nail apparatus is involved, the lunula or matrix is involved, in immunocompromised and in the elderly. Terbinafine, itraconazole and fluconazole are being used for the treatment of onychomycosis. Terbinafine 250 mg/day for 12 weeks (toe nails) and 6 weeks for finger nails, itraconazole 200 mg/day or 400 mg daily for 1 week per month for 2–3 months, fluconazole 150 mg/week for 6–12 weeks.
- Combination or sequential or supplementary therapy: Combining oral and topical antifungal or using two antifungal sequentially in a pulse regimen which act at different levels of ergosterol metabolism. Supplementary therapy refers to extended course of oral antifungal in patients found mycologically positive after conventional time periods.
- *Photodynamic therapy and lasers:* Neodymium-doped yttrium aluminum garnet (Nd:YAG) laser causes photoinactivation of the fungal pathogens at a depth below the nail tissue surface without causing collateral damage and leaves the surrounding tissue intact. Noveon dual-wavelength (using 870- and 930- nm light) near-infrared diode laser is also used and does not cause photoablation toxic plumes unlike Nd:YAG.
- *Surgical methods:* Partial or complete nail avulsion with matrixectomy followed by application of topical antifungal.

Q17. Terbinafine has better mycological cure than itraconazole in dermatophytic onychomycosis because:

a. It has shorter duration of treatment and better compliant
b. Lesser side effects profile
c. Achieves higher concentration in nail apparatus
d. Inhibits squalene epoxidase and thus inhibits fungi better than azole

Ans: c. Achieves higher concentration in nail apparatus. Its concentration in the nail is about 100-fold higher than its mean fungicidal concentration, while that of itraconazole is in the borderline between fungicidal and fungistatic concentrations.

Q18. What is BOAT and BATT?

Ans: BOAT and BATT

BOAT*:* Boosted-oral antifungals treatment therapy. A piece of SDA is secured on to the affected nail plate for 48 hours following the weekly pulse of itraconazole.

BATT*:* Boosted antifungal topical treatment. Topical amorolfine nail lacquer is applied weekly once, second day onwards. SDA piece is secured in place over nail for week, later removed and amorolfine nail lacquer is applied.

Mechanism of action: It targets chlamydospores and arthroconidia within the nail plate and produces sensitive hyphae which are less refractory to treatment with antifungals.

Disadvantage: Risk of over stimulation and systemic spread of fungi that are not susceptible to the antifungal agent.

Q19. What are the causes of treatment failure?

Ans: Treatment failure is due to:

- Incorrect diagnosis
- Inappropriate choice of drug or its delivery modality
- Dermatophytoma (a sequestered mass of dermatophytes invading and expanding the space between the nail plate and the nail bed, appears as a dense linear or round white area, it is impenetrable to systemic or topical antifungals)
- Drug interactions and drug resistance
- Local causes: Thick nail, extensive involvement of the entire nail unit, lateral nail disease, yellow longitudinal streaks or "spikes", mixed infection
- Coexisting diseases (psoriasis, lichen planus), concomitant disease (e.g. peripheral vascular disease, diabetes), and immunosuppression
- Noncompliance of patient to treatment protocol.

Q20. How would you differentiate a case of relapse from reinfection?

Ans: It is not possible to distinguish between relapse and reinfection. However, following clinical and mycological cure, recurrence of toe nail onychomycosis is more likely to be due to relapse if it has developed within 18 months of starting oral antifungal therapy, and reinfection if after that.

CHAPTER 94

Pityriasis Versicolor

Sankeerth V

Case study — Pityriasis Versicolor

Presenting Complaints

Doctor, I have been noticing a few small light-colored patches, appearing on my skin in the upper chest and upper back since last 2 months. They are not itchy or painful, but do look odd. I am getting worried as it has been slowly spreading.

Setting

Dermatology outpatient department

History of Present Illness

A 25-year-old man, presented with complaints of few light-colored patches over the skin on the upper chest and upper back since last 2 months. He comes from a place where the climate is predominantly hot and humid. Initially, there were 2–3 patches, but they are gradually increasing in number. These patches were not associated with any symptoms like itching, burning, or pain sensation.

There is no history of tightening of skin or similar lesions in any other family members.

General Physical Examination and Systemic Examination

No abnormality detected.

Dermatological Examination

Multiple, well-defined, hypopigmented, oval to round macules with fine branny scaling, few coalescing to form patches, distributed over the upper chest and upper back region of the body (Fig. 1).

Q1. What is the most likely diagnosis?

a. Pityriasis versicolor
b. Vitiligo
c. Progressive macular hypomelanosis
d. Seborrheic dermatitis

Ans: a. Pityriasis Versicolor

Q2. How do you diagnose Pityriasis versicolor?

Ans: Pityriasis versicolor is most often diagnosed on clinical grounds. The classical lesions are well-defined oval to round macules showing fine branny scaling. These lesions may be hypopigmented or hyperpigmented or slightly erythematous, distributed in seborrheic-rich areas.

In most cases, stretching of the lesion will make the scales prominent. This is known as "coup d'ongle sign" (scratch sign or besnier's sign).

Q3. How will you confirm the diagnosis?

Ans: Diagnosis can be confirmed by potassium hydroxide (KOH) mount, Wood's lamp and fungal culture.

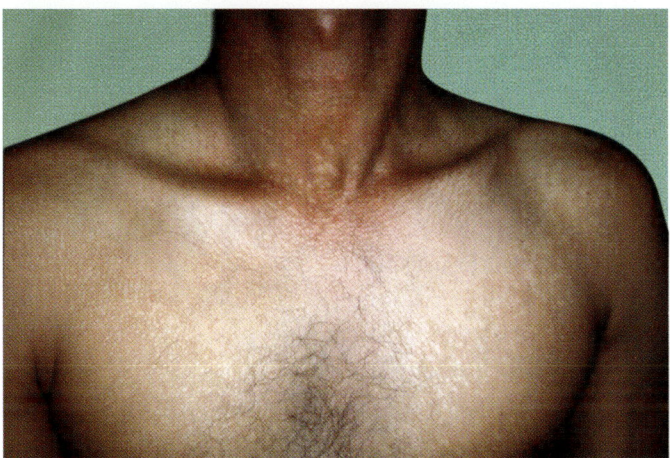

Fig. 1: Multiple, well-defined, hypopigmented, oval to round macules with fine branny scaling over the upper chest

- Potassium hydroxide preparation of skin scraping demonstrates the characteristic fungal spores and short cigar-butt hyphae. This appearance is called "Spaghetti and meatballs or banana and grape" appearance. Addition of methylene blue stain to KOH preparation may enhance the visualization of fungal elements.
- Wood's lamp: It shows orange-yellowish fluorescence over the involved skin, which is suspected to be due to a compound called Pteridine.
- Culture: It is rarely necessary and usually requires a lipid-containing medium (i.e. olive oil) to demonstrate the growth. Isolation of Malassezia species from the scrapings is of no diagnostic value as they are a part of the normal flora of the skin.

Q4. Which are the causative organisms in Pityriasis versicolor?

Ans: The causative organisms are lipophilic yeasts belonging to the genus *Malassezia*. They are described in Table 1.

Table 1: Causative organisms belonging to genus Malassezia

Malassezia globosa (most common)	*Malassezia furfur*
Malassezia sympodialis	*Malassezia restricta*
Malassezia obtuse	*Malassezia slooffiae*
Malassezia japonica	*Malassezia dermatis*
Malassezia nana	*Malassezia caprae*
Malassezia equine	*Malassezia yamotoensis*

Q5. Which are the most common sites involved in Pityriasis versicolor infections?

Ans: The seborrheic-rich areas like scalp, upper trunk, neck, axilla and flexures are usually involved.

Q6. What are the factors predisposing to development of Pityriasis versicolor infections?

Ans: Malassezia species are a part of the normal flora of the skin. They exist as saprophytic yeast. Infection sets in which they get converted into the parasitic mycelia form. The factors which predispose for this conversion are:
- Warm, humid environment
- Hyperhidrosis
- Poor hygiene
- Oral contraceptive use
- Systemic corticosteroid use
- Cushing's disease
- Immunosuppression
- Malnourished state.

Q7. What are the different types of presentations of Pityriasis versicolor?

Ans: Morphological variants:
- Hypopigmented variant
- Hyperpigmented variant
- Follicular variant
- Erythrodermic variant.

Other sites
- Inverse variant (involves flexures predominantly)
- Face may be involved in some cases (Fig. 2).

Q8. What are the synonyms for Pityriasis versicolor?

Ans: Synonyms:
- Tinea versicolor

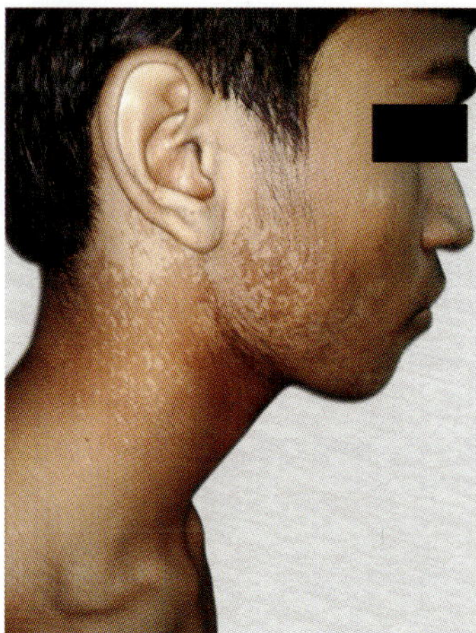

Fig. 2: Hypopigmented pityriasis versicolor lesions extending on to the face

- Dermatomycosis furfuracea
- Tinea flavea
- Liver spots
- Chromophytosis.

Q9. What are the different metabolites secreted by Malassezia?

Ans: Metabolites secreted by *Malassezia*:

- *Azelaic acid:* It is responsible for hypopigmentation, as it inhibits tyrosinase.
- *Malassezin:* It induces apoptosis of melanocytes.
- *Pityriacitrin:* yellow-compound that absorbs ultraviolet (UV) light.
- *Pityrialactone*
- *Pityriarubin:* It inhibits 5-Lipoxygenase activity.
- *Pteridine:* Responsible for orange-yellow fluorescence under Wood's lamp.

Q10. What is the differential diagnosis for Pityriasis versicolor?

Ans: Differential diagnosis:

- Pityriasis alba
- Vitiligo
- Pityriasis rosea
- Erythrasma
- Idiopathic guttate hypomelanosis
- Progressive macular hypomelanosis
- Seborrheic dermatitis
- Confluentand reticulated papillomatosis of Gougerot and Carteud
- Hypopigmented mycosis fungoides.

Q11. How do you treat a case of Pityriasis versicolor?

Ans: Several topical and systemic agents are effective in treating Pityriasis versicolor. These include:

- Topical treatment:
  - Ketoconazole 2%
  - Oxiconazole 1%
  - Miconazole 2%
  - Selenium sulfide 2.5%
  - Zinc pyrithione 1%
  - Ciclopirox olamine
  - Terbinafine 1%.

For extensive areas of involvement, lotions are preferred. Topical treatment should be continued for 3–4 weeks.

- *Systemic treatment:*
  - Oral Ketoconazole: 400 mg single dose or 200 mg daily for 7 days
  - Oral Fluconazole: 400 mg single dose
  - Oral Itraconazole: 400 mg single dose or 200 mg daily for 7 days.

Oral Itraconazole usually reserved for *recalcitrant cases*. Recovery usually 3–4 weeks, but however skin tone may take several months to return to normal.

Q12. Which are the other conditions wherein Malazzesia has etiological role?

Ans: Malassezia folliculitis, seborrheic dermatitis, neonatal cephalic pustulosis, confluent and reticulated papillomatosis, invasive fungal septicaemia in immunocompromised patients.

CHAPTER 95

Mycetoma Foot

Shilpa K

Case study Mycetoma Foot

Presenting Complaints

Doctor, my right foot is swollen since 9 months. Blood mixed with pus and powdery material is coming out through the swollen area since 6 months.

Setting

Dermatology outpatient department

History of Present Illness

A 38-year-old male patient, agriculturist by occupation presented with complaints of swelling of right foot since 9 months. History of penetrating injury with plant sticks present around 1 month prior to the onset of swelling. Since 6 months, there is discharge of pus mixed with blood from the swelling. On taking treatment from local doctor the lesion partially healed, however similar lesions started appearing in the adjacent skin to gradually involve entire right foot. He also gave history of black-colored powdery material being discharged through these lesions.

General Physical Examination and Systemic Examination

No abnormality detected

Dermatological Examination

1. Gross deformity of the right foot with multiple nodules, sinuses and healed scars (Fig. 1)
2. Induration, thickening and hyperpigmentation is present on skin of right foot
3. Black colored grains discharging through the sinuses.

Q1. What is the most likely diagnosis?

a. Eumycotic mycetoma
b. Actinomycotic mycetoma
c. Actinomycosis
d. Botryomycosis

Ans: a. Eumycotic mycetoma.

Gross swelling and deformity of the foot, with multiple nodules, sinuses discharging black-colored grains favor eumycotic mycetoma.

Mycetoma is a chronic subcutaneous infection caused by actinomycetes or fungi. This infection results in a granulomatous inflammatory response in the deep dermis and subcutaneous tissue, which can extend to the underlying bone. It is characterized by the formation of grains containing aggregates of the causative organisms that may be discharged onto the skin surface through multiple sinuses Mycetoma caused by microaerophilic actinomycetes is termed

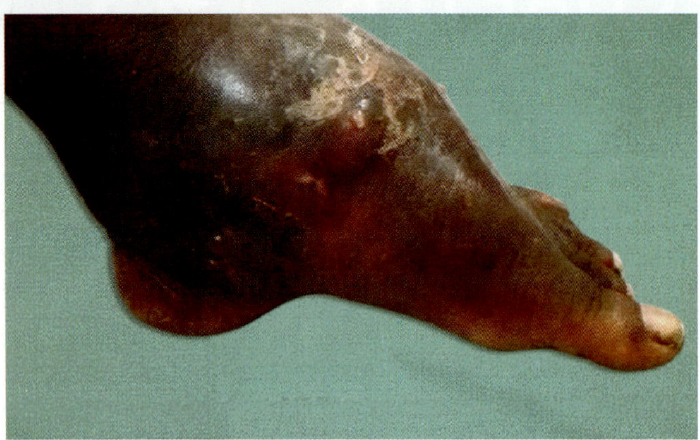

Fig. 1: Swelling of foot with nodules and discharging sinuses

actinomycetoma, and mycetoma caused by true fungi is called eumycetoma.

Q2. How do you diagnose this condition?

Ans: Mycetoma is diagnosed on clinical grounds. However the causative organisms can be confirmed through culture. The primary isolation media used should be Löwenstein-Jensen for actinomycetoma and Sabouraud's dextrose agar for eumycetoma. Other investigations include:

- *Biopsy or fine-needle aspiration cytology (FNAC):* Shows grains which are surrounded closely and sometimes infiltrated by neutrophils.
- *Bone radiography:* Shows, multiple lytic lesions or cavities, cortical thinning, cortical hypertrophy or periosteal proliferation giving a sunray appearance and a Codman triangle. Computed tomography (CT) scan provides a better detail of changes than conventional radiography.
- *Magnetic resonance imaging (MRI):* Shows dot-in-circle sign a highly specific MRI sign of mycetoma.
- *Serological:* Antibodies against the causative organisms can be detected via immunodiffusion, counterimmunoelectrophoresis (CIE), enzyme-linked immunosorbent assay, or Western blot.

Q3. Which are the organisms causing mycetoma?

Ans: The causative organisms have been described in Table 1.

Q4. What are grains?

Ans: Grains represent the microcolonies of the causative organisms which are diagnostic of the condition.

Q5. Red colored grain is produced by which etiological agent?

a. *Actinomadura pelletieri*
b. *Actinomadura madurae*
c. *Acremonium strictum*
d. *Aspergillus terreus*

Ans: a. *Actinomadura pelletieri*. Table 2 shows the different color of colonies produced by different organisms.

Q6. What are the common sites involved?

Ans: The most common site involved is foot (68.7%), followed by the leg (9.9%), trunk (6.1%), and arm (4.0%).

Q7. What are the complications associated with mycetoma?

Table 1: Organisms causing mycetoma

Actinomycetoma	*Eumycetoma*
• *Actinomadura madurae* • *Streptomyces somaliensis* • *Actinomadura pelletieri* • *Nocardia brasiliensis* • *Nocardia asteroides* • *Nocardia otidiscaviarum* • *Actinomyces israeli* • *Nocardia spp* • Unidentified actinomycetes	• *Madurella mycetomatis* • *Scedosporium boydii* • *Falciformispora senegalensis* • *Trematosphaeria grisea* • *Acremonium falciforme* • *Aspergillus fumigatus* • *Exophiala jeanselmei* • *Geotrichum candidum* • *Neotestudina rosatii* • *Medicopsis romeroi* • *Aspergillus flavus* • *Microsporum audouini* • *Cochliobolus lunatus* • *Rhinocladiella atrovirens* • *Aspergillus nidulans* • *Neoscytalidium dimidiatum* • *Fusarium spp.* • *Cladosporium spp.*

Table 2: Different organisms produce different color colonies.

Red grains	*Actinomadura pelletieri*
White or Yellow grains	*Acremonium strictum* *Actinomadura madurae* *Aspergillus nidulans* *Noetestudina rosatii* *Phaeoacremonium krajdenii* *Pseudallescheria boydii*
Black grains	*Aspergillus terreus* *Curvularia lunata* *Cladophialophora bantiana* *Exophiala jeanselmei* *Leptosphaeria senegalensis* *Leptosphaeria tompkinsii* *Madurella grisea* *Madurella mycetomatis* *Pyrenochaetaro meroi*

Ans: The complications associated with mycetoma are:

- Bone involvement
- Secondary bacterial infections can progress to full-blown bacteremia or septicemia, resulting in death
- Deformities and disabilities
- Amputation may result from neglected chronic infections
- Lymphatic obstruction and fibrosis can cause lymphedema
- Pulmonary mycetoma has been found to develop and progress more rapidly in individuals infected with HIV
- Drug toxicities due to prolonged therapy.

Q8. How do you differentiate between eumycotic and actinomycotic mycetoma?

Ans: Difference between eumycotic and actinomycotic has been described in Table 3.

Irrespective of the causal agent, the appearance of the mycetoma lesion is similar in both eumycotic and actinomycotic mycetoma except for few subtle differences.

Q9. What are the differential diagnoses of mycetoma?

Ans: This condition is to be differentiated from actinomycosis, which is an endogenous suppurative infection caused by *Actinomyces israelii* or other species of *Actinomyces* or related-bacteria, affecting the cervical-facial, thoracic, and pelvic sites. The branching bacteria that cause actinomycosis are non-acid-fast anerobic or microaerophilic bacteria. These bacteria are smaller than 1 μm in diameter, smaller than eumycotic agents. On the other hand, the agents that cause actinomycetoma are always aerobic and are sometimes weakly acid-fast.

Q10. What are the principles in treating a case of actinomyectoma?

Ans: In early lesions without bone involvement, surgical excision followed by chemotherapy as an adjunct is the best option available. In late lesions with bone involvement, chemotherapy is the first choice, which could be followed by surgical excision. Response to medical treatment is usually better in actinomycetoma than eumycetoma.

Current concept in the treatment of actinomycotic mycetoma is using a combination of drugs (Table 4).

Q11. How will you treat a case of Eumycotic mycetoma?

Ans: *Treatment of Eumycetoma:*

Eumycetoma is difficult to treat using current therapies. The common drugs regimes are:

- Ketoconazole: The dose is 400–800 mg daily.
- Itraconazole, has a good success and low recurrence rate given at 400 mg daily dosage. Treatment is continued till clinical clearance of lesions. It is usually stopped with clinical, serological, radiological and ultrasonic cure.

The criteria for cure are:

- Disappearance of the subcutaneous mass, healing of the sinuses and the skin return to normal.

Table 3: Difference between eumycotic and actinomycotic mycetoma

Organ	*Eumycotic mycetoma*	*Actinomycotic mycetoma*
Extent and progression	Compared to actinomycetoma it is well-circumscribed and progresses slowly	Less well-circumscribed and comparatively faster progression
Grain color	Black, red or yellow	Yellow, white or brown
X-ray	Cavities may be large and few in number with well-defined margins	Small and numerous with ill-defined margins
Ultrasonography	The hyper-reflective echoes are sharp, corresponding to the grains in the lesion	The hyper-reflective echoes are fine and closely aggregated and commonly settle at the bottom of the cavities
Histopathology	Organisms better stained with Gomori methenamine silver or periodic acid-Schiff stains. Brownish color with hematoxylin-eosin stain; black with a green-tinge with May-Grünwald-Giemsa stain	Organisms better stained with Gram stain. Homogenously eosinophilic with hematoxylin-eosin stain; blue in the center with pink filaments in the periphery with May-Grünwald-Giemsa stain. (Splendore-Hoeppli reaction thicker filaments, brown, oval or irregular granule with radiating hyphae and chlamydospores at the periphery surrounded by eosinophilic precipitate)
Primary isolation media	Blood agar	Löwenstein-Jensen
Treatment	Azole antifungals	Combination of antibiotics
Prognosis	Amputation may be required in neglected cases	Early and prolonged treatment has better prognosis

Table 4: Treatment of actinomycotic mycetoma is using a combination of the drugs

Regimen	*Intensive phase*	*Maintenance phase*
Welsh regimen	Amikacin 15 mg/kg/d IM 12 hourly in two divided doses and Tab sulfamethoxazole (35 mg/kg/d) and trimethoprim (7 mg/kg/d) equally divided in three doses for 21 days constituting one cycle. One to three such cycles are given at the interval of 15 days during which tablet sulfamethoxazole trimethoprim is given in same dose	Tab sulfamethoxazole-trimethoprim in same dose 2 weeks after last cycle
Modified-Welsh regimen	Amikacin 15 mg/kg/d in two divided doses + Tab sulfamethoxazole-trimethoprim 35 + 7 mg/kg/d + Cap rifampicin 10 mg/kg/d for 21 days constituting one cycle. One to three such cycles were given at interval of 15 days during which tab sulfamethoxazole-trimethoprim and cap. rifampicin in same doses were given	Tab sulfamethoxazole-trimethoprim 35 mg/kg/d + Cap. rifampicin 10 mg/kg/d after last cycle for 3 months
Ramam regimen	Crystalline penicillin 10 lakh units intravenous (IV) 6 hourly + Gentamicin 80 mg IV 12 hourly + Tab cotrimoxazole (80/400) two tablets twice daily (Duration–5–7 weeks)	Tab cotrimoxazole (80/400) two tablets twice daily + Tab amoxicillin 500 mg thrice daily for 2–5 months after disease becomes inactive
Modified two step Ramam regimen	Step 1: Gentamicin 80 mg IV 12 hourly + Tab cotrimoxazole(80/400 mg) two tablets twice daily (Duration—4 weeks)	Step 2: Cap doxycycline 100 mg twice daily + Tab cotrimoxazole (80/400 mg) two tablets twice daily (Duration-till 5–6 months after complete healing of all sinuses)

- Three consecutive negative CIE test 1-month apart.
- Bone regains its normal radiological appearance with remodeling.
- Absence of hyperreflective echoes and cavities on ultrasonic examination.
- No grains to be seen in *fine-needle aspiration* (FNA).

Surgery for eumycetoma: The goal of surgery in mycetoma is complete removal of the lesion or the reduction of size followed by medical treatment. Eumycetoma is well-encapsulated unlike actinomycetoma.

- Simple bone curettage and soft tissue excision is recommended for localized bony lesions. Margins of the lesion are first delineated and then excised. Later, the wound is covered with tincture of iodine to destroy any missed grains. Postoperative dressing is done using normal saline and Eusol solution.
- In advanced cases of mycetoma not responding to medical treatment for a prolonged period, amputation done. Extensive repeated excisions of the diseased tissue, including bone is carried out. This debulking procedure must be coupled with chemotherapy.
- In less advanced cases less mutilating surgery is advised for example, toe, mid tarsal or Syme's amputation. However, in inadequate surgery recurrence frequently occurs.

SECTION 18

Infections-2 (Viral and Parasitic)

Ruby Venugopal

CHAPTER 96

Chickenpox

Kirti S Jangid

Case study Chickenpox

Presenting Complaints

An 8-year-old girl presented with fever and fluid-filled lesions over body since 4 days.

Setting

Dermatology outpatient department

History of Present Illness

Patient was apparently asymptomatic, 4 days back when she developed running nose and mild fever which subsided with antipyretics. Two days after the onset of fever, patient noticed reddish elevated lesions which first appeared on face, gradually progressed in number and extent to involve trunk and extremities. These gradually converted into fluid-filled lesions. There were no systemic complaints. There was no history of similar skin findings or associated symptoms in siblings or parents. History of being exposed to child with similar findings in neighborhood was present.

General Physical Examination

Well-oriented to time, place and person
Pulse:80 BPM, BP:110/60 mm Hg, Respiratory rate: 13/min, Temperature:100°F

Systemic Examination

No abnormality detected

Dermatological Examination

On examination, she was found to have erythematous papules, vesicles and few crusted lesions distributed over face, trunk and extremities (Fig. 1). Oral mucosal examination revealed three shallow ulcers, about 0.3 cm in diameter over the buccal mucosa. Other mucosal examination was within normal limits. Nail, joints, palms and soles were within normal limits.

Q1. What is diagnosis?

a. Disseminated herpes simplex infection
b. Herpes zoster
c. Chickenpox
d. Eczema herpeticum

Ans: c. Chickenpox (Varicella-zoster). The distinctive features of varicella are the centripetal distribution, the polymorphism in each affected site and the rapid progression of the individual lesion from vesicle to crust.

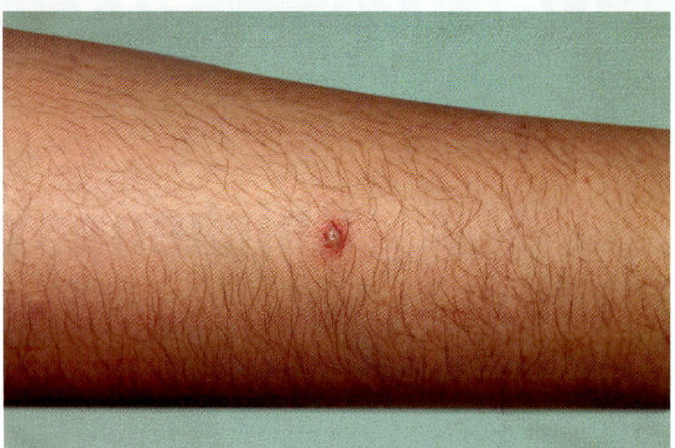

Fig. 1: Classical umbilicated vesicle on forearm

Q2. How will you confirm a diagnosis of chickenpox?

Ans: Tzanck smear from a vesicle will usually show characteristic multinucleate giant cells.

In difficult cases detection of Varicella zoster virus (VZV) antigen by direct fluorescent-antibody staining of a smear or of VZV DNA by polymerase chain reaction (PCR) in a scraping from the base of a vesicle offers an alternative method. Titration of complement-fixing antibody in acute and convalescent sera may be a useful test in atypical infections. PCR analysis can permit detection of VZV and is particularly useful in patients with suspected encephalomyelitis, in whom examination of the cerebrospinal fluid can lead to rapid diagnosis.

In skin biopsies, the VZV proteins can be detected by immunohistochemistry and the viral nucleic acid by in situ hybridization or PCR of extracted DNA. Since VZV grows poorly and slowly in the laboratory, viral culture is rarely indicated.

Q3. Name the virus causing chickenpox?

Ans: Chickenpox is caused by a virus, the VZV. VZV is a DNA virus, member of herpesvirus family. Other members of this family include herpes simple virus (HSV) 1 and 2, cytomegalovirus (CMV), Epstein-Barr virus (EBV), human herpes virus (HHV) 6, 7, and 8.

Q4. What is the incubation period of chickenpox?

Ans: The incubation period is 10–21 days (usually 14–15 days).

Q5. Explain the transmission of chickenpox?

Ans: Transmission is via the respiratory route and less commonly by direct contact with the lesions. A susceptible person may develop varicella following exposure to the lesions of herpes zoster. Infected persons are infectious from 5 days before the appearance of the eruption, and most infectious 1–2 days prior to the appearance of the rash. Infectivity ceases 5–6 days after the eruption appears in most cases. There is an initial viral replication in the nasopharynx and conjunctiva, followed by infection of the reticuloendothelial system (liver spleen) between days 4 and 6. A secondary viremia occurs at days 11–20, resulting in infection of the epidermis and the appearance of the characteristic skin lesions.

Q6. What are the clinical features of chickenpox?

Ans: Varicella is characterized by a vesicular eruption consisting of delicate "teardrop" vesicles on an erythematous base. The eruption starts with faint macules that develop rapidly into vesicles within 24 hours. Successive fresh crops of vesicles appear for a few days, mainly on the trunk, face, and oral mucosa. The vesicles quickly become pustular and umbilicated, then crusted. The lesions appear in crops with centripetal distribution.

Q7. Enumerate the differential diagnosis of Chicken pox.

Ans: Vesicular exanthems of coxsackie and echovirus, poxvirus infections, impetigo, insect bites, contact dermatitis, erythema multiforme, vesicular or pustular drug eruptions, disseminated herpes zoster, papular urticaria, scabies, dermatitis herpetiformis.

Q8. What are the differentials of umbilicated lesions?

Ans: Varicella, herpes zoster, Kaposi varicelliform eruption, molluscum contagiosum, cryptococcosis, coccidioidomycosis, histoplasmosis, penicillosis, aspergillosis, hydroa vacciniforme, acne necrotica and histioid leprosy.

Q9. What are complications of chickenpox?

Ans: Complications are more common in infants, adults and people with depressed immune systems:

- Secondary bacterial infection with *Staphylococcus aureus* or a streptococcal organism is the most common complication of varicella. Hemorrhagic vesicle may occur. Cutaneous gangrene ("varicella gangrenosa") may follow secondary infection. Rarely, it may be complicated by osteomyelitis, other deep-seated infections, or septicemia.
- Varicella pneumonia and hepatitis may occur.
- Encephalitis, often presenting with ataxia in less than one per 1000.
- Thrombocytopenic purpura, Rhabdomyolysis, viral arthritis, Reye's syndrome, Erythema multiforme, Stevens-Johnson syndrome occurring

as a consequence of varicella infection has been reported.

- Acute retinal necrosis syndrome may occur.
- Chronic varicella with persistent hyperkeratotic lesions and repeated attacks of varicella have also been observed.

Q10. What are the complications of Varicella during pregnancy?

Ans: Maternal infection with the VZV during the first 20 weeks of gestation may result in a syndrome of congenital malformations (congenital varicella syndrome), as well as severe illness in the mother. The risk for spontaneous abortion by 20 weeks is 3%; in an additional 0.7% of pregnancies, fetal death occurs after 20 weeks. The risk of preterm labor is 3-fold increased. Congenital varicella syndrome is characterized by a series of anomalies, including hypoplastic limbs (usually unilateral and lower extremity), cutaneous scars, and ocular and *central nervous system* (CNS) disease. Female fetuses are affected more commonly than males. The overall risk for this syndrome is between 1% and 2%. The highest risk is from maternal varicella between weeks 13 and 20 when the risk is 2%. Infection of the fetus in utero may result in zoster occurring postnatally, often in the first 2 years of life. This occurs in about 1% of varicella-complicated pregnancies and the risk for this complication is greatest in varicella occurring in weeks 25–36 of gestation.

If the mother develops varicella between 5 days before and 2 days after delivery, neonatal varicella can occur and be severe, as transplacental delivery of antivaricella antibody has been inadequate. These neonates develop varicella at 5–10 days of age.

Q11. What is the management of varicella during pregnancy?

Ans: Severe varicella and varicella pneumonia or disseminated disease in pregnancy should be treated with intravenous acyclovir. All varicella in pregnancy should be treated with oral acyclovir, 800 mg five times a day for 7 days (except perhaps during the first month, when a specialist should be consulted). In all women past 35 weeks of gestation or with increased risk of premature labor, admission and intravenous acyclovir, 10 mg/kg three times daily, should be recommended. The patient should be evaluated for pneumonia, renal function should be carefully monitored, and the patient should be switched to oral therapy once lesions stop appearing (usually in 48–72 hours).

Varicella zoster immune globulin (VZIG) should not be given once the pregnant woman has developed varicella. VZIG should be given for significant exposures within the first 72–96 hours to ameliorate maternal varicella and prevent complications.

Q12. What is Modified varicella-like syndrome?

Ans: Children immunized with live attenuated varicella vaccine may develop varicella of reduced severity on exposure to natural varicella. This has been called modified varicella-like syndrome (MVLS). The frequency of MVLS is between 0% and 2.7% per year. The illness occurs an average of 15 days after exposure to varicella and consists primarily of macules and papules with relatively few vesicles, number of lesions is about 35–50, compared with natural varicella, which usually has about 300 lesions. The majority of patients are afebrile and the illness is mild, lasting fewer than 5 days on average.

Q13. What is the treatment for chickenpox?

Ans: Both immunocompetent children and adults with varicella benefit from acyclovir therapy if started early (within 24 hours of the appearance of the eruption). Therapy does not appear to alter the development of adequate immunity to reinfection. Because the complications of varicella are infrequent in children, routine treatment is not recommended; therapeutic decisions are made on a case-by-case basis.

Varicella in the otherwise healthy child requires only symptomatic treatment. Some advocate the use of acyclovir in childhood chickenpox to reduce the severity and duration of the eruption. Soothing antiseptic applications may be helpful and secondary bacterial infection will require antibiotics.

An antiviral is indicated for varicella in adults and for severe disease at any age in the immunocompromised.

Treatment should be started as early as possible, preferably within the first 1 or 2 days. Typically Tab. Acyclovir 800 mg 5 times daily orally is the standard treatment given. Courses of 5, 7, and 10 days have been used. The dose in children is 20 mg/kg (maximum 800 mg per dose) four times a day for 5 days. Alternatively Tab. Valacyclovir 1 g TDS can be used for ease of administration.

Q14. Describe varicella in human immunodeficiency virus infected individuals?

Ans: In human immunodeficiency virus (HIV) infection, varicella may be severe and fatal. Atypical cases of a few scattered lesions without a dermatomal distribution usually represent reactivation of disease with dissemination. Persons with atypical varicella should be evaluated for the presence of pneumonia or hepatitis. Chronic varicella may complicate HIV infection, resulting in ulcerative (ecthymatous) or hyperkeratotic (verrucous) lesions. These patterns of infection may be associated with acyclovir resistance. Acyclovir-resistant varicella is treated with foscarnet, and in cases failing that agent, cidofovir.

Q15. Which are the vaccines available for chickenpox and what are the indications?

Ans: Two vaccines containing varicella virus are licensed for use:

1. Single-antigen varicella vaccine.
2. Combination measles, mumps, rubella, and varicella (MMRV) vaccine.

Both vaccines contain live, attenuated VZV derived from the Oka strain.

Children 12 months through 12 years old:

- Two doses (0.5 mL each) of varicella vaccine should be given subcutaneously, separated by at least 3 months
- MMRV vaccine is approved for healthy children in this age group.

Single-antigen vaccine and MMRV vaccine can be used for the routine 2-dose varicella vaccination.

1. First dose: 12 through 15 months
2. Second dose: 4 through 6 years.

People 13 years or older

- 2 doses (0.5 ml each) of the single-antigen varicella vaccine subcutaneously 4 to 8 weeks apart
- MMRV vaccine is not approved for people in this age group.

Q16. What is the duration of protection offered by vaccination?

Ans: Studies show that one dose of varicella vaccine was 97% effective in the 1st year after vaccination and 86% effective in the 2nd year. From the 2nd year to 8th year after vaccination, the vaccine effectiveness remained stable at 81–86%. Most vaccinated children who developed varicella during the 8 years after vaccination had mild disease.

Q17. What is the effectivity of this vaccine?

Ans: Vaccine effectivity:

Single dose of single-antigen varicella vaccine is—

- 85% effective at preventing any form of varicella
- Almost 100% effective against severe varicella.

Q18. What are the contraindications for the use of vaccine?

Ans: Contraindications for vaccine:

- History of anaphylactic or anaphylactoid reaction to gelatin, neomycin, or any other component of the vaccine
- Blood dyscrasias, leukemia, lymphomas, or malignant neoplasms affecting bone marrow or lymphatic system
- Receiving prolonged, high-dose systemic immunosuppressive therapy (≥2 weeks), including large doses of oral steroids (≥2 mg/kg of body weight or a total of 20 mg/day of prednisone or its equivalent for people who weigh >10 kg)
- Moderate or severe concurrent illness
- Received blood products (such as whole blood, plasma, or immunoglobulin) during the previous 3–11 months
- Family history (first degree relatives) of congenital hereditary immunodeficiency
- Pregnancy.

CHAPTER 97

Herpes Zoster

Ankur Talwar

Case study | Herpes Zoster

Presenting Complaints

Doctor, I am developing blisters on the right side of my abdomen since the past two days. These lesions are extremely painful and I have been unable to sleep since the past two days due to it. I am not even able to go to my office.

Setting

Dermatology outpatient department

History of Present Illness

A 52-year old man presented with extremely painful blisters on the right side of abdomen since the past two days. The lesions were abrupt and sudden in onset and were preceded by mild to moderate gnawing pain for 2 days prior to cutaneous eruption. There is no history of application of any irritant substance or any history suggestive of insect bite/ crawl. He is a known diabetic under treatment and his current sugar levels are well controlled.

General Physical Examination and Systemic Examination

No abnormality detected

Dermatological Examination

Multiple clear vesicular lesions grouped together in clusters on an erythematous base. Multiple such clusters were seen. Lesions are distributed unilaterally on the right abdomen along the T9-T10 dermatome on the front and back.

Q1. What is the most likely diagnosis?

a. Allergic contact dermatitis
b. Insect bite reaction
c. Chickenpox
d. Herpes zoster

Ans: d. Herpes zoster

The presence of characteristic clear vesicles on an erythematous base distributed in a dermatomal pattern is almost pathognomonic of herpes zoster (Fig. 1). The lesions stop abruptly at the midline of the limit of sensory coverage of the involved dermatome. Further, most lesions are preceded or accompanied by intense debilitating pain, as in this case.

Q2. How will you confirm the diagnosis?

Ans: Diagnosis of herpes zoster is predominantly clinical based primarily on the history and physical findings. In most patients, confirming the diagnosis via laboratory tests has no utility. In extremely doubtful cases, one of the least expensive and simplest laboratory diagnostic methods for varicella-zoster

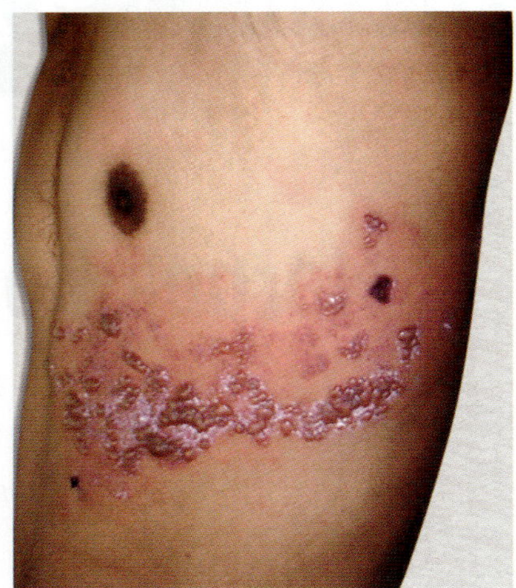

Fig. 1: Multiple grouped vesicles in dermatomal distribution

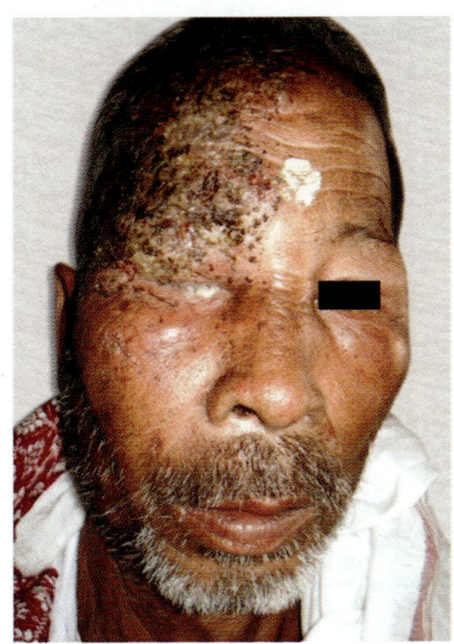

Fig. 2: Herpes zoster ophthalmicus

virus (VZV) is the Tzanck smear. This is performed by scraping the base of a fresh vesicular lesion after it has been unroofed and staining the resultant specimen with Giemsa. This is then evaluated for characteristic presence of multinucleated giant cells.

Q3. What is the cause of herpes zoster?

Ans: Herpes zoster is caused by the VZV. VZV infection gives rise to two distinct syndromes. The primary infection, chickenpox, is a contagious and usually benign febrile illness. After this infection resolves, viral particles remain in the dorsal root or other sensory ganglia, where they may lay dormant for years to decades. Reactivation of VZV that has remained dormant leads to herpes zoster. VZV reactivates when the host mechanisms fail to contain the virus.

Q4. Who are the candidates at increased risk for developing herpes zoster?

Ans: The risk appears due to impaired cell-mediated immunity to VZV. The risk factors include:

- Emotional stress
- Immunosuppressive therapy, e.g. oral steroids, anti-TNF-alpha agents, etc.
- Inflammatory bowel disease (IBD)
- Acute leukemia and other malignancies
- Immunosuppressive state, e.g. HIV, diabetes, etc.
- External re-exposure to the virus.

Q5. What is postherpetic neuralgia (PHN)?

Ans: PHN is defined as persistent or recurring pain lasting 30 or more days after the acute infection or after all lesions have crusted. The pain is confined to the area of original dermatomal involvement and can be extremely severe and incapacitating. The pain may persist for weeks to months followed by slow and gradual resolution.

Q6. Who develops postherpetic neuralgia?

Ans: PHN develops in:

- Older age appears to be the most significant risk factor for developing PHN. At age 60 years, approximately 60% of patients with herpes zoster develop PHN, and at age 70 years, 75% develop PHN.
- In addition, PHN is observed more frequently after cases of herpes zoster ophthalmicus (HZO) and in instances of upper-body dermatomal involvement.

Q7. What is herpes zoster ophthalmicus and what are the possible complications?

Ans: HZO develops when cranial nerve V (trigeminal nerve) is involved in viral reactivation. The cutaneous lesions may occur on the ipsilateral forehead, upper eyelid and ala of nose (Fig. 2). This is generally accompanied by severe orbital edema. The nasociliary branch involvement, characterized by vesicles at the tip of the nose, is an early sign of involvement of eye (the Hutchinson rule). The eye involvement poses a risk to vision and should be considered a medical emergency. Iritis, iridocyclitis, glaucoma, and corneal tissue ulcerations are possible in these cases. Other possible complications include conjunctivitis, scleritis, episcleritis, keratitis, iridocyclitis, Argyll-Robertson pupil.

Postherpetic neuralgia is more common in HZO than in other forms of zoster. PHN is observed in well over 50% of patients with HZO and can be severe and long-lasting.

Q8. Ramsay Hunt syndrome is a complication due to herpes zoster due to involvement of:

a. Facial nerve
b. Trigeminal nerve
c. Auditory nerve
d. Vagus nerve

Ans: a. Facial nerve

Ramsay Hunt syndrome is defined as an acute peripheral facial nerve neuropathy associated with herpes zoster rash over the ear canal/auricle (known as herpes zoster oticus). The patient may also complain of vertigo and ipsilateral hearing loss along with ipsilateral lower motor neuron facial paresis/palsy. Other symptoms may include otalgia, tinnitus, dysarthrias, etc.

Q9. What are the specific agents available for the management of herpes zoster?

Ans: The specific antivirals with action against VZV include:

- Acyclovir—800 mg PO every 4 hour while awake (5 times daily) for 7 days, 10 mg/kg IV 8 hourly in immunocompromised
- Famciclovir—500 mg PO 8 hourly for 7 days
- Valacyclovir—1 g PO 8 hourly for 7 days.

Their mechanism of action involves preventing VZV replication through inhibition of viral DNA polymerase. Usually, the earlier antiviral medications are started, the more effective they are in shortening the duration of zoster and in preventing PHN. Ideally, therapy should be initiated within 72 hours of symptom onset. Several studies found antiviral therapy to be capable of reducing zoster pain even when started beyond the 72-hour window.

Q10. What is the consensus regarding the use of oral corticosteroids in active herpes zoster?

Ans: Oral steroids have been used conventionally to reduce the acute pain associated with zoster by reducing inflammation in dorsal root ganglia and involved sensory nerves. However, in view of potential risk of dissemination of VZV, it has been suggested that they should be limited to cases of moderate to severe zoster pain or patients in which significant neurologic symptoms (e.g. facial paralysis) are seen. Further, steroids should be administered concurrently with antiviral therapy and the duration of steroid use should not extend beyond the period of antiviral therapy.

Q11. What agents are available for the management of postherpetic neuralgia (PHN)?

Ans: Agents available for the management of PHN are:

- Gabapentin, pregabalin
- Neuroactive agents (e.g. Tricyclic antidepressants)
- Anticonvulsant agents (e.g. Phenytoin)
- Narcotic and non-narcotic analgesics, both systemic (e.g. opioids) and topical
- Corticosteroids
- Dosage of gabapentin varies from 300 mg/day up to 1,800 mg/day. Doses more than 1,800 mg/day have demonstrated no additional benefit
- Dosage of pregabalin varies from 75 mg/day to 300 mg/day
- Dosage of amitriptyline/nortriptyline may vary from 25 mg/day to 75 mg/day
- Topical capsaicin cream can be helpful; it acts by depletion of substance P at involved nerve endings. However, it must be applied at least 5 times daily, and pain may increase upon application in the initial days as accumulated neurotransmitters are released. However, once neurotransmitter reserves have been depleted, any resultant pain relief is temporary.

Q12. What is Jaipur block?

Ans: This is a nerve block for the management of PHN in debilitating cases. This consists of local subcutaneous infiltration of 2% xylocaine, 0.5% bupivacaine and 4 mg/mL dexamethasone solution. The block may be repeated at 6 weeks intervals. In modified Jaipur block, the dexamethasone solution is replaced by methylprednisolone with other components remaining the same.

Q13. Is there any vaccine to prevent herpes zoster?

Ans: A live attenuated VZV vaccine named Zostavax is available. The US Food and Drug Administration (FDA) has approved Zostavax for prevention of herpes zoster in people aged 60 years and older. The vaccine reduced the incidence of herpes zoster by 61.1% and the incidence of PHN by 66.5% in individuals over the age of 60 years. The effective duration of this vaccination is not yet known. However, studies have demonstrated that benefits persist for at least 5 years after vaccination.

CHAPTER 98

Herpes Labialis

Sankeerth V

Case study Herpes Labialis

Presenting Complaints

Doctor, I have developed multiple tiny fluid-filled lesions at the corner of my mouth since last 2 days and they are associated with a lot of burning and itching sensation.

Setting

Dermatology outpatient department.

History of Present Illness

A 25-year old woman presented with complaints of fluid-filled lesions at the angle of the mouth since last 2 days. These lesions were associated with intense burning and itching sensation. The burning sensation started a day before the onset of the fluid-filled lesions. There was no history of fever or drug intake, no history of any trauma or application of any substance at the site.

General Physical Examination and Systemic Examination

No abnormality detected.

Dermatological Examination

Multiple, well-defined, grouped vesicles with clear fluid, overlying an erythematous base were noted near the angle of the mouth on the right side, partly involving the vermilion border of the upper lip.

Q1. What is the most likely diagnosis?

a. Herpes labialis
b. Insect bite reaction
c. Irritant contact dermatitis
d. Fixed drug eruption

Ans: a. Herpes labialis—presence of multiple grouped vesicles overlying an erythematous base involving the vermilion border, lesions associated with burning and itching sensation with presence of prodromal symptoms before the onset of skin lesions go in favor of herpes labialis (Fig. 1).

Q2. How will you confirm the diagnosis of herpes virus infections?

Ans: Herpes labialis is most often diagnosed on clinical grounds. The diagnosis can be supported and confirmed by the following tests:

- Tzanck smear test (bedside, not specific)
- Skin biopsy (not routinely done)
- Polymerase chain reaction (PCR)—*most sensitive*
- Viral culture (using human diploid fibroblast culture is "*Gold standard*")

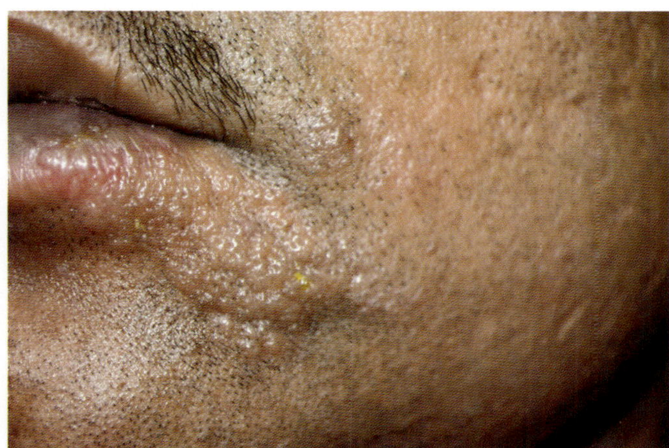

Fig. 1: Multiple grouped vesicles at the angle of the mouth

Serological testing for type-specific antibodies [helps to differentiate between herpes simplex virus type 1 (HSV-1) and HSV-2].

Q3. How is Tzanck smear performed?

Ans: It is a bedside investigation which is easy to perform. It helps to support the diagnosis and is not confirmatory. For Tzanck smear, a fresh vesicle of less than 4 days duration is preferred. The vesicle is gently deroofed and the base of the lesion is scraped gently with a scalpel/spatula. The specimen obtained is transferred onto a clean glass slide and is fixed using the formol-Zenker solution. The slide is then stained using the Giemsa stain and is visualized under the light microscope.

The classical changes seen in herpes infections are presence of multinucleated syncitial giant cells with a few acantholytic cells. The giant cells often have a bipolar, tadpole or irregular tear-drop shape with a smooth external contour.

Q4. What is the causative virus of herpes labialis infections?

Ans: The causative virus is HSV-1. It is a double-stranded DNA virus belonging to the family Herpesviridae.

Q5. Enumerate all the types of herpes viruses?

Ans:

- *Alpha herpesviridae:* Herpes simplex virus 1 and 2 (HSV1, HSV2), varicella zoster virus (VZV-Herpes virus 3)
- *Beta herpesviridae:* Cytomegalovirus (CMV)—herpes virus 5, human herpes virus 6 and 7 (HHV6, HHV7)
- *Gamma herpesviridae:* Epstein-Barr virus (EBV)—herpes virus 4, human herpes virus 8 (HHV-8 Kaposi sarcoma-associated virus).

Q6. What is the mode of transmission of herpes simplex virus infections?

Ans: HSV-1 infections are transmitted through direct contact or contaminated saliva. HSV-2 infections are transmitted through sexual contact and via transplacental route.

Q7. What do you mean by primary, nonprimary and recurrent herpes infections?

Ans:

- *Primary infection*: Individuals exposed to the HSV virus for the first time, either type 1 or type 2. These patients are seronegative initially but subsequently develop HSV-specific antibodies.
- *Nonprimary infection*: When an individual with already pre-existing antibodies to one type of HSV develops infection with the other HSV type, it is referred to as nonprimary infection, e.g. patients with antibodies to HSV-1 develop HSV-2 infection.
- *Recurrent infection*: When an individual with antibodies to one type of HSV develops infection with the same type of HSV again, it is referred to as recurrent infection. It is due to reactivation of latent virus in the sensory ganglion, which then migrates along the nerves to the site in the skin where the primary infection occurred. Most common sites for recurrences are lips, genitals and sacral area.

Q8. What is the incubation period for herpes simplex virus infections?

Ans: Incubation period is the time between the exposure and development of skin lesions. It is estimated to be around 3–14 days.

Q9. What are the different types of herpes simplex virus infections?

Ans: Different types of HSV infections are:

- *Herpes gingivostomatitis*
- *Herpetic keratoconjunctivitis*
- *Herpes labialis*
- *Herpes gladiatorum (scrumpox/mat pox/herpes rugbiorum)*
- *Herpetic whitlow (infection of the finger tips/pulp)*
- *Genital herpes (caused by HSV-2)*
- *Herpetic sycosis (infection of hair follicle)*
- *Eczema herpeticum (Kaposi's varicelliform eruptions seen in atopics)*
- *Neonatal herpes virus infections.*

Q10. What is asymptomatic shedding?

Ans: In some cases of recurrent infections, shedding of virus occurs even without the patient having any symptoms or lesions. This occurs most commonly in 1st year after the primary episode (more so in the first 3 months). These patients are a potential source for transmission of infection. It is more commonly seen in HSV-2 infections.

Q11. What are the complications of herpes simplex virus infections?

Ans: Complications are not very common in HSV infections. Patients with compromised immunity are more prone to develop complications.

- *Ocular complications*: Corneal ulcers, corneal opacities, visual loss, acute retinal necrosis
- *Neurological complications*: Meningitis, encephalitis, Guillain-Barre syndrome, radiculoneuropathy
- *Dermatological complications*: Eczema herpeticum, pigmentary changes in skin at site of lesions, scarring and recurrent herpes infections
- *In immunocompromised*: Hepatitis, pneumonitis, tracheobronchitis, pancreatitis, adrenal necrosis, transverse myelitis, cerebral angiitis, meningitis and encephalitis.
- *Others:* Pharyngitis, monoarticular arthritis, neonatal herpes infections.

Q12. What are the differential diagnoses of herpes virus infections?

Ans: Differential diagnosis:

- *For orolabial herpes infections*: Erosive lichen planus, aphthous ulcers, erythema multiforme, oral candididasis, mucous membrane pemphigus, Behcet's disease, herpangina, syphilis, insect bite reactions, irritant contact dermatitis.
- *For genital herpes*: Syphilis, chancroid, lymphogranuloma venereum, donovanosis, Behcet's disease, candidiasis, Crohn's disease, fixed-drug eruptions, traumatic ulcers.

Q13. What is the treatment for primary herpes infections?

Ans: Treatment for primary herpes infections:

- *Acyclovir (ACV)* 200 mg five times/day PO or 400 mg three times/day for 7–10 days. For pediatric patients, 15 mg/kg/dose for five times/day
- *Valacyclovir* 1 g twice daily PO for 7–10 days
- *Famciclovir* 250 mg thrice daily PO for 7–10 days.

Q14. What is the treatment for recurrent herpes infections?

Ans: The treatment for recurrent infections is in two phases namely episodic and suppressive.

Episodic

- *ACV* 200 mg five times/day or 400 mg three times/day PO for 5–7 days
- *Valacyclovir* 1 g daily PO for 5 days
- *Famciclovir* 125 mg twice daily PO for 5 days.
- Topical *Penciclovir* 1% cream or *Docosanol* 10% cream five times daily.

Suppressive—period of 9 months–1 year

- *ACV* 400 mg PO twice daily
- *Valacyclovir* 500–1000 mg PO daily
- *Famciclovir* 500 mg PO daily.

Q15. What is the drug of choice in acyclovir resistant cases?

Ans: For ACV resistant HSV infections, foscarnet, 40 mg/kg 8-hourly for up to 10 to 42 days is used.

Q16. What is the treatment for neonatal herpes simplex virus (NHSV) infections?

- Early therapy with intravenous (IV) ACV improves the prognosis for all three presentations of NHSV. Therefore, infants should be started on IV ACV before laboratory confirmation of NHSV, as soon as the infection is suspected clinically.
- *ACV* 20 mg/kg body weight, intravenous route, 8th hourly for 14 days (for skin and mucous membrane involvement only) or 21 days (for disseminated infections or CNS involvement) assuming renal function as normal. Oral ACV has limited bioavailability resulting in inadequate drug levels, hence parenteral route is ideal.
- For infants with CNS disease, CSF should be sampled near the end of a 21-day course of therapy. If the PCR remains positive, treatment should be extended with weekly CSF sampling and ACV stopped when a negative result is obtained
- In combination with parenteral ACV, neonates with ocular involvement should receive a topical ophthalmic agent such as trifluridine.
- Suppressive therapy with oral ACV (300 mg/m^2 per dose administered three times per day) should be given for 6 months to infants with CNS disease
- Follow-up is necessary to detect and manage adverse effects related to suppressive ACV treatment as well as for the neurodevelopmental sequelae of NHSV.

CHAPTER 99

Molluscum Contagiosum

Shruthi C, Sujala S Aradhya

Case study — Molluscum Contagiosum

Presenting Complaints

Doctor, my child has whitish eruptions on the face and hands since 2 months.

Setting

Dermatology outpatient department

History of Present Illness

A 5-year old male child, presented with multiple whitish, asymptomatic lesions over face, hand and abdomen for 2 months. On expression, a whitish cheesy material comes out. His elder brother is also affected with similar lesions over abdomen.

General Physical Examination and Systemic Examination

No abnormality detected

Dermatological Examination

Multiple, discrete, pearly white papules with central umbilication over the cheeks, nose, eyelids, dorsum of right hand and abdomen (Fig. 1). There was no mucosal involvement.

Q1. What is the most likely diagnosis?

a. Milia
b. Molluscum contagiosum (MC)
c. Wart
d. Fordyce spots

Ans: b. Molluscum contagiosum (Multiple, pearly white, dome-shaped, umbilicated papules).

Q2. What is molluscum contagiosum?

Ans: MC is a viral infection of skin caused by molluscum contagiosum virus (MCV), a DNA virus belonging to the Poxviridae family and the genera of Molluscipox virus. Four strains of MCV are detected—MCV1, MCV1a, MCV2, MCV3.

Q3. What are the points that aid in the diagnosis of molluscum contagiosum?

Ans: Diagnosis of MC:

- Solitary/multiple, discrete papules which are dome-shaped or hemispherical
- Papules are waxy, skin colored, pearly white or pinkish in color
- A central punctum (umbilication) visible in all well-formed lesions

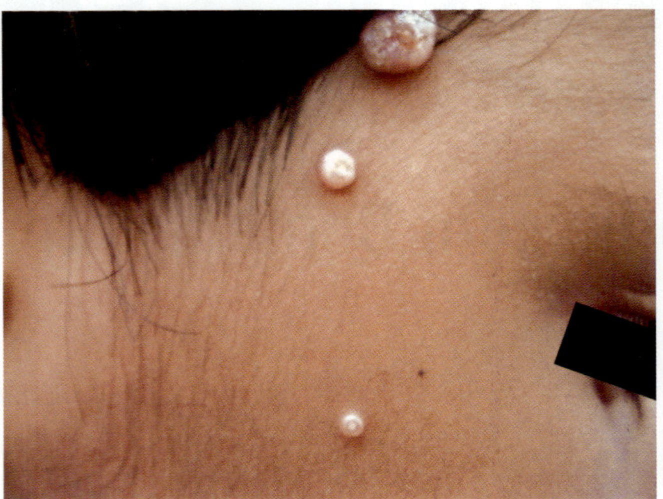

Fig. 1: Multiple, discrete, pearly white papules with central umbilication over the cheeks

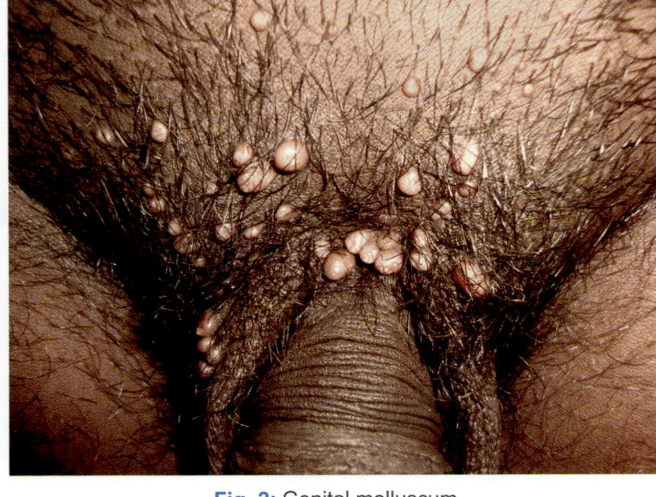

Fig. 2: Genital molluscum

- In children, lesions are usually distributed on the trunk and face but can occur at any body parts
- In young adults and adolescents, genital lesions are usually due to sexual transmission (Fig. 2)
- Uncommon sites of involvement include scalp, lips, tongue, buccal mucosa and soles
- MC has been seen on scars and in tattoos
- Linear lesions may be seen due to autoinoculation (pseudo-Koebner phenomenon)
- Large, multiple, widespread and facial lesions may indicate immunosuppression
- Lesions confined to hair follicles are also reported ("molluscum folliculitis").

Q4. What are the differential diagnoses for molluscum contagiosum? Differential dignosis of papular lesion with umbilication?

- Milia
- Epidermal nevi
- Keratoacanthoma
- Perforating disorder (Perforating folliculitis, reactive perforating collagenosis)
- Pyogenic granuloma
- Adnexal tumor like syringoma, trichoepithelioma
- Deep fungal infection like cryptococcosis, histoplasmosis, penicilliosis especially in immunocompromised setting.

Q5. What is the mode of spread for molluscum contagiosum virus?

Ans: It spreads by direct contact from person-to-person or by fomites (towels, clothing, parlor procedures like shaving, waxing, facial), sharing swimming pools, bath etc.

Q6. What is pseudo-Koebner's phenomenon?

Ans: Also known as pseudo-isomorphic phenomenon, it is characterized by the appearance of similar lesions at the site of injury in infective lesions due to inoculation of the microorganism at the site. Seen in molluscum contagiosum, warts, tuberculosis, etc.

Q7. What is Meyerson's phenomenon?

Ans: Also known as halo dermatitis, it is an eczematous reaction, possibly immune-mediated occurring around a molluscum lesions. It was first noted in congenital melanocytic nevus. This phenomenon is also noted in seborrheic keratosis, molluscum contagiosum, dermatofibromas, basal cell carcinoma (BCC), squamous cell carcinoma (SCC) and in dysplastic nevus. The condition responds to topical steroids or removal of initiating lesion.

Q8. What is the natural course of molluscum contagiosum?

Ans: Natural course:

- The incubation period of MC varies from 2 weeks to 6 months.
- A lesion starts as a tiny papule and progresses to a size of 5–10 mm in 6 to 12 weeks. Number varies from very few to innumerable.
- Small lesions may join to form a plaque ("agminate form").
- The presence of numerous and giant lesions in an adult suggests immunosuppression.

- In most cases, lesions resolve spontaneously over a period of 6–9 months; rarely persist for years.
- Resolution is heralded by inflammation, suppuration and crusting.
- They usually heal without forming a scar.

Q9. What are the complications of molluscum contagiosum?

Ans: Complications:

- Patchy eczema ("molluscum dermatitis") may develop around one or more of the lesions but this disappears as the infection resolves.
- Eyelid involvement leads to "toxic conjunctivitis". It may also lead to chronic conjunctivitis and superficial punctate keratitis.
- Depressed scars or anetoderma-like lesions can remain when mollusca clear.
- Dissemination (mostly in immunocompromised).

Q10. How do you diagnose the condition?

Ans: The diagnosis is clinical. It can be confirmed by a crush smear after needling out the lesion. Histopathology can confirm 100% of the lesions.

Q11. How is a crush smear done and what are the findings?

Ans: The curetted molluscum body is crushed between two microscopic slides and the material stained with Leishman or Geimsa stain. Tissue smear shows enlarged keratinocytes with the cytoplasm filled with large hyaline acidophilic granular mass known as *molluscum body or Henderson Patterson (HP) body* which pushes the nucleus to the edge of the cell. These bodies are present in large numbers in the cavity which appears near the surface at the center.

Q12. What are the other methods of diagnosis of molluscum contagiosum?

Ans: The other laboratory methods for diagnosis include detection of antibodies using ELISA and molecular analysis of DNA using hybridization or PCR techniques.

Q13. What are the modalities of treatment of molluscum contagiosum?

Ans: Modalities of treatment of molluscum contagiosum:

- Needling is the best, simple and nonexpensive method of treatment
- Curettage or diathermy can be done for large lesions
- Cryotherapy with liquid nitrogen (3–4 weekly intervals until complete clearance)
- Cantharidin 0.9% in flexible collodion is carefully applied by the physician to each lesion and washed off after 2–4 hours
- Potassium hydroxide 10% solution applied daily over the lesion
- Topical therapy with 0.5% podophyllotoxin
- Imiquimod can be applied 1–3 times a day for 3–7 days per week for 4–16 weeks
- The application under occlusion of a nitric oxide liberating cream containing 5% sodium nitrate combined with salicylic acid 5% was found to be effective in MC
- Topical wart paints, containing 15–20% salicylic acid in collodion or acrylate base, applied carefully to lesions once or twice weekly
- Oral cimetidine found to be effective in extensive MC in children.

CHAPTER 100

Eczema Herpeticum or Kaposi Varicelliform Eruption

Archana S

Case study: Eczema Herpeticum or Kaposi Varicelliform Eruption

Presenting Complaints

Informant: Mother: Doctor, my baby developed sudden fever which was followed by rashes all over the body which is different from his pre-existing eczema. He is itchy and irritable.

Setting

Dermatology outpatient department

History of Presenting Illness

A 3-year old male baby, known case of atopic dermatitis, was brought by his mother. He was apparently well one day ago, when he developed sudden fever with chills, fatigue and malaise followed by extensive itchy rashes all over the body which was rapidly progressive. The mother describes fluid-filled lesions as well. She also complained of recurrent itchy rashes over the neck, elbow folds, knee folds, forearms and legs which were on and off since the last 1 year. Child is immunized for age. Milestones attained normally. No significant birth history.

General Physical Examination

Child, ill looking, conscious and oriented to his surroundings:

- Temperature 101 °F. No pallor, icterus, clubbing, koilonychia, lymphadenopathy or edema.
- Weight and height normal for age.
- Pulse–88 bpm, respiratory rate–24 per minute

Systemic Examination

- No abnormality detected.

Dermatological Examination

- Extensive disseminated papulovesicular rash all over the body, occasional pustules present
- Erosions present
- Characteristic umbilicated vesicles seen
- Exaggerated lesions over active dermatitis.

Q1. What is the likely diagnosis?

a. Eczema herpeticum (EH)
b. Langerhans cell histiocytosis
c. Varicella
d. Gianotti-Crosti syndrome
e. Erythema multiforme

Ans: a. Eczema herpeticum. The appearance of explosive papulovesicular rash with umbilication on a background of atopic dermatitis suggests the diagnosis of eczema herpeticum.

Q2. What is the definition of eczema herpeticum?

Ans: Eczema herpeticum (EH) or Kaposi varicelliform eruption is a severe disseminated herpes simplex virus (HSV) infection that occurs in individuals with pre-existing dermatoses such as atopic dermatitis or other chronic skin diseases including pemphigus, Darier's disease, ichthyosis vulgaris, congenital ichthyosiform erythroderma, mycosis fungoides, Sezary syndrome, secondary degree burns and certain procedures such as dermabrasion as well as laser therapy.

Q3. Who described this condition?

Ans: EH was initially described by Kaposi in 1887 as a potentially life-threatening herpetic superinfection of a pre-existing skin disease. Further, Lynch in 1954 proposed the term eczema herpeticum for extensive HSV infection, complicating eczema and other dermatoses.

Q4. Which age group is affected by eczema herpeticum?

Ans: Children of all age groups are affected by EH. Adults having widespread dermatoses are also rarely affected.

Q5. What is the incubation period of eczema herpeticum?

Ans: Approximately 10 days (range 5–19 days).

Q6. Explain the etiopathology of eczema herpeticum.

Ans: Etiopathology of eczema herpeticum:

- All reported cases of childhood EH are due to HSV-1 and HSV-2.
- Single nucleotide polymorphisms in the interferon regulatory factor-2 (IRF2) gene confer higher risk of EH.
- Disruption of the skin barrier is the most common predisposing factor.
- History of herpes simplex in the family members or close contacts
- Immunosuppression most commonly secondary to the primary dermatoses also serves as a risk factor.

Q7. Enumerate the clinical features of eczema herpeticum.

Ans: Clinical features:

- Sudden deterioration of eczema
- Abrupt onset of fever, malaise
- Dramatic explosive extensive rapidly progressive papulovesicular, vesiculopustular lesions
- Intense itching and soreness present.
- Maybe discrete or appear in crops.
- The lesions progress to become hemorrhagic and painful crusted ulcers.
- May affect any part of the body
- More prominent in areas of active dermatitis. More accentuated over head, neck and trunk.
- Lesions are widespread and monomorphous.
- Characteristic umbilication of vesicles
- Maybe associated with anorexia, nausea, vomiting and dermatopathic lymphadenopathy.
- Complications include keratoconjunctivitis, secondary bacterial superinfection due to *Staphylococcus aureus*; beta hemolytic streptococci and pseudomonas, fluid loss, viremia.

Q8. What are the differential diagnosis of eczema herpeticum?

Ans: Differential diagnosis of eczema herpeticum:

- Eczema vaccinatum
- Eczema coxsackium
- Impetigo
- Gianotti-Crosti syndrome
- Varicella
- Langerhans cell histiocytosis
- Erythema multiforme.

Q9. What are the relevant investigations?

Ans: The diagnosis can be verified by:

- Tzanck smear and staining with Giemsa or Wright stain (look for multinuclear giant cells or balloon cells.)
- Direct fluorescent assay for antibodies against HSV 1 and 2
- Viral culture from fresh vesicle
- Routine histology helps with detecting viral infection but not with the virus typing.

Q10. What is the treatment for eczema herpeticum?

Ans: Treatment for EH:
- Topical corticosteroid and tacrolimus (for treating atopic eczema) has not affected the outcome of antiviral treatment
- Systemic acyclovir should be initiated
- Severe cases must be hospitalized and treated with intravenous acyclovir. Early administration of acyclovir has shown better outcomes for EH
- Systemic antibiotics must be administered if secondary bacterial infection is strongly suspected
- Empirical antibiotic should not be used
- Other synergistic yet important protocols include hydration, electrolyte balance and pain control
- Scrupulous skin care should be observed including gentle cleansers, bland emollients and antibiotics when required
- Ophthalmologic evaluation is required when extensive face involvement is noticed
- Patients with history of recurrent HSV 1 or 2 infections and a chronic skin disease must be offered prophylactic antiviral therapy.

Q11. What is the dose of acyclovir required?

Ans: Dose of acyclovir:
- Oral acyclovir 20 mg per kg per dose 5 times a day for 7 days
- 20 mg per kg per dose every 8 hourly IV for 14–21 days.

Q12. What is the prognosis of eczema herpeticum?

Ans: The prognosis is favorable in early diagnosed and treated cases.

Q13. What is the response to acyclovir?

Ans: The response to antivirals is dramatic.

Q14. What is the treatment for the underlying dermatosis?

Ans: Treatment of eczema or the underlying dermatosis can be done in the usual way. However, if acyclovir is being withheld for any reason, immunosuppressants like steroids should be used with caution till the viral infection subsides.

CHAPTER 101

Cutaneous Leishmaniasis

Piyush Kumar

Case study Cutaneous Leishmaniasis

Presenting Complaints

Doctor, my son has many ulcers on the face for the last 3 months.

Setting

Dermatology outpatient department

History of Present Illness

A 6-year-old boy from Bihar presented with painless well-defined ulcers over face for 3 months. They started as slow growing raised lesions, which enlarged over few months to form large lesions that ulcerated in a week's time to form ulcers. Lesions were painless throughout the course of the disease. There was no associated lymphadenopathy, fever, and weight loss was not marked.

General Physical Examination and Systemic Examination

No abnormality detected

Dermatological Examination

- Three ulcerated and crusted plaques with raised edges and surrounding dusky red skin.
- No lymphadenopathy.

Q1. What is the most likely diagnosis?

a. Cutaneous leishmaniasis (CL)
b. Atypical mycobacterial infection
c. Bacterial infection (pyoderma)
d. Lupus vulgaris

Ans: a. Cutaneous leishmaniasis. Presence of painless, indurated, crusted ulcer over face (exposed part) in a person residing in an endemic area suggests the diagnosis of CL. However, confirmation needs to be done.

Q2. What are the causative organisms of cutaneous leishmaniasis?

Ans: Leishmaniasis is a disease caused by different species of protozoa of the genus *Leishmania* that are transmitted by Phlebotomine sand flies. Tegumentary leishmaniasis (cutaneous and mucocutaneous forms) are prevalent in 82 countries, and most (90%) of the cases are reported in Africa (mainly in Morocco, Ethiopia and Tunisia), the Middle-East (mainly in Afghanistan, Pakistan, Iran, Iraq, Syria and

Saudi Arabia) and Latin America. As per Eurocentric worldview, dermotropic *Leishmania* parasites are divided into:

- *Old world CL* (Mediterranean basin, Middle East, Africa, Europe and the Indian subcontinent)—*L. major, L. tropica, L. aethiopica* (Ethiopia and Kenya), *L. infantum* (Europe)
- *New world CL* (Latin America)—*L. mexicana, L. braziliensis, L. chagasi.*

The Old World species cause self-limiting ulcers in most cases. New World species cause a syndrome called American tegumentary leishmaniasis comprising CL associated with a variety of other manifestations, such as mucocutaneous leishmaniasis (MCL) and the much rarer diffuse and disseminated cutaneous leishmaniasis (DCL).

Q3. Describe the pathogenesis of leishmaniasis in brief.

Ans: *Leishmania* species are obligate intracellular parasites that exist in two forms: the promastigote and the amastigote. In the gut of the sand fly, the organisms multiply as extracellular flagellated promastigotes. Following bite, the parasites are inoculated (in the promastigote form) into the skin and are rapidly engulfed by the host's phagocytes. There they transform into amastigotes (nonmotile form).

Further course of disease depends on amount of exposure, virulence of infecting species, and cell-mediated immunity response. Inadequate Th1 response [less interleukin-2 (IL-2) and interferon-γ (IFN-γ) production] or development of a Th2-type response (production of IL-4 and IL-10) is associated with progressing disease.

Q4. What are the clinical features of cutaneous leishmaniasis?

Ans: CL usually begins as a small papule at the site of bite (usually exposed sites) that may enlarge into a nodule or plaque, and then become ulcerated or verrucous. The lesions are often solitary but they may be multiple with the formation of satellites or lymphatic spread. The majority of acute cutaneous infections resolve spontaneously with scarring, but some may become chronic or disseminated. CL has been traditionally described as follows:

- *Old world cutaneous leishmaniasis*
  - *Wet or rural type*: It is usually caused by *L. major* and is characterized by multiple lesions, short incubation period (1 week to 3 months), rapid and mild course and good response to therapy. Lesion starts as an indurated papule which enlarges to form a nodule that ulcerates. Satellite lesions may develop and spread in nodular sporotrichoid fashion along the lymphatics. Spontaneous healing occurs in 6 months leaving a characteristic scar.
  - *Dry or urban type*: It is usually caused by *L. tropica* and is characterized by a longer incubation period, protracted course (potential to persist/progress, recur and visceralize) and by a worse response to therapy. It usually starts as an itchy brown papule gradually spreading to form an infiltrated plaque (Fig. 1), which finally ulcerates at the center. Ulcer heals with characteristic depressed cribriform scar over a year.
  - *Leishmaniasis recidivans (leishmania recidiva cutis):* It is a rare chronic CL caused mostly by *L. tropica* (sometimes by *L. braziliensis)* and is characterized by erythematous, scaly papules and plaques, often with apple jelly appearance at the borders of a completely or partially healed lesion.
- *New world cutaneous leishmaniasis*: Pure cutaneous forms resemble old world CL and verrucous or ulcerated papules, nodules and plaques are characteristic. It is less likely to spontaneously resolve and is associated with a greater risk for spread of the infection to mucous membranes or for systemic dissemination if it is left untreated.

Q5. What are the complications of cutaneous leishmaniasis?

Ans: Complications:

- Secondary bacterial infection
- Scarring and disfigurement

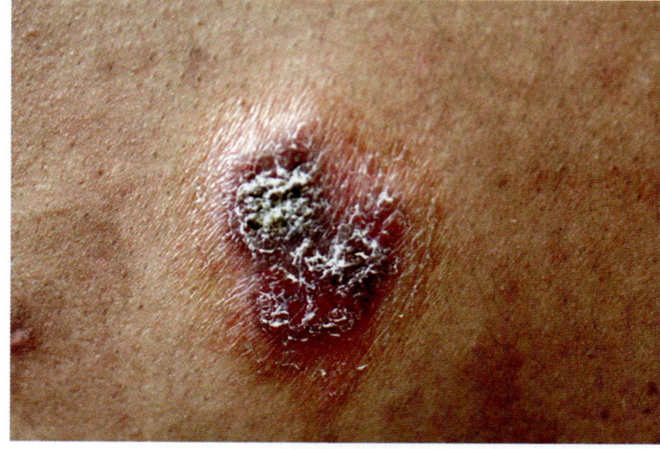

Fig. 1: Solitary plaque in dry type of cutaneous leishmaniasis

- *Chronic cutaneous leishmaniasis*: Lesions develop into chronic disfiguring nodules/plaques that exhibit variable degrees of scaling, ulceration, verrucosity and scarring.
- *Mucocutaneous leishmaniasis:* It results from direct extension or hematogenous/lymphatic spread to the upper respiratory tract and is associated with CL caused by *L. braziliensis* and *L. aethiopica*. It may present several years after resolution of the primary CL or rarely, while they are still present. Bony structures are spared and symptoms include epistaxis, corhyza, hyperemia, and nasal septum crusting and ulceration.
- *Diffuse cutaneous leishmaniasis (DCL)*: It is caused by *L. aethiopica and L. amazonensis* and is seen in persons with defective leishmania-specific cell-mediated immunity (anergy). As a result, there is uncontrolled parasite growth (seen as abundant LD bodies in smear). It closely resembles lepromatous leprosy and is clinically characterized by numerous nonulcerating nodules and plaques all over body. Mucous membranes are usually spared. Treatment response is usually poor and lesions may persist for years.
- *Disseminated cutaneous leishmaniasis*: It is usually seen in patients with HIV coinfection and is caused by *L. braziliensis* group and *L. mexicana*. Leishmanin skin test is strongly positive and parasite load is scanty in smears. Clinically, it is characterized by numerous papules and nodules. Lesions frequently ulcerate and mucosal involvement is common. Response to treatment is variable, but better than DCL.
- Visceral dissemination.

Q6. What are the differential diagnoses of cutaneous leishmaniasis?

Ans: Differential diagnosis:

- *Acute CL:* Arthropod bite, infections [pyoderma, dermatophyte (Majocchi) granuloma, tuberculosis, atypical mycobacterial and deep fungal infections], malignancy (basal cell/squamous cell carcinoma, keratoacanthoma), lymphoma/pseudolymphoma
- *Chronic CL*: Lupus vulgaris, sarcoidosis, discoid lupus erythematosus, lymphoma/pseudolymphoma, leprosy
- *Diffuse CL:* Lepromatous leprosy, xanthoma, lymphoma.

Q7. How will you confirm the diagnosis?

Ans: Confirmation of diagnosis:

- *Smear*: Air-dried smear (specimen collected by FNAC or scrapping) stained by Giemsa or Leishman stain shows Leishman Donovan bodies (LD bodies).
- Histology shows dense and diffuse mixed inflammatory cell infiltrate composed predominantly of histiocytes and scattered multinucleated giant cells, lymphocytes and plasma cells. LD bodies can be found both within histiocytes and extracellularly. Giemsa stain stains the parasite nonmetachromatically and the kinetoplast bright red.
- *Culture*: Novy-MacNeal-Nicolle (NNN) shows rapid growth but sensitivity is less.
- *Leishmanin test*: A delayed hypersensitivity skin test to promastigote form has been useful in making diagnosis of CL. But, this test cannot differentiate between current and past infection. Also, this test may be positive in up to 50% people in endemic area without any current or past disease.
- *Serology*: Indirect fluorescent antibody test, ELISA, complement fixation test and counter immunoelectrophoresis are some of the serological tests, but are of little importance because of low sensitivity and specificity.
- *Isoenzyme analysis*: It consists of enzyme electrophoresis of cultured promastigotes and allows species identification.
- *Molecular techniques*: Polymerase chain reaction (PCR) can detect organism by using species-specific oligonucleotide probes for kinetoplast DNA. Recombinant K39 (rK39) rapid dipstick test is an immunochromatographic assay to detect leishmania antibodies in serum. This is a qualitative test for diagnosis of visceral leishmaniasis as K39 is an epitope conserved on amastigotes of leishmania species causing visceral infection.

Q8. How to manage cutaneous leishmaniasis?

Ans: Spontaneous healing is very common and treatment is indicated in the following conditions:

- Risk of disabling or disfiguring scars, particularly on the face or ears or near joints
- Decrease the risk for mucosal dissemination/disease (In new world CL)
- Accelerate healing of the skin lesions
- Decrease the risk for relapse (clinical reactivation) of the skin lesions
- Involvement of mucous membranes or cartilage
- Large lesions and failure to heal spontaneously

- Control of disease in the population.

Common treatment modalities are:

Local treatment:

- Local heat—heating a sore to 37–43°C for 12 hours promotes healing
- Curettage—simple curettage in 4 weeks time with minimal scarring
- Cryosurgery—freezing with CO_2 snow or liquid nitrogen
- Intralesional injection of 5% mepacrine
- Intralesional administration of Sodium stibogluconate
- Topical paromomycin (15%)
- Photodynamic therapy (PDT) using porphyrin precursors as sensitizers
- CO_2 LASER

Systemic treatment:

- *Sodium stibogluconate (IM/IV)*: The standard dose is 20 mg/kg/day and the traditional duration of therapy is 20 days for cutaneous leishmaniasis (10 days may suffice in some settings) and 28 days for mucosal (and visceral) leishmaniasis.
- Amphotericin B and liposomal amphotericin B in case of *L. braziliensis* and *L. guyanensis*
- Intramuscular pentamidine in case of antimony resistant cases
- *Miltefosine*: Evidence for its use in CL is scarce. It has been used at a dose of 2.5 mg/kg/day (150 mg for an adult) for 28 days. Effectiveness has been variable in different geographic regions.

Other drugs including azoles (fluconazole, ketoconazole, itraconazole), dapsone, rifampicin, allopurinol, and levamisole have been tried with limited success.

Q9. Is there any vaccine available for cutaneous leishmaniasis?

Ans: Presently no human vaccine is commercially available. The main hindrance is the complexity of the cellular immune response in this disease, and the variety of parasite species responsible for visceral and tegumentary forms. More than 30 leishmania antigens have been or are being tested as candidate vaccines but none were able to provide consistent protection so far.

CHAPTER 102

Post-Kala-Azar Dermal Leishmaniasis

Piyush Kumar

Case study Post-Kala-Azar Dermal Leishmaniasis

Presenting Complaints

Doctor, I have been developing red raised lesions on my face and trunk for the last 3 years.

Setting

Dermatology outpatient department

History of Present Illness

An 18-year-old boy from rural Bihar presented with complaints of multiple asymptomatic red raised lesions on face and trunk for 3 years. The lesions were increasing in number and size. He gave a history of kala-azar 5 years back for which he was treated with injections (details not available with patient) at a district hospital.

General Physical Examination and Systemic Examination

No abnormality detected

Dermatological Examination

- Multiple nontender, erythematous, juicy papules and nodules on face (predominantly in perioral area) and upper trunk
- Multiple nonscaly, hypopigmented macules and patches on face and trunk (Fig. 1). The sensations over patches were intact
- No loss of sensation in acral areas
- Peripheral nerves were not thickened.

Q1. What is the most likely diagnosis?

a. Lepromatous leprosy
b. Mycosis fungoides
c. Post-kala-azar dermal leishmaniasis (PKDL)
d. Sarcoidosis

Ans: c. Post-kala-azar dermal leishmaniasis. History of kala-azar (visceral leishmaniasis) and juicy papules and nodules in perioral location (muzzle area of face) and hypopigmented macules on the trunk suggest the diagnosis of PKDL.

Q2. What is post-kala-azar dermal leishmaniasis (PKDL) and how is it related to visceral leishmaniasis?

Ans: PKDL is a cutaneous complication of visceral leishmaniasis (VL) caused by *Leishmania donovani*. PKDL is not associated with visceral leishmaniasis

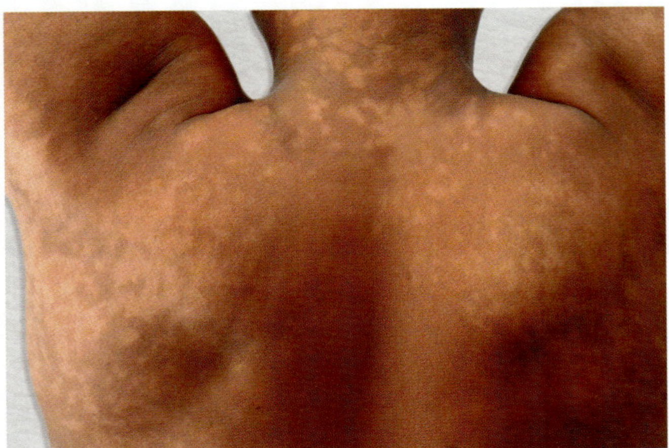

Fig. 1: Multiple nonscaly hypopigmented macules on the back

caused by other species and is geographically restricted to Indian subcontinent and East Africa (Kenya and Sudan). PKDL usually develops 2–3 years (range 6 months to 32 years) after apparent cure of VL. However, PKDL has been reported in cases without prior history of VL and in cases still on treatment for VL (Para kala-azar dermal leishmaniasis). In PKDL, parasite can be demonstrated in skin only. PKDL lesions, especially the papulonodules, are parasite-rich and therefore, these cases are considered to be a reservoir of infection and might play a pivotal role in the interepidemic transmission of VL.

Q3. Is there any predictor of post-kala-azar dermal leishmaniasis?

Ans: Some accepted predictors are:

- *Incomplete or inadequate treatment*: Patients who fail to complete treatment are more likely to develop PKDL.
- *High level of C-reactive protein (CRP)*: Patients who had high C-reactive protein levels (>40 µg/mL) at the time of VL had higher risk of developing PKDL.
- *High level of interleukin 10 (IL-10)*: High concentrations of IL-10 in the blood and the presence of this cytokine in normal-looking skin during VL are associated with PKDL.
- *Ultraviolet (UV) light*: UV light associated immunosuppression has been thought to play a role in development of PKDL. It explains predominance of skin lesions on sun-exposed areas and severe form of disease in young children (attributed to generalized ultraviolet light exposure since young children often walk about undressed).
- Severe PKDL has been found to be associated with shorter duration between VL and PKDL.

Q4. Describe clinical picture of post-kala-azar dermal leishmaniasis.

Ans: Two types of morphological lesions are seen—the early hypopigmented macules (coalesces to form patches) and later papulonodular/plaque lesions. The hypopigmented macules start as small pinpoint lesions appearing on face and then spread to involve trunk, upper limbs and thighs. An erythematous bat wing rash may be around the muzzle area, becoming prominent on exposure to sun. As the disease progresses, the hypopigmented lesions are replaced by soft, juicy and skin colored or erythematous papulonodular lesions and plaques. Involvement of mucous membrane of the tongue, palate and genitalia resembling lepromatous leprosy is common. Xanthomatous lesions on the axillary fold, cubital fossae, inner thigh and around outer canthus of the eye are the other morphological patterns.

Lymphadenopathy is usually absent in PKDL in Indian subcontinent.

Q5. What are the differential diagnoses of post-kala-azar dermal leishmaniasis?

Ans: Differential diagnosis:

- *Macular lesions*: Lepromatous leprosy, pityriasis versicolor, pityriasis alba, nutritional dyschromia, onchocerciasis
- *Nodular lesion*: Lepromatous leprosy, syphilis, mycosis fungoides, leukemia cutis, nodular lesions of neurofibromatosis, keloids and sarcoidosis
- *Plaque lesion*: Lepromatous leprosy, cutaneous tuberculosis, granuloma annulare, psoriasis, syphilis, sarcoidosis and mycosis fungoides.

Q6. How will you confirm the diagnosis?

Ans: Demonstration of *L. donovani* (LD) bodies is considered to be the gold standard for diagnosis. LD bodies can be demonstrated in slit skin smears, fine needle aspiration cytology (FNAC), histopathology or by culture of tissue. However, these methods are invasive, less sensitive, and difficult to perform at the periphery level.

Q7. Describe *Leishmania donovani* bodies.

Ans: LD bodies are tiny (2.5–7 µm), nonmotile amastigotes that cause disease in humans. Under microscope, each amastigote organism shows a tiny nucleus and a short rod-shaped mitochondrium called a kinetoplast, giving a characteristic "dot and dash" appearance.

Q8. What is the role of serological tests in the diagnosis of post-kala-azar dermal leishmaniasis?

Ans: Serological tests such as the direct agglutination test (DAT) and ELISA are of limited value in endemic areas as leishmanial antibodies after VL may persist for years. The importance of serological tests [including widely available rK39 strip test (rapid diagnostic ELISA)] lies in excluding other conditions and in cases where a history of visceral leishmaniasis is uncertain.

Q9. Describe histopathology of post-kala-azar dermal leishmaniasis.

Ans: Macules of PKDL show a minimal mixed chronic inflammatory infiltrate consisting of lymphocytes, histiocytes, and occasional plasma cells in the perivascular areas of the upper dermis. Nodules and plaques are characterized by a dense inflammatory infiltrate of mononuclear cells, histiocytes and plasma cells in the upper dermis and a narrow subepidermal grenz zone. LD bodies are seen in a fraction of cases. A few cases show granuloma—macrophage granuloma, epithelioid cell granuloma and even granuloma with predominant foam cells.

Q10. How to treat post-kala-azar dermal leishmaniasis?

Ans: PKDL patients show high rate of spontaneous healing and hence, milder cases are left untreated and are observed. Indian PKDL cases do not show spontaneous healing and are routinely treated. Commonly used drugs are:

- *Pentavalent antimony*: Dose and duration of treatment are higher than VL. Usual dose is 20 mg/kg and duration of treatment is up to 120 days *(National Vector Borne Disease Control Programme)*. Resistance to sodium stibogluconate is known and hence this drug is not preferred in endemic areas.
- *Amphotericin B*: This is now preferred drug in endemic areas. It is given at a dose of 1 mg/kg as IV infusion daily or alternate day for 60–80 infusions over 4 months.
- *Liposomal amphotericin B*: A short course of treatment with two doses of liposomal amphotericin B (5 mg/kg per dose) per week for 3 weeks (for a total dose of 30 mg/kg) is used under National Vector Borne Disease Control Programme.
- *Miltefosine*: Under National Vector Borne Disease Control Programme, it is given for 4 weeks to treat VL and is now considered first-line drug. For PKDL, recommended duration of treatment is 12 weeks. The dose recommended are 100 mg daily, 50 mg daily and 2.5 mg/kg/day for adults (>12 years) weighing more than 25 kg, adults (>12 years) weighing less than 25 kg and children aged 2–11 years, respectively. The drug is not to be used in the case of children below 2 years of age, pregnant and lactating women and women of reproductive age who refuse to use contraceptives during the treatment period and two months after completion of treatment and in HIV-positive patients.
- Other drugs like ketoconazole, itraconazole, fluconazole and rifampicin have been tried with limited success. However, these drugs are not recommended.

SECTION 19

Mucosal Disorders

Anupam Das

CHAPTER 103

White Lesions in Oral Cavity

Harish Prasad

Case study — White Lesions in Oral Cavity

Presenting Complaints

Doctor, there is a white colored patch inside my mouth since the last 3 years.

Setting

Dermatology outpatient department

History of Present Illness

A 41-year-old gentleman presented with complaints of a white patch in the oral cavity for last 3 years. The patch has gradually increased in size to attain the present status. He does not complain of any difficulty in swallowing or chewing food. There is no burning sensation or irritation while consuming hot and spicy food and liquids. There is a history of chewing gutkha throughout the day for last 10 years and the patient has been smoking 25–30 cigarettes per day for the past 5 years.

General Physical Examination and Systemic Examination

No abnormality detected

Dermatological Examination

- Irregular whitish patch in the buccal mucosa (left side) extending to the angle of the mouth (Fig. 1).
- The patch cannot be rubbed off with gauze.
- There is no reticulate pattern or involvement of occlusion line or amalgam fillings.

Q1. What is the most likely diagnosis?

a. Oral lichen planus
b. Oral submucous fibrosis
c. Oral leukoplakia
d. Oral candidiasis

Ans: c (Oral leukoplakia).

Presence of whitish patch in the buccal mucosa (which cannot be rubbed off) in a middle-aged man with a history of chewing tobacco and smoking cigarettes (25–30/day) for 5 years suggests a diagnosis of oral leukoplakia. No clinical or histopathological cause can be ascribed to, and is not associated with any physical or chemical causative agent except tobacco.

Q2. How do you classify white lesions in oral cavity?

Ans: Classification of white lesions in oral cavity:

- *Developmental or congenital*: Leukoedema, white sponge nevus, dyskeratosis congenita, Fordyce spots

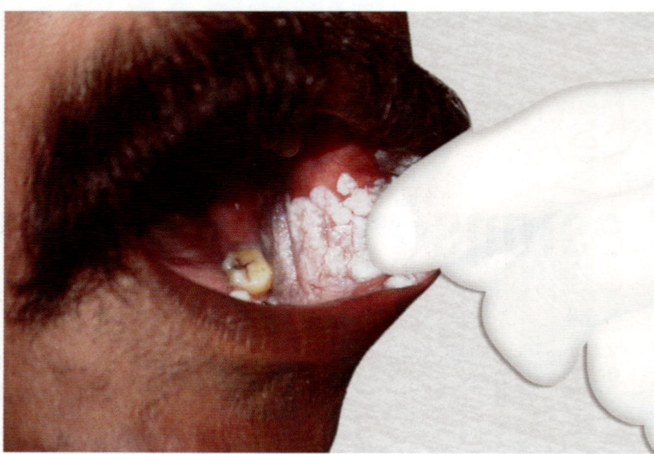

Fig. 1: Irregular whitish patch in the buccal mucosa (left side) extending to the angle of the mouth

- *Inflammatory/Reactive*: Morsicatio buccarum et labiorum, frictional, chemical and thermal keratosis, tobacco pouch keratosis
- *Infective*: Candidosis, oral hairy leukoplakia, warts, syphilitic mucous patches
- *Oral manifestation of systemic disorders*: Uremic stomatitis
- *Oral manifestation of dermatological disorders*: Lichen planus, keratosis follicularis, discoid lupus erythematosus, mucosal vitiligo
- *Premalignant*: Oral submucosal fibrosis, proliferative verrucous leukoplakia, florid oral papillomatosis, leukoplakia
- *Malignant*: Squamous cell carcinoma
- *Miscellaneous*: Mucosal retention cyst, graft versus host disease, drugs.

Q3. How do you approach to a patient with white lesions in oral cavity?

Ans: Approach to white lesions:

History

- Duration of the lesions help to differentiate congenital from acquired causes
- H/o using any form of tobacco, alcohol, other irritants
- Any form of immunodeficiency—infections
- Dental procedures and dentures, amalgam fillings, braces, habitual mucosal biting, irregularities in alignment of teeth, and habitual peeling of mucosa.

Examination

- Malignancy should always be suspected in long-standing and treatment-resistant cases.
- If one can rub off the lesions, take specimen for KOH preperations, brush biopsies as simple bedside tests
- Excision biopsy or wedge biopsy to be considered and subjected to histopathological examination if none of the simple tests leads to diagnosis
- Specific tests, if any, helps one to diagnose the pinpoint etiology for oral white lesions.

Q4. What is the prevalence and age and sex predilection of oral leukoplakia?

Ans:
- Prevalence is less than 1%
- Male:female = 2:1
- More than 80% of patients present after 40 years of age.

Q5. What is the natural history of oral leukoplakia?

Ans: Natural history:
- The earliest lesion is a nonpalpable translucent white discoloration, which on pressing from above retains the white color.
- Later, the lesion develops into an elevated, opaque, white plaque studded with fine granules.
- In the late stages, the lesion is a thick indurated plaque with fissuring and ulceration, which can progress to squamous cell carcinoma.

Q6. What are the clinical types of leukoplakia?

Ans:
- Homogeneous
- Nonhomogeneous (Speckled, verrucous and ulcerated).

Q7. What is the commonest site of oral leukoplakia?

a. Floor of the mouth
b. Behind oral commissure
c. Dorsum of tongue
d. Gingivobuccal sulcus

Ans: b (Behind oral commissure).

Q8. What are the red flag signs of oral leukoplakia?

Ans: Following are the red flag signs that are markers of impending progression to squamous cell carcinoma:
- Verrucous variant
- Erosive/ulcerative variant
- Presence of nodule within the lesion
- Induration in the periphery of the lesion
- Location in the anterior part of the floor of mouth and under surface of tongue.

Q9. How do you manage oral leukoplakia?

Ans:
- Leukoplakias have a relatively low risk of malignant transformation. Initial treatment

involves the elimination of all possible known risk factors, following which the patient should be re-examined 3 months later. If the lesion regresses, no further treatment is indicated. Persistent lesions warrant a biopsy.

- Regular follow-up of these lesions is of utmost importance.
- Surgery (scalpel or laser excision) is an obvious option for the management of leukoplakias with a high predisposition to malignant transformation.
- *Other treatment modalities*: Cryosurgery, retinoids, b-carotene, bleomycin, calcipotriol, photodynamic therapy and vitamin A.
- No definite measures have been devised for the prevention of development of leukoplakia or oral carcinoma. Avoidance of smoking and alcohol and consumption of fresh fruits and vegetables may have a protective effect. Oral cancer screening programs can help in early diagnosis of these lesions and improve the prognosis and treatment success.

Q10. What is the prognosis of oral leukoplakia?

Ans: Prognosis:

- 10% lesions progress into invasive carcinoma.
- Some cases of leukoplakia with dysplasia turn into malignancy, in spite of surgical excision.
- Many dysplastic cases regress spontaneously.

Q11. What are the various clinical forms of oral candidiasis?

Ans: Clinical forms of oral candidiasis:

- Acute pseudomembranous candidosis (oral thrush) presents with sharply defined superficial curd-like white patches covered by pseudomembrane, which when wiped off leaves an erythematous base. The buccal mucosa, gums or palate may be affected with extension to the pharynx or esophagus seen in severe cases.
- Chronic pseudomembranous candidosis is seen in immunocompromised patients.
- Acute erythematous candidosis (acute atrophic oral candidiasis; antibiotic sore tongue) is characterised by marked soreness and focal or diffuse areas of denuded atrophic erythematous mucosa, particularly on the dorsum of the tongue.
- Chronic erythematous candidosis (chronic atrophic candidiasis, denture sore mouth, denture stomatitis) presents as a variable bright-red or dusky area of erythema with a pebbly or velvety surface confined to the upper denture-bearing area, the palate and gums. There is often an associated angular cheilitis.
- Angular cheilitis presents as fissures or erosions, and crusting with underlying erythema developing at the commissures associated with soreness.
- Chronic hyperplastic candidosis (candidial leukoplakia) appears as firm, well-demarcated, white, thick, or verrucus plaques commonly on the cheek or the tongue that cannot be rubbed off easily.
- Chronic nodular candidosis is a rare form where the clinical appearance that usually affects the tongue is cobbled.
- Median rhomboid glossitis appears as an asymptomatic diamond- or oval-shaped erythematous depapillated area on the dorsum of the tongue. The surface is smooth or lobulated. It occurs more frequently in AIDS (acquired immune deficiency syndrome) patients.
- Chronic mucocutaneous form of candidosis is a heterogenous group that presents as persistent candida infection of the mouth, skin and nails, refractory to conventional topical therapy.

Q12. What are the factors predisposing to candidiasis?

Ans: Changes in the oral environment that predisposes or precipitates oral candidiasis include:

Local host factors

- Denture wearing
- Steroid inhaler use
- Reduced salivary flow (xerostomia)
- High sugar diet

Systemic host factors

- Extremes of age
- Endocrine disorders (e.g. diabetes)
- Immunosuppression
- Receipt of broad spectrum antibiotics
- Nutritional deficiencies.

Q13. How do you diagnose oral candidiasis?

Ans: Diagnosis:

- The diagnosis of this condition is by positive direct microscopy. On 10% potassium hydroxide (KOH) mount, pseudohyphae or budding cells consistent with the candida morphology can be demonstrated.
- A cytologic smear or biopsy can also be stained with periodic acid–Schiff. This method stains the abundant carbohydrates in the fungal cell walls. The organisms are identified easily by their bright magenta color.

- Definitive identification of the fungi is performed by culture on Sabouraud's dextrose agar.

Q14. How do you manage candidiasis?

Ans: Management:

- Identification and treatment of underlying predisposing factors.
- Topical antifungal therapy
- Systemic antifungals in unresponsive and chronic cases, such as those with hyperplastic candidosis, patients with AIDS or chronic mucocutaneous candidiasis. Combination antiretroviral therapy in AIDS patients improves the therapeutic outcome significantly. Triazoles (fluconazole and itraconazole) are commonly used for systemic treatment. The usual daily doses are itraconazole 100–200 mg and fluconazole 100–400 mg.
- In patients with chronic oral candidiasis, a biopsy may be justified to exclude leukoplakia.

CHAPTER 104

Oral Lichen Planus

Niharika Lal

Case study Oral Lichen Planus

Presenting Complaints

Doctor, I am experiencing painful ulcers in my oral cavity since last 3 months.

Setting

Dermatology outpatient department

History of Present Illness

A 32-year-old man presented to the dermatology outpatient department with complaints of painful ulcers in the oral cavity for the last 3 months. He also complained of difficulty in eating and drinking due to the ulcers. There was no history of fever or malaise with the onset of lesions. No history of drug intake prior to their eruptions. No photosensitivity or history of joint pain. There was a history of dental surgery few months back. Patient is a chronic smoker.

General Examination and Systemic Examination

No abnormality detected.

Dermatological Examination

Multiple erosions and ulcers on buccal mucosa, inner lip and gingiva. Presence of violaceous hue in buccal mucosa along the line of teeth occlusion (Fig. 1). Other mucosal surfaces such as penile and conjunctival mucosae were free from any involvement.

Q1. What is the provisional diagnosis?

a. Erosive variant of oral lichen planus (OLP)
b. Aphthous ulcer
c. Orolabial herpes
d. Mucosal lupus erythematosus

Ans: a (Oral erosive LP)

Q2. What are the other differential diagnoses?

Ans: a. Herpetic gingivostomatitis
b. Fixed drug eruption (FDE)
c. Discoid lupus erythematosus (DLE)
d. Oral pemphigus vulgaris
e. Cicatricial pemphigus.

Q3. What are the points in favor of your diagnosis?

Ans: Longstanding painful multiple ulcers with violaceous margins and history of amalgam filling.

Q4. How will you exclude other conditions clinically?

Ans: No causal relationship with drugs, persistence of lesions since 3 months and no preference for

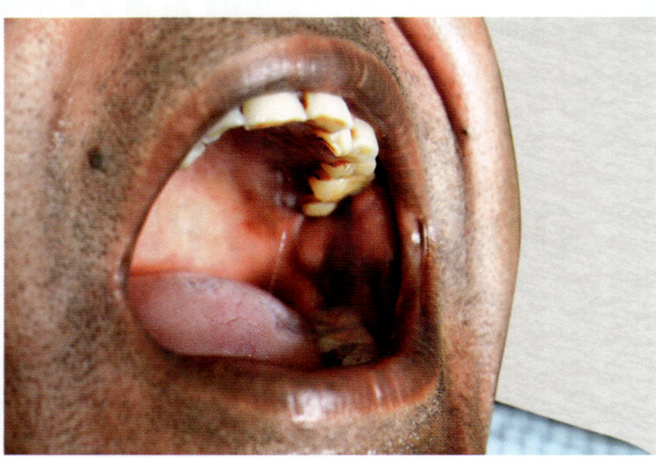

Fig. 1: Violaceous hue along occlusion line on buccal mucosa

keratinized mucosa make a diagnosis of FDE and herpetic gingivostomatitis unlikely. Mucosal DLE is painless. Also no history of photosensitivity, fever or joint pain exclude this condition.

Q5. How will you confirm your diagnosis?

Ans: *Bedside Examination*

Apart from a violaceous hue, a network of fine white lacy lines (Wickham's stria) can be appreciated over the lesions on close-up examination or dermoscopy.

Laboratory Examination

Tzanck smear: To demonstrate acantholysis and multinucleate giant cell in pemphigus and herpetic ulcers. Mucosal biopsy for histology and immunofluorescence.

Q6. What are the biopsy findings in OLP?

Ans:
- Parakeratosis with wedge-shaped hypergranulosis
- Saw toothing of rete ridges with liquefactive degeneration of basal layer and lymphocytic infiltration of dermoepidermal junction
- Plenty of plasma cells.

Q7. What is the etiology for OLP?

Ans: The exact etiology of OLP is unknown:
- Oral lichen planus is classified as an immunologically mediated disorder, but the origin of putative antigen (endogenous or exogenous) triggering the inflammatory response is unclear.
- Genetics, familial clustering, and human leukocyte antigen association, although initially implicated to play a role in the pathogenesis of OLP, are no longer considered critical factors.
- Polymorphisms and genetic variations in the expression of cytokines have been linked with the risk of developing lesions of OLP and govern whether lesions are limited to the oral cavity [IFN-γ (interferon gamma)] or skin [TNF-α (tumor necrosis factor alpha)].
- Various viruses such as varicella zoster virus, Epstein-Barr virus, cytomegalovirus, human herpes virus, human papilloma virus and hepatitis C virus (HCV) have been implicated in development of OLP, but only the role of HCV has been extensively studied. It is believed that the immune reaction mediated by HCV replication may cause damage to the basal layer cells and result in OLP lesions.
- Even though the association of dental amalgam with increased risk of OLP is reported, the exact mechanism leading to development of OLP is not clear; allergic and/or irritant reaction to mercury in amalgam is postulated.
- Stress, anxiety and depression are known to significantly influence the development of OLP.

Q8. What are the other variants of OLP?

Ans: Variants:
- *Reticular subtype:* This is the most common form of lichen planus. Characteristically, it presents as a network of small, raised, whitish-gray, lacy lesions known as Wickham striae, which may be surrounded by a discrete erythematous border. The buccal mucosa is most commonly involved. They may also be seen on the lateral border of tongue and less often on the gingiva and the lips.
- *Papular subtype:* This form presents as small white pinpoint papules about 0.5 mm in size. It is rarely seen, and due to the small size it is possibly overlooked during routine oral examination.
- *Plaque subtype:* This lesion resembles oral leukoplakia and occurs as homogenous white patches. The plaque-like form may range from a slightly elevated and smooth to an irregular form and may be multifocal. The primary sites are the dorsum of the tongue and the buccal mucosa.
- *Atrophic subtype:* The atrophic type has diffuse, red areas with white striae at the margins that radiate peripherally. The gingiva is often involved and the condition is commonly referred to as "chronic desquamative gingivitis". This condition can cause burning sensation particularly when in contact with certain foods.
- *Bullous subtype:* Appears as small bullae or vesicles that tend to rupture easily leaving behind an ulcerated painful surface. The bullous form is commonly seen on the buccal mucosa,

particularly in the posteroinferior areas adjacent to the second or third molar teeth. The next most common site is the lateral margin of the tongue.

- *Erosive subtype*: This is the second most common type. The erosions are often large, slightly depressed or raised with a yellow slough, and have an irregular outline. The surrounding mucosa is often erythematous and glazed in appearance. The periphery of the lesion is usually surrounded by reticular or finely radiating keratotic striae. Erosive LP frequently affects the dorsum and lateral borders of the tongue or the buccal mucosae on both sides.

Q9. What is vulvovaginal gingival syndrome?

Ans: Ulceration occurring in the mouth and gums as well as on the vulva and in the vagina is a severe variant of ELP (erosive lichen planus) in women known as the vulvovaginal gingival syndrome. Equivalent condition in men is penogingival syndrome.

Q10. What are the complications of OLP?

Ans:
- Difficulty in eating
- Dysphagia if esophageal involvement occurs
- Malignant transformation (longstanding ulcers, erosive and atrophic type, tobacco use).

Q11. What drugs can cause oral lichenoid eruptions?

Ans: Drugs causing OLP:
- Allopurinol
- ACE (angiotensin-converting-enzyme) inhibitors
- Cyanamide
- Dental restorative materials
- Gold salts
- Ketoconazole
- Nonsteroidal anti-inflammatory drugs
- Penicillamines
- Sulfonylurea.

Q12. How will you manage your patient?

Ans: Management:
- General measures:
  - Maintenance of oral hygiene
  - Stop smoking
  - Removal of amalgam and replacing it with inert composite
- Topical therapy:
  - Topical anesthetics
  - Topical steroids in gel or base
  - Chlorhexidine mouth wash
  - Anti-candidal medications may be needed during therapy
  - *For severe cases*: Intralesional steroids may be given
  - Topical retinoic acid (tretinoin/isotretinoin gel)
  - Topical cyclosporine wash
  - Topical tacrolimus
- Systemic therapy
  - Systemic steroids
  - Acitretin 30 mg/day
  - Isotretinoin 40 mg/day
  - Hydroxychloroquine 200–400 mg/day
  - Cyclosporine 3–10 mg/kg/day
  - Griseofulvin 200–400 mg/day.

CHAPTER 105

Oral Ulcer

Anupam Das

Case study Oral Ulcer

Presenting Complaints

Doctor, I am having a red and painful lesion inside my mouth, for the last 2 days.

Setting

Dermatology outpatient department

History of Present Illness

A 22-year-old gentleman presented with complaints of a painful red lesion in the oral cavity for the last 2 days. He complains of a burning sensation while consuming hot and spicy food and liquids. There is no history of any addiction or any drug history prior to the onset of the ulcer. He complains of similar lesions, at least three to four times a year.

General Physical Examination and Systemic Examination

No abnormality detected

Dermatological Examination

Solitary shallow round ulcer (1 cm in diameter) surrounded by an erythematous halo and edema. The floor of the ulcer is covered with yellowish pseudomembrane.

Q1. What is the most likely diagnosis?

a. Traumatic ulcer
b. Herpetic stomatitis
c. Aphthous stomatitis
d. Erythema multiforme

Ans: c (Aphthous stomatitis).

The acute onset of the ulcer and the classical clinical finding of shallow round ulcer surrounded by an erythematous halo clinch the diagnosis.

Q2. What is the etiology behind aphthous stomatitis?

Ans: T-lymphocyte mediated localized destruction of mucosa. Rarely, hereditary influence is suggested.

Q3. What are the predisposing factors?

Ans: Predisposing factors:

- Trauma
- *Food*: Cheese, tomato, lemon, pineapple, etc.
- *Drug induced*: NSAIDs (nonsteroidal anti-inflammatory drugs), chemotherapy, cytotoxic drugs, etc.
- Deficiency of iron, folic acid, vitamin B_{12}
- Stress
- Systemic mycoses
- HIV (human immunodeficiency virus) infection
- Behcet syndrome

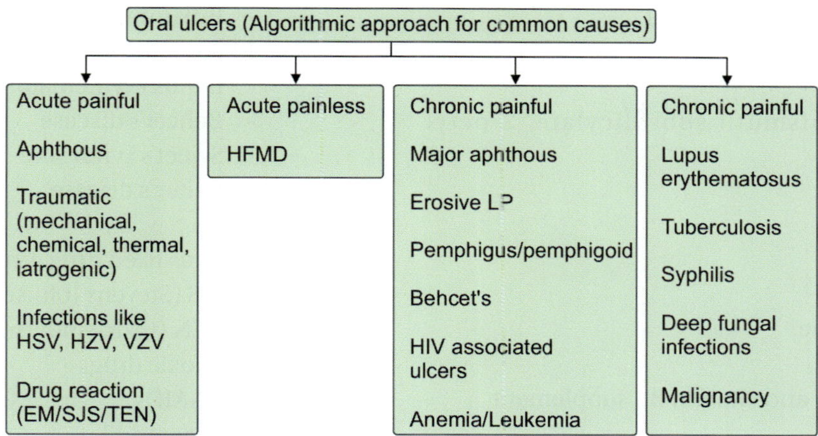

Fig. 1: Oral ulcers (algorithmic approach for common causes)

Abbreviations: HSV, herpes simplex virus; HZV, herpes zoster virus; VZV, varicella zoster virus; EM, erythema multiforme; SJS, Stevens Johnson syndrome; TEN, toxic epidermal necrolysis; HFMD, hand, foot and mouth disease; HIV, human immunodeficiency virus

- Sweet syndrome
- PFAPA syndrome (periodic fever, adenitis, pharyngitis, aphthous stomatitis)
- MAGIC syndrome (mouth and genital ulcers with inflamed cartilage)
- Celiac sprue
- Xerostomia.

Q4. What are the sites of involvement of oral ulcer?

Ans: Sites of involvement:

- Oral mucosa (lips, inner side of cheeks)
- Gingivae
- Floor of mouth
- Uvula and palate
- Tongue.

Q5. Which sites are classically spared in aphthous stomatitis?

Ans: Sites spared:

- Dorsum of tongue
- Unattached gingivae
- Mucosa over the hard palate.

Basically, keratinized mucosae are spared, except in HIV infection.

Q6. What are the types of recurrent aphthous stomatitis?

Ans: Types of recurrent aphthous stomatitis:

- *Minor*: Also known as Mikulicz ulcer. This is the commonest presentation, manifesting as multiple shallow round to oval ulcers surrounded by erythema and edema. The lesions heal within 1–2 weeks without scarring.
- *Major*: Also known as Sutton ulcer. These are usually single, larger in size, recurrent, more painful than minor ulcers, often have a raised border, heal within 10–30 days with scarring. They often appear in crops and can involve keratinized mucosae as well.
- *Herpetiform*: Usually found in elderly population. Appear as crops of painful ulcers on any part of the oral cavity. They coalesce to form large and irregular ulcers.

Q7. What are the differential diagnoses?

Ans: Differential diagnoses:

- Herpes simplex infection
- Erythema multiforme
- Pemphigus vulgaris
- Paraneoplastic pemphigus
- Hand, foot and mouth disease
- Drug-induced stomatitis
- Erosive lichen planus (LP).

Q8. What are the treatment options for oral aphthous ulcers?

Ans: Treatment options:

Topical

- Steroid paste or ointment (dexamthasone, triamcinolone, fluocinolone)
- *Tetracycline*: 250 mg capsule dissolved in 10 mL of water and gargled for 5 minutes, repeat 4 times a day
- H_2O_2 and water rinse
- Chlorhexidine mouth wash

- Lignocaine or benzocaine gel
- Amlexanox ointment
- Tretinoin
- Sucralfate, bismuth subsalicylate, 2-octyl cyanoacrylate

Systemic
- Steroids
- Thalidomide
- Dapsone
- Pentoxiphylline
- Montelukast
- Iron, folic acid and vitamin B_{12} supplement
- Colchicine
- *Immunosuppressive*: Azathioprine, levamisole
- Cevimeline and pilocarpine.

Q9. What are the causes of oral ulcers?

Ans: Causes:
- Traumatic
- Idiopathic—recurrent aphthous stomatitis
- Infective
  - Viral
    - Herpetic stomatitis
    - Chickenpox
    - Herpes zoster
    - Hand, foot and mouth disease
    - Herpangina
    - Infectious mononucleosis
    - HIV
  - Bacterial
    - TB
    - Syphilis
  - Fungi
    - Rare, mostly with systemic fungal diseases
- Associated with different diseases
  - Cutaneous diseases
    - Erosive LP and chronic ulcerative stomatitis
    - Pemphigus
    - Pemphigoid
    - Erythema multiforme
    - Dermatitis herpetiformis
    - Linear IgA disease
    - Epidermolysis bullosa
  - Blood disorders
    - Anemia
    - Leukemia
    - Neutropenia
  - Gastrointestinal
    - Celiac sprue
    - Inflammatory bowel disease
  - Rheumatic disease
    - Lupus erythematosus
    - Behcet's disease
    - Sweet's syndrome
    - Reiter's disease
- Drugs
  - Bullous fixed drug eruption
    - SJS (Stevens Johnson syndrome)
    - TEN (toxic epidermal necrolysis)
  - Cytotoxic drugs
    - NSAIDs
    - Nicorandil
    - Alendronate
- Neoplastic—squamous cell carcinoma
- Disorders of uncertain pathogenesis:
  - Angina bullosa hemorrhagica
  - Hypereosinophillic syndrome
  - Eosinophillic ulcer
  - Necrotizing sialometaplasia.

Q10. What are the causes of acute-onset oral ulcers?

Ans:
- Recurrent aphthous stomatitis
- Herpes simplex
- Drug rash
- Following dental or medical procedures
- Chemical burns
- Thermal burns
- New ill fitting dentures.

Q11. What are the causes of chronic oral ulcers?

Ans:
- Lichen planus (LP)
- Pemphigus, pemphigoid
- Gastrointestinal diseases such as celiac sprue, ulcerative colitis, Crohn's disease
- Connective tissue disorders
- Nutritional deficiencies
- Carcinomas.

Q12. Classify the causes of oral ulcers on the basis of presence or absence of pain.

Ans:
- Painless
  - DLE (discoid lupus erythematosus)
  - SLE (systemic lupus erythematosus)
  - Syphilis
  - Carcinoma.
- Painful
  - Trauma
  - Idiopathic
  - Infections

- Erosive LP
- Chronic ulcerative stomatitis
- Pemphigus
- EM (erythema multiforme)
- TEN.

Q13. What are the predominant sites of involvement of various oral ulcers?

Ans: Sites of involvement:

- *Recurrent aphthous stomatitis*: Nonkeratinized surface
- *Erosive LP*: Buccal mucosa, dorsa of tongue
- *Pemphigus*: Hard palate, gingiva
- *Paraneoplastic pemphigus*: Lips
- *Nutritional deficiency (glossitis and angular cheilitis)*: Tongue
- *Locally advanced CA (carcinoma)*: Posterolateral border of tongue
- *DLE*: Hard palate
- *Necrotizing ulcerative gingivitis*: Interdental and marginal gingiva.

Q14. What are the causes of oral ulcers with induration?

Ans: Oral ulcers with induration:

- *Infections*: Fungal, syphilitic chancre
- *Extensive deep ulcers with indurated borders located in hard or soft palate*: Necrotizing sialometaplasia
- *Longstanding, nonhealing, indurated ulcer with firm infiltration beneath the mucosa*: Malignancy.

Q15. What are the treatment options for various oral ulcers?

Ans: Treatment options

- Traumatic ulcers
  - Removal of traumatic factors
  - Topical steroids may be used for a short time
  - Antiseptic—anesthetic mouth gel
- Aphthous ulcers (discussed already)
- Viral infections
  - Supportive care (antipyretics, analgesics, hydration)
  - Severe forms treated with valacyclovir or acyclovir
  - Treatment for secondary bacterial infections (Streptococcus)
- Oral candidiasis
  - *Mild*: Clotrimazole mouth paint
  - *Refractory/immunocompromised*: Fluconazole, IV amphotericin B± fluconazole
- Erythema multiforme
  - Supportive measures
  - Topical lidocaine
  - *Topical ± oral antibiotics*: prevent secondary infection
  - Topical steroids
- Oral lichen planus
  - Topical lignocaine
  - Topical steroids/tacrolimus
  - Treatment for oral candidiasis
  - Cyclosporine mouth wash for 4–8 weeks
  - *Severe disease*: Systemic steroids, azathioprine, retinoids, dapsone
- Lupus erythematosus
  - *Oral lesions*: Generally no treatment required
  - *Topical corticosteroids*: Improve lesions
  - *Steroid resistant cases*: Methotrexate
- Immunobullous diseases
  - Systemic steroids
  - Steroid sparing immunosuppressive agents
  - *Monoclonal antibodies*: Rituximab
  - Intravenous immunoglobulins
  - Dapsone, tetracyclines
  - Plasmapheresis
- Squamous cell carcinoma
  - Surgery
  - Chemotherapy
  - Radiotherapy
  - Oral retinoids
  - *Sirolimus*: Organ transplant recipients.

Q16. What are the investigations which should be done in a case of oral ulcer: common to rare?

Ans:

- Complete blood count
- Serum iron, ferritin, vitamin B_{12} levels
- Tzanck smear
- Blood for antinuclear antibody
- HIV and VDRL (venereal disease research laboratory) serology
- Biopsy followed by suitable staining
- *Direct and indirect immunofluorescence*: In relevant cases
- Pathergy test
- Patch test, if required
- Serum antiendomysial antibody and transglutaminase assay
- Colonoscopy.

CHAPTER 106

Red Lesion on Penis

Amit Bahuguna

Case study Red Lesion on Penis

Presenting Complaints

Doctor, I have a red painless lesion on the penis since 1 year.

Setting

Dermatology outpatient department

History of Present Illness

A 46-year-old male presented with complaints of painless, slightly itchy red rash over the penis, present for the preceding 1 year. To start with, the lesion was small in size which gradually progressed to the present state. There was a history of frequent episodes of itching over glans penis for last few years, even before this rash had appeared. Besides, he gave a history of transient improvement with topical antifungal and steroid creams. There is no history of bleeding/discharge, phimosis, dysurea or urinary obstruction.

General Physical Examination and Systemic Examination

No abnormality detected

Dermatological Examination

A solitary, well-defined, erythematous, moist glistening plaque over the glans penis, 2 cm × 2.5 cm in size (Fig. 1). Cayenne pepper stippling (yellowish hue with minute purpuric spots) was noted. Scaling, fissures or ulceration were absent. Prepucial sac, penile shaft and urethral meatus were absolutely normal. No inguinal lymphadenopathy.

Q1. What is the most likely diagnosis?

a. Erythroplasia of Queyrat
b. Zoon's balanitis
c. Psoriasis
d. Candidiasis

Ans: b (Zoon's balanitis)

The classical cutaneous findings of a solitary well-defined erythematous moist plaque over the glans penis along with the presence of cayenne pepper stippling clinch the diagnosis.

Q2. What are the sites of involvement of Zoon's balanitis?

Ans: Glans penis, vulva, mouth, lips and epiglottis.

Q3. What are the possible etiological factors in the pathogenesis of Zoon's balanitis?

Ans:
- Chronic friction and heat
- Trauma to the genitalia
- Poor hygienic condition
- Mycobacterium smegmatis infection

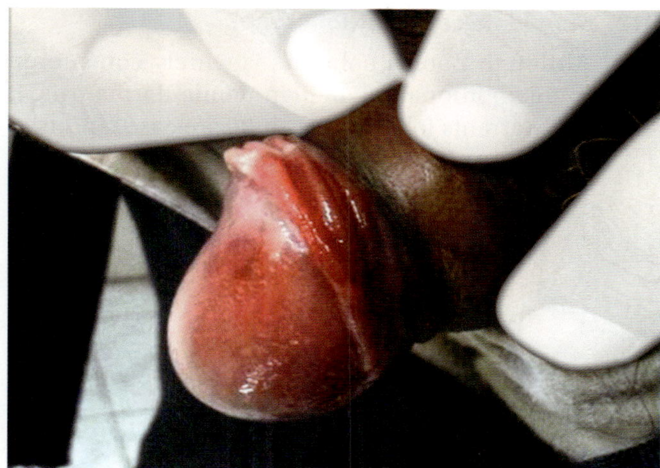

Fig. 1: A solitary, well-defined, erythematous, moist glistening plaque over the glans penis

- IgE (immunoglobulin E) antibody-mediated hypersensitivity
- Hypospadias.

Q4. What are the differential diagnoses for this condition?

Ans:
- Erosive lichen planus (histology shows basal layer degeneration and band-like infiltrate of lymphocytes)
- Erythroplasia of Queyrat (clinically shows a velvety surface and histology is consistent with squamous cell carcinoma in situ)
- Psoriasis (histology shows parakeratosis, Munro's microabscesses, neutrophils in stratum corneum)
- Fixed drug eruption (definite history of drug intake, recurrence of lesion in the same site and resolution on stoppage of the drug)
- Contact dermatitis (history of application of irritant antiseptics, cleansers, etc. present)
- Candidiasis (history of diabetes may be present)
- Lichen sclerosus et atrophicus (histology shows epidermal atrophy, follicular plugging, papillary dermal edema, basal layer degeneration)
- Pemphigus vulgaris (erosions and flaccid blisters may be found in other parts of body, histology shows suprabasal acantholysis).

Q5. What is the closest differential diagnosis of Zoon's balanitis?

Ans: Erythroplasia of Queyrat.

Q6. How do you diagnose Zoon's balanitis?

Ans: Zoon's balanitis is diagnosed on clinical suspicion and confirmed by distinctive histologic findings.

Q7. All are found in the histopathology of Zoon's balanitis except:

a. Hemosiderin deposition
b. Lozenge keratinocytes
c. Lichenoid subepidermal infiltrate
d. Squamous eddies

Ans: d (Squamous eddies).

Squamous eddies are not seen in Zoon's balanitis. Histopathology findings of Zoon's balanitis depend on the duration of the disease. Initially, the epidermis is slightly thickened with patchy lichenoid infiltrate of lymphocytes, parakeratosis and few plasma cells. Diamond-shaped suprabasal keratinocytes referred to as "lozenge keratinocytes" are found, along with "watery spongiosis". As the disease progresses, the lichenoid subepidermal infiltrate becomes more dense, composed largely of plasma cells. Capillaries are dilated, and erythrocyte extravasation and hemosiderin deposition are also noted.

Q8. Where do you see cayenne pepper spots?

a. Purpura annularis telangiectodes
b. Schamberg's disease
c. Zoon's balanitis
d. All of the above

Ans: d (All of the above).

The cayenne pepper spots are actually not the hallmark of Zoon's balanitis, in fact they are seen in other conditions also which have hemosiderin deposition.

Q9. What are the variants of Zoon's balanitis?

Ans:
- Histology showing predominance of lymphocytes and pronounced dermal edema
- Erosive type
- Hypertrophic type.

Q10. What are the various modalities in treating a case of Zoon's balanitis?

Ans.
- Medical
  - Topical steroids
  - Antifungals
  - Tacrolimus and pimecrolimus
  - Fusidic acid cream 2%
- Surgical
  - Circumcision
  - Erbium:YAG (yttrium aluminum garnet) laser/ CO_2 (carbon dioxide) ablation
- Supportive
  - Good hygiene and emollient creams.

Q11. What is considered as curative for Zoon's balanitis?

a. Ablation with CO_2 laser
b. Ablation with Erbium:YAG laser
c. Circumcision
d. Topical pimecrolimus

Ans. c (Circumcision)

Circumcision is considered as treatment of choice for Zoon's balanitis.

Q12. Should there be any follow up?

Ans: Although Zoon's balanitis is widely considered to be an idiopathic, benign penile dermatosis. It still warrants follow up as there are case reports of squamous cell carcinoma developing at the same site.

SECTION 20

Nutritional Disorders

Priyadarshini Kharge

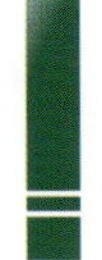

CHAPTER 107

Acrodermatitis Enteropathica

Bhumika S

Case study Acrodermatitis Enteropathica

Presenting Complaints

Doctor, my child is having loose and frequent stools and is very irritable since 10 days. She has also developed redness and dry skin lesions around the anal and mouth areas thereafter. The pediatrician referred me to a skin doctor after I met them today.

Setting

Dermatology outpatient department

History of Present Illness

An anxious mother, who was referred by the pediatrician, brought her irritable 5-month-old infant who had foul-smelling diarrhea since 10 days. Child had also become very irritable, restless, inactive, poorly responsive and poorly feeding since then. Thereafter, the child developed redness and dry skin around her mouth and pelvic areas. The redness is also seen around the nose, eye, hands and feet now. Thinning of scalp hair has also been noticed suddenly. The baby, who was normal since birth, had been weaned off breast milk 2 weeks before. No significant obstetric or family history was present.

General Physical Examination

- An irritable and listless child who has a weight for age less than 2nd percentile.
- Child is afebrile with no signs of pallor, icterus or lymphadenopathy. All other parameters were within normal limits.

Systemic Examination

No abnormality detected

Dermatological Examination

- Bilateral, symmetrical, well-defined psoriasiform and eczematous lesions present over perioral, periorbital, perinasal, perineal (Fig. 1) regions and extensor surfaces of elbows, knees, hands and feet.
- A few vesicles and erosions with honey-colored crusts seen over perioral (Fig. 2) and perineal region.
- Nonscarring alopecia of scalp was seen.

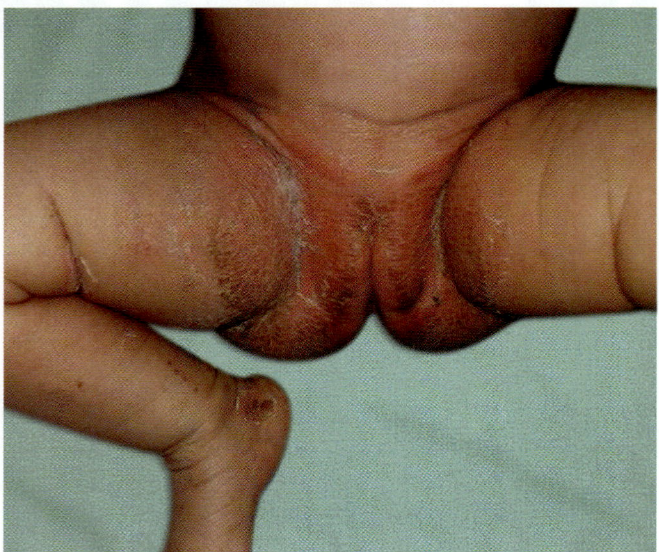

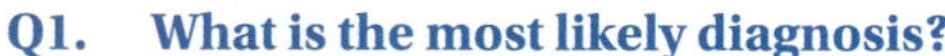
Fig. 1: Psoriasiform lesions in perineal region

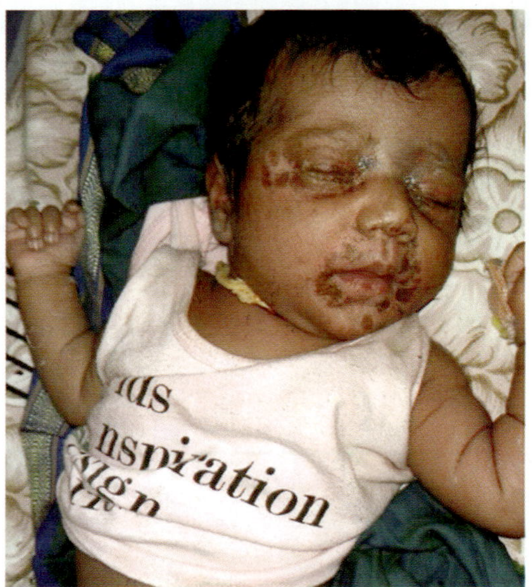

Fig. 2: Honey-colored crusts in perioral region

Q1. What is the most likely diagnosis?

a. Acrodermatitis enteropathica
b. Biotinidase deficiency
c. Epidermolysis bullosa
d. Langerhans cell histiocytosis

Ans: a (Acrodermatitis enteropathica).

Presence of periorificial and acral psoriasiform and eczematous dermatitis, diarrhea, failure to thrive and diffuse alopecia of scalp after the start of weaning suggests diagnosis of acrodermatitis enteropathica (inherited type).

Q2. What is the definition of acrodermatitis enteropathica?

Ans: Acrodermatitis enteropathica is a biochemical disease of metal metabolism due to zinc deficiency. There is an inability to absorb sufficient zinc from the diet. Though it was first described by the Swedish dermatologist Thore Brandt in 1936, the term acrodermatitis enteropathica was coined by Danbolt and Cross in 1942.

Q3. What is the role of zinc in biological functions?

Ans:
- Zinc is a component of more than 100 enzymes required for degradation of lipids, proteins and nucleic acid.
- Required for cell division and growth, DNA (deoxyribonucleic acid) and RNA (ribonucleic acid) synthesis, stabilization of biomembranes, protection against free radical damage, male sex hormone development, fetal development and metabolism of neurotransmitters
- Mobilization of vitamin A from the liver
- Maintaining both cellular and humoral immunity.

Q4. What are the types of zinc deficiency?

Ans: Zinc deficiency may be:
- Genetic
- Acquired
  - The genetic disorder has an autosomal recessive inheritance.
  - Acquired zinc deficiency is seen in individuals receiving long-term parenteral nutrition, undergone intestinal bypass procedures, as a complication of Crohn's disease, HIV (human immunodeficiency virus) infections, cystic fibrosis, chronic alcoholics, anorexia nervosa, zinc-deficient vegetarian diets, and in patients with low pancreatic enzyme levels resulting in poor intestinal absorption.

Q5. When will acrodermatitis enteropathica first manifest?

Ans: The condition first manifests days to weeks after birth if bottle-fed and shortly after weaning if breast-fed.

Q6. What is the genetic mutation causing this condition?

Ans: The disorder results from mutations in *SLC39A*, which encodes an intestinal zinc transporter ZIP4.

Q7. Can a breast-fed baby develop zinc deficiency with signs mimicking acrodermatitis enteropathica?

Ans: Yes. In addition to the classic inherited disease, zinc deficiency with signs mimicking acrodermatitis enteropathica may also occur in babies who are breast-fed. This abnormality results from inadequate secretion of zinc in maternal milk. Maternal mutations in *SLC30A2* [ZnT-2 (zinc transporter-2)], which encodes a protein required for zinc secretion, have been found.

Q8. What is the classical triad of acrodermatitis enteropathica?

a. Dermatitis, diarrhea, dementia
b. Dermatitis, diarrhea, alopecia
c. Dermatitis, diarrhea, failure to thrive
d. Diarrhea, dehydration, dizziness

Ans: b (Dermatitis, diarrhea, alopecia)

This triad consists of acral and periorificial skin lesions, intractable diarrhea and diffuse partial alopecia.

Q9. Enumerate the clinical features of acrodermatitis enteropathica?

Ans: Clinical features:

- *Cutaneous features*: Erythematous, scaly, crusted, psoriasiform, eczematous or vesiculobullous eruption, localized around the body orifices (mouth, nose, ears, eyes and perineum) and symmetrically located on the buttocks and extensor surface of major joints (elbows, knees, hands and feet), scalp, fingers and toes (hence the term acrodermatitis). On the face, the eroded and crusted peribuccal plaques may appear impetiginized, and secondary infection with *Candida albicans* is common.
- *Nail changes*: Marked erythema and swelling of the digits is noted, often with subsequent nail deformity.
- *Hair changes*: Progressive alopecia of the scalp, eyelashes and eyebrows.
- *General features*: Many infants have frequent crying episodes, irritability and restlessness. Failure to thrive is significantly noted sooner than later. Children stop smiling early in the disease and this is always the first sign noticed when the child starts to improve.
- *Diarrhea*: Frothy, bulky, foul-smelling loose stools are present.
- Other findings may include conjunctivitis, photophobia, stomatitis, perlèche, recurring candidal or bacterial infections.

Q10. What are the differential diagnoses of acrodermatitis enteropathica?

Ans: The differential diagnoses of acrodermatitis enteropathica include:

- Napkin dermatitis, napkin psoriasis, candidiasis, severe seborrheic dermatitis, langerhans cell histiocytosis and epidermolysis bullosa in children. Alcoholic pellagrins who are zinc deficient and nutritional dermatoses in older age groups.
- Acrodermatitis enteropathica-like dermatitis reported in metabolic disorders such as arginine deficiency syndrome, methylmalonic acidemia, multiple carboxylase deficiency syndrome, essential fatty acid deficiency, biotin deficiency and cystic fibrosis.
- An acrodermatitis enteropathica-like symptom complex is reported in association with AIDS (acquired immunodeficiency syndrome).

Q11. What are the relevant investigations required?

Ans: The diagnosis is based on the clinical features along with:

- Serum zinc levels of 50 μg/dL or lower
- Low serum alkaline phosphatase levels (even when serum zinc level is normal).
- Low serum lipid levels
- Skin biopsy is not diagnostic, but may help in certain cases. Features showing psoriasiform epidermal hyperplasia and spongiosis, pallor of upper part of epidermis along with ballooning of keratinocytes and parakeratosis. Spongiform pustules and microabscesses are not seen.
- Zinc levels can also be measured in maternal milk.

Q12. Does the condition have a good prognosis?

Ans: The prognosis is completely resolved if identified early, but is poor in unrecognized or untreated infants, with progressive deterioration of health, and death in 4–5 years. Hence, a pediatric and dermatologist have to work together for an early diagnosis.

Q13. What is the recommended daily allowance (RDA) for zinc?

Ans:

- *Adult*: 15.5 mg
- *Less than 6 months infant*: 3–5 mg
- *6 months to 1 year*: 5 mg
- *Children*: 10 mg
- *Pregnant and lactating women*: 20–25 mg.

Q14. What is the treatment of choice in acrodermatitis enteropathica?

a. 2 mg/kg/day of oral zinc sulfate given for 2 weeks
b. 2 mg/kg/day of oral zinc sulfate given lifelong
c. 5 mg/kg/day of oral zinc sulfate given for 2 weeks
d. 5 mg/kg/day of oral zinc sulfate given lifelong

Ans: b (2 mg/kg/day of oral zinc sulfate given lifelong—is the treatment of choice).

Q15. Describe the response to treatment with zinc supplementation?

Ans:
- Improvement in temperament, especially the smile response and decrease in irritability noted within 1 or 2 days.
- Appetite improves in a few days.
- Diarrhea and skin lesions begin to respond within 2 or 3 days.
- Hair growth begins after 2–3 weeks of therapy.
- Improvement in growth of the infant generally occurs within 2 weeks.

Q16. What are the dietary sources of zinc?

Ans: Seafood, liver, eggs, meat, legumes, nuts, whole grain and leafy vegetables are good sources of zinc.

CHAPTER 108

Pellagra

Parul Thakur

Case study Pellagra

Presenting Complaint

Doctor, I have got dark rashes on my face, neck and forearms since 3 months with blistering over my chest since 5 days.

Setting

Dermatology outpatient department

History of Presenting Illness

A 30-year-old male, bus driver by occupation, came with chief complaints of rashes over the face and forearms since 3 months and blistering over chest since 5 days. Patient was apparently well 3 months back when he developed red areas over the nose, cheeks and hands, associated with photosensitivity. These lesions slowly progressed to become brown, thickened and scaly. He complains of redness over the V area of neck and upper chest since past week and developed blistering over the same area 5 days back. On further enquiry, he also complains of burning sensation in the mouth since past 2–3 months and difficulty in eating spicy food. Patient has mild diarrhea on and off since 3 months, with a frequency of 4–5 small motions per day. There is no history of blood in stools or weight loss. Patient follows a vegetarian diet with rice and jowar being his staple foods. He has been consuming alcohol since 23 years of age, consuming about 2–3 pegs (60–90 mL) of alcohol a day.

General Physical Examination

- Well oriented to time, place and person
- BMI: 16 kg/m^2
- Pulse: 80 bpm, mildly icteric conjunctival mucosa.

Systemic Examination

No abnormality detected.

Dermatological Examination

Patient has a well-defined area of hyperpigmentation over the bridge of nose and malar areas with sparing of the nasolabial folds (Fig. 1). Symmetrical involvement of dorsum of both hands with well-demarcated hyperpigmented scaly plaques can be seen (Fig. 2). The flexural aspect of upper extremities was characteristically spared. There is diffuse erythema over the presternal area with vesicles and bullae also present (Fig. 3). Desquamation surrounded by an area of hyperpigmentation can be seen adjacent to the blistered area. Lower lip and buccal mucosa show erosions. Tongue is erythematous with flattening of papillae. No genital involvement seen.

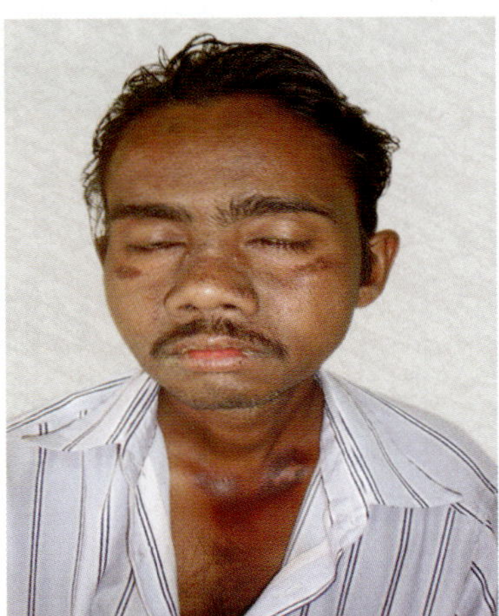

Fig. 1: A 30-year-old male with well-defined hyperpigmented plaques over bridge of nose and malar area

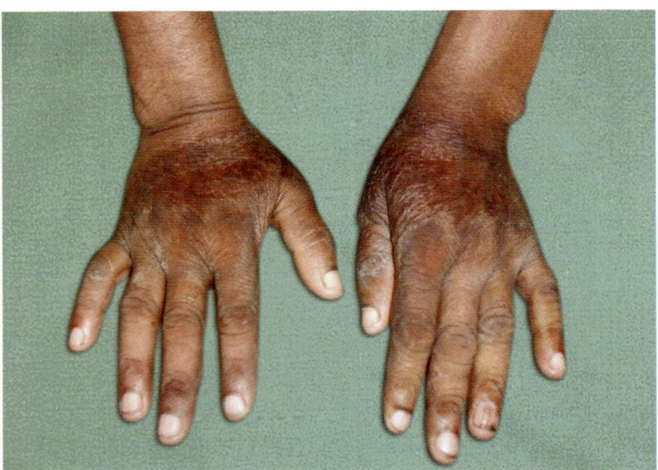

Fig. 2: Similar lesions over hands

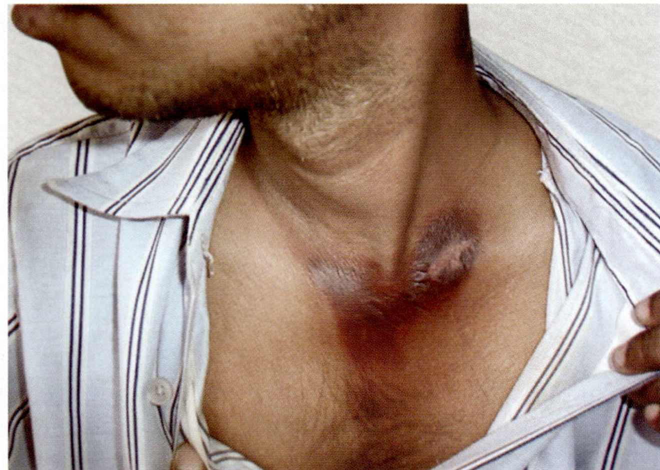

Fig. 3: Blistering over presternal area
Courtesy: Dr. Dipak Kulkarni, Alok clinic, Panvel, Mumbai, Maharashtra

Q1. What is the most likely diagnosis?

a. Pellagra
b. Porphyria cutanea tarda
c. Phototoxic reaction
d. Systemic lupus erythematosus

Ans: a (Pellagra)

Presence of photosensitive rash can be seen in all the above conditions. However, well-demarcated photodistributed hyperpigmented plaques, concomitant diarrhea and oral involvement are suggestive of pellagra. The patient is a chronic alcoholic and also consumes jowar on a regular basis which increase the possibility of pellagra.

Q2. What causes pellagra?

a. Deficiency of niacin
b. Deficiency of tryptophan
c. Disorders of malabsorption
d. All of the above

Ans: d (All of the above).

Pellagra is a disease of malnutrition involving deficiency not only of the "vitamin B3" i.e. niacin, but also its precursor tryptophan. This deficiency can be primary due to reduced intake of niacin, tryptophan along with other B vitamins in diet, or it can be secondary due to reduced absorption of niacin or its increased consumption.

Q3. What are the dietary factors leading to pellagra?

Ans: Various indirect dietary factors can also lead to deficiency of niacin and tryptophan leading to pellagra.

- Consumption of diet with excess of leucine such as jowar can lead to pellagra as leucine inhibits a step in conversion of tryptophan to niacin (conversion of quinolinic acid to nicotinic acid). Leucine also inhibits tryptophan uptake. Pellagra is more common in populations whose staple diet is maize or jowar. Maize is a poor source of tryptophan while the nicotinic acid present in maize is a bound form that is not assimilated by human gastrointestinal tract.

  Indian millet (jowar) contains adequate amounts of tryptophan and niacin; however, it also contains a high amount of leucine, which interferes with the conversion of tryptophan to nicotinic acid in the niacin pathway, thus leading to its deficiency.
- Inadequate intake of vitamins B2, B6 and proteins also increase the risk of developing pellagra.
- Diet grossly lacking in proteins, food faddism, anorexia nervosa can also lead to pellagra.

Q4. What are the secondary causes of pellagra?

Ans: Secondary deficiency of niacin can occur in:

- Malabsorption
  - Conditions such as jejunoileitis, Crohn's disease, gastroenterostomy, subtotal gastrectomy and chronic diarrhea
  - Cirrhosis of liver and chronic alcoholism are other common causes of pellagra.
- Hartnup's disease
  - Impaired absorption of amino acids (including tryptophan)
- Carcinoid syndrome
  - Excess synthesis of serotonin and nearly 60% of dietary tryptophan is diverted for synthesis of the same. This leads to reduced niacin production and thus, pellagra.
- Prolonged therapy with drugs such as isoniazid, pyrazinamide, azathioprine, 6-mercaptopurine, 5-fluorouracil, sulfonamides, anticonvulsants (carbamazepine, phenobarbital and hydantoins) and antidepressants. Isoniazid interferes with pyridoxine, which is a coenzyme in tryptophan metabolism, thus indirectly leading to niacin deficiency. 6-Mercaptopurine inhibits NAD (nicotinamide adenine dinucleotide) production by interfering with NAD phosphorylase, while 5-fluorouracil inhibits conversion of tryptophan to niacin, thus leading to pellagra.

Q5. How does alcohol cause pellagra?

Ans: Alcoholism contributes to pellagra through the associated malnutrition, vitamin B and zinc deficiencies and impaired absorption and processing of nutrients.

- Alcohol impairs conversion of tryptophan to niacin, leading to its deficiency. It also leads to inactivation of pyridoxal 5' phosphate leading further to decreased formation of niacin.
- Alcohol leads to disturbances of glutamate and GABA (gamma-aminobutyric acid) neuronal activity further aggravating the psychosis in pellagra.
- Liver dysfunction leads to improper metabolism of niacin.
- Increased alcohol intake also leads to increased empty calories which further increase the requirement of nicotinic acid.
- Alcoholics usually have poor appetite due to gastritis and hence a poor intake of nutritious diet. Severe alcohol dependence can also make it difficult for a person to afford a healthy nutritious diet.

Q6. What are the various systems involved in pellagra?

Ans: Classically, pellagra is described as 3**Ds**—**d**ermatitis, **d**iarrhea and **d**ementia. A 4th **D**—**d**eath, describes the final outcome if it is left untreated. The systems involved include gastrointestinal system and central nervous system, apart from the cutaneous and mucosal manifestations.

Q7. What are the characteristic skin changes in pellagra?

Ans: The classical photodermatitis of pellagra initially begins with erythematous patches over the photoexposed areas, which are painful and/or pruritic on sun exposure. The skin becomes progressively erythematous and blisters may develop, which rupture with formation of erosions and crusting.

Over a period of time, the skin thickens, developing into well-demarcated reddish brown hyperpigmented, scaly, rough plaques. Desquamation occurs after several weeks or months leaving areas of hypopigmentation with a characteristic hyperpigmented border. Painful fissuring over palms and soles may occur. The photosensitive rash may involve the dorsum of the hands (gauntlet of pellagra), chest and neck (Casal's necklace), elbows, knees, and the dorsum of the feet, depending upon the clothing used. A butterfly distribution maybe seen on the face. Redness and maceration over the intertriginous areas may be seen.

Mucous membranes, including oral, vaginal, urethral mucosa may be involved. Dry fissured lips, angular stomatitis, oral ulcerations maybe seen. The entire tongue, gingival and buccal mucosa may become inflamed, swollen and ulcerated giving a scarlet appearance. The tongue appears red and smooth with erosions, ulcers and fissures. There is atrophy of the filiform papillae with or without hypertrophy of fungiform papillae (scarlet glossitis). Vulvitis, vaginitis, perirectal sores and scrotal dermatitis have also been reported.

Q8. Enumerate the systemic involvement and what are the investigations that should be done to evaluate them?

Ans: Systemic involvement:

- *Gastrointestinal system*: Gastrointestinal symptoms include pain, diarrhea and achlorhydria in 50% of cases. The gastrointestinal disturbance of pellagra may begin with burning sensation in the mouth, dyspepsia along with constipation or diarrhea. Changes may occur throughout the tract starting from parotid gland swelling and increased salivation to intestinal bleeding. The esophagus, stomach and colon are usually affected. In severe forms, anorexia, dyspepsia, nausea, vomiting and abdominal pain may occur. Diarrhea may be bloody because of gastrointestinal mucosal involvement.

- *Central nervous system involvement*: This usually presents late. Early involvement may go unnoticed or present as depression, anxiety or restlessness. In relatively advanced pellagra, it may exhibit a plethora of neuropsychiatric manifestations ranging from disorientation to apathy, insomnia, delusions, impairment of memory and psychosis. Encephalopathic syndrome, with clouding of consciousness, cogwheel rigidity of extremities, involuntary sucking and grasping reflex may be seen. Myelitis, peripheral neuropathy, incoordination are occasionally encountered. Deep tendon reflexes are exaggerated in almost all patients of pellagra.

Q9. What are the differential diagnoses?

Ans: Porphyria (porphyria cutanea tarda, variegate porphyria and hereditary coproporphyria), Hartnup's diseases, phototoxic reaction, sunburn, systemic lupus erythematosus are the common differential diagnosis. All these conditions may present with photosensitive rash.

Q10. How will you confirm the diagnosis?

Ans: The diagnosis of pellagra is primarily clinical. Dramatic response to vitamin supplementation confirms the diagnosis. Laboratory testing is usually not required; however, measurement of urinary metabolites of niacin, i.e. *N*-methylnicotinamide and pyridine may be used to aid in the diagnosis.

Q11. What does the treatment in pellagra entail?

a. Diet only
b. Diet and medications
c. Diet, medications and lifestyle modifications
d. Medications only

Ans: c (Diet, medications and lifestyle modifications).

As pellagra encompasses a multitude of causative etiological factors, all of the above modalities of treatment are important in the affected individual.

Q12. What is the main principle in treating a case of pellagra?

Ans: Treatment principles:

Nutritional supplementation: The recommended daily allowance of niacin is 0.66 mg per 1,000 kcal (approximately 10–20 mg per day). Since niacin can cause headache and flushing, niacinamide is preferred for therapy. Treatment with 300-500 mg/day or niacinamide given orally in divided doses is recommended. When oral therapy is precluded, intramuscular injections of niacinamide can be given (100 mg three times a day). Severe neuropsychiatric involvement calls for a higher dose of niacinamide (1,000 mg orally in addition to 100–200 parentally). Neuropsychiatric symptoms usually show improvement after 24–48 hours of treatment. Skin erythema, mucosal lesions and diarrhea respond in a few days. Skin lesions often take 3–4 weeks to clear completely.

Pyridoxine and riboflavin supplementation is also recommended especially in case of neurological manifestations. Thiamine supplementation will help in correction of alcoholic encephalopathy, often found concomitantly in patients suffering from pellagra due to chronic alcoholism. Proteins, iron and zinc should also be given in adequate amounts. A balanced diet should be prescribed.

Nutrition education: Adequate intake of food rich in niacin and tryptophan and avoidance of total dependence on maize and jowar can prevent pellagra in endemic regions. Avoiding or reducing alcohol intake is important. Treatment of any underlying cause and avoidance of drugs causing pellagra is necessary.

Whole grain cereals, pulses, peanuts, yeast, eggs, bran, peanuts, poultry, fish, red meat are good sources of niacin and tryptophan. Although poor in nicotinic acid, milk is rich in tryptophan and is effective in preventing pellagra.

Symptomatic treatment: Topical therapy with zinc oxide ointment and sunscreens has to be advised as it is a photosensitive condition.

SECTION 21

Autoimmune Connective Tissue Disorders

Nirmal Krishna B

CHAPTER 109

Systemic Lupus Erythematosus

Govind Mittal

Case study Systemic Lupus Erythematosus

Presenting Complaints

Doctor, I have a rash over my cheeks and forearms for the last 1-week. I have also noticed weight loss and loss of hair since the last 6 months.

Setting

Department of outpatient dermatology

History of Presenting Illness

A 22-year-old lady presented with a rash on the cheeks and forearms since 1 week. She had gone for a beach holiday with her friends to Goa 1-week prior to the onset of these lesions. She has also noticed increased hair loss since the last 6 months. She also complained of recurrent episodes of fever and also pain and swelling in her joints. She admitted to have noticed bluish discoloration of fingers and toes with mild pain and discomfort, on exposure to cold. She complained that she had lost about 2 to 3 kg in the last 6 months.

General Physical Examination

Pulse rate: 82/min, BP: 130/80 mm Hg, Temperature: 100.3°F, Pallor: present.

Dermatological Examination

Erythematous plaques in a butterfly distribution noted over the malar area (Fig. 1). Similar erythematous papules and plaques were noted over the upper limbs. Hair was thin, lusterless, and fine hair was noted along the frontal area. Oral mucosa showed erythema and erosions over the central arch of the hard palate.

Systemic Examination

No significant finding was noted on systems review. Swelling of the right ankle and right wrist joint was noted.

Q1. What is the most likely diagnosis?

a. Viral fever with rash
b. Dermatomyositis
c. Systemic lupus erythematosus (SLE)
d. Drug hypersensitivity reaction

Ans: c. SLE. It is a multifactorial autoimmune rheumatological disorder involving multiple organs. Highest incidence is seen in women of reproductive age group. Points in favor of diagnosis:

- Characteristic generalized rash of acute cutaneous lupus erythematosus (ACLE)
- History suggestive of photosensitivity, hair loss,
- Characteristic hard palate involvement, and
- Fever with arthritis.

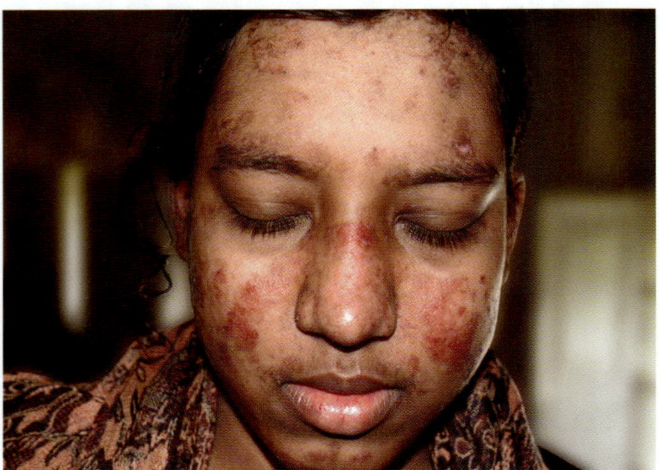

Fig. 1: Erythematous plaques in a butterfly distribution noted over the malar area

Q2. How do you diagnose systemic lupus erythematosus? How can this be confirmed?

Ans: The diagnosis of SLE requires reasonable clinical suspicion. Confirmation of diagnosis can be made by using the American College of Rheumatology (ACR) criteria: a person is defined as having SLE if any 4 or more of the 11 criteria are present, serially or simultaneously, during any interval of observation (Table 1).

Q3. Does the newer systemic lupus international collaborating clinics criteria offer any advantage over the older criteria?

Ans: Systemic lupus international collaborating clinics (SLICC) classification criteria: Patient should have biopsy proven lupus nephritis with antinuclear antibody (ANA) or anti-dsDNA, or patient should satisfy four criteria including at least one clinical and one immunological criteria

- *Clinical criteria*
  - Acute cutaneous lupus: all variants of ACLE and subacute cutaneous lupus erythematosus (SCLE)
  - Chronic cutaneous lupus: all variants
  - Oral ulcers or nasal ulcers
  - Nonscarring alopecia
  - Synovitis: Two or more joints, tenderness in two or more joints, at least 30 minutes of morning stiffness
  - Serositis: Typical pleural or pericardial involvement
  - Renal: Urine protein to creatinine ratio (or 24-hour urine protein) representing 500 mg protein/24 hours or red blood cell casts
  - Neurologic: Seizures, psychosis, mononeuritis multiplex, myelitis, peripheral or cranial neuropathy, acute confusional state
  - Hemolytic anemia
  - Leukopenia (<4,000/mm^3) or lymphopenia (<1,000/mm^3)
  - Thrombocytopenia (<10,000/mm^3).
  - All of the above in the absence of other causes.
- *Immunologic criteria*

Table 1: The American College of Rheumatology–1982 revised criteria for classification of systemic lupus erythematosus

S.No.	*Criterion*	*Characteristic features*
1	Malar rash	Tending to spare the nasolabial folds
2	Discoid rash	Adherent keratotic scaling, follicular plugging and atrophic scarring
3	Photosensitivity	Unusual reaction to sunlight, by history or observation
4	Oral ulcers	Oral or nasopharyngeal ulceration, usually painless
5	Arthritis	Nonerosive arthritis involving two or more peripheral joints
6	Serositis	Pleuritis, pericarditis
7	Renal disorder	Persistent proteinuria >0.5 g/day or cellular casts
8	Neurological	Seizures, psychosis
9	Hematological	Hemolytic anemia, reticulocytosis, leukopenia <4,000/mm, lymphopenia < 1,500/mm^3, thrombocytopenia < 100,000/mm^3
10	Immunological disorder	1. Positive anti-DNA antibody 2. Presence of anti-Smith nuclear antigen 3. Positive finding of antiphospholipid antibodies
11	Antinuclear antibodies (ANA)	An abnormal titer of ANA by immunofluorescence

- ANA positivity
- Anti-dsDNA antibody positivity
- Anti-Smith antibodies
- Antiphospholipid antibody positivity: lupus anticoagulant, false-positive rapid plasma regain, anticardiolipin antibody, anti-beta-2-glycoprotein 1
- Low complement: low C3, low C4, low CH50
- Direct Coombs' test in the absence of hemolytic anemia

Q4. What are the cutaneous manifestations of systemic lupus erythematosus?

Ans: Gilliam and Sontheimer classification of LE-associated skin lesions

- *Histopathologically specific (LE-specific) skin lesions*
  - ACLE: Localized ACLE, Generalized ACLE, Toxic epidermal necrolysis-like ACLE
  - SCLE: Annular, Papulosquamous, Mixed patterns
  - Chronic cutaneous LE- Classic DLE (a) Localized (b) Generalized, hypertrophic (verrucous) DLE, lupus erythematosus panniculitis or profundus, Mucosal LE, LE tumidus, Chilblain LE, DLE–lichen planus overlap
- *Histopathologically nonspecific (LE nonspecific) skin lesions*
  - Cutaneous vascular disease- Vasculitis, vasculopathy, periungual telangiectasia, livedo reticularis, thrombophlebitis, Raynaud's phenomenon, Erythromelalgia
  - Alopecia (nonscarring)- Lupus hair, telogen effluvium, alopecia areata
  - Sclerodactyly
  - Rheumatoid nodules
  - Calcinosis cutis
  - LE nonspecific bullous lesions: Epidermolysis *bullosa* acquisita (EBA)-like bullous LE, dermatitis herpetiformis (DH)-like bullous LE, Pemphigus erythematosus, bullous pemphigoid, porphyria cutanea tarda
  - Urticaria
  - Papulo-nodular mucinosis
  - Anetoderma or cutis laxa or mid-dermal elastolysis
  - *Acanthosis nigricans* (type B insulin resistance)
  - Erythema multiforme (Rowell's syndrome)
  - Leg ulcers
  - Lichen planus.

Q5. What are the phases in etiopathogenesis of systemic lupus erythematosus ?

Ans: The phases on etiopathogenesis of SLE are:

- Susceptibility phase: Inheritance of susceptibility genes
- Induction phase: Induction of autoimmunity
- Expansion phase: Expansion of autoimmune process
- Injury phase: Immunological injury

Q6. What are the drugs that have been implicated in induction of systemic lupus erythematosus?

Ans: Procainamide, isoniazid, hydralazine, minocycline, phenytoin, chlorpromazine.

Q7. What is the differential diagnosis of malar rash?

Ans: Differential diagnosis of malar rash:

- Dermatomyositis
- Acne rosacea
- Seborrhoeic dermatitis
- Polymorphous light eruption
- Drug-induced photosensitivity (generalized ACLE)
- Photoallergic contact dermatitis
- Pemphigus erythematosus.

Q8. Describe the oral lesions in systemic lupus erythematosus?

Ans: Oral ulcers may occur in about 26% of patients with SLE, and exhibit site specificity for hard palate involvement in about 80% of cases. Other sites involved are gingiva and buccal mucosa. Ulcers are characteristically painless and may be erythematous, purpuric or have a superficial dirty yellowish-slough. Patients may also have acute lip involvement in the form of edema, cracking, and crusting.

Q9. What are the various systems involved in systemic lupus erythematosus?

Ans: Systemic involvement in SLE:

- Musculoskeletal: Myalgia, myopathy, tendon rupture, avascular bone necrosis, arthralgia, arthritis (nonerosive, nondeforming, symmetric)
- Renal: 50–75% of patients with SLE have renal involvement. Glomerulonephritis of mesangial, focal and segmental proliferative, diffuse proliferative or membranous types, nephrotic syndrome, renal amyloidosis, renal vein thrombosis, lupus cystitis
- Pulmonary: Pulmonary hypertension, pulmonary hemorrhage, lupus pneumonitis, shrinking lung or vanishing lung syndrome, fibrosing

alveolitis, pleuritis, pleural effusion and hilar lymphadenopathy

- Central nervous system (CNS) or neuropsychiatric: Mild cognitive dysfunction (most common), neuropsychiatric abnormalities, seizures, cranial nerve abnormalities, cerebrovascular events, severe headache or lupus headache, choreoathetosis, extrapyramidal features, peripheral neuropathy
- Cardiac: Hypertension, pericarditis, atrial fibrillation, heart block and other conduction defects, Libman-sacks endocarditis, coronary arteritis
- Gastrointestinal (GI) and hepatic: Painless oral and nasal mucosal erosions, esophageal ulcerations, dysphagia, vasculitis of abdominal vessels, GI motility disorders, pancreatitis, ulcerative colitis, colonic perforation, peritoneal serositis, mesenteric lymphadenopathy, hepatic veno-occlusive disease, hepatitis, liver failure, hepatic infarction, lupoid hepatitis
- Eye-conjunctivitis, subconjunctival hemorrhages, lacrimal hyposecretion, episcleritis, scleritis, uveitis, retinal cytoid bodies, central retinal artery occlusion, retinal hemorrhages, lupus retinopathy
- Endocrine: Autoimmune thyroiditis
- Reticuloendothelial and glandular: Lymphadenopathy, splenomegaly, swelling of salivary and lacrimal glands.

Q10. List the investigations that may be required at initial evaluation of a case of systemic lupus erythematosus.

Ans: Investigations in SLE:

- Complete blood count
- Liver function test, blood urea, serum creatinine
- Blood sugar, 24-hour urine for protein and creatinine, urinalysis
- Erythrocyte sedimentation rate, C-reactive protein
- Antinuclear antibody, Anti-dsDNA antibody
- Chest X-ray, electrocardiography (ECG) and echocardiography (if cardiac involvement suspected)
- Others which can be done:
  - Anti-Smith [and anti-ribonucleoprotein (RNP)] antibody, anti-Sjögren's-syndrome-related antigen A (Anti-SSA/Ro) antibody, anti-SSB/La antibody, anticardiolipin antibodies (IgG, IgM, IgA), anti-beta-2 glycoprotein 1 antibodies
  - Prothrombin time or International normalized ratio (INR), partial thromboplastin time
  - Lupus anticoagulant, Coombs' test, C3, C4, homocysteine, fibrinogen
  - Thyroid studies, fasting lipid panel.

Q11. How would you assess a patient with systemic lupus erythematosus on follow up?

Ans: On follow up, apart from analyzing the symptoms (for specific cutaneous and system involvement) and clinical evaluation, it is important to perform the following investigations on follow-up visits:

- Erythrocyte sedimentation rate or C-reactive protein (ESR/CRP) (CRP levels may not be reliable in all cases since patients with SLE can have anti-CRP antibodies)
- Hemoglobin and blood counts
- Anti-dsDNA, C3, C4 levels
- Urine routine examination (look for hematuria, proterinuria and pyuria).

The serology may be done at less frequent intervals if clinical assessment and other basic investigations are within normal limits.

Q12. Which are the specific serological parameters for diagnosis of systemic lupus erythematosus?

Ans: ANA is used to screen for SLE; presence of anti-dsDNA, anti-Smith antibody are confirmatory and specific for SLE (Anti-dsDNA is more sensitive among the two, while anti-Smith antibody is more specific).

Q13. What are the various patterns of antinuclear antibody?

Ans: Using Hep-2 cells, the staining patterns and antibodies include:

- Homogenous: Histone
- Speckled: U1-RNP, Sm, Ro, La
- Peripheral: DNA
- Nucleolar: U3-RNP, RNA polymerase-1, Pm-Scl
- Ground glass: Scl-70
- Centromere: Calcinosis, Raynaud phenomenon, esophageal dysmotility, sclerodactyly, and telangiectasia (CREST) syndrome.

Q14. What is seen in histopathology of cutaneous lupus erythematosus and how do you differentiate acute from chronic cutaneous lupus erythematosus?

Ans: *Histopathological features*:

- Epidermal atrophy and relative hyperkeratosis with follicular plugging
- Basal cell liquefactive degeneration
- Thickening of basement membrane
- Edema, hyalinization and fibrinoid changes in the dermis

- Patchy dermal lymphocytic infiltrates around appendages and blood vessels.

Acute cutaneous lupus erythematosus has more epidermal atrophy, basal cell liquefactive degeneration, dermal edema and less hyperkeratosis and dermal infiltrates.

Q15. What is lupus band test?

Ans: Lupus band refers to the linear band of deposition of immune reactants along the basement membrane zone and is considered positive when one or more of the immune reactants are positive (IgG, IgM, IgA, C3). When three or more reactants are present in nonlesional sun-protected site, the possibility of SLE is high.

Q16. What are the bullous lesions of lupus erythematosus?

Ans: Bullous lesions of LE can be classified as:

- *Specific*:
  - Toxic epidermal necrolysis-like acute cutaneous LE (acute syndrome of panepidermolysis)
  - Toxic epidermal necrolysis-like SCLE
  - Vesiculobullous annular SCLE
  - Bullous discoid LE
- *Nonspecific*
  - Bullous systemic LE
  - SLE-associated bullous disorders: Bullous pemphigoid, DH, Pemphigus erythematosus, Porphyria cutanea tarda.

Q17. What is bullous systemic LE?

Ans: Bullous systemic LE is a nonspecific bullous lesion of LE characterized by bullous lesions resembling erythema multiforme over face, neck, upper trunk not limited to sun-exposed skin associated with glomerulonephritis and hypocomplemententemia (Fig. 2). Histopathology is characterized by subepidermal blister and neutrophilic upper dermal infiltrate resembling dermatitis herpetiformis. Direct immunofluorescence (DIF) shows linear deposition of IgA, IgG, IgM and to a lesser extent C3 along the basement membrane zone.

Q18. What are treatment principles while treating a case of systemic lupus erythematosus?

Ans: Treatment principles include:

Genetic counseling and general measures

- In acute cases: bed rest
- Undue exposure to sun to be avoided (use broad brimmed hats/caps full length clothing/ regular sunscreen application)

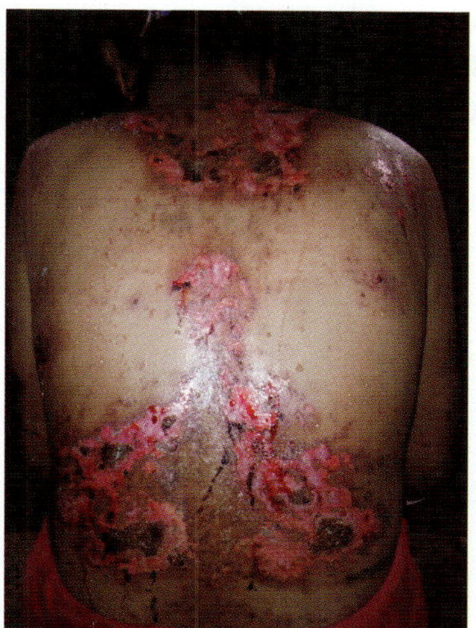

Fig. 2: Bullous systemic lupus erythematosus

- Mental stress, physical over-exertion, secondary infection to be avoided.

Topical treatment

- Sun protection: Broad spectrum sunscreen, Preferably SPF30 or more, photo-stabilized avobenzone, micronized titanium dioxide, micronized zinc oxide
- Topical steroid: Milder steroids like hydrocortisone, desonide, fluticasone for face. Clobetasol preparations may be used for nonfacial lesions, for shorter duration
- Calcineurin inhibitors: Pimecrolimus 1%, Tacrolimus 0.1%.

Systemic therapy

- Antimalarials help in reduction of cutaneous and systemic disease, and also reduce photosensitivity. Hydroxychloroquine 6 mg/kg body wt/day for 8–12 weeks (Ophthalmological screening and monitoring check-ups are necessary while using antimalarials)
  a. Other systemic agents especially in skin specific disease- Thalidomide, dapsone, isotretinoin, acitretin, clofazimine.
  b. Short course of oral steroids.
  c. Renal involvement: Prednisolone 1 mg/kg/day tapered over 3–6 months or pulsed methylprednisolone (dose may be altered based on severity of disease).
  d. Immunosuppressive therapy: Steroid sparing or in addition to steroids or for long-term use or for patients not responding to steroids. Azathioprine, Cyclophosphamide (conventional or pulsed), methotrexate 7.5 mg/

week for steroid-resistant cases (those without CNS and renal involvement).

e. Other supportive treatment:
   - Nonsteroidal anti-inflammatory drugs (NSAIDs)—arthralgia and arthritis
   - Antihypertensives: hypertension
   - Diuretics may be needed in nephrotic syndrome and cardiac failure
   - Anticonvulsants: Epilepsy
   - Chlorpromazine: Psychosis.

CHAPTER 110

Discoid Lupus Erythematosus

Malcolm Pinto, Akshi Bansal

Case study Discoid Lupus Erythematosus

Presenting Complaints

Doctor, I have itchy patches on my scalp along with hair loss since 2 years. I also have dark raised lesions on my face since 2 months.

Setting

Dermatology outpatient department

History of Present Illness

A 36-year-old lady, presented to dermatology outpatient department with complaints of dark lesions on her scalp since 2 years associated with burning and itching. Hair loss was present in these patches. There is history of similar lesion present on right ear since 1-year. She also has developed dark lesions on cheeks since 2 months. She gives history of aggravation of symptoms on sun exposure. No history of associated systemic complaints.

General Physical Examination and Systemic Examination

No abnormality detected.

Dermatological Examination

1. Multiple hyperpigmented plaques with thick, adherent scale and crusting present over scalp (Fig. 1). Carpet-tack sign positive on removal of scale. Few depigmented areas found within these patches and few depigmented macules present in adjoining areas of scalp. Alopecia present in the patches.
2. Hyperpigmented plaque with scaling present on cheeks (Fig. 2) and similar lesions but with central depigmentation present in concha of right ear.

Q1. What is the most likely diagnosis?

a. Pemphigus vulgaris
b. Lichen planus
c. Discoid lupus erythematosus (DLE)
d. Squamous cell carcinoma

Ans: c DLE. Presence of depigmented plaques with adherent scales showing carpet-tack sign, associated cicatricial alopecia and history of photo-aggravation of symptoms suggest a diagnosis of DLE. The lesions on cheeks add to the characteristic presentation. DLE is also known as chronic cutaneous LE (CCLE) presently.

Q2. How will you confirm the diagnosis?

Ans: Diagnosis is confirmed by skin biopsy. The histopathologic features include:

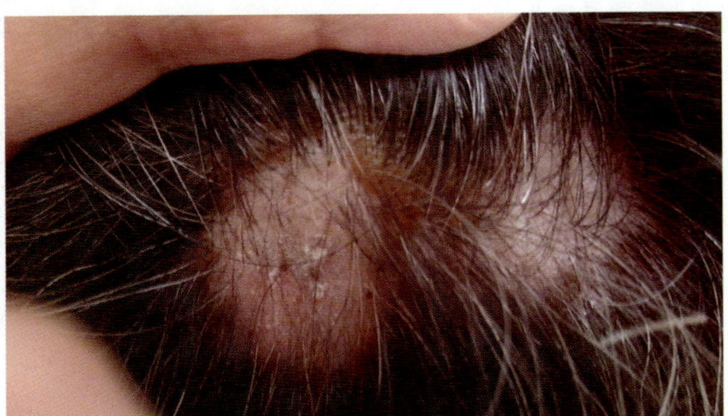

Fig. 1: Hyperpigmented plaques with scaling, depigmented areas and alopecia on scalp

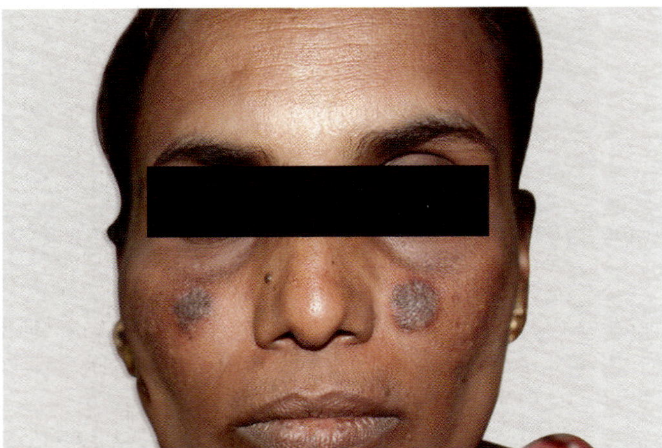

Fig. 2: Hyperpigmented symmetrical plaques on cheeks

- Orthohyperkeratosis with atrophy of stratum malpighi
- Keratotic follicular plugging
- Hydropic degeneration of basal cells
- Colloid bodies which are rounded, homogenous, eosinophilic structures
- Thickened basement membrane
- Lymphocytic infiltration at dermo-epidermal junction and in a perivascular and peri-adnexal distribution
- Interstitial mucin deposition

Direct immunofluorescence can be used adjunctively in cases where histopathology is not conclusive.

Q3. What are the histopathological differential diagnosis of discoid lupus erythematosus?

Ans: DLE must be differentiated from other conditions in which lymphocytic infiltration of dermis can occur.

- Lichen planus
- Jessner's lymphocytic infiltrate
- Polymorphic light eruption
- Lymphocytic lymphoma
- Lymphocytoma cutis
- Benign lymphocytic infiltration.

Q4. What are the immunopathology findings in discoid lupus erythematosus?

Ans: In more than 80% of skin lesions older than 6 weeks, immunohistology shows the presence of IgG, IgM, IgA and complements at dermo-epidermal junction. Homogenous, granular and thread patterns can be seen. However, they do not occur in uninvolved skin, unlike systemic lupus erythematosus (SLE) cases.

Q5. Enumerate all the clinical variants of chronic cutaneous lupus erythematosus?

Ans: Clinical variants of CCLE:

- Classic discoid LE
  - Localized DLE
  - Generalized DLE
- Hypertrophic or verrucous DLE
- Lupus profundus or lupus panniculitis
- Mucosal DLE
  - Oral DLE
  - Conjunctival DLE
- Lupus tumidus (Urticarial plaques of LE)
- Chillblain LE
- Lichenoid LE (Lupus planus)
- LE telangiectaticus
- Linear LE
- Others: Rosaceous LE, Acneiform LE, pigmented-macular type, Dego's like lesions of CCLE, LE hypertrophicus et profundus, LE vermiculatus.

Q6. What are the clinical signs seen in discoid lupus erythematosus?

Ans: Clinical signs are:

- *Carpet-tack or tin-tack or cat's tongue sign:* DLE is characterized by partially adherent scales entering patulous hair follicles. On lifting the scale, keratotic spikes similar in appearance to carpet-tacks are seen to project from the undersurface of scale. Also seen cases of Pemphigus foliaceus and seborrheic dermatitis.
- *Shuster's sign*: Scarring of concha due to lesions of DLE. Positive in 30% cases of DLE.

Q7. Name the other dermatological conditions characterized by follicular plugging.

Ans: Follicular plugging:

- Phrynoderma
- Keratosis pilaris

- Follicular lichen planus
- Pityriasis rubra pilaris
- Acne
- Seborrheic keratosis.

Q8. What is Kaposi-Irgang disease?

Ans: Also called as lupus panniculitis or lupus profundus, it is an unusual variant of CCLE in which cutaneous infiltrate occurs primarily in deeper portions of corium, giving rise to firm, sharply-defined nodules, lying beneath clinically normal skin. Frequently affected sites include cheeks, proximal arms, chest, buttocks and thighs. Lupus panniculitis confined to the breast is called as lupus mastitis.

Q9. Which is the most photosensitive variant of chronic cutaneous lupus erythematosus?

Ans:
- Chillblain lupus
- Classic DLE
- Lupus tumidus
- Lichenoid LE

Ans: c (Lupus tumidus). Characterized by succulent, edematous, urticarial-like plaques with little surface changes. Typically responds to antimalarials.

Q10. How do you differentiate chillblain lupus erythematosus from idiopathic chilblains?

Ans: Persistence of lesions beyond the cold months, positive antinuclear antibody (ANA) and presence of one of the American College of Rheumatology (ACR) criteria for SLE at the time of diagnosis of chillblain lesions helps to distinguish chillblain LE from idiopathic chilblains.

Q11. What percentage of discoid lupus erythematosus patients subsequently progress to systemic lupus erythematosus?

Ans: 5% of localized and 20% of generalized DLE patients subsequently develop SLE. Risk factors for development of SLE are:

- Females less than 40 years old with HLA-B8 histocompatibility
- Presence of LE nonspecific skin lesions
- Generalized lymphadenopathy
- Raynaud's phenomenon
- Periungual nail fold telangiectasia
- Arthralgia
- Laboratory abnormalities: Unexplained anemia, leukopenia, biological false-positive test for syphilis, persistent high titers of ANA (>1:320), depressed serum-compliment levels and elevated-gamma globulins.

Q12. What percentage of discoid lupus erythematosus patients show antinuclear antibody positivity?

a. 30–40%
b. 50–60%
c. 80–90%
d. Greater than 95%

Ans: a 30–40%. ANA is positive in low titers in 30–40% of patients with DLE. However, less than 5% patients have ANA levels characteristic of overt SLE (>1:320). Other autoantibodies in patients of DLE include: Anti-ss-DNA antibodies (20%), Anti-Smith antibody (<5%), anti-dsDNA antibodies, anti-Ro or La antibodies (1%) and decreased complements C3, C4.

Q13. How will you manage a case of discoid lupus erythematosus?

Ans: *Investigations:*

- Complete blood count
- Chemistries [Blood urea nitrogen (BUN), Creatinine]
- Urinalysis
- Erythrocyte sedimentation rate
- ANA with profile
- Complement levels (C3, C4)
- Skin biopsy for histopathology and direct immunofluorescence.

Treatment:

- Local therapy:
  - Sun protection
  - Topical and intralesional steroids
  - Topical calcineurin inhibitors
  - Topical retinoids
- Systemic therapy:
  - Antimalarials: Hydroxychloroquine (6.5 mg/kg/day), chloroquine (3.5–4 mg/kg/day)
  - Retinoids (isotretinoin, acetretin)
  - Systemic corticosteroids
  - Thalidomide (50–100 mg bd to qid)
  - Dapsone
  - Clofazamine
  - Sulfasalazine
  - Immunosuppressive agents (e.g. azathioprine).
- Physical and surgical modalities like laser, cryotherapy and dermabrasion for resistant cases.

CHAPTER 111

Scleroderma

Shekhar Neema

Case study Scleroderma

Presenting Complaints

Doctor, my fingers and toes become blue on cold exposure since the last 3 years and my skin is becoming dark and tight since the last 2 years.

Setting

Dermatology outpatient department

History of Present Illness

A 28-years-old lady, presented with complaints of episodic discoloration of toes and fingers on exposure to cold for last 3 years and insidious onset gradually progressive, darkening and tightening of skin over face, upper trunk and extremities since 2 years. She also complains of difficulty in swallowing solid food, weight loss, anorexia and breathlessness on exertion. There is no history of photosensitivity, oral ulcers or joint pains. She has regular menstrual cycles and two healthy children.

General Physical Examination

BMI: 16 kg/m^2, Pulse: 80 BPM, Pallor: Present

Systemic Examination

Respiratory: Chest expansion reduced bilaterally.

Dermatological Examination

1. Mask-like facies, mouth opening is two fingers wide (Fig. 1)
2. Sclerodactyly (tapering of digits and thickening of skin of fingers) present (Fig. 2)
3. Induration, thickening and hyperpigmentation is present on skin of forearm, arm, and trunk.

Q1. What is the most likely diagnosis?

a. Scleroderma: Diffuse systemic sclerosis
b. Scleroderma: Limited systemic sclerosis
c. Morphea
d. Systemic lupus erythematosus

Ans: a. Scleroderma: Diffuse systemic sclerosis. Presence of Raynaud's phenomenon, sclerodactyly and proximal scleroderma suggests diagnosis of diffuse systemic sclerosis.

Q2. How do you diagnose scleroderma?

Ans: Scleroderma is diagnosed on clinical grounds. The American College of Rheumatology (ARA) criteria for diagnosis of scleroderma is as follows:

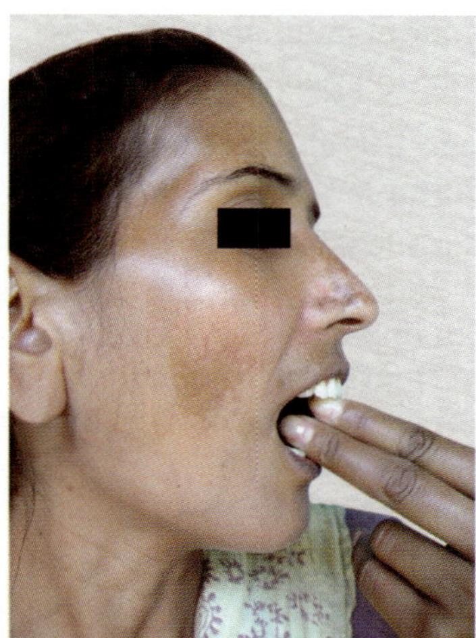

Fig. 1: Mask-like facies, mouth opening is two fingers wide

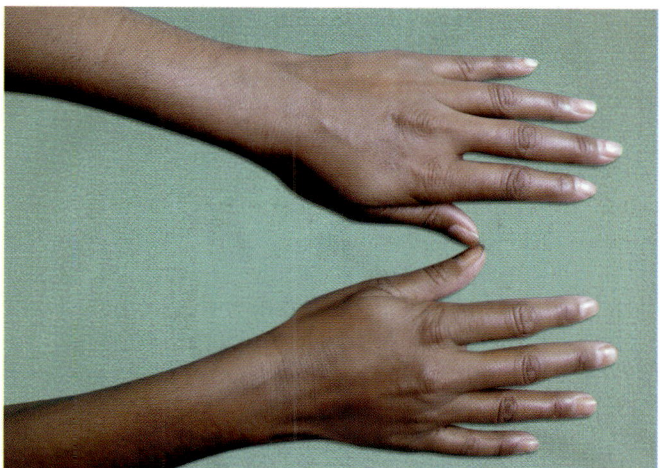

Fig. 2: Sclerodactyly (tapering of digits and thickening of skin of fingers) present

- *Major criteria:* Scleroderma (Tightening of skin): proximal to digits [Metacarpophalangeal (MCP joints)] affecting limbs, face, neck or trunk.
- *Minor criteria*
  - Sclerodactyly
  - Digital-pitted scars
  - Bibasilar pulmonary crackles

Presence of one major or two minor criteria suggests a diagnosis of scleroderma with 97% sensitivity and 98% specificity.

Q3. Is there any recent criteria to diagnose scleroderma?

Ans: The European League Against Rheumatism (EULAR) criteria for diagnosing scleroderma (Table 1) has come into being since 2013.

Q4. How will you confirm the diagnosis?

Ans: Diagnosis is made on clinical grounds. Laboratory evaluation is required mainly to diagnose cases with atypical presentations, to assess severity of disease and systemic involvement.

Q5. Which of these antibodies is the best indicator of diffuse scleroderma?

a. Anti-Scl-70
b. Anti-centromere
c. Antinuclear antibody
d. None of the above

Ans: a (Anti-Scl-70). This antibody is present in approximately 30% of cases of diffuse scleroderma and these patients have high risk of pulmonary disease. Anti-centromere antibody is present in 40–50% cases of limited scleroderma. These antibodies maintain fidelity in specific subsets and are useful in classification of disease in diffuse and limited variety. ANAs are present in approximately 90% of the patients of scleroderma, however it is not specific for the disease.

Table 1: The European league against rheumatism criteria for scleroderma

Category	*Subcategory*	*Weightage*
Skin thickening proximal to metacarpophalangeal (MCP) joint		9
Skin thickening of fingers (max 4)	Puffy fingers	2
	Sclerodactyly	4
Fingertip lesions (max 3)	Digital- tip ulcers	2
	Fingertip pitting scars	3
Telangiectasia		2
Abnormal nail fold capillaries		2
Pulmonary arterial hypertension/ Interstitial lung disease		2
Raynaud's phenomenon		3
Autoantibodies	Anti-centromere 3, Anti-topoisomerase I, Anti RNA Polymerase III (renal crises)	3

Note: Score greater than or equal to 9= definite Scleroderma (addition of max weightage in each category)

Q6. What are the various organ systems involved in scleroderma?

Ans: Scleroderma involves almost all major systems and that is why it is also known as systemic sclerosis or total tissue dystrophy. However gastrointestinal (GI)

system, respiratory system, kidney and heart are majorly affected.

Q7. Enumerate the systemic involvement and what are the investigations that should be done to evaluate them?

Ans: The systemic involvement and investigations are:

- *GI involvement:*
  - Esophagus: Most common (75% cases). Dysphagia, reflux, stricture, hiatus hernia, peristalsis or rarely carcinoma esophagus
  - Stomach: Carcinoma stomach, telangiectasia leading to hematemesis
  - Duodenum: Ulcers, dilatation
  - Intestine: Obstruction, volvulus, stricture, bacterial overgrowth, steatorrhea, malabsorption
  - Colon: Constipation, diarrhea, diverticula, perforation, rectal prolapse
  - Hepatic: Rarely cirrhosis, portal hypertension.

  Investigation: Barium swallow and upper GI endoscopy- all cases. Rest like barium meal follow through and colonoscopy depending on involvement.
- *Pulmonary involvement:*
  - Lung involvement: most important predictor of mortality-interstitial lung disease, diffuse pulmonary fibrosis, pulmonary hypertension.

  Investigations: Chest X-ray, Pulmonary function tests and high-resolution computed tomography (HRCT)- all cases. Echocardiography- for pulmonary hypertension.
- *Renal:*
  - Scleroderma renal crisis: rapid rise in blood pressure, declining renal function, and/or of heavy proteinuria.

  Investigations: Urine routine and microscopic examination, blood urea and serum creatinine.
- *Cardiac:*
  - Arrhythmias, right heart failure.

  Investigations: Electrocardiography (ECG) and echocardiography
- *Muskuloskeletal:*
  - Arthralgia, myalgia, joint flexion contractures, tendon friction rubs, carpul tunnel syndrome, muscle weakness.

Q8. What are the three phases in cutaneous changes of scleroderma?

Ans: The three phases in cutaneous changes of scleroderma:

1. Early edematous phase
2. Sclerotic or indurated phase
3. Atrophic phase.

Q9. What are the characteristic skin changes in scleroderma?

Ans: Characteristic skin changes are:

- *Face*: Mask-like face, pinched nose, decreased mouth opening, lower eyelid cannot be pulled down (Ingram sign), longitudinal beading and ridging of neck (neck sign- Barnett's sign), mat like telangiectasia
- Calcinosis cutis
- *Pigmentary abnormalities*: Generalized hyperpigmentation, salt and pepper pigmentation (hyperpigmentation and hypopigmentation interspersed)
- *Generalized pruritus*
- *Digital pitted-scars*
- *Nails*: Onycholysis, onychorrhexis, pterygium inversus unguis, ragged cuticles, nail fold capillaries- dilatation and drop out. Mizutani's sign- disappearance of peaked contour on fingerpads.

Q10. How do you differentiate between diffuse and limited cutaneous scleroderma?

Ans: The difference between diffuse and limited cutaneous scleroderma has been described in Table 2.

Q11. How do you assess severity of skin involvement?

Ans: The severity of skin involvement can be assessed as:

1. Modified Rodnan skin score
2. Ultrasound
3. Durometer.

Table 2: Difference between diffuse and limited cutaneous scleroderma

Organ	*Diffuse*	*Limited*
Skin induration	Above elbow/knee	Sclerodactyly
Raynaud's phenomenon	At onset of disease	Precedes involvement of systems by 5–10 years
Gastrointestinal tract (GIT)	Entire GIT can be involved	Esophagus
Lungs	Interstitial lung disease	Pulmonary hypertension
Renal	Renal crisis	Usually not involved
Cardiac	Arrhythmias	Usually not involved
Liver	Usually less involved	Primary biliary cirrhosis
Nails	Capillary dropouts	Capillary dilatation
Serology: antibodies	Anti-scl-70 (40% cases)	Anti-centromere (60% cases)

Q12. What are the differential diagnosis of scleroderma?

Ans: These are also known as sclerodermoid or pseudo-sclerodermatous conditions:

- Genetic: Phenylketonuria, Progeria, Werner syndrome
- Environmental and occupational: Vibration syndrome, polyvinyl chloride use, silicosis
- Metabolic: Congenital porphyria, porphyria cutanea tarda, scleredema
- Immunologic: Chronic graft versus host disease, scleromyxedema
- Drugs: Bleomycin, pentazocine
- Malignancy: Carcinoid syndrome, metastatic melanoma
- Radiation dermatitis.

Q13. What is the CREST syndrome?

Ans: CREST is limited cutaneous systemic sclerosis characterized by:

C- Calcinosis

R- Raynaud'sphenomenon

E- Esophagial hypomotility

S- Sclerodactyly

T- Telangiectasia.

Q14. What are the complications of Scleroderma?

Ans: Digital infarctions, wound infections, pulmonary hypertension, renal failure, myositis.

Q15. What is the main principle in treating a case of Scleroderma?

a. Organ-specific treatment

b. Immunomodulation

c. Antifibrotic therapy

d. Combining all three above

Ans: d. Combining all three above.

Q16. Describe treatment modalities in scleroderma.

Ans: The treatment modalities in scleroderma are:

- *Supportive therapy*
  - Counseling
  - Avoid smoking, caffeine, emotional stress and beta-blockers
  - Physical: Warm water bath, massage, range of motion exercise, warm clothing
  - Topical therapy: Emollients, antibacterial for digital ulcers
- *Organ-specific treatment*
  - Vascular component: Intravenous prostacyclines, calcium-channel blockers, phosphodiesterase 5 inhibitors (Sildenafil), bosentan, ambrisentan
  - Pulmonary fibrosis: Cyclophosphamide, Bosentan
  - Pulmonary arterial hypertension: Sildenafil tadalafil, iloprost, bosentan
  - GI involvement: Frequent small meals, proton pump inhibitors
  - Renal involvement: Angiotensin-converting enzyme (ACE) inhibitors
  - Calcinosis cutis: Minocycline, rituximab, surgery.
- *Immunomodulation*
  - Methotrexate, mycophenolate mofetil-1st line
  - Cyclophosphamide, corticosteroids, cyclosporine, azathioprine, hydroxychloroquine.
  - Anti-fibrotic: D-penicillamine, methotrexate, mycophenolate mofetil, allogenic bone marrow transplantation
  - Recent advance: Interleukin-6 (IL-6) receptor antagonist—tocilizumab, rituximab.

CHAPTER 112

Morphea

Lekshmipriya B

Case study Morphea

Presenting Complaints

Doctor, I have developed few dark-colored sunken hard patches on various parts of my body since last 6 months.

Setting

Dermatology outpatient department

History of Present Illness

A 36-year-old lady, presented with complaints of insidious onset multiple sunken dark colored patches over her trunk and limbs. The patches were initially swollen and red in color, later on flattened to form very hard patches. She also complained of occasional joint pains. There is no history of photosensitivity, oral ulcers or any menstrual complaints. Her obstetric history is unremarkable.

General Physical Examination and Systemic Examination

No abnormality detected

Dermatological Examination

1. Several, well-circumscribed, hyperpigmented, oval to round, firm indurated plaques of varying sizes seen over chest, abdomen, lower limbs and back (Fig. 1)
2. Alopecia seen over the plaques.
3. Few plaques are smooth, ivory colored, with atrophy of the central area.

Q1. What is the most likely diagnosis?

a. Morphea: Localized
b. Morphea: Generalized
c. Scleroderma: Diffuse systemic sclerosis
d. Systemic lupus erythematosus

Ans: b. Morphea: Generalized. Presence of multiple indurated hyperpigmented plaques with an atrophic surface involving multiple areas on the trunk suggests the diagnosis of generalized morphea.

Q2. What are the different forms of morphea? What are the characteristic features of various types of morphea?

Ans: Different types of morphea:

- *Plaque morphea*: Indurated round or oval ivory-colored smooth shiny plaques with a lilac border.
- *Bullous morphea*: Tense subepidermal bulla overlying typical morphea lesion.

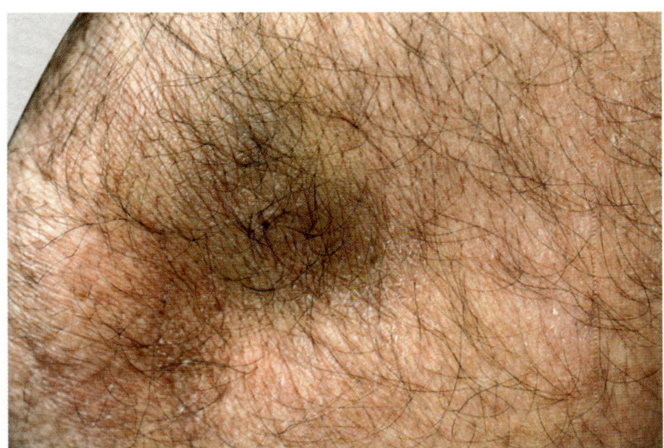

Fig. 1: Hyperpigmented indurated-plaque with an atrophic surface

- *Linear morphea*: Single and unilateral lesions usually occurring on limbs.
- *Deep morphea (Morphea profundus):* Ill-defined sclerotic plaques fixed to the underlying structures. They are characterized by fibrosis, hyalinization of collagen fibers and a deep-dermal and subcutaneous inflammatory infiltrate.
- *Generalized morphea*: Multiple enlarging plaques usually appear on trunk, rapidly coalesce, progress to involve the entire trunk and extend to involve the extremities resulting in disabling contractures.
- *Pansclerotic morphea*: Severe, mutilating form of morphea involving the dermis, fat, fascia, muscle and bone. Deep sclerotic lesions involving trunk and extremities.
- *Atrophoderma of pasini and pierini*: Small slightly depressed hyperpigmented patches with a sharp border seen symmetrically distributed over trunk and upper extremities.

Q3. How will you confirm the diagnosis?

Ans: Diagnosis is made mainly on clinical grounds. Investigations are done to confirm the diagnosis and to assess the severity and systemic involvement.

- Eosinophilia
- Erythrocyte sedimentation rate (ESR) raised
- Hypergammaglobulinemia
- Antinuclear antibody (ANA): 40% (homogenous pattern)
- Anti-ssDNA antibodies
  - Plaque—25%
  - Linear—50%
  - Generalized—75%
- Rheumatoid arthritis (RA) factor positive- 40%
- Antihistone antibody
  - Localized—50%
  - Generalized—85%
- Skin biopsy
- High frequency B-scan ultrasonography (USG).

Q4. What are the systemic involvements in morphea?

Ans: Systemic involvement is uncommon, seen mainly in deep morphea and localized scleroderma of children.

- Arthralgia
- Colicky abdominal pain
- Spinal abnormalities: Spina bifida, scoliosis, kyphosis, sacralization of lumbar vertebrae
- Neurologic: Epilepsy, migraine, peripheral neuropathy.

Q5. What is the differential diagnosis of morphea?

Ans: The differential diagnosis of morphea :

- Systemic scleroderma
- Panniculitides
- Eosinophilic fasciitis
- Eosinophilia myalgia syndrome
- Lichen sclerosis
- Lipodermatosclerosis
- Chronic graft versus host disease
- Morpheaform sarcoidosis
- Sclerosis at injection sites.

Q6. How do you differentiate between generalized morphea and scleroderma?

Ans: The difference between generalized morphea and scleroderma has been described in Table 1.

Table 1: Difference between generalized morphea and scleroderma

	Generalized morphea	*Scleroderma*
Distribution of lesion	Trunk more frequently involved	Face, hands and feet are more commonly involved
Raynaud's phenomenon	Uncommon	Almost always present
Systemic involvement	Less common	Almost all systems involved- GIT, pulmonary, cardiac, renal, hepatic and musculoskeletal
Serology: antibodies	Anti-ssDNA antibodies (75% cases)	Anti-Scl-70 (40% cases)
Prognosis	Usually improves over the years	Generally progressive

Q7. What are the modalities of treating a case of morphea?

a. Topical
b. Systemic
c. Phototherapy
d. Supportive management
e. All of the above

Ans: e. All of the above. Various modalities of management of morphea and their effectiveness based on level of evidence are as follows:

a. *Topical*
   - Topical calcineurin inhibitors- tacrolimus, pimecrolimus
   - Topical steroids
   - Topical vitamin D3 analogs-calcitriol, calcipotriol imiquimod cream 5%.

b. *Systemic*
   - Corticosteroids
   - Methotrexate
   - Mycophenolate mofetil
   - Cyclosporine
   - D-pencillamine
   - Cyclophoshamide
   - Azathioprine
   - Antimalarials
   - Salazopyrine
   - Colchicine
   - Phenytoin
   - Etretinate and acitretin
   - Potassium para-aminobenzoate
   - Griseofulvin.

c. *Phototherapy*
   - Ultraviolet A-1 (UVA-1) therapy
   - Psoralen and ultraviolet A radiation (PUVA)
   - Narrowband ultraviolet B (NBUVB)
   - Extracoporeal photochemotherapy (Photopheresis).

d. *Supportive Management*
   - Passive and active physical therapy
   - Regular lymph drainage

Flowcharts 1A to C: Treatment algorithms

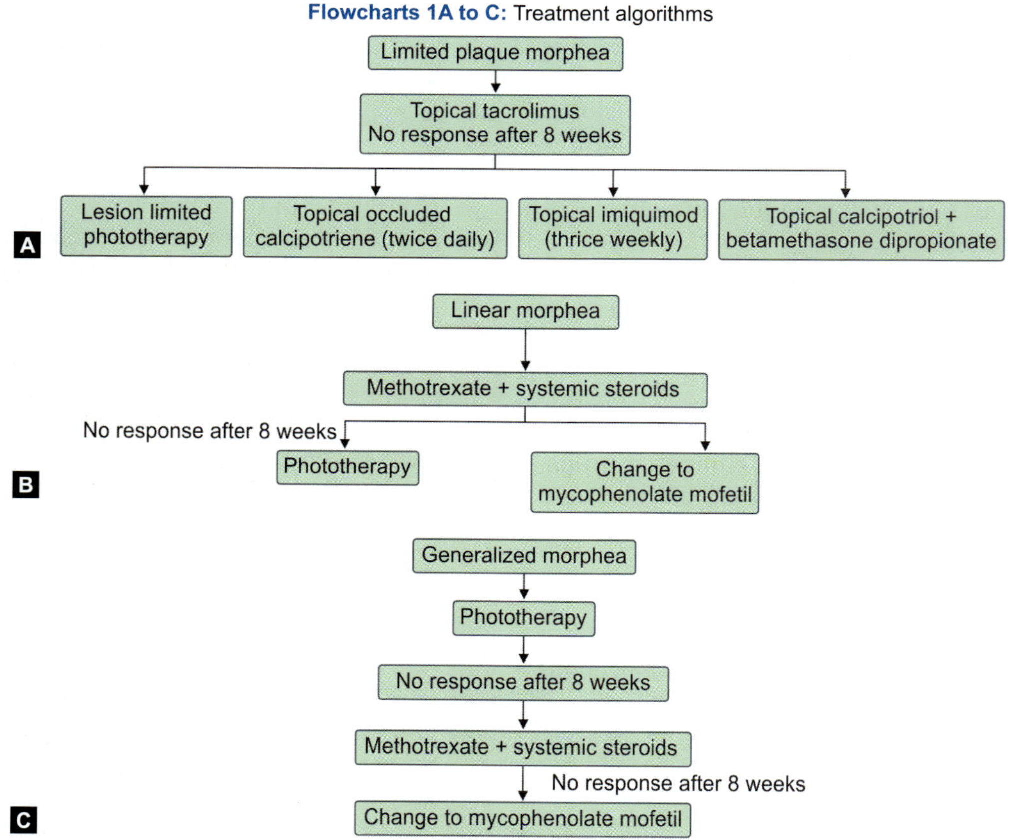

- Surgery for releasing contracture, scar revision surgeries, limb lengthening procedures
- Reconstructive surgeries.

Q8. What is the prognosis of morphea?

Ans: Circumscribed plaques of morphea tend to resolve spontaneously after 3–5 years. Linear and deep subtypes persist longer and cause considerable morbidity in the form of joint contractures, atrophy and limb length discrepencies. Generalized morphea has a worse prognosis with the disease process lasting for many years. Progression to systemic sclerosis is rare.

CHAPTER 113

Dermatomyositis

Nirmal Krishna B

Case study **Dermatomyositis**

Presenting Complaints

Doctor I have difficulty in getting up from sitting position and combing my hairs since 1 week. I have also noticed a red-rash around my eyes since a month.

Setting

Dermatology outpatient department

History of Presenting Illness

A 36-year-old female presented with history of difficulty in getting up and doing activities with her arms since 1 week. She gave history of difficulty in swallowing food since the last 2 days. On detailed history taking, she also gave history of having noticed a red rash around her eyes since 1 month. There was no history of breathlessness, urinary complaints, photosensitivity or weight loss.

General and Physical Examination

Vitals: Within normal limits (WNL), General examination: WNL.
Muskuloskeletal examination: Proximal muscle weakness present with power 3/5 both upper and lower limbs.

Dermatological Examination

Violaceous to erythematous rash around both eyelids (Fig. 1). Violaceous to hyperpigmented discoloration present over both shoulders (Fig. 2).

Q1. What is the clinical diagnosis?

a. Scleroderma
b. Dermatomyositis (DM)
c. Systemic lupus erythematosus (SLE)
d. Mixed connective tissue disease

Ans: b. Dermatomyositis.

Q2. What is dermatomyositis?

Ans: DM is a genetically determined autoimmune disorder characterized by a combination of proximal muscle weakness and inflammatory skin changes (also known as Wagner-Unverricht disease).

Q3. What is idiopathic inflammatory dermatomyopathy?

Ans: Idiopathic inflammatory dermatomyopathy (IIDM) is a heterogenous group of disorders that target skeletal muscle and/or skin comprising DM, polymyositis (PM) and inclusion body myositis (IBM).

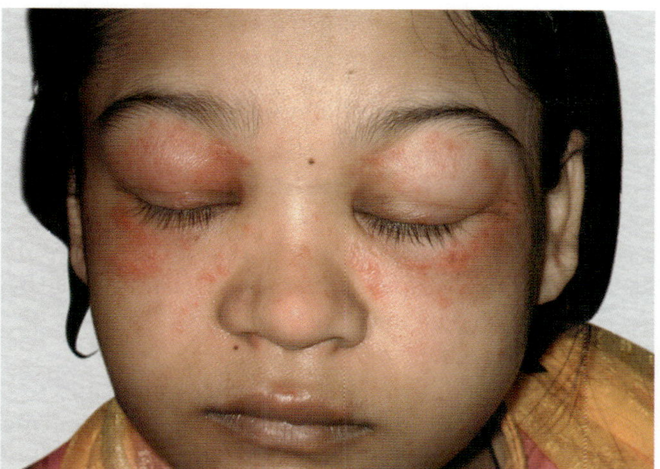

Fig. 1: Violaceous to erythematous rash around both eyelids
Courtesy: Dr Vishalakshi Vishwanath

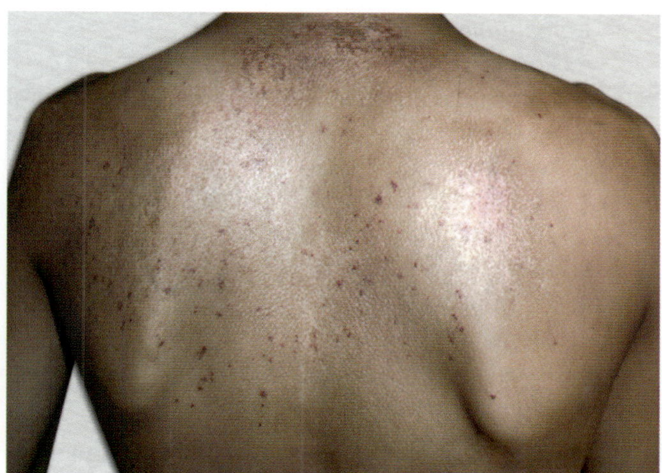

Fig. 2: Violaceous to hyperpigmented discoloration present over both shoulders
Courtesy: Dr Vishalakshi Vishwanath

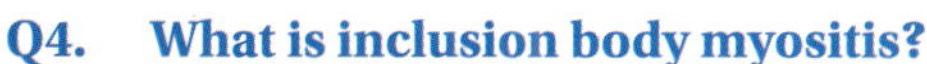

Q4. What is inclusion body myositis?

Ans: IBM is a pathologically distinct steroid-resistant disorder asymmetrically involving distal muscles.

Q5. What is clinically amyopathic dermatomyositis?

Ans: Clinically amyopathic dermatomyositis (CADM) is a term used to include amyopathic DM (DM sine myositis) and hypomyopathic DM.

- Amyopathic DM is biopsy confirmed cutaneous DM in the absence of clinical and laboratory signs of myositis for at least 6 months after the onset of skin disease, after excluding systemic steroid therapy for at least two consecutive months and drugs-causing DM-like changes.
- Hypomyopathic DM is similar to amyopathic DM in the absence of clinical evidence of myositis but have laboratory evidence of myositis.

Q6. What is the pathogenesis of idiopathic inflammatory dermatomyopathy?

Ans: IIDM pathogenesis has four sequential phases:

1. *Susceptiblity: Genetic*-human leukocyte antigen (HLA) DR3, DRW52-associated with anti-synthetase antibodies, TNFα 208A single nucleotide polymorphism-associated with disease chronicity and calcinosis cutis.
2. *Induction:* UV light, infections [Coxsackie virus, Parvo virus B19, Epstein-Barr virus (EBV), human immunodeficiency virus (HIV), human T-lymphotropic virus (HTLV-1), Toxoplasma]
3. *Expansion*: Loss of immune regulation leads to auto antibody formation and auto-reactive T-cell expansion
4. *Injury:* Antibody or immune-complex-mediated injury in DM and HLA class 1- dependent CD8+ T-cell mediated injury in PM and IBM.

Q7. What is the age of onset and sex predominance of DM?

Ans: DM has a bimodal distribution with smaller peak in children and larger peak in adults (40–65 years). Females out number males in both adult and childhood DM, ratio being 2:1 and 5:1, respectively.

Q8. What are the cutaneous manifestations of dermatomyositis?

Ans: *Pathognomonic:*

- Gottron papules: Flat-topped lichenoid papules over distal interphalangeal (DIP), proximal interphalangeal (PIP), metacarpophalangeal (MCP) joints of hands. When these papules are present over palms, they are known as inverse Gottron papules.
- Gottron sign: Symmetric confluent macular violaceous erythema (CMVE) involving dorsal aspect of DIP, PIP, MCP joints, olecranon process, patella, medial malleolus.

Characteristic:

- Periorbital CMVE (Heliotrope rash) and lid edema
- CMVE involving extensor aspect of forearms and arms, deltoid, posterior shoulder, nape of neck, V-area of neck, upper chest (Shawl sign), hips and lateral thigh (Holster sign)
- Hyperkeratosis of radial aspect of hands and feet (Mechanic's hands)
- Periungual telangiectasia

Compatible:
- Poikiloderma atrophicans vasculare
- Calcinosis cutis- involving shoulder girdle, elbows and hands

Other findings:
1. Sub-epidermal vesicle or bullae-seen with extensive cutaneous inflammation
2. Flagellate erythema
3. Purpura over Gottron sign
4. Alopecia
5. Panniculitis
6. Cutaneous ulceration.

Q9. How is the rash of dermatomyositis different from lupus erythematosus?

Ans: DM rash:
- Involves nasolabial fold
- Pruritic
- Accompanied by edema
- Has a violaceous hue
- Rash on the fingers are present only on the knuckles and PIP joints spares the skin in between
- Involves eyelids more than malar eminences.

Q10. Why is violaceous hue seen in rash of dermatomyositis?

Ans: Violaceous hue is seen in rash of DM because:
- Edema-associated with DM displaces hyperemic cutaneous vasculature deep into the dermis.
- Deoxygenation of blood flowing through abnormal dermal microvasculature.

Q11. What is Keining sign?

Ans: Tender or painful to touch cuticles in DM is called Keining sign.

Q12. What is Wong-type of dermatomyositis?

Ans: DM with pityriasis rubra pilaris-like lesions presenting with follicular hyperkeratosis and destruction of hair follicles is called Wong-type of DM.

Q13. Describe the nail fold capillaroscopy in dermatomyositis.

Ans: Scleroderma-DM pattern with at least two of the following in at least 2 nail folds (Maricq criteria)
1. Enlargement of capillary loops
2. Budding or bushy capillaries
3. Enlarged-twisted capillaries
4. Capillary hemorrhages (more than two punctuate hemorrhages per finger or confluent hemorrhage areas)
5. Loss of capillary loops (avascular areas)
6. Disorganization of capillary loops.

Q14. What is the histopathology of dermatomyositis?

Ans: Histopathology of DM:
- Earliest change is thickening of basement membrane.
- In acute DM, changes resemble subacute cutaneous lupus erythematosus characterized by:
  - Cell poor interface dermatitis
  - Prominent dermal mucin
  - Vasculopathy of dermal microvasculature.
- Late lesions of DM resembles scleroderma and shows: epidermal atrophy, effacement of rete ridges, increased pigmentation of basal layer, dermal collagen showing thickening, homogenization, sclerosis and thickening of vessel walls.
- Direct immunofluorescence shows IgM, IgG and C3 at the dermoepidermal junction in 50% of the cases.

Q15. Describe muscle involvement in dermatomyositis.

Ans: Muscle changes in DM include: insidious onset proximal muscle weakness manifesting as difficulty in climbing stairs and brushing hair, muscle atrophy and contracture, muscular calcification.

Q16. Describe the respiratory system involvement in dermatomyositis.

Ans:
- Interstitial pneumonitis characterized by dry cough, exertional dyspnea, fine late inspiratory crepitations
- Respiratory muscle weakness
- Aspiration pneumonia.

Q17. What are the other systems involved in dermatomyositis?

Ans: The other systems involved in DM are:
- Cardiovascular system (CVS)—Cardiomyopathy, conduction defects
- Gastrointestinal tract (GIT)—Dysphagia, large bowel infarction or perforation secondary to vasculopathy
- Eye—Retinopathy.

Q18. Describe the malignancies associated with dermatomyositis.

Ans: Risk for malignancy in DM is 20–25% and polymyositis is 3–10%. Common malignancies seen in:
- Males: Lung, GIT

- Females: Ovary, breast
- Asians: Naso-pharyngeal carcinoma.

Q19. What are the risk factors of malignancy in dermatomyositis?

Ans: Risk factors for malignancy:

- Elderly age group
- Severe skin disease
- Dysphagia
- Diaphragmatic weakness
- Anti-transcriptional intermediary factor 1-gamma (Anti-TIFγ), nuclear matrix protein (NXP2) antibodies.

Q20. What are the causes of death in dermatomyositis?

Ans: The causes of death in DM are:

- Childhood DM: Bowel or central nervous system (CNS) vasculopathy
- Adult DM: Occult malignancies, cardiac and pulmonary complications.

Q21. What are the specific features of overlap syndrome?

Ans: Specific features of overlap syndrome are:

- Associated with high titers of anti-RNP antibodies
- Characterized by high incidence of Raynaud phenomenon, sclerodactyly, inflammatory myositis, interstitial pneumonitis and pulmonary hypertension.

Q22. What are the specific features of anti-synthetase syndrome?

Ans: The specific features of antisynthetase syndrome are:

- Associated with Histidyl t-RNA synthetase (anti-Jo-1), anti-threonyl-tRNA synthetase (anti PL-7), anti PL-12 antibodies
- Characterized by high incidence of Raynaud phenomenon, arthritis, inflammatory myositis, interstitial lung disease, fever and mechanic's hands.

Q23. What are the specific features of clinically amyopathic dermatomyositis?

Ans: The specific features of CADM:

- Associated with anti-melanoma differentiation associated protein (anti MDA-5) antibodies
- Despite absence of myositis, they have an increased risk to develop interstitial lung disease and malignancy.

Q24. What are the specific features of childhood or juvenile dermatomyositis?

Ans: Specific features of childhood or juvenile DM are:

- No increased risk of malignancy
- Characterized by high incidence of calcinosis cutis (6–50%), acquired lipodystrophy (10%) and cutaneous ulceration due to infarctive vasculopathy.

Q25. What are the two types of childhood or juvenile dermatomyositis?

Ans: The two types of childhood or juvenile DM are:

1. Brunsting type: Slow course, progressive weakness, calcinosis cutis, steroid responsive
2. Banker type: Rapid onset, severe weakness, vasculitis of muscle and GIT, steroid unresponsive.

Q26. What are the forms of cutaneous calcification in childhood or juvenile dermatomyositis?

Ans: The forms of cutaneous calcification in childhood or juvenile DM:

- Superficial cutaneous or subcutaneous calcification
- Intramuscular tumorous calcification
- Calcification of myofacial planes
- Extensive encasing calcinosis (Exoskeleton).

Q27. What are the drugs causing dermatomyositis-like features?

Ans: Drugs causing DM-like features-

- Hydroxyurea
- Statins
- Penicillamine
- Diclofenac
- Phenytoin
- Tryptophan
- Practolol.

Q28. What are the antibodies in dermatomyositis and its associations?

Ans: *Myositis specific antibodies (MSA):*

- Anti-Jo-1 : PM greater than DM, Raynaud, arthritis, inflammatory myositis, interstitial lung disease, fever, mechanic's hands
- Anti-Mi-2 (Helicase nuclear protein): Classic cutaneous DM
- Anti-SRP (Signal recognition particle) : PM greater than DM, cardiac involvement
- Anti-MDA-5: CADM, interstitial lung disease (ILD), vasculopathic ulcers, painful red papules
- Anti TIF-1γ: Increased risk of malignancy
- Anti NXP-2: Childhood or Juvenile DM
- Anti- SUMO-1 activating enzyme (Anti-SAE) : Dysphagia

- Anti-hydroxy-methylglutaryl-CoA reductase (Anti-HMGCR): Necrotizing myopathy especially not exclusively with statins

Myositis Associated Antibodies (MAA):

- Anti 52kd Ro: Most prevalent MAA in IIDM
- PM-Scl: SSc-PM overlap
- Anti Ku: LE-PM overlap
- Anti RNP: MCTD.

Q29. What are the investigations in dermatomyositis?

Ans: Investigations in DM:

- Antinuclear antibody (ANA): Positive in 80% cases of DM in low titer, nuclear pattern-speckled or nucleolar
- Creatine phosphokinase: Most sensitive and specific marker of myositis
- Aldolase: Less sensitive, more useful in childhood or juvenile DM
- Electromyography shows—
  - Small polyphasic potential during contraction
  - Spontaneous fibrillation with positive sharp waves
  - Bizzare high frequency discharges during mechanical stimulation
- Magnetic resonance imaging with short T1 interval resonance (STIR) shows edema which is suggestive of muscle inflammation but not confirmatory.
- Muscle biopsy—
  - Perivascular and perimysial B-cell inflammation in DM
  - Endomysial CD8+ T cell infiltrate in PM
  - Granular vacuoles in muscle fibers in IBM
- Plain X-ray: to detect calcinosis cutis
- Lung function test: Restrictive pattern in interstitial lung disease
- High resolution computed tomography (CT) scan chest: To detect interstitial lung disease
- CT neck, thorax, abdomen, pelvis, positron emission tomography (PET) scan: To screen for malignancy.

Q30. What are the treatment options in dermatomyositis?

Ans: Management of DM is multispecialty involving dermatology, rheumatology and respiratory medicine. The management in classic DM is aggressive to prevent complications while CADM is conservative.

Classic DM:

- Systemic corticosteroids: 0.5–1 mg/kg
- Pulse IV methyl prednisolone: 0.5–1g/day for 3 days in life-threatening severe disease
- Steroid sparing drugs:
  - Methotrexate 10–20 mg/week
  - Mycophenolate mofetil 500–1500 mg twice daily
  - Cyclosporine 3–5 mg/kg/day
  - Oral Tacrolimus
- Intravenous immunoglobulin—especially in patients with dysphagia
- Rituximab: 1g 2 -weeks apart

CADM:

- Topical corticosteroids
- Topical tacrolimus
- Hydroxychloroquine sulfate
- Methotrexate.

Q31. How do you differentiate steroid-induced myopathy from a flare of myositis in dermatomyositis?

Ans:

- If steroids are withdrawn, strength improves in steroid-induced myopathy but worsens in the latter.
- Increased urine creatinine is seen in steroid-induced myopathy but not in the latter.

SECTION 22

Connective Tissue Disorders

Navya Handa

CHAPTER 114

Lichen Sclerosus

Navya Handa

Case study Lichen Sclerosis

Presenting Complaints

Doctor, I have severe itching over my vulva during the last 6 months and pain during intercourse since 2 months.

Setting

Dermatology outpatient department

History of Present Illness

A 50-year-old lady, presented with complaints of severe itching over her vulva since 6 months. Itching was severe in intensity causing her physical and psychological discomfort. Patient also complains of pain during intercourse since 2 months.

General Physical Examination and Systemic Examination

No abnormality detected

Dermatological Examination

Vulvar hypopigmentation with thin wrinkled and atrophic skin, telangiectasia and follicular plugging on the surface in a "figure of 8" distribution around vulva and anus-like a cigarette-paper appearance (Fig. 1).

Q1. What is the most likely diagnosis?

a. Genital lichen sclerosus et atrophicus (LSA)

b. Vitiligo

c. Lichen simplex chronicus

d. Morphea

Ans: a. Genital LSA: Classical symptoms and signs of genital LSA are present in this case.

- Vitiligo: Clinically, lesions of vitiligo are asymptomatic and chalky-white in comparison to lesions of LSA which are porcelain white with cigarette-paper appearance. Patients with LSA may be asymptomatic or may present with itching, burning, bleeding, dysuria, difficulty in intercourse. On histopathology LSA has thickened epidermis initially, followed by atrophy and follicular hyperkeratosis. There is hydropic degeneration of basal cells, alteration in collagen and a band of lymphocytic infiltrate, which is absent in vitiligo.
- LSC also looks porcelain white but it can be differentiated from LSA as itching is the primary symptom and it lacks characteristic histopathological features of LSA.

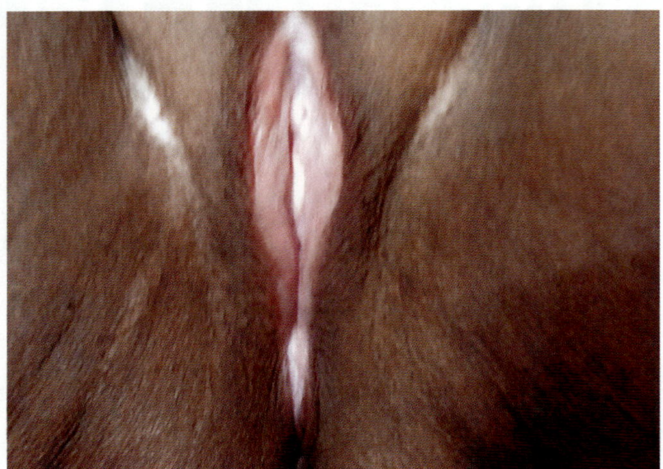

Fig. 1: Vulvar hypopigmentation with thin wrinkled and atrophic skin

Q2. What are the synonyms of lichen sclerosus et atrophicus?

Ans: Kraurosis vulvae, balanitis xerotica obliterans, white-spot disease.

Q3. Which are the sites affected by lichen sclerosus et atrophicus?

Ans: Sites affected:

1. Extragenital: Skin, oral mucosa
2. Genital: *Male*—Penis, foreskin; *Female*—Vulva, perineal skin.

Q4. What is the etiology of lichen sclerosus et atrophicus?

Ans: Etiology of LSA:

- Genetic predisposition
  - HLA A29, HLA B44, HLA DQ7
- Mutation in extracellular matrix 1 (ECM)
- Hormonal factors
  - Ten times more common in females
  - Onset around menopause
  - Spontaneous resolution in girls after puberty.
- Chronic infections, irritation, friction
  - Implicated infectious agents: *Borrelia burgdorferi*, human papilloma virus, ebstein-barr virus associated with autoimmune diseases.

Q5. In what all conditions is cigarette-paper appearance seen?

Ans: LSA, striae distensae, poikiloderma atrophicans vasculare, healed lesions of secondary syphilis.

Q6. What are the complications of lichen sclerosus et atrophicus?

Ans: *Male*: Phimosis, paraphimosis, urethral meatal stenosis, recurrent balanitis, rectal bleeding, constipation, cosmetic disfigurement and development of squamous cell carcinoma (SCC).

Female: Shrinkage of vulva, labial fusion, small introitus and development of SCC.

Q7. What are the risk factors for development of squamous cell carcinoma?

Ans: It is more common in females. Hypertrophic vulvar lesion and age older than 60 years increase the chances of development of SCC.

Q8. What is the differential diagnosis of lichen sclerosus et atrophicus?

Ans: Differential Diagnosis:

Extragenital: Morphea, atrophic lichen planus (LP), idiopathic guttate hypomelanosis, atrophoderma of Pierini and Pasini, vitiligo, pityriasis versicolor

Genital: Vitiligo, LSC, genital LP, extramammary Paget disease.

Q9. How do you differentiate histopathologically between morphea and lichen sclerosus et atrophicus?

Ans: The difference between morphea and LSA has been described in Table 1.

Q10. What are the dermoscopic findings of lichen sclerosus et atrophicus?

Ans: A halo, with a well-defined border and comedone-like openings.

Q11. What is the treatment of lichen sclerosus et atrophicus?

Ans: *Genital*

- Treat the superadded infection

Table 1: Histopathological difference between morphea and lichen sclerosus et atrophicus (LSA)

	Morphea	*LSA*
Epidermis	Relatively normal No follicular plugging	Thinning of rete pegs Follicular plugging+
Dermo-epidermal Junction	No hydropic degeneration Subepidermal separation rare	Hydropic degeneration+ Sub-epidermal bulla+
Dermis	Homogenized collagen Elastin+	Marked edema Elastic fibers absent
Subcutaneous fat	Inflammation Fibrosis	No inflammation No fibrosis

- Minimize soap substitution, avoidance of urinary contact
- Very potent topical steroids, e.g. clobetasol ointment twice daily
- Moisturization with emollients (maintenance phase)
- Calcineurin inhibitors
- Oral stanozolol and topical testosterone may be helpful
- CO_2 laser
- Frenuloplasty, meatotomy, circumcision
- Fenton procedure—in case of distortion of vulvar architecture
- Photodynamic therapy.

Extragenital

- Topical calcipotriol
- Phototherapy—Narrowband ultraviolet B (NB-UVB), ultraviolet A1 (UVA1)
- Mycophenolate mofetil.

CHAPTER 115

Atrophoderma and Anetoderma

Rajesh Kumar Mondal

Case study — Atrophoderma and Anetoderma

Presenting Complaints

Doctor, I have these brown sunken patches on my body for last 3 years. To start with there were few such patches on my back but slowly they have increased in number. I do not have any symptoms associated with them, but they look ugly.

Setting

Dermatology outpatient department

History of Present Illness

A 20-year-old boy presented with complaints of depressed brownish patches over his back for last 3 years. Initially, there were only few patches, but in the last 2 years numerous such patches appeared over his back, abdomen and thighs. There were no associated symptoms. There was no history of any trauma or infection at the sites. None of his family member has such disease.

General Physical Examination and Systemic Examination

No abnormality detected.

Dermatological examinations

Multiple well-defined ovoid hyperpigmented patches with central depression over back of trunk, abdomen and thighs. They have a cliff-drop border. The lesion is soft and nonindurated (Fig. 1).

Q1. What is your diagnosis?

a. Morphea

b. Atrophoderma of Pasini and Pierini

c. Lichen sclerosus et atrophicus (LSEA)

d. Anetoderma

Ans: b (Atrophoderma of Pasini and Pierini).

Asymptomatic hyperpigmented depressed ovoid nonindurated patches with normal overlying and surrounding skin with a cliff-drop border suggests atrophoderma of Pasini and Pierini.

Q2. What are the differential diagnosis of atrophoderma of Pasini and Pierini?

Ans: Anetoderma, morphea and LSEA are the closest differential diagnosis.

- Presence over site of previous dermatoses, depressed or pouch-like atrophic macule or patches with inward herniation on palpation and absence of cliff-drop border suggests anetoderma.
- Presence of lilac border, overlying skin atrophy and sclerosis are characteristic points of morphea whereas atrophoderma of Pasini and Pierini lacks

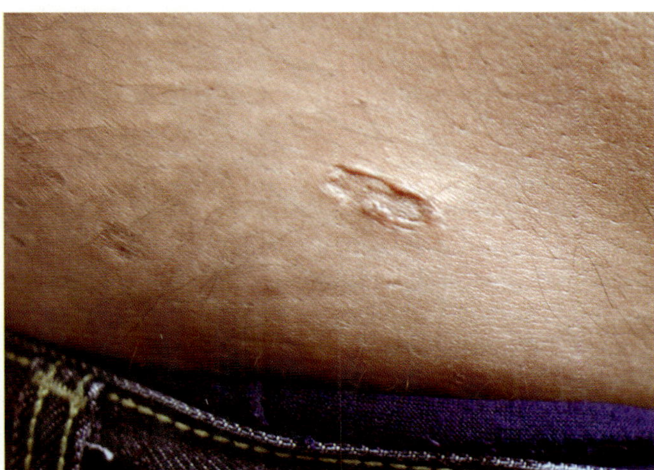

Fig. 1: Multiple well-defined ovoid hyperpigmented patches with central depression over back of trunk, abdomen and thighs. The closest lesion highlights the cliff-drop border

sclerosis, and lesions commonly coalesce over time, producing a moth-eaten appearance.
- Pearly white color, follicular plugging and overlying atopic skin are suggestive of LSEA.

Q3. How will you confirm your diagnosis?

Ans: Atrophoderma of Pasini and Pierini is diagnosed clinically and the histological and imaging findings are only additional inputs and are mainly done only to rule out other diseases.
- Enzyme-linked immunosorbent assay to detect anti-*B. burgdorferi* antibodies
- Antinuclear antibody, anti-topoisomerase II alpha antibody to rule out morphea
- *Ultrasonography or magnetic resonance imaging*: To measure the thickness of the dermis and subcutis for diagnosis and follow-up.

Q4. What are the histologic findings of atrophoderma of Pasini and Pierini?

Ans: Histologic findings:
- Normal or slightly atrophic epidermis
- Flattened rete pegs
- Increased melanin in basal layer
- Mild perivascular lymphohistiocytic infiltration
- Collagen bundles may be altered and clumped with normal appendages.

Q5. What are the treatment options for atrophoderma of Pasini and Pierini?

Ans: There is no definitive treatment. There is reported benefit with topical steroids, antimalarials, antibiotics, especially doxycycline (in cases associated with *B. burgdorferi* antibody positivity). Excessive sun exposure can lead to darkening of lesions, therefore sun protection is advised.

Q6. What is the prognosis?

Ans: It is a benign, asymptomatic condition that runs a protracted course over 10–20 years and may resolve on its own. Follow-up for the development of new lesions is advised.

Q7. What is anetoderma?

Ans: Anetoderma is a benign condition characterized by well-defined atrophic macules and patches with distinct inward herniations on palpation with surrounding normal skin. It is caused by loss of mid-dermal elastic tissue resulting in well-defined areas of pouch-like herniations of flaccid skin.

Q8. How will you classify anetoderma?

Ans: Anetoderma can be classified as follows:

a. *Primary anetoderma:* There is no history of any pre-existing skin disease. This type can be further subdivided into Jadassohn-Pellizzari type and Schweninger-Buzzi type. The first one is preceded by clinical inflammation or urticaria and the later occurs on healthy skin.

b. *Secondary anetoderma:* It occurs on site of previous dermatoses. The common dermatoses associated are acne vulgaris, varicella, prurigo nodularis, Hansen's disease, urticaria pigmentosa, B-cell lymphoma, syphilis, juvenile xanthogranuloma, granuloma annulare, molluscum contagiosum, congenital melanocytic nevus, cutaneous tuberculosis and nodular amyloidosis.

c. *Drug-induced anetoderma:* Penicillamine.

d. *Familial anetoderma:* It usually has an autosomal dominant inheritance.

e. *Congenital anetoderma:* It is mainly reported in premature infants with gestational age of 24–29 weeks.

Q9. All are true for anetoderma except:

a. Penicillamine may cause anetoderma

b. Cliff-drop appearance present

c. Loss of elastic tissue in dermis

d. Can occur on normal skin

Ans: b. "Cliff-drop" appearance is seen in atrophoderma of Pasini and Pierini.

Q10. What is the differential diagnosis of anetoderma?

Ans: Differential diagnosis:
- Atrophoderma of Pasini and Pierini

- Morphea
- LSEA
- Cutis laxa
- Mid-dermal elastolysis
- Connective tissue nevus
- Focal dermal hypoplasia
- Nevus lipomatosus superficialis
- Perifollicular atrophoderma
- Atrophic scars
- Granulomatous slack skin
- B-cell lymphoma
- Striae distensae.

Q11. What are the histological changes in anetoderma?

Ans: Normal or atrophic epidermis. Complete loss of elastic fibers in papillary and reticular dermis. Periadnexal lymph-plasma histiocytic infiltration may be present.

Q12. How to treat anetoderma?

Ans: No definitive treatment available. The treatment modalities available with variable reported efficacy are: surgical excision, cryotherapy, intralesional steroids, colchicine, hydroxychloroquine, vitamin E, oral penicillin G, dapsone, aspirin and phenytoin.

CHAPTER 116

Keloids and Hypertrophic Scars

Nidhi Sharma, Shekhar Neema

Case study Keloids and hypertrophic scars

Presenting Complaints

Doctor, I have a raised lesion over my chest since 4 months. It is slowly increasing in size and there is some pain and itching over it.

Setting

Dermatology outpatient department

History of Present Illness

A 20-year-old male presented with complaints of a pinkish, firm, raised lesion over his chest since 4 months. The lesion was initially small, but is gradually increasing in size and becoming paler. The lesion is associated with mild pain and itching. There is no history of preceding trauma or surgery. He is otherwise healthy.

General Physical Examination and Systemic Examination

No abnormality detected.

Dermatological Examination

Solitary large pink, plaque with a smooth and glistening surface and multiple crab-like projections situated over presternal region (Fig. 1). It is firm, indurated and tender on palpation.

Q1. What is the most likely diagnosis?

a. Hypertrophic scar
b. Keloid
c. Dermatofibroma
d. Morphea

Ans: b (Keloid: presternal).

Presence of gradually progressing lesion over chest, associated pain and pruritus and claw-like projections at the periphery suggests diagnosis of keloid.

Q2. What are the differential diagnoses?

Ans: The various differential diagnoses are as follows:

- Hypertrophic scar
- Dermatofibroma
- Lobomycosis (keloidal blastomycosis)
- Keloidal morphea
- Sarcoidosis.

Q3. How do you differentiate between keloid and hypertrophic scar?

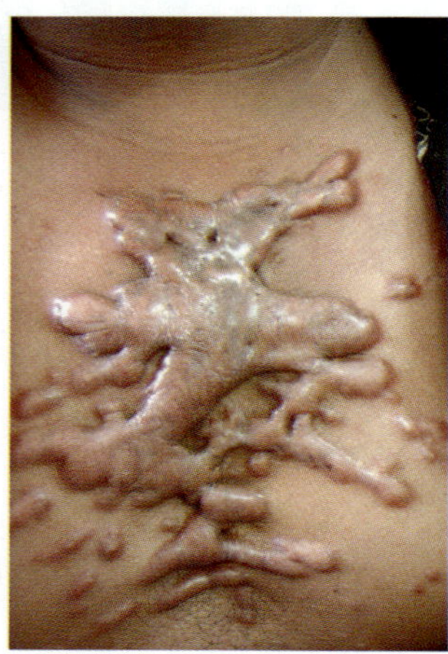

Fig. 1: Solitary large pink, plaque with a smooth and glistening surface and multiple crab-like projections situated over presternal region

Ans: The differences between keloid and hypertrophic scar are discussed in Table 1.

Q4. What are the anatomic sites prone to development of keloids?

Ans: Keloids usually occur over sites of increased skin tension or over bony protuberances that stretch the skin like:

- Presternal area
- Upper back
- Upper arms
- Deltoid area
- Earlobes (dumbbell keloids)
- Rare over face, palms and soles.

Table 1: Differentiation between keloid and hypertrophic scar

Feature	*Keloid*	*Hypertrophic scar*
History of trauma	Not always, can be spontaneous	Always
Onset	Delayed	Sudden
Race	More common in Blacks and Asians	No racial predilection
Familial tendency	Present	Absent
Symptoms	Itching and pain usually present	Itching and pain present sometimes
Anatomic sites	High-risk sites such as sternal area, upper back, upper arms	Anywhere on the body
Confinement to wound margin	No	Yes
Spontaneous resolution	Rare	Sometimes
Response to treatment	Poor	Good

Q5. What are the factors predisposing to keloid and hypertrophic scar formation?

Ans: Table 2 depicts the factors predisposing to keloid and hypertrophic scar formation.

Q6. What is the pathogenesis of keloids and hypertrophic scars?

Ans:

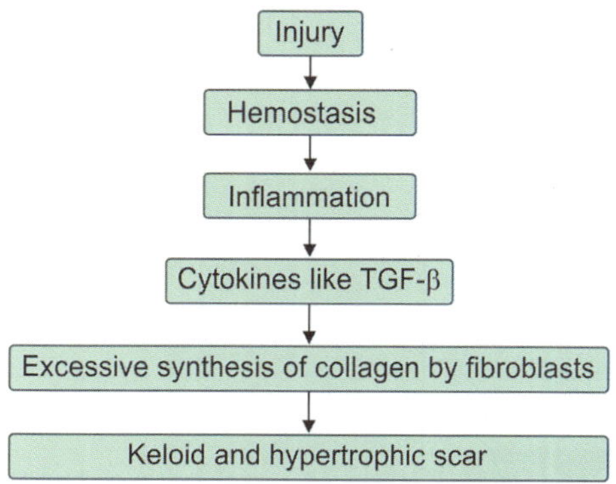

Q7. What are the histopathological features of keloids and hypertrophic scars?

Ans: Histopathological examination reveals large, thick collagen bundles in both keloids and hypertrophic scars. As compared to normal skin there is increased vascularity and connective tissue. There is an absence of adnexal structures. However, there are a few differences between them (Table 3).

Q8. What is the treatment of keloids?

Ans: Treatment of keloids:

- Intralesional steroid injections (ILS)
  - Injection triamcinolone 10–40 mg/mL given at 4–6 week interval
  - Maximum dose is 40 mg in one sitting
  - Injection can be diluted with lignocaine to reduce pain
  - Works by inhibiting fibroblast growth

Table 2: Predisposing factors for keloid and hypertrophic scar formation

Predisposing factors for keloids	*Predisposing factors for hypertrophic scar*
Race: Blacks and Asians Familial tendency Regional variation of skin-sternal area, upper back, upper arms Diseases such as Ehler-Danlos syndrome, osteogenesis imperfecta Types of injury: keloids are commoner in thermal burns where there is severe tissue damage	Poor approximation of wound edge Poor surgical technique Wound infection Tension while closing Foreign body or wound dehiscence

Table 3: Histopathological features of keloids and hypertrophic scars

Feature	*Keloid*	*Hypertrophic scar*
Dermis	Thick, hyalinized, homogenous collagen bundles oriented haphazardly throughout the dermis. Relatively few fibroblasts	Replaced by hypertrophic collagen bundles and increased fibroblasts
Dermal vessels	Very few vertically oriented blood vessels	Vertically oriented, i.e. perpendicular to skin surface
Myofibroblasts	Increased, but not within collagen nodules	Increased and present within collagen nodules

 - *Adverse effects*: Telengiectasia, dermal atrophy, pain.
- Cryotherapy
 - Usually combined with intralesional steroid injection
 - Results in tissue edema, hence larger dose of steroid can be injected
 - More effective than ILS alone
 - 3–4 weeks interval
 - *Adverse effect*: Pigmentary abnormalities, blistering.
- 5 Fluorouracil (5-FU)
 - Generally used in combination with ILS
 - 5-FU (50 mg/mL) + Triamcinolone (40 mg/mL) in ratio of 9:1, weekly for 8 weeks
 - *Adverse effects*: Pain, hyperpigmentation, ulceration.
- Silicone gel sheet
 - Apply 12–24 hours per day
 - Minimize transepidermal water loss, results in tissue edema.
- Laser
 - *Pulse dye laser*: decreases vascularity
 - *Long pulse Nd:YAG*: decrease vascularity.
- Other treatment options
 - Topical potent corticosteroids under occlusion
 - Intralesional bleomycin: used in doses of 1.5 IU/mL
 - Intralesional INF-alpha 2b
 - Intralesional verapamil
 - *Surgical excision*: best for ear keloid followed by ILS
 - Radiation therapy has good results, but has safety issues
 - Topical tacrolimus, imiquimod, tretinoin
 - Botulinum toxin A.

Q9. What are the treatment options for hypertrophic scars?

Ans: The treatment options for hypertrophic scars are:
- Intralesional steroid injection
- Silicone gel sheet
- Allium cepae extract
- Surgical excision
 - Should be done after 1 year as scar matures and improves till 1 year
 - Decrease wound tension or reorientation by Z-plasty.

Q10. What are the modalities for prevention of keloid and hypertrophic scars?

Ans: Preventive measures:
- *Good surgical technique*: Good wound approximation, closure without tension and aseptic procedure
- Intralesional steroid in wound edges (1–2 mg/mL)
- Silicone gel sheet after suturing
- Immobilization of the part after suturing.

SECTION 23

Granulomatous Disorders

Meenaz Khoja

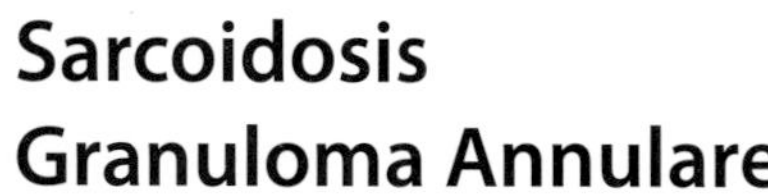

CHAPTER 117

Sarcoidosis

Ishad Aggarwal

Case study **Sarcoidosis**

Presenting Complaints

Doctor, I have these red patches on my skin and nose since 3 years along with breathlessness, cough and fatigability.

Setting

Dermatology outpatient department

History of Presenting Illness

A 42-year-old lady presented with mildly pruritic, slowly progressive lesions of insidious onset of 3 years duration on face, nose, back and trunk. There is no numbness over these patches. There is no fever or history of joint pains. The patient complained of progressive cough, dyspnea and fatigue. No history of any other systemic involvement. No significant drug or family history. Patient is neither a known hypertensive nor diabetic.

General Physical and Systemic Examination

Vitals: stable
Respiratory system examination revealed bilateral crepitations.

Dermatological Examination

Multiple erythematous papules and nodules seen over the cheeks, nose, back and trunk. No sensory deficit is revealed. There is no peripheral nerve thickening. Mucosa and nails were normal.

Q1. What is the most likely diagnosis?

a. Sarcoidosis
b. Post-kala-azar dermal leishmaniasis
c. Hansen's disease
d. Cutaneous T-cell lymphoma

Ans: a. (Sarcoidosis)

Presence of multiple papules and nodules on face, nose and trunk with progressive cough and dyspnea gives a clue to the diagnosis of sarcoidosis. There is no sensory deficit or peripheral nerve thickening. Therefore, there is less possibility of Hansen's disease which may form the closest differential.

Q2. How will you work up this case?

Ans: Following investigations should be carried out to establish the diagnosis:

- Biopsy from skin lesions
- Chest X-ray posteroanterior (PA) view

Following investigations are supportive:

- Serum angiotensin-converting enzyme (ACE) levels (60% patients have raised ACE levels)

- Serum erythrocyte sedimentation rate (ESR)
- Serum calcium levels
- Intradermal Kveim test (part of spleen from a known case of sarcoidosis is injected intradermally and test is positive if noncaseating granulomas develop within 4–6 weeks)
- Slit lamp and ophthalmoscopic examination (10–20% of patients with sarcoidosis have eye involvement)
- Sputum acid-fast bacillus (AFB) (to rule out pulmonary Koch's).

Following investigations should be done to assess the pulmonary system:

- Chest X-ray PA view
- Pulmonary function test [decreased forced vital capacity (FVC) and diffusing capacity for carbon monoxide (DLCO), restrictive changes in advanced pulmonary disease]
- High-resolution computed tomography scan chest
- 67 Gallium scan
- Bronchoscopic bronchial alveolar lavage and lung biopsy (CD4/CD8 ratio >3.5)
- F-fluorodeoxyglucose positron emission tomography (FDG-PET) scan
- Cardiopulmonary exercise testing (for lung and heart involvement).

Q3. How common is skin involvement in sarcoidosis?

Ans: Between 10% and 35% of patients with systemic sarcoidosis have skin lesions, but cutaneous sarcoidosis can also occur without systemic disease.

Q4. What are the typical histopathological features of sarcoidosis?

Ans: Histopathological hallmarks of sarcoidosis are superficial and deep dermal noncaseating epitheloid granulomas with sparse or no cuff of lymphocytic infiltrates (so called "naked granulomas") which stain negatively for fungus and mycobacteria. Multinucleate Langhans (more commonly seen in older lesions) or foreign body giant cells are usually present but not invariably so. Giant cells may contain inclusion bodies which may be stellate (eosinophilic inclusions showing open-umbrella appearance asteroid bodies) or rounded (basophilic Schaumann). These inclusion bodies, however, are not specific to sarcoidosis.

Q5. What are the clinical variants of cutaneous sarcoidosis?

Ans: Traditionally cutaneous sarcoidosis was classified as specific (with characteristic histology, "apple jelly" appearance is appreciated on diascopy, deeper subcutaneous involvement and poor prognosis) and nonspecific lesions (like erythema nodosum). A more practical morphological classification is generally followed.

Classical types

- Maculopapular and erythematous
- Papular (seen commonly over the knees) (Figs 1 and 2)
- Nodular
- Brocq-Pautrier angiolupoid type
- Annular type
- Lupus pernio
- Erythema nodosum
- Plaque type (Fig. 3)
- Scar sarcoidosis/tattoo sarcoidosis (Fig. 4)
- Subcutaneous sarcoidosis (presenting as lobular panniculitis).

Unusual types

- Alopecia (sarcoidosis involving the scalp with scarring alopecia similar to pseudopelade of Brocq
- Bony cysts of terminal phalanx (when nails are involved)
- Atrophic forms
- Erythrodermic sarcoidosis
- Lichenoid variety
- Ichthyosiform
- Hypopigmented form
- Pseudotumor
- Psoriasiform
- Pruriginous
- Verrucous
- Ulcerative
- Necrobiosis lipoidica like
- Morphea like.

Q6. What is lupus pernio?

Ans: This is a distinctive variant of cutaneous sarcoidosis in which infiltrated nodules and plaques are seen more or less symmetrically on nose, ears, lips, forehead, cheeks, fingers and toes. The papules and nodules are painless, rarely ulcerate and have a very doughy consistency. Cheeks show prominent telangiectasia.

Q7. What is Darier-Roussy disease?

Ans: It is also known as sarcoid panniculitis as it almost only affects the subcutaneous fat. Painless nodules without epidermal change are seen over the extremities and trunk.

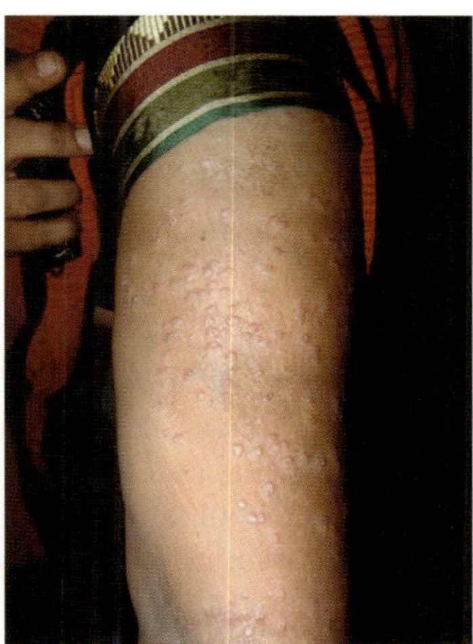

Fig. 1: Characteristic red-brown papules of papular sarcoidosis distributed over extremities
Photo courtesy: Dr Piyush Kumar, Associate Professor, Dermatology, Katihar Medical College, Dalan, Bihar, India

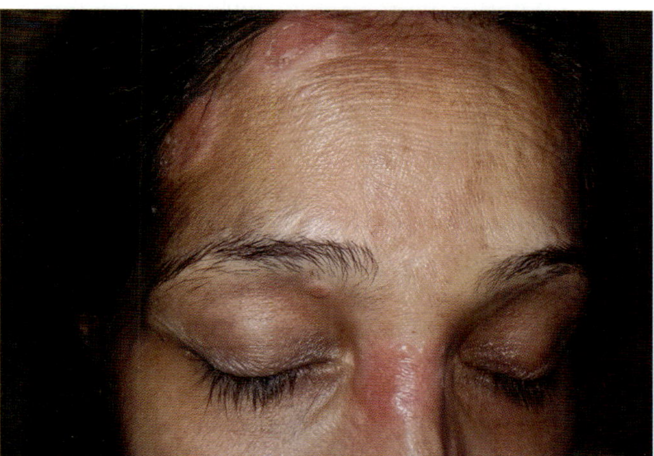

Fig. 3: Erythematous plaques of sarcoidosis seen over forehead, nose and just below right eyebrow
Photo courtesy: Dr Dependra Timshina, Consulting Dermatologist, Siliguri, West Bengal, India

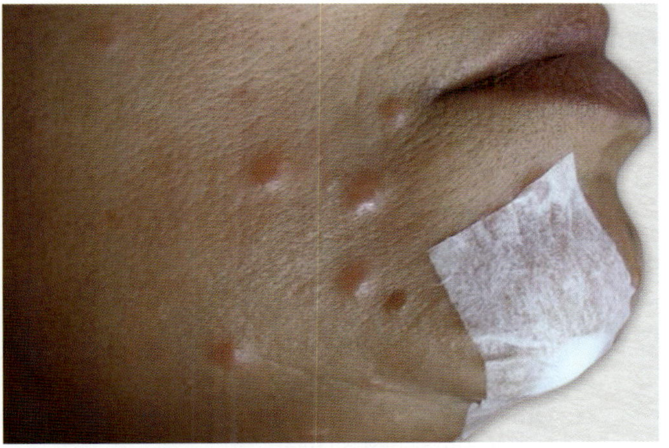

Fig. 2: Multiple, erythematous shiny papules of sarcoidosis over the face
Photo courtesy: Dr Anil Patki, Consulting Dermatologist, Pune, Maharashtra, India

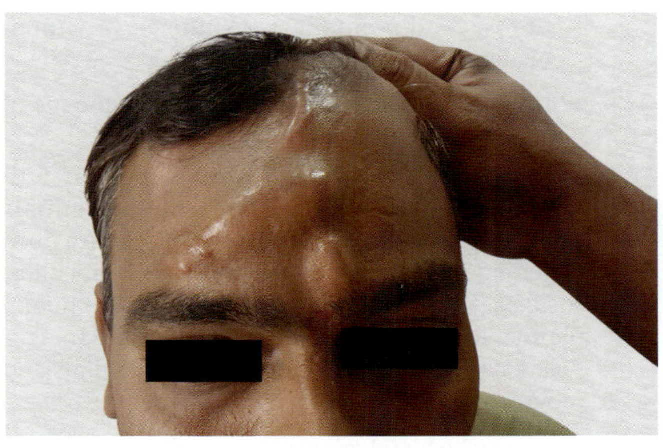

Fig. 4: Scar sarcoidosis
Photo courtesy: Dr Pradyumna Vaidya, Consulting Dermatologist, Pune, Maharashtra, India

Q8. What is the relevance of erythema nodosum in sarcoidosis?

Ans: It is the commonest nonspecific lesion of sarcoidosis. It is associated with acute and subacute sarcoidosis and is a good prognostic sign.

Q9. What is Heerfordt-Waldenström syndrome?

Ans: Also known as "uveoparotid fever": presents with fever, parotid gland enlargement, anterior uveitis, facial nerve palsy, meningism, papilledema, lethargy and neurological changes.

Q10. What is Löfgren syndrome?

Ans: Löfgren syndrome:

- Acute sarcoidosis
- Erythema nodosum
- Adenopathy (bilateral hilar and right paratracheal)
- Acute iritis
- Migrating polyarthritis
- Fever.

This form has an excellent prognosis although may have high recurrence.

Q11. What are the other syndromes associated with sarcoidosis?

Ans: Other syndromes associated with sarcoidosis are as follows:

- *Blau syndrome:* Presents in childhood, positive family history, no pulmonary involvement.

Arthritis, uveitis and granulomatous dermatitis are features.

- *Mikulicz syndrome:* bilateral enlargement of parotid, lacrimal, submental and sublingual glands secondary to sarcoidosis.

Q12. What are the chest radiographic features of pulmonary sarcoidosis?

Ans: Chest radiographic features can be seen in four stages:

- Stage 0: 5–10% of patients with sarcoidosis have a normal chest radiograph
- Stage I: Bilateral hilar lymphadenopathy alone—seen on the presenting radiograph of 35–45% of patients
- Stage II: Bilateral hilar lymphadenopathy with parenchymal lung involvement of fine "fluffy" or coarse type
- Stage III: Late stage of pulmonary infiltration with fibrosis and pulmonary insufficiency without bilateral hilar lymphadenopathy.

Q13. What are the clinical differential diagnoses of cutaneous sarcoidosis?

Ans: Sarcoidosis is one of the "great imitators" in dermatology. It may have various differentials depending up on the clinical presentation. Differentials include Hansen's disease, panniculitis, rosacea, lupus erythematosus, psoriasis, lichen planus, tinea corporis, cutaneous leishmaniasis, post-kala-azar dermal leishmaniasis, syphilids and tuberculides, deep fungal infections, etc.

Q14. What are the histological differentials of cutaneous sarcoidosis?

Ans: Histological differentials of cutaneous sarcoidosis:

- Foreign body granuloma [differentiated on polarization and special stains like periodic acid-Schiff (PAS), Grocott methenamine silver (GMS), Ziehl-Neelson (ZN), Gram and Wade Fite]
- *Lupus vulgaris*: Shows epitheloid cell granulomas with caseation necrosis
- *Tuberculoid Hansen's disease*: Epitheloid granulomas surrounded with cuff of lymphocytic infiltrate, granulomas elongated along the nerves along with nerve damage, acid fast bacilli detected.
- Leishmaniasis, deep fungal infections, suppurative granulomas, etc.

Q15. What are the associations of sarcoidosis?

Ans: Patients with sarcoidosis show an increased risk of Hodgkin lymphoma, autoimmune diseases like Sjögren syndrome, rheumatoid arthritis, vasculitis, systemic sclerosis, psoriasis, Hashimoto thyroiditis, Grave's disease, pyoderma gangrenosum and Sweet syndrome. Various organisms like *Propionibacterium acnes, Rickettsia helvetica, Borrelia burgdorferi, Mycobacterium tuberculosis, Chlamydia pneumonia, Histoplasma capsulatum, Epstein-Barr virus,* etc. are known to be associated.

Q16. How is cutaneous sarcoidosis treated?

Ans: It should always be kept in mind that sarcoidosis can resolve spontaneously, therefore expectant management may be given. Treatment options include:

- *Topical therapy for mild disease*: Potent topical corticosteroids
- *For extensive cutaneous involvement*: Oral corticosteroids are usually given in a dose of 30–40 mg/kg/day tapered gradually. Intralesional steroids can be given for resistant lesions.
- Other drugs like antimalarials, methotrexate and tetracyclines can be used.
- Isotretinoin, pentoxifylline, tacrolimus, apremilast, melatonin, allopurinol and PUVA therapy may be used.
- Role of cyclosporine is still controversial.
- Other drugs like immunosuppressants, biologics like tumor necrosis factor (TNF) antagonists (infliximab and adalimumab) can be tried if systemic corticosteroids are contraindicated.

CHAPTER 118

Granuloma Annulare

Meenaz Khoja

Case study Granuloma Annulare

Presenting Complaints

Doctor, I have these raised ring-like lesions almost over my entire body for the past 2 months. I have hypothyroidism and I am taking regular medicines. It does not bother me except for an occasional itch but I do not like the appearance of it because it is on the exposed areas.

Setting

Dermatology outpatient department

History of Present Illness

A 35-year-old female with hypothyroidism presented with complaints of occasionally itchy rashes over her hands, forearms, chest, back, neck and legs since 2 months. She has taken treatment from a general doctor for fungal infection with no relief.

General Physical Examination and Systemic Examination

Within normal limits.

Dermatological Examination

Multiple skin-colored to slightly erythematous papules coalescing to form annular plaques over both the forearms (more over the dorsal areas than the volar aspect), chest, back and lower legs. Body folds like groins and axillae are relatively spared. Sun-exposed areas are more involved than the covered areas.

Q1. What is the most likely diagnosis?

a. Tinea corporis
b. Id eruption
c. Lupus erythematosus
d. Granuloma annulare (GA)

Ans: d. Granuloma annulare.

Q2. How do you diagnose GA?

Ans: Granuloma annulare is mainly a clinical diagnosis and is characterized by an asymptomatic (sometimes itchy) rash over the exposed areas (usually in the localized variant), or generalized to involve the entire body. Characteristic morphology of GA is skin-colored to erythematous papules coalescing to form annular plaques. Rarely, lesions may have a violaceous hue.

Q3. What is the most common site for GA?

a. Dorsae of hands
b. Feet

c. Trunk
d. Face

Ans: a. (Dorsae of hands)

Granuloma annulare commonly affects exposed areas such as dorsae of hands, wrists, knuckles, feet, face and V-area of neck (actinic GA). It can also involve other areas such as the chest, back, lower extremities, genitals, ears and mucosae [especially in human immunodeficiency virus (HIV)].

Q4. What are the age groups and races affected?

Ans: All age groups are equally affected. However, it is rarely seen in infancy. Females have a stronger predilection, male to female ratio of occurrence being 1:2. There is no racial predominance per se except for the perforating variant which is seen commonly in the ethnic Hawaiians.

Q5. What are the various types of GA?

Ans: Granuloma annulare may present as the following types:

- *Localized GA:* This is the commonest form (3/4th cases), seen more commonly in children. Predilection for the dorsae of hands, knuckles, fingers, feet, ankles and lower limbs. Acral lesions tend to enlarge as nodules rather than as annular plaques (Fig. 1)
- *Generalized GA (also known as disseminated GA):* Makes up to 10–15% of cases. This type occurs predominantly in adults, occurrence in females being twice as common. The trunk (flanks and abdomen) usually involved, as well as the neck, extremities (Fig. 2), face, scalp, palms and soles. This type usually presents with itching or burning and is the commonest form of GA seen in HIV patients. Interestingly, previous vaccination sites are spared in disseminated GA.
- *Subcutaneous GA (benign rheumatoid nodules, deep GA and pseudorheumatoid nodules):* It is seen predominantly in children. Subcutaneous GA presents with individual lesions (5 mm to 4 cm in diameter), firm or hard, usually painful nodules in the deep dermis or subcutaneous tissues. They are usually seen over the anterior tibial aspect of legs, scalp, ankles, dorsal feet, buttocks and hands. It can also involve periorbital areas, eyelids, penis, subperiosteal areas and mucosae (in HIV patients).
- *Perforating GA:* This is a rare variant seen in adults as well as children. Perforating GA is usually localized to the dorsae of hands and fingers or may be generalized on the trunk and extremities. It is characterized by superficial umbilicated papules that heal with hypopigmented or hyperpigmented scarring.

Q6. What are the other reported variants of GA?

Ans: Other variants:

- Papular umbilicated "follicular pustulous GA" which is seen on dorsae of hands in children. Histopathology of these lesions shows palisading necrobiotic granuloma occurring in a perifollicular distribution.
- *Pustular generalized GA*: Dense infiltrate of neutrophils within the areas of necrobiosis seen on histopathology.

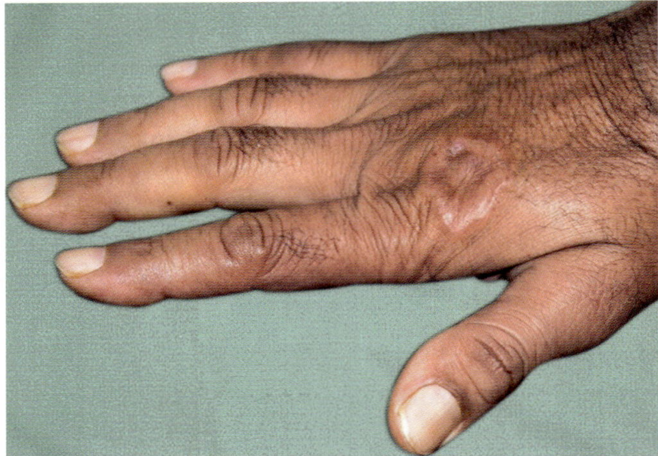

Fig. 1: *Localized granuloma annulare*: Typical skin-colored to erythematous annular plaque with raised and indurated rim over dorsum of right hand
Courtesy: Dr Sanjay Khare, Consulting Dermatologist, Indore, Madhya Pradesh, India

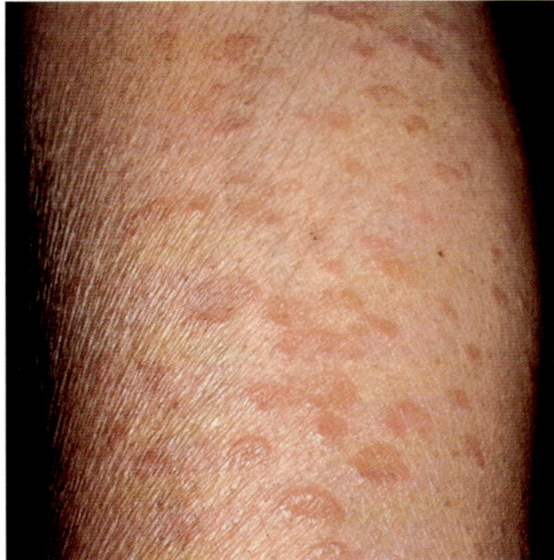

Fig. 2: Multiple erythematous annular plaques over extremities in disseminated granuloma annulare
Courtesy: Dr Sanjay Khare, Consulting Dermatologist, Indore, Madhya Pradesh, India

- *Linear GA*: May be an example of interstitial granulomatous dermatitis.
- *Patch GA*: Presenting with erythematous patches over trunk and limbs. May represent interstitial granulomatous form of drug reaction.
- *Arcuate dermal erythema*: This is an uncommon form of GA that manifests as infiltrated erythematous patches that may form large, hyperpigmented rings with central clearing.
- *Actinic granuloma*: Considered to be a subset of GA, occurring on sun-exposed sites (Fig. 3).
- *GA in HIV*: Diffuse and atypical forms of GA may occur in addition to the localized and generalized GA. Molluscoid lesions and violaceous lesions mimicking Kaposi's sarcoma may be seen. Uncommon sites such as penis, periocular and mucosal areas may be involved.

Q7. What are the common associations of GA?

Ans: Common associations:

- *Autoimmune diseases*: Systemic Lupus erythematosus, rheumatoid arthritis and Addison's disease
- *Sun exposure and phototherapy*: Commonly associated
- *Thyroid disease*: Localized and generalized GA is associated with thyrotoxicosis in women and thyroid adenoma (plummer disease)
- *Diabetes*: May be associated but this association has not been confirmed as yet
- *Malignancies*: Atypical GA, especially in the elderly is associated with malignancies such as myeloid or lymphoid neoplasms

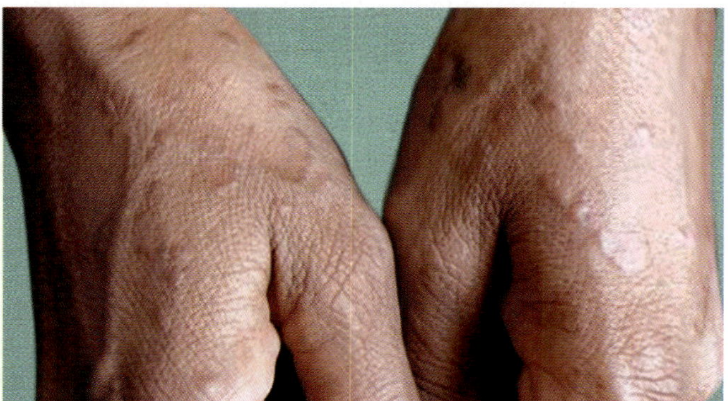

Fig. 3: *Actinic granuloma annulare*: multiple skin-colored papules coalescing to form plaques typically distributed over sun-exposed areas such as dorsae of hands and feet
Photo courtesy: Dr Sharad Mutalik, Head, Dermatology Department, Maharashtra Medical Foundation Joshi Hospital, Pune, Maharashtra, India

- Psoriasis, uveitis, hyperlipidemia and insulin resistance have been recently found to be associated
- *HLA Bw35*: There is an increased prevalence of HLA Bw35 in patients of generalized GA as compared to those of localized GA and controls
- *Morphea, sarcoidosis, necrobiosis lipoidica*: Coexistence of GA with these conditions has been reported
- *Infections*: A variety of infections and infestations such as scabies, hepatitis C, Epstein Barr-virus (EBV), mycobacterium tuberculosis, HIV, human papilloma virus (HPV), varicella zoster virus (VZV) and Borellia burgdorferi.

Q8. What is the pathogenesis of GA?

Ans: The exact pathogenesis of GA is not known but it is accepted to be a reaction pattern to a variety of stimuli. Proposed pathogenic mechanisms include cell-mediated immunity, delayed hypersensitivity and an immunoglobulin-mediated vasculitis as a reaction to underlying infection with VZV, HPV, EBV, HIV, etc. GA has been reported postimmunization, tuberculin skin testing (Mantoux), tattooing (especially the red ink), saphenectomy and insect and animal bites.

Localized GA over the exposed sites has been attributed to sun exposure and generalized GA has been noted after oral psoralens and UVA (PUVA).

Q9. How often is Koebner phenomenon seen in GA?

Ans: Granuloma annulare exhibits isotopic phenomenon, Koebner and reverse Koebner phenomenon.

Isotopic phenomenon: One disease may be responsible for the localization of another disease. For instance, GA appearing at sites of herpes zoster.

Koebner phenomenon: Suggests disease appearing at sites of minor trauma such as scratch or abrasions. For instance, psoriatic plaques appearing at sites of abrasions.

Reverse Koebner phenomenon: The disappearance of disease after trauma or scarification. For example, GA lesions resolving after biopsy at a distant site.

Q10. Which drugs are commonly implicated in the causation of GA?

Ans: The following drugs are reported causes of GA:

- Tumor necrosis factor alpha (TNF α) blockers
- Topiramate
- Allopurinol
- Calcium channel blockers
- Angiotensin converting enzyme inhibitors.
- Lipid-lowering agents

- Anticonvulsants and antidepressants
- Beta blockers
- Antihistamines
- Subcutaneous injection therapies for desensitization in type I allergy patients.
- Zalcitabine (ddC) for highly active antiretroviral therapy.

Q11. What are the histological features of GA?

Ans: Necrobiosis literally means death and life. This term applies to granulomatous disorders wherein the dermal connective tissue becomes homogenized and loses its normal architecture (outline is maintained) resulting in mucinous, fibrinoid or sclerotic alteration with a peripheral zone of epitheloid histiocytes arranged in a parallel fashion.

The characteristic histological features of GA are a normal epidermis and an anuclear dermis with collagen degeneration (necrobiotic granuloma) with palisading epitheloid histiocytes and mucin deposits.

Q12. Which other conditions present with necrobiosis?

Ans: Necrobiosis is also seen in necrobiosis lipoidica, acne agminata and rheumatoid nodule.

Q13. What are the investigations performed to clinch the diagnosis of GA?

Ans: The diagnosis of GA is mostly clinical. Biopsy is usually needed in cases of subcutaneous, perforating, generalized and atypical GA. Biopsy with or without special stains such as Alcian blue and colloidal iron confirms the diagnosis. Dermoscopy exhibits an orange to reddish structureless peripheral linear erythema as the only recognizable dermoscopic feature.

Q14. What are the differential diagnoses of GA?

Ans: *Differential diagnoses of GA:* Tinea corporis, erythema multiforme, annular lichen planus, erythema annulare centrifugum, erythema migrans of Lyme disease, tuberculides, annular sarcoidosis, papular syphilids, tertiary syphilis, subacute cutaneous lupus erythematosus, early inflammatory phase of morphea, eruptive syringomas, leukemia cutis, annular elastolytic giant cell granuloma and mycosis fungoides. Necrobiotic xanthogranuloma is a histological differential.

Differentials for perforating GA: Elastosis perforans serpiginosa, molluscum contagiosum, perforating disorders, sarcoidosis and papulonecrotic tuberculid.

Differentials for subcutaneous GA: Perniosis, callosities, rheumatoid nodules and epitheloid sarcoma.

Q15. What are the complications of GA?

Ans: Secondary anetoderma, mid-dermal elastolysis may occur as a sequel to GA. Loss of elastic fibers leading to development of open comedones on the rim of sun-exposed GA lesions may be observed.

Q16. What are the principles of treatment of GA?

Ans: Granuloma annulare is usually asymptomatic and self-limiting and reassurance usually suffices. Recurrence of GA after few years is not uncommon. For those patients with cosmetic concern, various treatment modalities have been tried with variable success. The trauma of skin biopsy occasionally leads to disappearance of lesions. Treatment modalities for localized GA include:

- *Steroids*: Mainstay. Topical potent or superpotent steroids, oral steroids and intralesional steroids
- *Cryotherapy*: Permanent scarring and atrophy may occur as a side effect of cryotherapy
- Electrodessication
- Low-dose recombinant interferon γ injections are found to be useful
- Imiquimod, photodynamic therapy (with 5-aminolevulenic acid or methyl aminolevulinate) and oral isotretinoin (0.5–1 mg/kg/day)
- Topical tacrolimus 0.1% ointment and pimecrolimus 1% cream applied twice a day
- *Lasers*: Pulsed dye laser, neodymium yttrium-aluminum-garnet (Nd:YAG), carbon dioxide and excimer laser
- *Subcutaneous GA lesions*: Left to be resolved spontaneously
- Despite the above treatments, GA lesions may recur after a few years.

Treatment modalities for generalized GA include:

- Initially above modalities used for localized GA can be tried
- *First line*: Dapsone, doxycycline, hydroxychloroquine, methotrexate, cyclosporine, retinoids, photochemotherapy and anti-TNF α agents
- *Second line*: Low-dose chlorambucil, pentoxyfylline, clofazimine, nicotinamide, topical vitamin E, combination of vitamin E and a 5-lipoxygenase inhibitor (zileuton), defibrotide and oral calcitriol
- *Rifampicin, ofloxacin and minocycline (ROM) therapy*: Rifampin (600 mg), ofloxacin (400 mg) and minocycline hydrochloride (100 mg) once daily for 3–6 months has shown resolution of GA lesions in some cases.

SECTION 24

Pruritic Conditions

Gopikrishnan Anjaneyan

CHAPTER 119

Generalized Pruritus

Brijesh C

Case study Generalized Pruritus

Presenting Complaints

Doctor, I am a housewife and I am suffering from terrible itching all over the body mostly over trunk and limbs since last 6 months.

Setting

Dermatology outpatient department

History of Present Illness

A 36-year-old lady, presented with complaints of generalized itching since last 6 months which was insidious in onset, slowly progressive and associated with no exacerbating and relieving factors. There was no seasonal variation noticed. The itching was disturbing her day-to-day activities and she was feeling stressed out. There was no history of intake of medicines except antihistamines and creams prescribed by general practitioners, no family history of skin problems and no personal history of asthma and allergies. The face and scalp were spared. The lady also gave history of aggravation of itch when she used to have wheat products like rotis, chapatis, etc. in place of her normal predominant rice diet. She also gave history of occasional diarrheas which used to last for 1–2 days and was watery, without any blood in stools or febrile episodes.

General Physical Examination

Mild pallor but well oriented to time, place and person:

- Body mass index (BMI): 19 kg/m^2
- Pulse: 80 beats/min (bpm).

Systemic Examination

No abnormality detected.

Dermatological Examination

- Excoriated pruritic grouped papules over axillae, buttocks, trunk and proximal limbs including elbows and knees
- These papules spared palms, soles, distal limbs, face, scalp and genitalia
- Post inflammatory pigmentation was present on healing areas.

Q1. What is the most likely diagnosis?

a. Transient acantholytic dermatosis
b. Uremic pruritus
c. Cholestatic pruritus
d. Dermatitis herpetiformis (DH)

Ans: d. (Dermatitis herpetiformis)

Dermatitis herpetiformis is a blistering skin disease, which is regarded as an extraintestinal manifestation of celiac disease. DH is an itchy, blistering autoimmune skin disease exacerbated by gluten diet of wheat barley, rye and oats most often affecting the elbows, knees and buttocks. Diagnosis of DH is based on the clinical picture and demonstration of granular immunoglobulin A (IgA) deposits in the papillary dermis. DH and celiac disease share the same genetic background, having a strong association with HLA-DQ2.

Q2. How can we treat DH?

Ans: In DH, both the rash and enteropathy respond to a gluten-free diet (GFD). It takes several months on a GFD until the DH rash clears, and therefore patients with an active rash require additional treatment with dapsone (4,4-diaminodiphenylsulfone). The initial dose is usually 25–50 mg/day and, on a strict GFD, it takes approximately 2 years until dapsone can be stopped.

Q3. What is the etiological classification of generalized pruritus?

Ans: Etiological classification of generalized pruritus:

- *Dermatological*: Arising from "diseases of the skin", such as psoriasis, atopic dermatitis, dry skin, scabies and urticaria
- *Systemic*: Arising from "diseases of organs" other than the skin, such as liver (e.g., primary biliary cirrhosis), kidney (e.g., chronic renal failure), blood (e.g., Hodgkin's disease) and certain multifactorial (e.g., metabolic) states or drugs
- *Neurological*: Arising from "diseases or disorders of the central or peripheral nervous system", e.g., nerve damage, nerve compression and nerve irritation
- Psychogenic/psychosomatic
- Mixed, overlapping and coexistence of several diseases
- Other undetermined origin.

Q4. What are the common dermatological diseases associated with chronic pruritus?

Ans: Dermatological conditions with chronic pruritus:

- *Inflammatory dermatoses:* Atopic dermatitis, psoriasis, contact dermatitis, dry skin, drug reactions and "invisible dermatoses"
- *Infectious dermatoses:* Mycotic, bacterial and viral infections and folliculitis, scabies, pediculosis, arthropod reactions and insect bites
- *Autoimmune dermatoses:* Bullous dermatoses, especially DH, bullous pemphigoid, dermatomyositis and systemic lupus erythematosus
- *Genodermatoses:* Darier's disease, Hailey-Hailey disease, Sjögren-Larsson syndrome and epidermolysis bullosa pruriginosa
- *Dermatoses of pregnancy:* Polymorphic eruption of pregnancy, pemphigoid gestationis and prurigo gestationis
- *Neoplasms:* Cutaneous T-cell lymphoma (especially erythrodermic variants), cutaneous B-cell lymphoma and leukemic infiltrates of the skin.

Q5. What are the common systemic diseases associated with chronic pruritus?

Ans: Systemic conditions with pruritus:

- *Endocrine and metabolic diseases:* Chronic renal failure, liver diseases with or without cholestasis, hyperthyroidism, malabsorption, perimenopausal pruritus and hypothyroidism
- *Infectious diseases:* Human immunodeficiency virus (HIV) infection, helminthosis and parasitosis
- *Hematological and lymphoproliferative diseases*: Iron deficiency, polycythemia vera, Hodgkin's disease, non-Hodgkin's lymphoma and plasmocytoma
- *Visceral neoplasms*: Solid tumors of the cervix, prostate, or colon, carcinoid syndrome
- *Pregnancy:* Pruritus gravidarum with and without cholestasis
- *Drug-induced pruritus:* Opioids, angiotensin converting enzyme (ACE) inhibitors, amiodarone, hydrochlorothiazide, estrogens, simvastatin, hydroxyethyl starch and allopurinol
- *Neurogenic origin (without neuronal damage):* Hepatic itch with increased endogenous μ-opioids
- *Neuropathic diseases (neuronal damage causes itch):* Multiple sclerosis, neoplasms, abscesses, cerebral or spinal infarcts, brachioradial pruritus, nostalgia paresthetica, post-herpetic neuralgia, vulvodynia and small fiber neuropathy

- *Somatoform pruritus:* Psychiatric/psychosomatic diseases, depression, anxiety disorders, obsessive-compulsive disorders and schizophrenia.

Q6. What is the general history to be taken in a case of generalized itch?

Ans: History in generalized itching:
- Onset of the itch
- Severity and quality of the itch
- Timing of the itch
- Relieving/exacerbating factors
- Bathing/skin care history
- Previous treatments
- Itchy contacts
- Pets
- Recent travel or exposures
- Previous history of itch and/or rash
- Past medical history
- Medication history
- Social history
- Family history
- Review of systems.

Q7. How can we broadly classify generalized itchy disorders in elderly?

Ans: Itching disorders in elderly:
- *Generalized itch with rash:* Psoriasis, lichen planus, asteatotic eczema, airborne contact dermatitis, phytophotodermatitis (parthenium), atopic dermatitis (adult), mastocytosis, mycosis fungoides, urticaria/symptomatic dermographism, bullous pemphigoid, DH, scabies, animal mites, bed bugs and parasitic disease.
- *Generalized itch without rash:* Xerosis, thyroid disease, iron deficiency, renal failure, liver diseases, lymphomas, leukemia, multiple myeloma, paraproteinemia, polycythemia vera, carcinoid tumor, HIV, hepatitis C, Sjögren syndrome, dermatomyositis, drug hypersensitivity, aquagenic pruritus of the elderly and neurodermatitis.

Q8. What are the drugs that are known to cause generalized pruritus?

Ans: Drugs causing generalized pruritus:
- *Antihypertensives:* ACE inhibitors, angiotensin II antagonists, calcium channel blockers, beta blockers, methyldopa, sildenafil, hydrochlorothiazide and furosemide.
- *Antiarrhythmics:* Amiodarone and quinidine
- Anticoagulants: Ticlopidine and unfractionated heparins
- *Antidiabetic drugs*: Biguanides and sulfonylureas
- *Hypolipemic drugs:* Statins and nicotinic acid derivatives
- *Antibiotics*: Penicillin, cephalosporins, macrolides, carbapenems, monobactams, quinolones, tetracyclines, lincosamides, streptogramins, metronidazole, rifampicin, co-trimoxazole, antimalarials, vancomycin and erythromycinestolate
- *Psychotropic drugs:* Selective serotonin reuptake inhibitor (SSRI), tricyclics, neuroleptics, phenothiazines, lithium and benzodiazepines
- *Antiepileptics:* Phenytoin, carbamazepine, oxcarbazepine and topiramate
- *Cytostatics:* Chlorambucil, paclitaxel, tamoxifen and bleomycin
- *Biologicals*: Granulocyte-macrophage colony-stimulating factor (GM-CSF), interleukin-2 (IL2), lapatinib, matuzumab and interferon
- *Volume expanders:* Hydroxyethyl starch
- *Others:* Thyroxine, antithyroid drugs, nonsteroidal anti-inflammatory drugs (NSAIDs), sex hormones, opioids, xanthine oxidase inhibitors, aspirin, gold, penicillamine, iodinated contrast media and anabolic steroids.

Q9. What is the minimum basic screen for generalized pruritus of chronic nature?

Ans: Basic screening for chronic pruritus:
- Complete blood counts with differential
- Erythrocyte sedimentation rate with C-reactive protein
- Peripheral blood smear + marrow aspirate/biopsy if anomaly detected
- Absolute eosinophil count
- Thyroid-stimulating hormone, T4
- Blood urea, creatinine
- Alkaline phosphatase, bilirubin
- Glucose
- Chest X-ray posteroanterior and lateral views
- Age-appropriate cancer screening
- Tests for HIV, hepatitis B virus, hepatitis C virus
- Stool for ova and parasites
- Therapeutic trial of antiscabietic preparations
- Biopsy of lesion + direct immunofluorescence if rash exists
- Urinary 5-hydroxyindoleacetic acid (carcinoids): optional

- Serum protein electrophoresis (SPEP)/immune protein electrophoresis (IPEP): Optional
- *All causes ruled out*: Think occult malignancy, evolving connective tissue disease, drug-induced pruritus, psychogenic pruritus and then label idiopathic.

Q10. What are the basic measures to be advised for patients suffering from generalized pruritus?

Ans: Basic measures:

- Frequent liberal application of thick bland emollients, especially after bathing
- Avoid hot and prolonged showers
- Use unscented bath oils (coconut oil)
- Avoid irritating soaps (including herbal soaps), and all soaps except to apocrine-gland-bearing areas
- Avoid friction from washcloths
- Consider using a humidifier
- Treat inflamed, dry skin with mild topical steroids
- Using moisturizers or barrier creams regularly (ideally with low pH)
- Applying moisturizers immediately following bathing will ensure a higher retention of moisture
- Keeping finger nails short
- Wearing light and loose clothing
- Maintaining a comfortable temperature
- Using an air conditioner in the summer
- Restricting time in the shower or bathtub
- Showering/bathing in cool or lukewarm water, as hot water can be drying
- Avoiding cleansers with a high pH or those containing alcohol.

Q11. What is the therapeutic ladder for cholestatic pruritus?

Ans: *TIER I*

- *Cholestyramine*: 4–16 g PO (give 30 minutes before and after breakfast & 30 minutes before lunch) or cholestipol 5–30 g daily
- *Rifampicin*: 300 mg thrice a week or 150–300 mg bid
- *Naltrexone*: 25–50 mg daily
- Oral antihistamines
- *Ursodeoxycholic acid*: 10–20 mg/kg daily or silymarin 140 mg daily.

TIER II

- *Sertraline*: 75–100 mg daily
- *Paroxetine*: 20 mg daily
- Ultraviolet phototherapy
- *Naloxone*: intravenous (IV) bolus 0.4 mg, then 0.2 μg/kg/m

TIER III

- *Phenobarbital*: 2–5 mg/kg daily
- *Lidocaine*: 100 mg IV daily
- *Butorphanol nasal spray*: 1–2 mg daily
- IV propofol (in conjunction with anesthetist)
- Bright light therapy
- Molecular adsorbent recirculating system (albumin dialysis) for severe acute itch crisis
- Liver transplant.

Q12. Describe the therapeutic ladder for renal pruritus.

Ans: *TIER 1*

- Emollients, moisturizers
- Oral antihistaminics
- Increase dialysis frequency and efficiency
- Change dialysis chemical if needed
- *Hyperphosphatemic itch*: Sevelamer/lanthanum carbonate
- *Capsaicin*: 0.025–0.1% 4–5 times daily.

TIER II

- *Gabapentin*: 100–300 mg PO three times a week or post dialysis
- *Doxepin*: 10 mg bid
- Broadband ultraviolet B thrice a week
- Gamma linolenic acid cream.

TIER III

- *Tacrolimus*: 0.1% locally bid
- *Thalidomide*: 100 mg daily
- *Activated charcoal*: 6 g daily
- *Nicergoline*: 5 mg IV during dialysis
- *Granisetron*: 1 mg bid
- Nalfurafine: 5 μg after dialysis
- Aprepitant
- Renal transplant.

CHAPTER 120

Scabies

Gopikrishnan Anjaneyan, Brijesh C

Case study Scabies

Presenting Complaints

Doctor, I am a student staying in a hostel and have developed itching along with reddish raised lesions all over the body.

Setting

Dermatology outpatient department

History of Present Illness

An 18-year-old boy presented with complaints of itching for the last 20 days which was sudden in onset, which started from right hand, slowly spreading all over the body. The nocturnal exacerbation of itching was disturbing his sleep. His hostel roommates had similar complaints.

General Physical Examination and Systemic Examination

No abnormality detected.

Dermatological Examination

- Excoriated pruritic papules over web spaces, sides of fingers, wrist, nipples, axillae and trunk (Fig. 1)
- Multiple erosions over the trunk
- Multiple erythematous papulonodules are present over glans penis and groins.

Q1. What is the most likely diagnosis?

a. Atopic dermatitis
b. Scabies
c. Allergic contact dermatitis
d. Dermatitis herpetiformis

Ans: b. (Scabies)

Presence of acute onset, pruritus usually sparing the face in adults with nocturnal exacerbation, similar history in close contacts, typical distribution of excoriated papules in a characteristic distribution suggests a diagnosis of scabies.

Q2. What is the causative organism?

Ans: Scabies is caused by an arthropod mite of the order Acarina called Sarcoptes scabiei variety hominis.

Q3. How many pair of legs does an adult Sarcoptes scabiei mite has?

a. Two
b. Three
c. Four
d. Five

Ans: c. (Four)

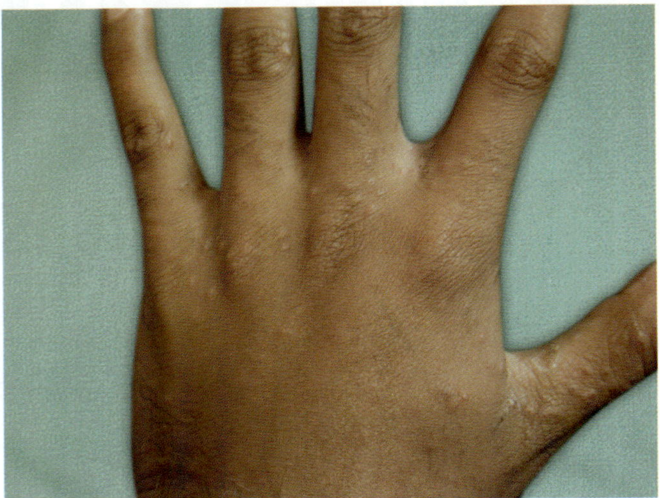

Fig. 1: Multiple excoriated papules over finger webs

The adult female mite measures 0.4 mm long by 0.3 mm broad, and the male measures 0.2 mm long by 0.15 mm broad. They have four pairs of legs.

Q4. What is the incubation period of scabies?

Ans: It takes approximately 2–6 weeks for pruritus to start after host immune system gets sensitized to the mite in first-time infestation. A reinfestation is usually recognized much earlier by the host and pruritus starts within 1–2 days.

Q5. What is the circle of hebra?

Ans: Circle of hebra is an imaginary circle intersecting the main sites of involvement, i.e., axillae, elbow flexures, wrists and hands and genitals.

Q6. Which is the pathognomonic lesion of scabies?

a. Excoriated papule
b. Lichenified scaly plaque
c. Burrow
d. Subungual hyperkeratosis

Ans: c. (Burrow)

It represents the tunnel that a female mite excavates below stratum corneum while laying eggs. It is 1–10 mm in length and is thread-like, grayish-white to skin colored. It is rarely seen in early cases and after patients have excoriated the affected sites.

Q7. Enumerate various investigations to confirm the diagnosis.

Ans: A classical history and examination of the patient and history of close contact is usually diagnostic. Following investigations are seldom required for diagnosis or for academic purposes:

- A burrow is gently scraped off and the material placed in oil on a slide under the microscope and the presence of mites, eggs or scybala confirms the diagnosis. A drop of India ink or gentian violet is applied to the infested area and then removed with alcohol. Thin thread-like burrow retains the ink.
- In adhesive tape test it is applied on a scabietic skin lesion, then pulled off and contents transferred directly onto a slide for microscopy.
- Dermoscopy is useful picturing the mites in its burrow resembling a "jet-with-contrail" or hang glider sign.
- Skin biopsy shows nonspecific changes but is diagnostic if a mite or its parts can be identified.
- Enzyme-linked immunosorbent assays, polymerase chain reaction and confocal microscopy, specific immunoglobulin E directed toward major mite components have been used in some studies.

Q8. Does using 10% potassium hydroxide for skin scraping give better results on microscopy for scabies?

Ans: Potassium hydroxide can dissolve mite pellets so should never be used for microscopic diagnosis of scabies.

Q9. Enumerate the various treatment options available for scabies.

Ans: Following are the scabicidal agents used:

- Permethrin cream 5%
- Crotamiton lotion or cream 10%
- Sulfur (5–10%) ointment
- Lindane lotion 1%
- Benzyl benzoate 25% ointment
- Oral ivermectin as 200 μg/kg/dose.

Ideally, clothes and bed linens coming in contact within 2–3 days of application of topical scabicidal agents should be machine washed with warm water and aerosolized insecticide should be used for materials that cannot be washed.

Moisturizers and oral antihistaminics are often prescribed with the above medications for symptomatic relief. All close contacts or family members ought to be treated together for effective management of scabies.

Q10. Why is lindane not the first line of treatment for scabies?

Ans: Lindane also known as gamma benzene hexachloride is an organochlorine compound which received an

FDA (Food and Drug Administration) "black box warning" in 2003. Overuse or accidental swallowing of lindane can be toxic to central nervous system. It should be used in patients who cannot tolerate other lesser toxic medications.

Lindane should not be used to treat premature babies, infants, people weighing less than 50 kg, pregnant or breastfeeding women, elderly patients and people with a seizure disorder or with extensive erosions leading to percutaneous absorption.

Q11. Ivermectin is available in which formulation?

Ans: Oral ivermectin is available as 6 mg tablets and given in the dose of 200–400 µg/kg. It is usually administered twice, 1–2 weeks apart.

Topical ivermectin is also available now as a 1% cream and it is also available as 0.5% lotion for pediculosis capitis.

Q12. What is the role of sulfur in scabies?

Ans: Precipitated sulfur is available as 5–10% paste which is applied over the body and kept overnight for 3 consecutive days. It is relatively safe for infants even less than 2 months of age, pregnant and breastfeeding women. It is messy to apply, has bad odor, may cause skin irritation and has questionable efficacy.

Q13. What is crusted scabies?

Ans: Crusted scabies also known as Norwegian or hyperkeratosis scabies is a rare and highly contagious severe form of the disease, characterized by the infestation of up to millions of mites, and hence may be the source of an outbreak of common scabies. It results in development of hyperkeratosis crusts over the skin frequently involving the acral areas and rarely trunk (Fig. 2). The thick scaly plaques can be misdiagnosed as psoriasis, eczema, Darier's disease or ichthyosis.

Crusted scabies occurs commonly in immunocompromised patients or debilitated patients, including those with neurologic disorders, Down's syndrome, organ transplants, graft versus host disease or leprosy.

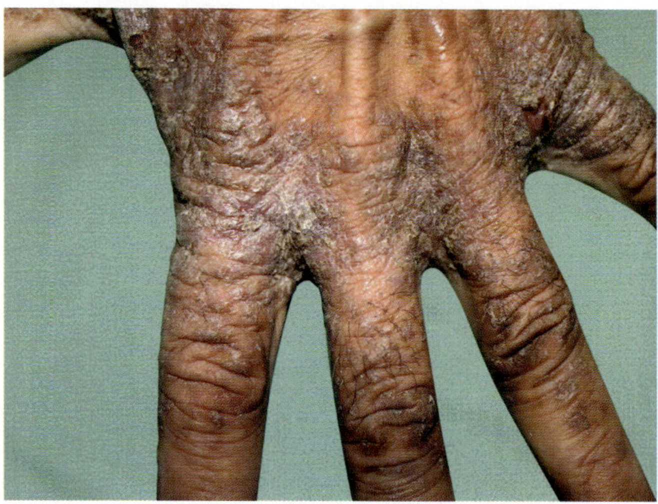

Fig. 2: Crusted lesions in the web spaces in Norwegian scabies

Q14. What is nodular scabies?

Ans: Nodular scabies represents a hypersensitivity reaction to mite antigens presenting as erythematous pruritic nodules often located in the groin, axillae and male genitalia. These lesions may persist for weeks or months even after successful treatment with scabicidal drugs. Topical steroids and crotamiton creams are sometimes given for complete resolution of the nodules.

Q15. When does the pruritus stop after successful treatment of scabies?

Ans: Itching may persist several weeks after successful treatment of scabies with scabicidal, so it should be thoroughly explained to the patient. Emollients may be helpful in cutaneous irritation, overtreatment or mild eczematization. The persistence of itching after 4 weeks must be reinvestigated for treatment failure, psychogenic pruritus or other causes and managed accordingly.

CHAPTER 121

Urticaria

Shruthi C

Case study **Urticaria**

Presenting Complaints

Doctor, I have itchy rashes on the body on and off since 5 days. They disappear after few hours to reappear again at a different place.

Setting

Dermatology outpatient department

History of Present Illness

A 35-year-old lady presented with complaints of itchy, red rashes all over the body since 5 days following a vacation. Symptoms are more at night and rashes subside over few hours but only to reappear elsewhere on the body. No history of preceding medications or known allergies. Itching is intense to hamper her daily activities and feels relief on rubbing or scratching the lesions.

General Physical Examination and Systemic Examination

No abnormality detected

Dermatological Examination

- Erythematous wheals on the scalp, face, trunk, limbs, palms and soles (Fig. 1)
- Few excoriations on the thighs
- No edema of the lips or genitals.

Q1. What is the most likely diagnosis?

a. Urticaria
b. Insect bite reactions
c. Erythema multiforme
d. Tinea corporis

Ans: a. Urticaria (transient nature of erythematous wheals on history, absence of punctum or targetoid lesions).

Q2. What is urticaria?

Ans: Urticaria is a cutaneous reaction pattern consisting of raised, erythematous skin lesions (wheals) that are markedly pruritic, evanescent and generally worsened by scratching and caused by a multitude of factors. It can be due to both immunologic and nonimmunologic mechanisms.

Q3. Which are the points that aid in the diagnosis of urticaria?

Ans: Important characteristics:

- Itchy, erythematous, raised lesions (wheals) of various sizes and shapes
- Transient (lasting for few hours)

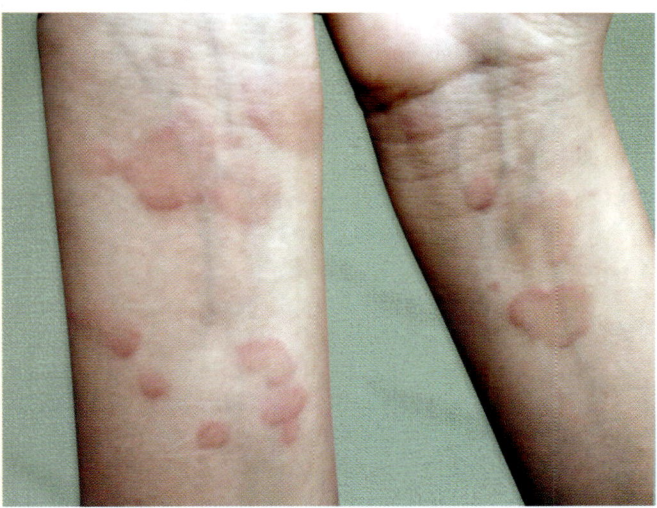
Fig. 1: Erythematous wheals over the forearms

- Patients tend to rub than scratch
- Can occur anywhere on the body
- May be preceded by systemic symptoms of malaise, vomiting, headache, abdominal pain, diarrhea
- Positive dermographism (in chronic and physical urticaria)
- Absence of edema of lips or labia majora (suggestive of angioedema).

Q4. How do you classify urticaria?

Ans: Classification of urticaria:

- Ordinary urticaria:
  - Acute (less than 6 weeks of continuous activity)
  - Episodic (acute and chronic intermittent)
  - Chronic (more than 6 weeks of continuous activity)
- Physical urticaria:
  - Mechanical stimuli:
    - Dermographism
    - Pressure urticaria
    - Vibratory angioedema
  - Temperature-related stimuli:
    - Heat and stress (cholinergic urticaria, localized heat contact urticaria)
    - Stress urticaria
    - Cold urticaria
  - Exercise-induced urticaria
  - Solar urticaria.
  - Aquagenic urticaria.
- Urticarial vasculitis
- Contact urticaria
- Angioedema without wheals
- Syndromes resembling urticaria or angioedema, or with urticaria as a component
  - Muckle-Wells syndrome
  - Familial Mediterranean fever
  - Systemic capillary leak syndrome.

Q5. What are the causes for ordinary acute urticaria?

Ans: Causes of acute urticaria:

- Idiopathic
- Infections:
  - Upper respiratory tract infection
  - Streptococcal infection
  - Hepatitis B infection
  - Anisakiasis
- Allergy (immediate hypersensitivity):
  - Foods
  - Drugs
  - Inhalants
- Nonallergic: Histamine liberators (e.g. codeine, atracurium)
- Pseudoallergens:
  - Aspirin and other nonsteroidal anti-inflammatories
  - Dietary (food additives, natural salicylates)
  - Radiocontrast media.

Q6. What are the causes for chronic urticaria?

Ans: Causes:

- Idiopathic
- Autoimmunity: Functional autoantibodies (50% cases)
- Pseudoallergens: Salicylates, food colors, preservatives, antioxidants
- Infections
  - Bowel parasites
  - *Helicobacter pylori*
  - Candidiasis of the bowel
  - Chronic sepsis (e.g. dental abscess).

Q7. How do you approach a patient with urticaria?

Ans: Approach to urticaria:

Initial workup:

- History taking:
  - Time of onset (time of day, time of year)
  - Duration of urticaria (acute or chronic)
  - Duration of individual lesion
  - Enquiry for food, food additives, drugs, infection
  - Enquiry for home and work environment
  - Family history of thyroid and other autoimmune diseases
  - History of atopy
  - History of dental diseases
- Physical examination:
  - Morphology of lesion (small papules, plaques, combination of lesions)

- Distribution (localized, generalized, sun exposed skin, other sites)
- Tests for physical urticaria (stroke, exercise, ice cube test)
- Features of systemic involvement (fever, arthralgia)
- Clinical evidence of infection (dental caries, sinusitis, cystitis, vaginitis)

Laboratory workup and special tests:

- Initial screening tests:
  - Complete blood count, differential, erythrocyte sedimentation rate, platelet count
  - Liver function tests
  - Thyroid function tests
  - Urinalysis
  - Serology for infections
  - Stool for ova and parasites
- Disease-specific focused tests:
  - Physical urticaria: Challenge tests
  - Contact urticaria: Open patch test, prick test, scratch test, use test, in vitro radioallergosorbent test (RAST)
  - Autoimmune urticaria: Autologous serum skin test (ASST), basophil release test
  - Urticarial vasculitis: Complement 3, total complement activity (CH50), skin biopsy
  - Thyroid diseases: Thyroid antibodies
  - Hepatic diseases: Hepatitis-associated antigens and antibodies
  - Collagen vascular diseases: Antinuclear antibodies and other disease-specific tests.

Q8. What is urticaria activity score?

Ans: The urticaria activity score (UAS) consisted of the sum of the wheal number score and the itch severity score. The wheal numbers and itch severity are graded from 0 to 3 in Table 1.

Table 1: Urticaria activity score

Score	*Wheals*	*Pruritus*
0	No	No
1	Mild (less than 20 wheals in a day)	Mild (Not troublesome)
2	Moderate (20–50 wheals in a day)	Troublesome but does not disturb sleep
3	Severe (more than 50 wheals in a day or large confluent areas of whealing)	Severe pruritus disturbing sleep and normal daily activity

One has to add both these scores, viz., for both the number of wheals and the severity of itch, on a given day for each of the days in a given week to get the weekly UAS. The possible weekly aggregate UAS, thereby, ranged from 0 to 42.

Q9. How is autologous serum skin test carried out and what is its interpretation?

Ans: Autologous serum skin test is a test to differentiate autoimmune urticaria (subset of chronic urticaria) from chronic idiopathic urticaria. Autoimmune urticaria patients exhibit functional autoantibodies against immunoglobulin E (IgE) and/or its high-affinity receptor (FcεRI).

Method: Approximately 0.05 mL, each of autologous serum, histamine diphosphate and sterile physiological saline is injected separately intradermally over volar aspect of the left forearm. After 30 minutes (15 minutes for histamine), the wheal formed at each injection site is measured. Positive ASST is the one with serum-induced wheal which has both redness and a diameter of more than or equal to 1.5 mm as compared to the saline-induced wheal at 30 minutes.

The reported prevalence of ASST positivity in patients of chronic urticaria varies from 35% to 58% in various studies. Despite being the most accessible and useful test for demonstrating endogenous vasoactive factors in the patient's blood with chronic idiopathic urticaria, a positive ASST is not synonymous to autoimmune urticaria.

Q10. What are the other tests for autoimmune urticaria?

Ans:
- Autologous serum skin test
- Peripheral basophil count (to document basopenia by a sensitive assay)
- Functional release assays with basophils and mast cells
- Immunoassay.

Q11. What are the tests for physical and cholinergic urticaria?

Ans: Tests for the diagnosis of physical and cholinergic urticaria are given in Table 2.

Q12. How do you differentiate urticaria from urticarial vasculitis?

Ans: Differences are listed in Table 3.

Q13. How do you treat a case of urticaria?

Ans: Treatment:

General measures:

- Identify and avoid trigger factors when there is a known cause (Foods, drugs, physical causes)

Table 2: Tests for the diagnosis of physical and cholinergic urticaria

Physical urticaria	*Challenge test*
Dermatographism	Itchy wheals occur in minutes lasting less than 1 hour after: • Firm stroking of the skin with a smooth blunt object • A calibrated dermographometer set at 36 g/mm² or less
Delayed pressure urticaria	Sustained pressure is applied to the back, shoulder or thigh: • 4.5 kg weighted rods with 1.5 cm diameter applied for 15 minutes • Dermographometer set at 100 g/mm² pressed against the back of the shoulder for 70 seconds, read after 2–6 hours and next day • Hanging a weight 15 lbs (7 kg) by a broad strap from a shoulder results in a wheal, often painful, at the application site 4–6 hours later, lasting from several hours up to 24 hours
Cholinergic urticaria	Raising the core body temperature by 0.7–1.0°C by exercise in a hot environment or a hot bath (42°C) for 15 minutes induces itching within minutes, with widespread small wheals
Cold urticaria (contact)	Application of a melting ice cube in a thin plastic bag for up to 20 minutes results in an itchy wheal at the site within minutes of removal
Cold urticaria (generalized)	Placing the patient (with supervision) in a cold room at 4°C for 30 minutes induces widespread small wheals; the ice cube test is negative
Solar urticaria	Exposure to sunlight or solar simulator induces redness, itchy wheals at site of exposure within a few minutes lasting less than 1 hour
Vibratory angioedema	Application of a laboratory vortex resting on the forearm or finger for 1–5 minutes results, within minutes, in a red swelling of the vibrated area, lasting less than 1 hour
Aquagenic urticaria	Exposure of skin to water at body temperature in a bath for 15 minutes induces small itchy wheals on the immersed site within minutes

- Treat underlying cause (Infections, infestations)
- Antipruritic, cooling skin lotions such as calamine lotion or 1% menthol in aqueous cream may help to relieve itching.

First-line therapies:

- H1 antihistamines: Cetirizine, chlorpheniramine, levocetirizine, hydroxyzine, loratadine, fexofenadine

Table 3: Differentiation between urticaria and urticarial vasculitis

	Ordinary urticaria	*Urticarial vasculitis*
Duration	Few hours	24–72 hours
Symptoms	Itchy wheals, transient, resolve without hyperpigmentation	Burning and pain more than itching, fixed for 3–5 days and resolve with post inflammatory pigmentation
Systemic symptoms	Occasionally present	More frequent: Fever, malaise, arthritis, conjunctivitis, pain in abdomen, glomerulonephritis
Cause	Immunologic (type I hypersensitivity) and nonimmunologic causes	Type III hypersensitivity reaction with cutaneous vasculitis
Histopathology	Edema of the dermis or subcutaneous tissue, dilatation of venules but no evidence of vascular damage. Mast cell degranulation	Edema of dermis with vasculitis: Perivascular inflammation, fibrinoid necrosis, leukocytoclasis
Association	Infections, drugs, food, atopy	Autoimmune disorders: Systemic lupus erythematosus, Sjögren's syndrome Infections: Hepatitis B, hepatitis C, Epstein-Barr virus Malignancies: Multiple myeloma, carcinoma colon

- Combination of H1 and H2 antihistamines

Second-line therapies:

- Systemic corticosteroids
- Leukotriene receptor antagonists: Montelukast, zafirlukast
- Omalizumab
- Other immunosuppressants: Cyclosporine, mycophenolate mofetil

Third-line therapies:

- Plasmapheresis
- Intravenous immunoglobulin)

Other interventions:

- Thyroxine has been tried in euthyroid patients with positive thyroid autoantibodies
- Stanozolol in glucocorticoid-dependent urticaria

- *Helicobacter pylori* eradication therapy in chronic idiopathic urticaria
- Nifedipine as an adjunctive therapy with H1 antihistamines
- Hydroxychloroquine, colchicine, dapsone and indomethacin have been tried in urticarial vasculitis with apparent success
- Tolerance induction by graduated exposure to stimuli
- Phototherapy and photochemotherapy
- Autologous serum therapy (Autoimmune urticaria).

Step-wise approach

- Step 1: Use nonsedating H1 antihistamine
- Step 2: Increase dose of the antihistamine up to four times or add another antihistaminic
- Step 3: Add leukotriene inhibitor or other second-line agents like Cyclosporine, Omalizumab.

CHAPTER 122

Angioedema

Gopikrishnan Anjaneyan

Case study Angioedema

Presenting Complaints

Doctor, I have been getting repeated episodes of swelling of the lips and genitals, sometimes accompanied by light headedness, dizziness and vomiting since past 5 years.

Setting

Dermatology outpatient department

History of Present Illness

A 16-year-old girl presented with complaints of recurrent episodes of swelling of the lips and/or genitals since the last 5 years. She has never got skin lesions over any part of the body. There is an increase in frequency and severity during her menstruation periods and school examinations. These episodes are sometimes accompanied by dizziness, abdominal cramps and vomiting. There is no history of breathing difficulty. Her father has a history of similar but milder lip-swelling episodes. She has no other comorbidities and is not on any medications.

General Physical Examination

Well oriented to time, place and person
Body mass index: 17 kg/m^2, pulse: 90 bpm, lip edema ++, no pedal edema

Systemic Examination

No abnormality detected

Dermatological Examination

- Both lips are edematous. Rest of oral cavity normal.
- No skin lesions over other parts of the body
- Genital examination: normal

Q1. What is the most likely diagnosis?

a. Granulomatous cheilitis
b. Hereditary angioedema
c. Chronic spontaneous urticaria
d. Episodic angioedema with eosinophilia (Gleich syndrome)

Ans: b. Hereditary angioedema (HAE)

Repeated episodes of angioedema without urticaria with gastroenterological symptoms in a patient in 2nd decade without any other significant aggravating factors suggest a diagnosis of HAE.

Q2. What is hereditary angioedema?

Ans: Hereditary angioedema is an autosomal dominant disorder caused by low levels of the acute phase protein C1 inhibitor (C1 esterase inhibitor or C1-INH) in plasma. It is characterized by recurrent episodes of angioedema, without urticaria or pruritus affecting the mucosae of the upper respiratory and gastrointestinal tracts.

Q3. What are the types of hereditary angioedema?

Ans: There are three types of HAE:

- HAE type I (85%) is the result of mutations in the genetic code that cause decreased transcription of the gene coding for C1-INH.
- HAE type II (15%) occurs due to genetic defect that allows for the transcription of a functionally defective C1-INH protein. This results in normal or slightly elevated quantitative but decreased functional levels of C1-INH.
- HAE type III has similar clinical findings but with normal C1-INH levels. It is seen mostly in women with some patients having factor XII defect.

Q4. The gene coding for the C1 esterase inhibitor is located on which chromosome?

a. Chromosome 5
b. Chromosome 9
c. Chromosome 11
d. Chromosome 17

Ans: c. Chromosome 11

SERPING1 gene coding for C1 esterase inhibitor is located on long arm q of chromosome 11.

Q5. Which is the single recommended screening test for C1-INH deficiency?

a. C4 level
b. C3 level
c. Quantitative C1-INH
d. C1q level

Ans: a. C4 level

Serum C4 level is suggested as a screening test for C1-INH deficiency.

In HAE, the C4 level is less than 30% of mean normal.

If the C4 level is low, then C3 level and function of C1-INH should be measured.

Q6. How do you classify a case of angioedema without wheals?

Ans: Angioedema without wheals can be divided into two broad categories: mast cell mediator induced (histaminergic) and bradykinin induced (non-histaminergic).

Mast cell mediator induced includes ordinary (spontaneous) urticaria and physical (inducible) urticaria (which very rarely causes only angioedema)

Bradykinin-induced urticaria includes HAE and acquired angioedema (Fig. 1).

Q7. How will you investigate and diagnose a case of angioedema without wheals?

Ans: Diagnosis is primarily made clinically based on a suggestive history and physical findings. Detailed clinical history and review of systems will help in identifying underlying causes.

Routine investigations to rule out inflammatory or infectious disorders are complete blood count with differential counts, liver function tests, renal function tests, urine routine microscopy, C-reactive protein and erythrocyte sedimentation rate.

Complement 4 is a good screening blood test for HAE types I and II, especially during attacks. It should be less than 30% of mean normal in affected patients.

If the C4 level is low, then level and function of C1-INH should be measured.

A low C1-INH level and function is suggestive of HAE type I.

If the C1-INH level is normal but the function is low, then it is likely to be hereditary angioedema type II.

Both C4 and C1-INH will be normal in type III HAE.

In acquired C1-INH deficiency, C4 and functional C1-INH are low and C1q is also reduced.

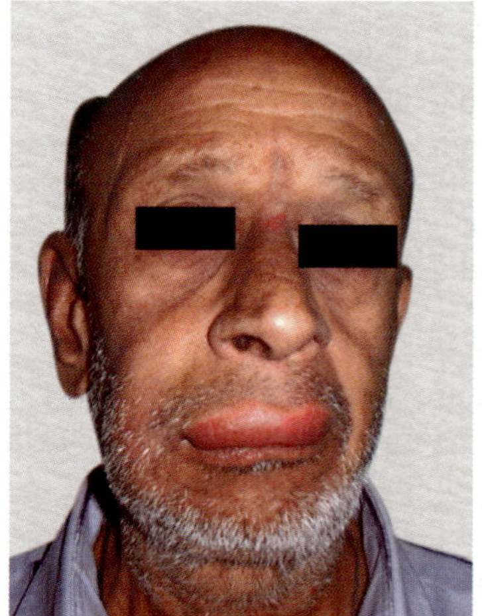

Fig. 1: Acquired angioedema

Q8. What are the treatment principles for angioedema?

Ans: Treatment of histaminergic angioedema:

- *For mild cases:* Antihistamines, usually second-generation drugs up to even four times the standard dosage can be preferred, if required. Steroids, immunomodulators (like cyclosporine) and omalizumab are other treatment options.
- *Moderate to severe cases:* Parenteral diphenhydramine and hydrocortisone is to be given and the patient is to be kept under close monitoring.
- *Severe cases with airway obstruction:* Airway should be secured and intubation or tracheostomy, if necessary, is performed. Injection epinephrine (1:1000) is given and repeated every 10 minutes till response. Patient should be admitted for observation for at least 24 hours.

Treatment of HAE is divided into three categories as follows:

- *Treatment for acute attacks:* Airway should be secured. One of the following options should be considered according to the availability, cost and patient compliance:
  - C1 inhibitor concentrate (derived from human plasma)
  - Recombinant human C1 inhibitor
  - Human plasma or fresh frozen plasma
  - Icatibant (a synthetic bradykinin B2-receptor antagonist)
  - Ecallantide (a recombinant plasma kallikrein inhibitor)
- *Short-term prophylaxis:* Short-term prophylaxis is indicated if invasive procedures, oral surgery or general surgery is planned and it is done using plasma-derived C1-INH.
- *Long-term prophylaxis*: Long-term prophylaxis consists of using plasma-derived C1-INH, fibrinolytics (tranexamic acid), anabolic steroids (danazol, stanozolol).

Q9. What are the differential diagnoses of angioedema?

Ans: Differential diagnoses:

- Allergic dermatitis
- Cellulitis and erysipelas
- Gleich syndrome (episodic angioedema with eosinophilia)
- Ascher syndrome (swelling of lips, blepharochalasis, and nontoxic thyroid enlargement)
- Cheilitis granulomatosa (Miescher's cheilitis) and Melkersson-Rosenthal syndrome
- Autoimmune conditions including systemic lupus, dermatomyositis, scleroderma and Sjogren's syndrome
- Hypothyroidism (cause skin changes mimicking angioedema)
- Muckle-Wells syndrome (urticaria-deafness-amyloidosis syndrome)
- Venous obstructive diseases (superior vena cava syndrome, deep vein thrombosis)
- Facial lymphedema
- Parasitic infections (Trichinella spiralis can cause periorbital edema).

Q10. What is the complement level profile of patients with angioedema?

Ans: Complement profile testing for different causes of angioedema:

- C1-INH: Decreased-HAE Type 1, acquired angioedema
- C4: Decreased- HAE Type 1, 2 and acquired angioedema
- C1Q: Decreased only in acquired angioedema.

Q11. Can angiotensin-converting enzyme inhibitor-induced angioedema occur after many months or years?

Ans: Yes, though the majority of angioedema cases occur in the first few weeks following start of angiotensin-converting enzyme (ACE) inhibitor, it can occur at any time and cases have been reported even after prolonged use for months to years.

Q12. Can patients having history of angioedema to angiotensin-converting enzyme inhibitor be started on angiotensin receptor blockers?

Ans: Angiotensin receptor blockers (ARBs) have also been very rarely reported to cause angioedema; hence, its safety after an episode of ACE inhibitor-induced angioedema is not well established.

Though controversial, if no other substitute is available then ARBs can be started in such patients after properly educating the patient regarding the possibility of ARB-induced angioedema. A fact to be considered is that ARBs have cardioprotective actions and hence are a preferred choice over other antihypertensives.

Q13. How does danazol work in prophylaxis of hereditary angioedema?

Ans: Danazol is used for long-term prophylaxis of HAE and works by increasing the hepatic synthesis of C1-INH. It is also thought to cause an increased synthesis of aminopeptidase P, another major enzyme responsible for the breakdown of bradykinin. Danazol is started in the dose of 100–200 mg daily.

Q14. What is the role of tranexamic acid in hereditary angioedema?

Ans: Antifibrinolytics like tranexamic acid are generally preferred over androgens for long-term prophylaxis in children and pregnant women due to their side-effect profile.

The mechanism of action of tranexamic acid in HAE is not well understood. It is an antifibrinolytic (protease inhibitor) which inhibits the conversion of plasminogen to plasmin and also inhibits activated plasmin. These fibrinolysis steps are also inhibited by C1-INH. Tranexamic acid possibly helps in treating HAE due to a sparing effect on C1-INH, which is the natural inhibitor.

It is given as 2–4 g in two divided doses daily.

SECTION 25

Miscellaneous Disorders

Harish Prasad

CHAPTER 123

Lichen Planus

Indrashis Podder

Case study Lichen Planus

Presenting Complaints

Doctor, I have developed these itchy, dark colored lesions around both my ankles and wrists since the last 4 months.

Setting

Dermatology outpatient department of a tertiary medical center

History of Present Illness

A 38-year-old man presented to us with the complaints of developing dark colored, elevated, itchy lesions around his ankles and wrists for the last 4 months. Initially, they developed around the ankles and were few in number, which have gradually increased. He also complains of burning sensation in the mouth at the time of food intake (especially spicy foods) for the last 2.5 months. Drug history and family history are unremarkable.

General Examination and Systemic Examination

Within normal limits

Dermatological Examination

- Presence of violaceous, flat-topped, polygonal papules and plaques with scanty adherent scales; average diameter ranging from 0.5–1 cm
- Sites: Bilateral distribution, around the ankles and on the volar aspect of both wrists
- Grayish or whitish streaks present on the surface of lesion in a crisscross fashion (Wickham's striae)
- Lesions show evidence of Koebner phenomenon
- Some lesions have healed leaving behind hyperpigmented macular areas
- Oral mucosa: White, lacy rash on the buccal mucosa (opposite the molars); bilateral distribution. Genital mucosa and conjunctiva are spared
- Nails: All finger and toe nails show hyperkeratosis and longitudinal ridging; the right index finger nail shows pterygium.

Q1. What is the most probable diagnosis?

a. Lupus erythematosus
b. Lichenoid drug eruption
c. Lichen planus
d. Lichenoid dermatitis

Ans: c. Lichen planus (LP).

Q2. What are the points in favor of your diagnosis?

Ans: Diagnosis:

- Presence of pruritic, polygonal, violaceous or purple (Fig. 1), plane (flat-topped) papules and plaques (6 Ps)
- Presence of Wickham's striae

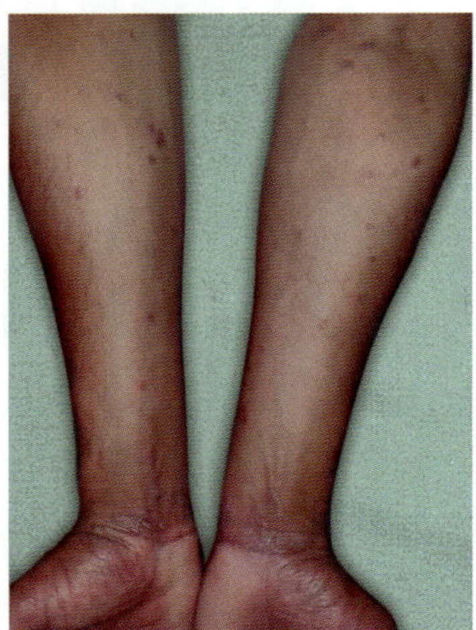

Fig. 1: Multiple violaceous papules on the forearm

- Presence of Koebner phenomenon
- Characteristic of oral mucosal lesion: whitish, lacy, reticulate rash on the posterior aspect of buccal mucosa (bilaterally symmetrical distribution)
- Characteristic nail involvement: 20 nails involvement, nail pterygium
- Old lesions heal with characteristic hyperpigmentation.

Q3. What are the common areas of predilection for development of lichen planus?

Ans: The common sites of predilection for LP include flexor aspect of the wrists, around the ankles, trunk, medial thighs, shins, dorsal hands and glans penis. It rarely occurs on the face, eyelids or lips.

Q4. How will you confirm your diagnosis?

Ans: Although, clinical picture suggests the diagnosis, a histopathological examination (HPE) is necessary to confirm the diagnosis.

Q5. Mention the classical histopathological picture of lichen planus.

Ans: The classical HPE finding of LP is given below:

Epidermis:
- Orthokeratotic hyperkeratosis
- Wedge-shaped hypergranulosis (clinically manifested as Wickham's striae)
- Saw-toothed rete ridges with irregular acanthosis
- Diffuse vacuolar degeneration of the basal layer
- Presence of Civatte bodies or colloid bodies (degenerated basal cells).

Dermis:
- Presence of Max-Joseph space (artefact created below the basal layer due to its degeneration)
- Band like lymphohistiocytic infiltration along the basement membrane (interface dermatitis).

Q6. What is the direct immunofluorescence finding in a case of lichen planus?

Ans: Classically, direct immunofluorescence (DIF) demonstrates the deposition of fibrin along the dermoepidermal junction (DEJ), which is classical for LP.

Q7. How will you treat such a patient?

Ans: The treatment is described in Figure 2:

Topical therapies:
- Topical corticosteroids is the mainstay of topical therapy.
- Topical tacrolimus or pimecrolimus have been found to be useful in oral LP.
- Intralesional corticosteroid in severe cases (nail LP, lichen planus hypertrophicus (LPH), etc.)

Systemic therapies:
- Systemic corticosteroids (0.5–1 mg/kg a day, long-term maintenance at lowest possible dose for about 8–12 weeks may be necessary to maintain remission)
- Other systemic immunosuppressives: cyclosporine, azathioprine, mycophenolate mofetil, etc.
- Systemic retinoids (isotretinoin, acitretin) and oral antimalarials like hydroxychloroquine for oral LP.
- Anecdotal reports: Metronidazole (400 mg twice daily for 6 weeks), griseofulvin, low-molecular-weight heparin (3 mg subcutaneous injection once a week)
- Newer therapies: Biologicals (alefacept).

Physical therapies:
- Narrowband ultraviolet B (NB-UVB)
- UVA1
- Psoralen with ultraviolet A (PUVA).

Q8. What are lichenoid disorders?

Ans: Lichenoid disorders are a group of cutaneous disorders characterized by diffuse lymphohistiocytic infiltration along the DEJ. The infiltrate is dense enough to obscure the DEJ.

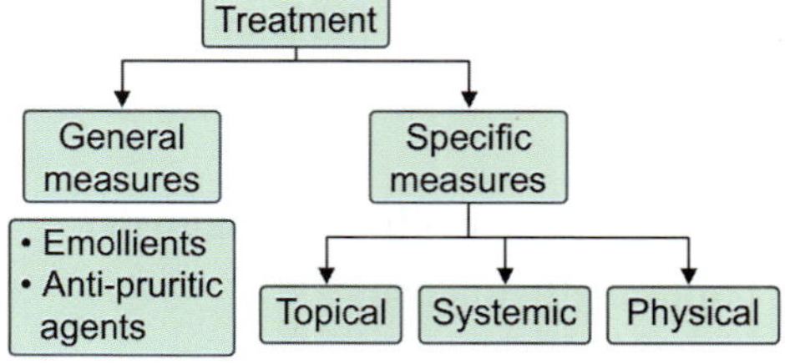

Fig. 2: Treatment in lichen planus

Q9. Name some common lichenoid disorders.

Ans: Some common lichenoid disorders are listed below:
- Lichen planus and its variants
- Lupus erythematosus
- Cutaneous lymphoma
- Polymorphic light eruption
- Hansen's disease.

Q10. What is Koebner phenomenon?

Ans: The Koebner (isomorphic) phenomenon is the development of similar pathological lesions in uninvolved skin along the line of trauma. This phenomenon was described by Heinrich Koebner.

Q11. Which of the following diseases do not show Koebner phenomenon?

a. Lichen planus
b. Psoriasis
c. Vitiligo
d. Viral warts (verrucae)

Ans: d. Viral warts (verrucae)
It shows pseudo-Koebner phenomenon. Molluscum contagiosum also shows pseudo-Koebner phenomenon.

Q12. Enumerate the various types of lichen planus.

Ans: The common variants of LP are listed below:
- Actinic LP
- Eruptive LP
- Annular LP
- Atrophic LP
- Bullous LP and lichen planus pemphigoides (LPP)
- Hypertrophic LP or LPH
- Inverse LP
- Lichen planus pigmentosus
- Lichen planopilaris
- Linear LP
- Lupus eythematosus-LP overlap syndrome
- Nail LP
- Oral LP
- Ulcerative LP or perforating LP
- Vulvovaginal LP
- Lichenoid drug eruption
- Palmoplantar LP.

Q13. Explain bullous lichen planus and lichen planus pemphigoides.

Ans: Bullous LP refers to development of vesicles or bullae only over preexisting LP lesions. When vesiculobullous lesions also develop on uninvolved skin, the condition is called LPP.

Q14. What are the common nail changes in lichen planus?

Ans: Common nail changes:
- Longitudinal ridging and splitting
- Onycholysis and red lunula
- Pterygium formation is very characteristic (the proximal nail fold fuses with the proximal portion of the nail bed)
- Subungual hyperkeratosis and onychopapilloma (in nail bed LP).

Q15. Mention some drugs causing lichen planus.

Ans: There are several drugs that may cause lichenoid eruption, some of the important drugs are listed below:
- Antitubercular drugs (rifampicin)
- Anticonvulsants (phenytoin)
- Antipsychotics (carbamazepine)
- Diuretics (thiazide diuretics)

Table 1: The differentiating features of drug-induced lichenoid eruption and classic lichen planus

Features	*Lichenoid drug eruption*	*Classic LP*
Distribution of skin lesions	More generalized, often spares the 'classic' sites of LP (viz. flexor wrists)	Flexor aspect of the wrist and forearm, lower legs, genitalia, etc.
Clinical appearance	More scaly (eczematous or psoriasiform)	Shiny, flat-topped, violaceous papules with minimal scaling
Wickham's striae	Uncommon	Present
Photodistribution	Frequent	Unusual
Mucosal involvement	Rare	Often involved (oral >genital)
Histology	Focal parakeratosis, eosinophilic and/or plasma cell infiltrate	No parakeratosis, dense band-like lymphohistiocytic infiltrate at DEJ, eosinophils/plasma cells uncommon

Abbreviations: LP, lichen planus; DEJ, dermoepidermal junction

- Nonsteroidal anti-inflammatory drugs (ibuprofen)
- Oral hypoglycemics (sulphonylurea)
- Antimalarials (chloroquine) (Antimalarials are also used for the treatment)
- Heavy metals (gold)
- Sildenafil
- Griseofulvin (also used in the treatment).

Q16. How can you differentiate drug-induced lichenoid eruption and classic lichen planus?

Ans: The differentiating features are given in Table 1.

CHAPTER 124

Annular Erythema

Akhilesh Shukla

Case study Annular Erythema

Presenting Complaints

Doctor, I have been having these red, raised, round lesions since last 18 months on my buttocks, trunk and thighs. Sometimes, there is slight itching on these lesions and white flakes at the margins.

Setting

Dermatology outpatient department

History of Presenting Complaints

A 42-year-old male presents with complaints of recurrent round, red lesions over trunk, buttocks, thighs, arms and legs for the last 18 months. The eruption began as small, red, raised lesions that joined together into ring-like lesions. Most of the lesions had flaking at margins. Occasionally, there is mild itching. The course of disease is relapsing and remitting. Some lesions disappear spontaneously with no treatment, while similar lesions occurred in the adjacent skin. There is no history of drug intake prior to these lesions. No family history of similar complaints.

General Physical Examination and Systemic Examination

Within normal limits

Dermatological Examination

There are multiple well-defined erythematous, annular or arcuate plaques with polycyclic borders present symmetrically over trunk, thighs, buttocks, legs and arms. There is also presence of small erythematous papules, few of them coalescing into annular plaques with central clearing and centrifugal spread. Most of the lesions show scale on the inner part of the raised border (Fig. 1). Face, hands and foot are spared. His hair, nails and mucosa are normal.

Q1. What is the most likely diagnosis?

a. Erythema annulare centrifugum
b. Urticarial vasculitis
c. Erythema migrans
d. Tinea corporis

Ans: a. Erythema annulare centrifugum (EAC).

Q2. What is erythema annulare centrifugum?

Ans: Erythema annulare centrifugum is an annular erythema that is typically characterized by annular, polycyclic and erythematous plaques with scaling behind the advancing edge.

Q3. How do the lesions in erythema annulare centrifugum progress?

Ans: Lesions first appear as erythematous indurated papules that slowly enlarge to form a ring as the

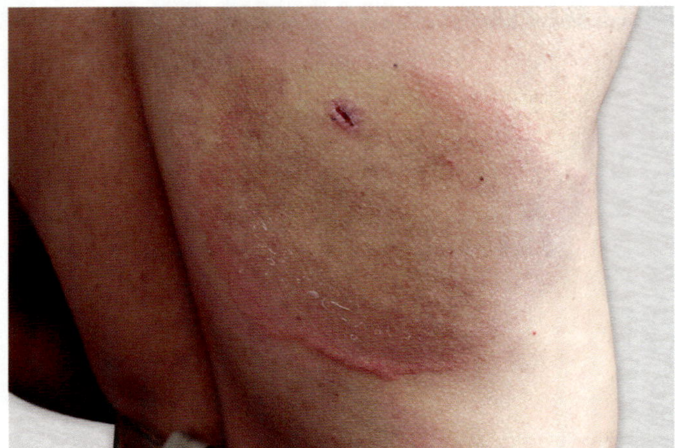

Fig. 1: Large erythematous annular plaque with trailing scale inside the margins

central area flattens and fades. The lesions may be static, have a varied rate of expansion (typically 2–3 mm/day), and the extension may be irregular producing arciform segments.

Q4. Describe the other clinical features of erythema annulare centrifugum?

Ans: Lesions may be solitary or, more often, multiple and last from a few days to months or years. Itching is variable, but seldom intense. The commonest sites are the buttocks, thighs and upper arms, but any area may be involved. Purpura and pigmentation may rarely occur within the lesions. There is no age or sex predilection for EAC. EAC may be of variable duration, lasting from days to decades, with a mean of 2.8 years.

Q5. Which of the following can be a cause of erythema annulare centrifugum?

a. Drugs
b. Infection
c. Malignancies
d. All of the above

Ans: d. All of the above

Erythema annulare centrifugum is a reactive process which may be precipitated by drugs, infection or malignancy. The commonest underlying association is concurrent infection, and most commonly this is within the skin with dermatophytosis being implicated in up to 48% of the cases. However, in most of the cases, the underlying cause is not identified. Table 1 describes the causes and associations of EAC.

Table 1: Causes and associations of erythema annulare centrifugum

Causes	*Associations*
Fungal infections	Dermatophytoses, candida
Bacterial infections	Mycobacteria, streptococci, *Escherichia coli*, syphilis, *Pseudomonas*, septicemia
Viral infections	Epstein-Barr virus, HIV, herpes simplex, herpes zoster, Molluscum contagiosum, viral hepatitis
Parasitic infections	Ascaris, lumbricoides, Phthirus pubis
Drugs	Acetazolamide, amitriptyline, ampicillin, cimetidine, co-trimoxazole, finasteride, gold, hydrochlorothiazide, nonsteroidal anti-inflammatory drugs, penicillin, salicylates, spironolactone, chloroquine and hydroxychloroquine
Endocrine	Hyperthyroidism, pregnancy
Infantile	Annular erythema of infancy
Autoimmune	Autoimmune hepatitis, lupus erythematosus, polyglandular autoimmune disease type I, relapsing polychondritis, Sjögren syndrome
Paraneoplastic	Lymphoproliferative malignancies, solid tumors including prostate adenocarcinoma, non-small cell lung cancer, breast cancer and malignant carcinoid tumor of the bronchus

Q6. What are the types of erythema annulare centrifugum?

Ans: Two types of EAC are traditionally distinguished in the literature: a *superficial type* (pruritic and scaling) with trailing scale on the inner border of the erythematous lesions and a *deep type* with infiltrated non-scaly plaques (non-pruritic and non-scaling). Scaling is the main distinguishing clinical sign of superficial EAC. Histology, in addition to confirming the depth of the inflammatory infiltrate, makes evident other differences between the superficial and deep forms (Table 2).

Q7. List the differential diagnoses of erythema annulare centrifugum.

Ans: Erythema annulare centrifugum must be differentiated from other annular erythematous lesions. They include:

- Transient lesions: urticaria, erythema marginatum
- Lesions for more than 24 hours: urticarial vasculitis, annular erythema of infancy, erythema migrans, Wells syndrome
- Granulomatous lesions: Leprosy (Borderline tuberculoid or tuberculoid leprosy), granuloma annulare, sarcoidosis
- Papulosquamous lesions: Tinea corporis, pityriasis rosea, annular lupus erythematosus, annular

Table 2: Clinicopathological variants of erythema annulare centrifugum		
Histologic findings	*Superficial erythema annulare centrifugum*	*Deep erythema annulare centrifugum*
Acanthosis	Occasionally	Absent
Parakeratosis	Present	Absent
Spongiosis	Focally present	Absent
Dyskeratosis	Absent	Occasionally
Dermoepidermal involvement	Absent	Present focally in almost 50% cases
Depth of inflammatory infiltrate	Superficial	Superficial to deep
Dermal edema	Occasionally	Absent

psoriasis, erythema gyratum repens, secondary syphilis.

Q8. How can you classify figurate lesions?

Ans: Figurate lesions can mimic each other clinically and might be very difficult to ascertain the exact diagnoses. Pathologically, the lesions can be classified depending on the principal component of the inflammatory cells (Table 3).

Q9. How do you confirm the diagnosis of erythema annulare centrifugum?

Ans: Investigations are aimed at excluding alternative diagnoses and identifying an underlying cause. As fungal infections are the commonest cause of EAC, a potassium hydroxide (KOH) mount of the scale is helpful. Additionally, a culture of affected skin and nails should be undertaken if a dermatophyte infection is suspected.

Biopsy of lesional skin and direct immunofluorescence will help to confirm the diagnosis and to exclude differential diagnoses. A spectrum of nonspecific histological findings is seen in EAC and it is critical to have clinicopathological correlation.

The characteristic histological feature in EAC is a perivascular 'sleevelike' lymphohistiocytic infiltrate which may be mainly superficial, mainly deep or mixed.

Additional investigations would include a full blood count, liver and thyroid function tests, abdominal ultrasound and chest X-ray. An antinuclear antibody profile, serum angiotensin-converting enzyme and HIV serology should also be checked; if a malignancy is suspected, positron emission tomography and computed tomography scanning should be undertaken.

Q10. How do you treat a case of erythema annulare centrifugum?

Ans: The goal of management is to identify and treat the underlying cause. The first-line topical management for EAC is medium potent to potent topical steroids and topical calcipotriol. The second-line treatment options are topical tacrolimus and phototherapy. In severe and recalcitrant patients, systemic steroids, chloroquine and hydroxychloroquine can be prescribed. Emollients help in alleviating the scaling and allow better penetration of the above said medications.

Table 3: Figurate lesions: classification according to the principal component of the inflammatory infiltrate			
Lymphocytic	*Neutrophilic-eosinophilic*	*Granulomatous*	*Plasma cells*
• EAC, superficial form • EAC, deep form • Polymorphous light eruption • Lupus erythematosus tumidus • Subacute lupus erythematosus • Chronic erythema migrans • Indeterminate leprosy • Erythema gyratum repens • Necrolytic erythema • Erythema multiforme • Erythrokeratodermia variabilis • Mycosis fungoides	• Annular psoriasis • Sneddon-Wilkinson syndrome • IgA pemphigus • Linear IgA dermatosis • Bullous pemphigoid • Leukocytoclastic vasculitis • Eosinophilic vasculitis • Urticarial vasculitis • Eosinophilic dermatosis • Erythema marginatum rheumatica • Annular erythema of infancy • Eosinophilic erythema annulare • Neutrophilic figurate erythema	• Granuloma annulare • Sarcoidosis • Borderline leprosy • Tuberculoid leprosy	• Secondary syphilis

Abbreviations: EAC, erythema annulare centrifugum; IgA, immunoglobulin A

Topical antipruritics and sedating antihistamines can be prescribed if there is associated pruritus. Even in the absence of an identifiable cause, some authors have advocated the empiric use of antibiotics or antifungal agents. Although systemic corticosteroids can induce a clinical remission, recurrences are common when the medication is discontinued.

There are recent reports of improvement in resistant cases of EAC with tumor necrosis factor α inhibitors–etanercept in 50 mg weekly dosage.

CHAPTER 125

Erythema Multiforme

Anju George

Case study Erythema Multiforme

Presenting Complaints

Doctor, I have been having painful ulcers in my mouth for the past 2 weeks and reddish, raised lesions on my hands and legs for the past 1 week. I have fever with severe body ache too.

Setting

Dermatology outpatient department

History of Present Illness

A 30-year-old male patient presented with complaints of painful ulcers in the oral cavity for 2 weeks duration. One week back, he had developed low grade fever and myalgia, and almost 2 days after the onset of fever, he noticed reddish raised asymptomatic lesions on the body. The skin lesions initially appeared on the hands and legs, and soon progressed to involve the forearms, thighs and trunk, with individual lesions gradually increasing in size. There is no history of photosensitivity, joint pain or weight loss and no history of prior drug intake. However, he gave history of similar episodes of oral ulceration, twice over the past 6 months, which subsided with medications.

General Examination

Moderately built and nourished; well oriented to time, place and person
Palpable cervical lymph nodes present, no pallor or pedal edema
Pulse: 90/min, Temperature: 101.6° F

Systemic Examination

No significant abnormality detected

Dermatological Examination

- Multiple, mostly discrete erythematous and edematous papules and plaques, distributed almost bilaterally symmetrically on both upper and lower extremities and anterior trunk. Most of the plaques have three zones, a central dark area surrounded by a pale middle zone and an outer erythematous border (Figs 1 and 2).
- Similar plaques present on the palms and soles
- Oral mucosa: Multiple confluent erosions with a scalloped border involving the buccal mucosae, lips and soft palate (Fig. 3)
- Eyes: Mild conjunctival congestion present
- Genital mucosa: Normal.

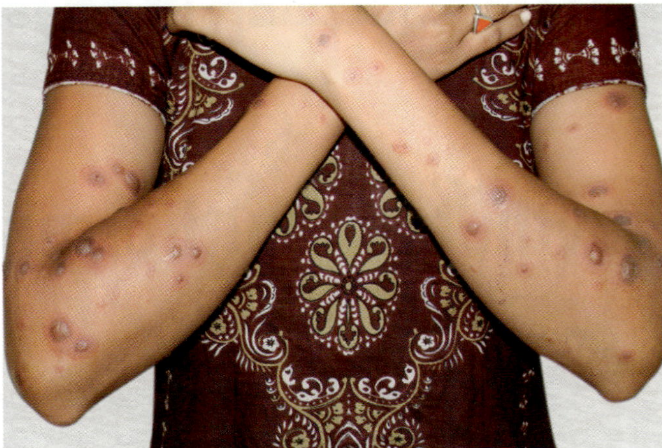

Fig. 1: Target lesions on both forearms

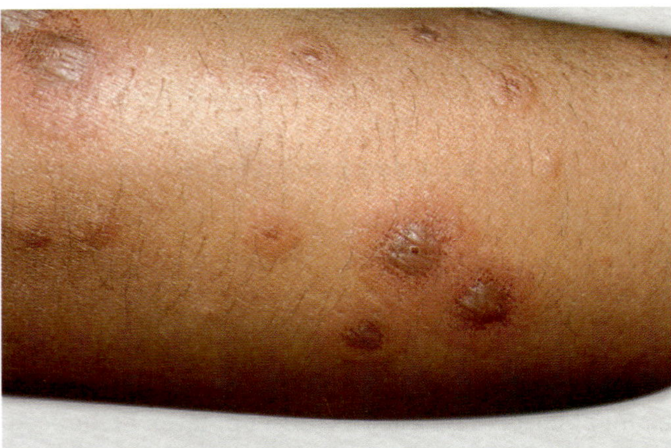

Fig. 2: Close up of the target lesions

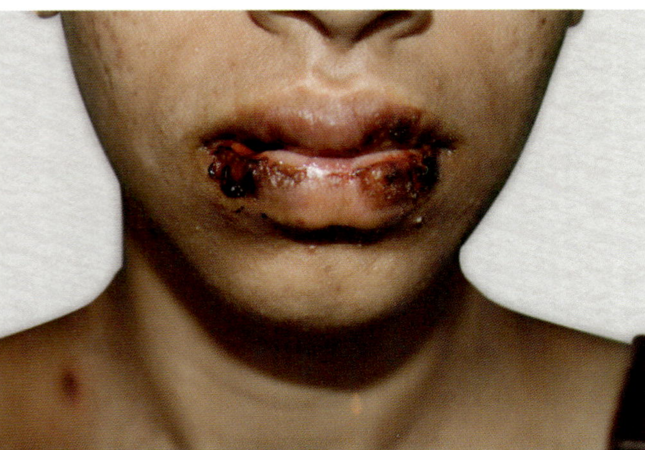

Fig. 3: Hemorrhagic crusts on lips

Q1. What is the most likely diagnosis?

a. Erythema multiforme major
b. Erythema multiforme minor
c. Stevens-Johnson syndrome
d. Rowell's syndrome

Ans: a. Erythema multiforme (EM) major

Presence of skin lesions having three characteristic zones, referred to as typical targets, along with fever and mucosal involvement points to a diagnosis of EM major.

Q2. What is erythema multiforme?

Ans: Erythema multiforme is an acute, self-limited, usually mild and often relapsing mucocutaneous syndrome, characterized by abrupt onset of symmetric, fixed erythematous papules which evolve into typical or atypical target lesions.

Q3. What do you think is the most likely cause for erythema multiforme in this scenario?

a. Drug-induced
b. Herpes virus infection
c. Systemic lupus erythematosus
d. Behcet's disease

Ans: b. Herpes virus infection

Infections account for more than 90% cases of EM, the most common being herpes virus infection (HSV 1). EM eruptions begin on an average of 7 days after a recurrence of herpes.

Q4. What are the different causes of erythema multiforme?

Ans: Causes:

- Infections (>90%)
  - Herpes simplex virus (mostly HSV 1)
  - *Mycoplasma pneumoniae*
  - Other viruses: Orf virus, *Varicella-zoster* virus, parvovirus B19, hepatitis B and C viruses
  - Bacterial: *Rickettsia*, *Chlamydia*, *Salmonella*, mycobacteria
  - Fungal: Histoplasma
- Drugs (<10% cases—nonsteroidal anti-inflammatory drugs, penicillin, sulfa drugs, tetracycline, phenytoin, etc.)
- Topical sensitizers (poison ivy, Primula obconica, nickel, rubber, etc.)
- Systemic diseases (inflammatory bowel disease, lupus erythematosus (LE), Behcet's disease, malignancies)

- Idiopathic (neither HSV nor any other cause can be identified).

Q5. How do you diagnose erythema multiforme?

Ans: Diagnosis is based on the history and clinical features. Patient will give history of a mild prodrome and history suggestive of usually HSV infection or drug intake prior to onset of lesions. The classical skin lesion of EM is known as *typical target or iris lesion.* These are plaques, less than 3 cm in diameter, with raised regular round shape and well-defined borders, having at least three different zones—a central dusky red zone/blister/purpura, a pale intermediate zone and an outer erythematous zone or halo. They appear almost symmetrically and show an acral distribution, on the extensor surfaces of extremities and face. They are usually asymptomatic. Severe disease shows mucous membrane erosions, and a history of previous attack is present in one-third of patients.

Q6. In a person with herpes simplex virus infection and erythema multiforme, are all episodes of erythema multiforme preceded by clinically-evident herpes simplex virus infection?

Ans: No. Not all episodes are preceded by clinically-evident EM and not all HSV episodes are followed by EM. Episodes of recurrent HSV infection may precede the development of HSV-related EM by many years.

Q7. Why the term 'multiforme' is used?

Ans: There are usually lesions of varying morphology coexisting, hence the term erythema 'multiforme'.

Q8. What is the cause for typical target or iris lesion?

Ans: The inflammatory activity may regress or relapse, leading to concentric rings of color.

Q9. What are the other skin lesions of erythema multiforme besides iris lesions?

Ans: Other skin lesions:

- Raised atypical targets: display two rings only
- Livid vesicles may occur. Larger lesions may have a central bulla and a marginal ring of vesicles, known as 'herpes iris of Bateman'
- Giant targets may occur
- Duration of individual lesion is less than 2 weeks
- Residual pigmentation may remain for months without any scarring.

Q10. Describe mucous membrane involvement in erythema multiforme.

Ans: Seen in almost 70% cases and mostly involves the oral cavity.

- Lips (cutaneous and mucosal aspect), buccal mucosae, ventral tongue and non-attached gingivae are involved
- Hard palate and attached gingivae are usually spared
- Erosions with fibrinous deposits are seen; occasionally intact vesicles or bullae are noted
- Eyes: Begins with pain, bilateral conjunctivitis, vesicles and erosions
- Nasal, urethral, anal mucosae may be inflamed
- Ectodermosis pluriorificialis: Severe involvement of two or three mucosal sites in the absence of skin lesions.

Q11. How do you classify the spectrum from erythema multiforme to Stevens-Johnson syndrome and toxic epidermal necrolysis?

Ans: Classification was proposed by Bastuji-Garin et al. in 1993 and revised in 2002 (Table 1).

Q12. What is the difference between erythema multiforme major and erythema multiforme minor?

Ans: Differences:

- *Erythema multiforme minor:* Skin lesions without mucosal involvement; no systemic involvement and is mostly due to infections.
- *Erythema multiforme major:* Skin lesions and mucosal involvement; systemic involvement is present and may be due to infections and drugs.

Table 1: 2002 Classification of Stevens-Johnson syndrome, toxic epidermal necrolysis and erythema multiforme

Erythema multiforme major	Epidermal detachment (ED) <10% body surface area (BSA), typical targets (TT) or raised atypical targets (RAT), acral distribution
SJS (Stevens-Johnson syndrome)	ED <10% BSA, blisters on macules, flat atypical targets (FAT), widespread erythematous macules
SJS-TEN (toxic epidermal necrolysis) overlap	ED 10–29% BSA, blisters on macules, FAT, widespread erythematous macules
TEN with spots	ED >30% BSA, blisters on macules, FAT, widespread erythematous macules
TEN without spots	ED >10% BSA, no discrete lesions, widespread large erythematous areas.

Q13. How do you confirm the diagnosis?

Ans: Diagnosis can be confirmed by histopathologic examination of the lesion, which will rule out other possibilities. Vacuolar interface dermatitis with necrosis of individual keratinocytes or satellite cell necrosis in the basal layer is the *hallmark of EM*.

Q14. What are the other relevant investigations?

Ans: Relevant investigations:

- Complete blood count with erythrocyte sedimentation rate (ESR). In severe cases, raised ESR and leukocytosis occur
- Serology for HSV
- Direct immunofluorescence, antinuclear antibodies—in suspected LE
- Tzanck smear in bullous EM, shows lymphocytes
- Chest X-ray and polymerase chain reaction assay of throat swab—to rule out *M. pneumoniae.*

Q15. What of the following conditions present with erythema multiforme like skin lesions?

a. Paraneoplastic pemphigus
b. Lupus erythematosus
c. Sarcoidosis
d. All of the above

Ans: d. All of the above conditions can present with EM-like skin lesions.

Q16. What are the clinical differential diagnoses?

Ans: Differential diagnoses:

- Urticaria
- Maculopapular drug eruption
- Bullous pemphigoid
- Paraneoplastic pemphigus
- Urticarial vasculitis
- Stevens-Johnson syndrome
- Rowell's syndrome (cutaneous LE with lesions resembling EM).

Q17. How will you treat erythema multiforme?

Ans: Treatment:

- Symptomatic treatment
- Avoid all drugs (in drug-induced EM)
- Management of ocular complications
- In herpes-associated EM: Acyclovir 400 mg thrice daily for 1 week
- Suppressive therapy: Acyclovir 400 mg twice daily for up to 1 year (>6 episodes a year)
- Episodic treatment given accordingly
- Role of systemic steroids is controversial. Prednisolone 30–60 mg/day tapered over 1–4 weeks tried in severe disease
- Thalidomide: In recurrent EM

Other drugs: Dapsone, azathioprine, mycophenolate mofetil, cyclosporine.

CHAPTER 126

Pruritic Urticarial Papules and Plaques of Pregnancy

Indrashis Podder

Case study Pruritic Urticarial Papules and Plaques of Pregnancy

Presenting Complaints

Doctor, I am 7 months into pregnancy, and recently I have developed these itchy bumpy lesions over my abdomen, thighs, buttocks and breasts.

Setting

Dermatology outpatient department (OPD) of a tertiary medical center

History of Present Illness

A 29-year-old primigravida was referred to us from the Gynecology Department with complaints of severe itching for the last few days. On enquiry the lady revealed that she was 7 months into pregnancy, and developed these itchy lesions since the last 2 weeks. These lesions started over her abdomen, most conspicuous over her striae. Gradually, similar lesions also appeared over her thighs, buttocks and breasts.

General Examination

Alert, conscious, cooperative, vitals → stable, mild pallor present.

Systemic Examination

Within normal limits.

Dermatological Examination

- Urticarial papules and plaques scattered over the abdomen (lesions are present over the striae) (Fig. 1), thighs, breasts and buttocks
- A few purpuric, vesicular and polycyclic lesions also noted
- Discrete, pruritic, excoriated papules were observed, some of them being crusted
- The lesions were perifollicular in distribution
- Her genital region, fingerwebs and flexures were spared
- Hair, nail, mucosa → spared.

Q1. What is the most probable diagnosis?

a. Scabies
b. Atopic dermatitis
c. Pruritic urticarial papules and plaques of pregnancy (PUPPP)/polymorphic eruption of pregnancy
d. Cholestasis of pregnancy

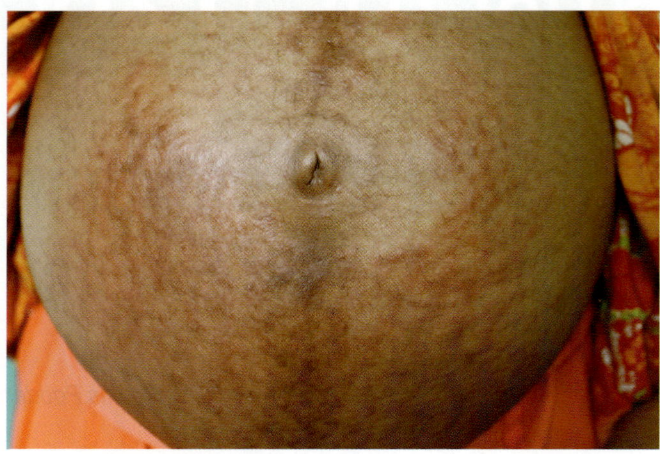

Fig. 1: Erythematous papules, wheals and plaques on the striae

Ans: c. PUPPP/polymorphic eruption of pregnancy.

Q2. What are the points in favor of your diagnosis from history?

Ans: Points in favor of diagnosis from history:

- Onset in the later part of pregnancy
- Primigravida (PUPPP occurs exclusively in primigravidae)
- Absence of generalized pruritus, sparing of fingerwebs and genitalia rules out scabies.
- Absence of flexural involvement and signs of atopy rules out atopic dermatitis.
- Absence of constitutional symptoms, sparing of palms and soles help us to rule out cholestasis of pregnancy.

Q3. How will you confirm your diagnosis?

Ans: Usually this is a clinical diagnosis. Proper history, temporal association with late pregnancy, typical distribution over the striae is sufficient to make this diagnosis. Biopsy and histopathological examination (HPE) may be needed to rule out other dermatoses of pregnancy, viz. impetigo herpetiformis, pemphigoid gestationalis. PUPPP shows hyperkeratosis, acanthosis and papillomatosis on skin HPE.

Q4. How will you treat this patient?

Ans: Proper counseling regarding the disease is of utmost importance in managing this patient. Topical antipruritic agents are prescribed along with systemic antihistamines in severe cases. Amongst antihistamines, loratadine is the first choice. Recently it has been shown that all antihistamines can be prescribed, except hydroxyzine during pregnancy. However, it is recommended to avoid systemic medications, especially during the early part of pregnancy, unless it becomes an absolute necessity. Topical corticosteroids can be used in severe cases.

Q5. What are the pregnancy dermatoses?

Ans: Pregnancy is a physiological state characterized by altered endocrine, metabolic and immunological milieus. These alterations result in multiple cutaneous changes, both physiological and pathological, collectively called the pregnancy dermatoses.

Q6. What are the physiologic skin changes seen during pregnancy?

Ans: Some of the important physiological cutaneous changes during pregnancy are given below:

- Pigmentary skin changes:
  - Diffuse hyperpigmentation
  - Selective hyperpigmentation (genitalia, axillae)
  - Secondary areolae
  - Linea nigra (hyperpigmented line from pubic symphysis to xiphoid process of sternum)
  - Melasma
  - Darkening of ephelides and melanocytic nevi
- Hair:
  - Hirsutism
  - Thickening of scalp hair
  - Postpartum telogen effluvium
  - Postpartum androgenetic alopecia
- Nail:
  - Subungual hyperkeratosis
  - Distal onycholysis
  - Transverse grooving
  - Brittleness
- Glandular:
  - ↑ Eccrine gland function: Miliaria, dyshidrotic eczema
  - ↑ Sebaceous function: Montgomery's tubercle, seborrheic dermatitis
  - ↓ Apocrine function (improvement of hidradenitis suppurativa)
- Structural changes:
  - Striae distensae/striae gravidarum (areas most prone to stretch → abdomen, thighs, buttocks and breasts)
  - Acrochordons/skin tags
- Vascular changes:
  - Spider angioma
  - Palmar erythema
  - Carpal tunnel syndrome
  - Non-pitting edema

  - Varicosities
  - Livedo reticularis
  - Dermatographism
  - Purpura
  - Pyogenic granuloma
  - Hemangiomas
- Mucosae:
  - Gingivitis
  - Jacqueimer Chadwick sign (bluish discoloration of vagina and cervix)
  - Goodell's sign (cervical softening).

Q7. Classify the pathological dermatoses, which may develop during pregnancy.

Ans: Several pathological dermatoses may develop during the course of pregnancy. These pathological dermatoses can be classified in the following pattern:
- Atopic eruption of pregnancy
- Eczema in pregnancy
- Prurigo of pregnancy (early onset)
- Pruritic folliculitis
- Polymorphic eruption of pregnancy (late-onset prurigo)/Besnier's prurigo (previously called PUPPP)
- Pemphigoid gestationis/herpes gestationis
- Prurigogravidarum/intrahepatic cholestasis of pregnancy
- Impetigo herpetiformis/pustular psoriasis of pregnancy.

Q8. What is pemphigoid gestationis?

Ans: Pemphigoid gestationis also known as herpes gestationis is an intensely pruritic, vesiculobullous eruption arising in the 2nd/3rd trimester of pregnancy and immediately postpartum.
- Clinical feature (CF) → This condition is characterized by the development of tense vesicles and bullae, initially periumbilical in distribution, gradually progressing to involve the trunk, abdomen, back and extremities. Sparing of face, mucosae, palms and soles is characteristic. These lesions heal with residual scarring.
- Fetal risk → This condition may be associated with fetal risks, viz. low-birth weight, preterm delivery and neonatal pemphigoid gestationalis.
- Investigations → Skin histopathology shows well-circumscribed subepidermal blister. Direct immunofluorescence (DIF) shows immunoglobulin G (IgG), immunoglobulin M (IgM) and/or complement (C3) deposition in the basement membrane zone.
- Differential diagnoses (DD) → Polymorphic eruption of pregnancy (PUPPP), erythema multiforme, drug reaction, bullous scabies, dermatitis herpetiformis.
- Treatment → Topical corticosteroids with antihistamines is the mainstay of treatment, in severe cases systemic treatment may be needed (corticosteroids, dapsone) after evaluating the risk-benefit ratio.
- Prognosis → The disease may resolve spontaneously in the later part of pregnancy, only to flare up at the time of delivery. There may no recurrence with successive pregnancies. However, recurrence has been reported in 5–10% cases with menstruation and/or oral contraceptive pill (OCP) use.

Q9. What are the features of impetigo herpetiformis?

Ans: Impetigo herpetiformis also known as pustular psoriasis of pregnancy is characterized by the formation of discreet, sterile pustules in a pregnant female.
- Onset → This condition arises in the 3rd trimester of pregnancy.
- CF → Erythematous, scaly patches and plaques with discreet, subcorneal (superficial) pustules at their margins.
- Distribution → This condition begins in the flexures, and gradually spreads centrifugally.
- Risk → There is fetal risk in the form of stillbirth resulting from placental insufficiency.
- Course → There is rapid resolution of symptoms after delivery; however, recurrences in subsequent pregnancies are common and more severe.
- DD → Pustular drug eruption (acute generalized exanthematous pustulosis), pemphigoid gestationis, subcorneal pustular dermatosis, generalized impetigo, etc.
- Investigations → Skin HPE shows subcorneal pustules with dense neutrophilic aggregation.
- Treatment → Topical corticosteroids, systemic corticosteroids, symptomatic treatment.

Note: Impetigo herpetiformis is the only type of psoriasis where systemic corticosteroids form the first-line of treatment.

Q10. What are the distinguishing features of cholestasis of pregnancy?

Ans: This condition also known as obstetric cholestasis, intrahepatic cholestasis of pregnancy, prurigo gravidarum and icterus gravidarum occurs due to elevated level of bile acid in the blood resulting from hormonal alteration.

- Onset and course → Occurs in the 3rd trimester of pregnancy, when the hormonal levels are maximum; there is spontaneous resolution following delivery.
- CF → Moderate-to-severe pruritus leading to excoriated papules which may be either generalized or localized to palms and soles. Constitutional symptoms, like fatigue, nausea and vomiting, may be present. The condition may progress to clinical jaundice, dark-colored urine or light-colored stools.
- Laboratory investigations → Degree of pruritus correlates with the bile acid concentrations, and it is the most sensitive indicator.
- Treatment → Cholestyramine, ursodeoxycholic acid (UDCA), narrowband ultraviolet B (NB-UVB) have been found to be beneficial along with symptomatic treatment in the form of bland emollients and antipruritic agents.
- Risks →
  - Fetal: Preterm delivery, fetal distress, fetal death may occur due to anoxia and aspiration of meconium stained fluid.
  - Maternal: Increased chance of postpartum hemorrhage (PPH) due to depletion of vitamin K, development of cholelithiasis/gallbladder disease.

Q11. Which of the pregnancy dermatoses is not associated with increased fetal risk?

a. Pemphigoid gestationis
b. Cholestasis of pregnancy
c. Polymorphic eruption of pregnancy/PUPPP
d. Impetigo herpetiformis

Ans: c. Polymorphic eruption of pregnancy/PUPPP.

CHAPTER 127

Erythema Nodosum

Sherina Laskar

Case study Erythema Nodosum

Presenting Complaints

Doctor, I have been having painful reddish swellings on my lower legs for the past 2 weeks and I also feel slightly feverish and unwell.

Setting

Dermatology outpatient department.

History of Present Illness

A 30-year-old lady presented with complaints of sudden onset of painful reddish swellings over her legs for the last 2 weeks. She also had mild fever on-and-off and accompanied malaise. She remembers having fever and sore throat a week before developing these lesions. There is no personal or family history of tuberculosis, and no history of diarrhea, joint pain, or skin lesions elsewhere on the body. Her menses are regular and she is not on oral contraceptive or any other medication.

General Physical Examination

The patient is well oriented in time, place and person

- Temperature: 98.6°F
- Pulse rate: 96 beats/min
- Blood pressure: 110/70 mm Hg
- Multiple, discrete, mildly tender submandibular lymph nodes: 1.5–2.0 cm in greatest diameter.

Systemic Examination

No abnormality detected.

Dermatologic Examination

- Multiple, slightly tender, bilaterally symmetrical, dusky erythematous, nodules and plaques on the shins, sized 1–5 cm (Fig. 1)
- Overlying skin is warm to touch
- Contusion-like color changes present over flattened lesions.

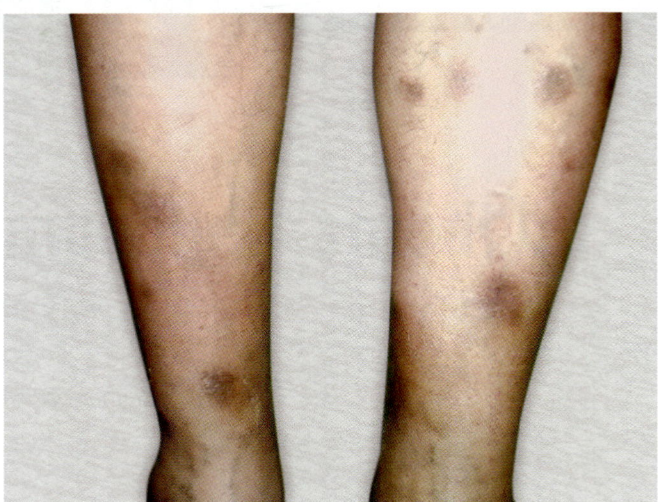

Fig. 1: Multiple nodules with hyperpigmented surface on anterior aspect of both legs

Q1. What is the most likely diagnosis?

a. Sweet's syndrome
b. Erythema nodosum (EN)
c. Erythema induratum
d. EN leprosum

Ans: b. Erythema nodosum. Bilaterally symmetrical, tender nodules and plaques of recent onset on the extensor aspect of the lower extremities, with associated bruise-like color changes over subsiding lesions in a young female patient suggest this diagnosis. A history of fever, malaise and sore throat are contributory, but not essential to the diagnosis. Absence of ulceration also helps differentiate it from other conditions, such as erythema induratum.

Q2. What other sites may be affected by EN?

Ans: Thighs, extensor aspects of the arms, neck, or face may occasionally be affected.

Q3. What are the possible extracutaneous manifestations of EN?

Ans: Extracutaneous manifestations:

- Constitutional: Fever (38–39°C), malaise, arthralgia, headache
- Gastrointestinal: Abdominal pain, diarrhea, vomiting, hepatosplenomegaly
- Ocular: Episcleritis, phlyctenular conjunctivitis
- Other: Lymphadenopathy, pleuritis.

Q4. What are the clinical variants of EN?

Ans: Clinical variants of EN:

- Erythema nodosum migrans (subacute migratory nodular panniculitis): Individual lesions, which appear almost exclusively on the leg, are similar to classic EN, but they appear to migrate due to central clearing and appearance of new lesions at the periphery of existing ones. There is a marked female predominance (9:1) of this subtype.
- Chronic EN: Lesions are clinically indistinguishable from classic EN, but persist for months to years.

Q5. What are the causes and disease associations of EN?

Ans: Causes:

- Infections (28–48%): Streptococcal sore throat, tuberculosis, atypical mycobacterial infections, brucellosis, diarrhea caused by *Yersinia enterocolitica*, *Salmonella*, and *Shigella*, viral infections including human immunodeficiency virus (HIV), hepatitis C virus (HCV), hepatitis B virus (HBV), Epstein-Barr virus (EBV), *Chlamydia* and deep fungal infections including histoplasmosis, blastomycosis, coccidioidomycosis and sporotrichosis.
- Systemic diseases: Sarcoidosis (11–25%), Behçet's disease, Sweet syndrome, lupus erythematosus, Sjögren's syndrome, inflammatory bowel disease (1–4%), immunoglobulin A (IgA) nephropathy, adult-onset Still's disease.
- Pregnancy: Seen in 4.6% of pregnant women.
- Drugs: Antibiotics, oral contraceptives, halides, sulfonamides, hepatitis B vaccine, granulocyte colony stimulating factor (G-CSF), infliximab, BRAF inhibitors.
- Malignancy (paraneoplastic EN): Hodgkin's disease, leukemia, lymphoma and solid tumors.

Q6. How would you investigate the case in question?

Ans: Investigations:

- Complete blood count and erythrocyte sedimentation rate
- Urinalysis
- Antistreptolysin O (ASO) titer
- Mantoux test and/or an interferon gamma (IFN-γ) release assay
- Chest X-ray
- Throat swab culture
- Stool culture
- Serology for suspected infectious etiology: Antibodies against chlamydia, coxsackie, mycoplasma, rickettsia, Yersinia. HIV, HBV, HCV serology.
- Skin biopsy: To confirm the diagnosis.

Q7. What is the ideal type of biopsy that you would perform in a case of suspected panniculitis?

Ans: To have the subcutaneous fat adequately represented, a deep incisional biopsy is required. A punch biopsy does not provide adequate tissue for histopathological assessment of the panniculitides.

Q8. Which of the following best describes the histopathological presentation of EN?

a. Septal panniculitis without vasculitis
b. Septal panniculitis with vasculitis
c. Lobular panniculitis without vasculitis
d. Lobular panniculitis with vasculitis

Ans: a. Septal panniculitis without vasculitis. EN is the prototype of septal panniculitis without vasculitis, although frank vasculitis may rarely be encountered, affecting the small veins. In the early stages, the septae between the fat lobules are widened and edematous and contain an acute inflammatory infiltrate of neutrophils and occasional eosinophils. The infiltrate often spills over onto the adjacent fat lobules, but fat necrosis does not occur as in the lobular panniculitides. The infiltrate is soon replaced by lymphocytes and histiocytes. Granulomatous inflammation with giant cells later develops, but without the caseation seen in nodular vasculitis. The overlying dermis shows a perivascular and periadnexal chronic inflammatory infiltrate.

- Miescher's granuloma is a characteristic, but not unique, feature of EN and consists of aggregates of histiocytes surrounding a cleft-like space.
- Older lesions show septal fibrosis and residual granulomatous inflammation.

Q9. What are the common types of panniculitis encountered in clinical practice?

Ans: The classification of panniculitis is quite extensive, but the common types that are usually encountered may be classified as in Table 1.

Table 1: Classification of panniculitis

Panniculitis	*Septal*	*Lobular*
Without vasculitis	Erythema nodosum Necrobiosis lipoidica Deep morphea	Lupus panniculitis Lipodermatosclerosis
With vasculitis	Polyarteritis nodosa	Erythema induratum/ nodular vasculitis

Q10. How would you manage a patient of EN?

Ans: Management of a patient of EN includes:

- Supportive therapy: Limitation of physical exercise, bed rest, limb elevation and cool wet compresses.
- Analgesia: Nonsteroidal anti-inflammatory drugs (NSAIDs), like aspirin, indomethacin, naproxen and ibuprofen. NSAIDs are contraindicated in inflammatory bowel disease.
- Potassium iodide: 400–900 mg/day in persistent cases
- Corticosteroids: Systemic corticosteroids may be used in refractory cases, but only after excluding infectious etiology. Intralesional triamcinolone acetonide 10 mg/mL is an option for single, persistent nodules.
- Colchicine: 0.6–1.2 mg/day
- Hydroxychloroquine: 200 mg twice daily.
- Tumor necrosis factor-alpha (TNF-α) inhibitors: Adalimumab and infliximab have been tried in chronic, refractory EN associated with inflammatory bowel disease, including pediatric Crohn's disease. However, EN itself may be precipitated by these agents.
- Others: Dapsone, thalidomide and methotrexate have also been tried.

CHAPTER 128

Cold-related Conditions: Chilblains, Frostbite and Raynaud's Phenomenon

GK Singh, RS Grewal

Case study 1 Chilblains

Presenting Complaints

Doctor, I have developed redness, sores and itching on my few toes from last 3 days.

Setting

Dermatology outpatient department

History of Present Illness

A 24-year-old young male who has recently inducted into high-altitude region presented with multiple reddish patches on the feet mostly on the dorsum of toes from last 3 days. These lesions, over 2 days formed flaccid vesicles and burst to form superficial raw areas. There was no history of similar episodes in the past. He is a smoker; however, other dietary habits are normal. There was no history of any oral ulcer, photosensitivity or joints pain, bluish discoloration of hands or feet during exposure to cold water or cold weather, substance abuse or drugs intake.

General Physical Examination and Systemic Examination

No abnormality detected.

Dermatological Examination

Bilaterally-symmetrically polysized, irregular-shaped erosions on the dorsum of most of the toes, margins of feet with areas of hyperpigmentation around them (Fig. 1). All peripheral pulses were felt and sensation was intact.

Q1. What is your provisional diagnosis?

a. Chilblains
b. Frostbite
c. Raynaud's phenomenon
d. Scleroderma

Ans: Chilblains (pernio). However, frostbite and Raynaud's phenomenon require exclusion.

Q2. What differentials you will consider at this stage?

Ans: Although history and clinical examination is quite characteristic of chilblains. Differentials include:

- *Early frostbite:* Erythema is more pronounced and associated with pain. Itching is never found, associated history of exposure to freezing temperature is always present.
- *Chilblain lupus erythematosus:* Often it has positive antinuclear antibody (ANA) or rheumatoid factor (RF) positivity. Histopathological and immunofluorescent evidence of lupus is present in the skin lesions. 50% of the patients have associated facial discoid lupus lesions, and 15% likely to develop systemic lupus erythematosus.

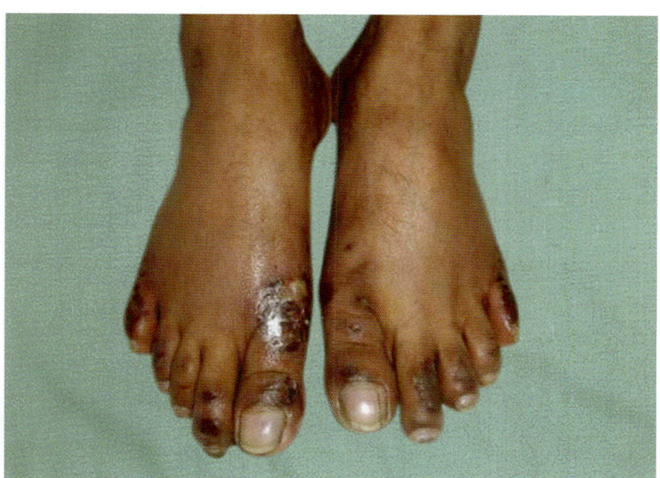

Fig. 1: Bilaterally symmetrically polysized, irregular-shaped erosions on the dorsum of toes

- *Acrocyanosis:* Bilateral, dusky, mottled discoloring of the entire hands, feet, and sometimes the face that is persistent and accentuated by cold exposure.
- *Erythrocyanosis:* It is a cyanotic discoloration that occurs over areas with a thick layer of subcutaneous fat.
- Cold erythema, cold urticaria and cold panniculitis are other effects of cold on the body tissues but the distribution are different and so is the presentation.
- *Raynaud's phenomenon:* History of bluish discoloration with exposure to cold water.
- Polycythemia vera.

Q3. How will you confirm the diagnosis?

Ans: Chilblains are usually clinically diagnosed; however, following tests shall be done to rule out few conditions which have got systemic and long-term impact:

- Complete blood count (CBC) and erythrocyte sedimentation rate (ESR): To rule out associated leukemia
- Antinuclear antibody: To rule out of lupus erythematosus
- Histopathological examination: Punch biopsy is advised to rule out other inflammatory processes in difficult chronic cases. Epidermal spongiosis or necrosis, intense papillary dermal edema, superficial and deep perivascular lymphocytic infiltrate which is described as "fluffy edema" of vessel walls may be present. Lymphocytic vasculitis may be present.
- Antiphospholipid antibody panel: To rule out incidence of antiphospholipid antibody syndrome.
- Cryoglobulins, cryofibrinogen and cold agglutinin testing: These generally are absent and not required, but should be considered as part of the laboratory evaluation in a patient with chronic chilblains. Because of occasional false-negative cryoprecipitate screening results, consider hepatitis C antibody screening or even RF as a marker for cryoglobulinemia in select cases.
- Serum protein electrophoresis (SPEP) and quantitative immunoglobulins: Dysproteinemias and macroglobulinemia, causing increased serum viscosity, may be associated with chilblains.

Q4. What are the risk factors to develop chilblains?

Ans: Young- or middle-aged women, children, smokers, hyperhidrosis, low body mass index and history of recurrence are the known risk factors for development of chilblains.

Q5. What is Chilblain? What is likely pathophysiology?

Ans: Chilblains (pernio) is an inflammatory skin condition presenting after exposure to nonfreezing temperature as pruritic and/or painful erythematous-to-violaceous acral lesions. Pathophysiology of chilblains is obscure; however, it may be due to an abnormal vascular response to cold exposure. It is usually idiopathic but may be secondary to an underlying disease.

Q6. Enumerate the systemic conditions which can present with chilblains as cutaneous features.

Ans: Chronic chilblains may be secondary to various systemic diseases as follows:

- Chronic myelomonocytic leukemia
- Antiphospholipid antibody syndrome
- Raynaud's disease
- Anorexia nervosa
- Dysproteinemias
- Cryoglobulinemia, cryofibrinogenemia and cold agglutinins
- Celiac disease
- Macroglobulinemia.

Q7. What preventive measures will you advise the patient to avoid chilblains in future?

Ans: Preventive measures to avoid chilblains in future:

- Proper foot care and keep extremities warm and dry
- Frequent changing of clothing and to wear multiple layers of warm clothing
- Exercise of extremities in pinned-down positions
- Recognition of symptoms of cold injury by health education

- Buddy aid treatment in remotely located place, more applicable to soldiers/adventurers
- Maintaining adequate hydration and nutritional status
- Cease smoking.

Q8. Is there any specific drug available for treatment of chilblains?

Ans: Chilblains is mainly a preventable disease. Oral nifedipine is still being considered as the most effective drug for chilblains. Topical emollient and topical aloe vera cream have been found effective. Other modalities, which have been tried with variable results, are rewarming of the affected parts of the body, ultraviolet rays, topical minoxidil, topical nitroglycerine, topical salbutamol, prazosin, topical antipruritic, iontophoresis and hydroxychloroquine.

Case study 2 Frostbite

Presenting Complaints

Doctor, I have developed painful blisters on my toes from last 2 days when I got exposed to extreme cold temperature during my trekking expedition.

Setting

Emergency department

History of Present Illness

A 22-year-old young trekker who has recently inducted into snow-bound region, presented with blisters on the toes from last 2 days. These lesions, started with redness, associated with pain and developed blister on toes over 10–12 hours. He has been trekking in snow-bound areas from last 2 days. There was no history of similar episodes in the past. He is a nonsmoker, does not consume alcohol, and dietary habits are normal. There was no history of any oral ulcer, photosensitivity or joints pain, bluish discoloration of hands or feet during exposure to cold water or cold weather, substance abuse or drugs intake.

General Physical Examination and Systemic Examination

No abnormality detected.

Dermatological Examination

It revealed tense bullae with surrounding erythema and edema present over the tip of toes even encircling the plantar aspect of toes and extending to dorsal aspect of forefeet; more pronounced on right than left foot (Fig. 2). There were few hemorrhagic bullae on left foot. These lesions were tender. All peripheral pulses were felt.

Q1. What is your clinical diagnosis?

Ans: Considering the history and examination findings, diagnosis of second-degree frostbite of both feet is apparent.

Q2. How do you differentiate between early frostbite and other cold injuries, like frostnip, trench foot and chilblains?

Ans: Points of differentiation amongst the above conditions are tabulated in Table 1.

Q3. What are frostbite and its mechanism of tissue damage?

Ans: Frostbite is defined as the freezing and crystallizing of fluids in the interstitial and cellular spaces as a consequence of prolonged exposure to freezing temperatures.

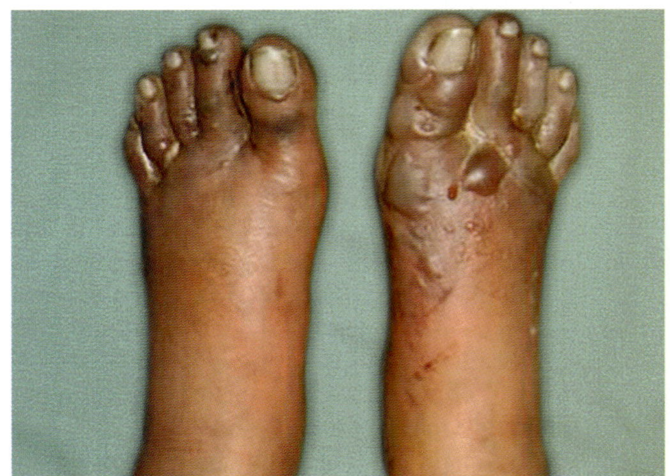

Fig. 2: Tense bullae with surrounding erythema and edema present over the tip of toes and extending to dorsal aspect of forefeet

Mechanisms of frostbite injury include the following:

- Direct cold damage to cells
- Direct cell damage from ice crystals, which includes protein and lipid disruption and electrolyte shifts
- Indirect cell damage from intracellular dehydration caused by the presence of extracellular ice crystals
- Microvascular stasis, thrombus formation, embolic events in the microvasculature and ischemia
- Reperfusion inflammatory injury.

Table 1: Differentiation amongst frostnip, trench foot, chilblains and early frostbite

Conditions	*Diagnostic considerations*
Frostnip	Blanching of the skin with transient numbness and paresthesias that resolves with rewarming
Trench foot	It results from prolonged exposure to a wet nonfreezing cold environment that produces peripheral neurovascular damage. It presents as pain, paresthesia, pallor, pulselessness and paralysis. Reversible if diagnosed and treated early. Better prognosis than patients with frostbite
Chilblains	Less severe than trench foot but mechanism is same; inflammatory reaction to dry nonfreezing temperature presenting as erythema, pigmentation, vesicles, nodules or superficial ulcers. Usually associated with itching in initial stage
Early frostbite	Most severe out of all four which is due to exposure to freezing temperature for long time leading to ice crystal formation and tissue damage. It presents initially as numbness followed by stinging, burning and throbbing sensation. Finally large blister develops. Superficial frostbite can be reverted back if timely action taken

Q4. What are the risk factors to develop frostbite?

Ans: Risk factors for frostbite are following:

- Inadequate or constrictive clothing
- Wind chill factor of high altitude
- High altitude with ambient freezing temperature
- Prolonged exposure to cold
- Inadequate shelter/homelessness
- Winter season with freezing temperature
- Prolonged exposure to moisture
- Immobilization
- Malnutrition and exhaustion
- Past history of cold injury
- Unacclimatized person
- Improper behavioral response to cold ambient temperature
- Extremes of age
- Altered mental status (e.g. from head trauma, ethanol or illicit drug abuse, or psychiatric illness)
- Exposure to drugs with vasoconstrictive effects (e.g. nicotine).

Q5. What are the disease conditions which may predispose the person to develop frostbite?

Ans: The following underlying conditions may predispose to frostbite:

- Infection
- Peripheral vascular disease/atherosclerosis
- Arthritis
- Diabetes
- Thyroid disease
- Stroke.

Q6. How frostbite is differentiated based upon degrees?

Ans: The descriptions are as followed in Table 2.

Q7. What are the sequelae of frostbite?

Ans: Healing of frostbite can take 6–12 months. Long-term sequelae may include the following:

- Paresthesias and sensory deficits
- Cold sensitivity
- Desquamation of skin
- Onycholysis
- Hyperhidrosis or anhydrosis
- Muscle atrophy
- Premature closure of epiphyses
- Decreased mineralization of bone
- Joint stiffness
- Tremor
- Phantom pain of amputated extremities
- Abnormal color changes indicative of vasospasm.

Q8. What are the complications of frostbite?

Ans: Complications are proportional to the degrees of frostbite. These are enumerated down below:

- Wound infection (most common almost to 30% of patients), usually caused by *Staphylococcus aureus*, β-hemolytic streptococci, Gram-negative bacilli, or anaerobes and may present with the increased pain, edema, extending erythema, pus discharge and fever
- Tissue loss and gangrene
- Sepsis
- Lymphedema
- Fascial compartment syndrome
- Irreversible growth plate injury leading to growth deformities and postinjury arthritis

Table 2: Differentiated frostbite based upon degrees

Degree	*Depth of involvement*	*Clinical appearance*	*Symptoms*	*Prognosis*
First	Partial thickness skin	Hard white waxy plaque with surrounding erythema, mild edema	Variable: Initial numbness followed by transient tingling/burning sensation	Excellent, complete recovery without tissue loss
Second	Full thickness skin	Blister formation with surrounding erythema and edema	"Pins and needles" followed by numbness, replaced by throbbing on rewarming	Good, heal over 3–4 weeks
Third	Full thickness skin and subcutaneous tissue	Hemorrhagic blisters. Hard black eschars in 2 weeks	Early throbbing or aching, later becomes insensate	Poor, tissue loss inevitable
Fourth	Full thickness skin and subcutaneous tissue with underlying muscle, tendon and bone	Deep purple or red, woody and mummified appearance. Little edema, late small hemorrhagic blisters	Initial decrease in sensation, later insensate	Extremely poor, loss of fingers and toes

- Reflex sympathetic dystrophy (autonomic dysfunction)
- Altered thermal perception at the injury site, especially cold sensitivity
- Hyperesthesia
- Hyperhidrosis
- Squamous cell carcinoma development at the frostbitten area
- Hyperglycemia
- Acidosis
- Refractory dysrhythmias
- Tetanus
- Death, in very rare cases.

Q9. What is role of investigation in the case of frostbite?

Ans: Frostbite is a clinical diagnosis. Although laboratory studies are not important in the initial diagnosis and management of frostbite, they may be helpful in identifying delayed systemic complications, such as wound infection with sepsis or complications of underlying hypothermia. Baseline laboratory studies to consider include CBC, electrolytes, blood urea nitrogen (BUN), creatine, glucose level and liver function tests (LFTs). Urinalysis may be used to detect evidence of myoglobinuria. Gram stains and cultures from suspected frostbite wound infections.

Q10. Is there any role of radiography or imaging studies in diagnosing the extent of tissue damage?

Ans: Role of radiography or imaging studies:

- Routine imaging studies are rarely helpful in determining the extent and amount of tissue damage. Because of transitory vascular instability in the affected tissues which may last for 2–3 weeks after the frostbite injury, no imaging technique (e.g. thermography, angiography, plethysmography and radioisotope bone scanning) reliably predicts tissue demarcation during the initial frostbite presentation.
- However, radiographs can identify clinically suspected fractures or dislocations, predicting long-term complications, such as osteomyelitis.
- Technetium-99m (^{99m}Tc) scintigraphy is sensitive and specific for tissue injury. Some authors recommend using it early in the management of frostbite (48 hours after injury) to aid in directing earlier debridement of nonviable soft tissue. Magnetic resonance imaging (MRI), when combined with physical findings, may also be helpful in the early determination of margins of tissue viability.

Q11. What additional preventive measures shall be explained to the patient of frostbite?

Ans: Apart from the measures as explained in the Section of Chilblains (Case Study 1), the following additional measures shall be adopted in the case of frostbite:

- Deinduct the patient from cold areas as soon as possible.
- If it is not possible to deinduct immediately, preplanning and use of appropriate clothing are mandatory. Follow weather forecasts, with special attention to both predicted temperature as well as wind-chill temperature index.
- Do not rub affected areas; this causes further damage.
- Do not use dry heat to thaw frostbitten areas; moist heat is better because it allows a more complete thaw.
- Do not allow the injury to thaw then refreeze; therefore, hospital rewarming is favored over field rewarming.

- In remote areas, use a buddy system to help prevent cold injury; have a system for rapid evacuation, if needed.

Q12. What is the principle of medical treatment for the frostbite?

Ans: The principle of medical management is to rewarm the injury as quickly as possible, provide pain control during rewarming, reduce reperfusion injury, prevent frostbite complications, and decrease long-term sequelae.

Q13. What are essential steps in the management of frostbite?

Ans: Essential steps in the management of frostbite:

- Preventive measures as discussed for any cold injuries. Remove the patient from cold. Replace wet and constrictive clothing with dry loose clothing. Remove jewelry from the affected area. Dress the extremity in a manner that minimizes mechanical trauma. Use of circulating water at 40–42°C without allowing too hot or too cold water. Avoid premature termination of the rewarming process. Nonsteroidal anti-inflammatory drugs (NSAIDs) for pain.
- Rewarming: Rapidly rewarm the affected area in circulating water at 37–39°C for 15–30 minutes or until thawing is, by clinical assessment, complete. Thawing takes about 20–40 minutes for superficial injuries and as long as 1 hour for deep injuries. NSAIDs for pain.
- Post-rewarming Management: protect the area from further injury and re-exposure to cold. Elevate the limb, dressing of wound. Monitor for any sign of infection in the area and splint the extremity. Sterile, nonadherent dressings should be applied; Oral/injection antibiotics, injection tetanus toxoid prophylactically.

Q14. What are the recent advances in the treatment of frostbite?

Ans: Recent advances in the treatment of frostbite:

- Tissue plasminogen activator (tPA): When administered within 24 hours of thawing, it has been shown to decrease amputation rates. Thrombolysis should only be performed after a careful risk-benefit analysis.
- Other ancillary modalities, which are helpful but have not been proven in well-controlled human trials, include the following:
  - Buflomedil (an α-blocker) to increase peripheral blood flow
  - Hyperbaric oxygen
  - Subatmospheric pressure therapy
  - Pentoxifylline
  - Vitamin C
  - Superoxide dismutase
  - Nifedipine.

Q15. What are the indications for early surgery in the case of frostbite?

Ans: Early surgery usually is contraindicated in frostbite, because of the time the nonviable tissue takes to demarcate. This process normally takes 6–8 weeks. However, there are conditions which require urgent surgical attentions:

- Post-thaw compartment syndrome warranting fasciotomy
- Wet gangrene is treated by urgent surgical excision of the affected area.

Case study 3 Raynaud's Phenomenon

Presenting Complaints

Doctor, I develop recurrent episodes of whitish to bluish, red discoloration associated with pain when I come in contact with cold water from the last 2 years.

Setting

Dermatology outpatient department

History of Present Illness

A 25-year-old lady, housewife, is presented with recurrent episodes of whitish, bluish and red discoloration of fingers and toes from last 2 years. It was sudden in onset gradually increasing in frequency and intensity. The discoloration of finger and toes are accompanied by moderate intensity of pain which hamper daily routine life. There is no history of oral ulcer, joint pain, photosensitivity or any drug intake. Her symptoms are aggravated in winter and on contact with cold water. There is no such history in the family. She is nonsmoker and consumes mixed diet. Her menstrual cycles are regular. She has one boy child: 2-year-old delivered normally. Her antenatal and postnatal periods were uneventful.

General Physical Examination and Systemic Examination

No abnormality detected.

Dermatological Examination

All peripheral pulses were felt and sensation was intact. Nail-fold capillary examined by ophthalmoscope did not reveal any abnormality of capillaries. Ice water challenge done on the patient; the fingers and toes turned bluish on contact, i.e. test was positive.

Q1. What is your diagnosis?

Ans: Clinically, she is a case of Raynaud's phenomenon. However considering clinical situation, there are many disease conditions which may mimic this and require exclusion through investigations.

Q2. What is Raynaud's phenomenon?

Ans: Raynaud's phenomenon (primary Raynaud's disease) is recurrent vasospasm of the fingers and toes and usually presents as pallor, bluish and red discoloration in sequence or without it which occurs in response to stress or cold exposure without any association to underlying disease.

Q3. What are the diagnostic criteria of Raynaud's phenomenon?

Ans: Diagnostic criteria for primary Raynaud's phenomenon are following:

- Attacks triggered by exposure to cold and/or stress
- Symmetric bilateral involvement
- Absence of necrosis
- Absence of a detectable underlying cause
- Normal capillaroscopy findings
- Normal laboratory findings for inflammation
- Absence of antinuclear factors.

Q4. What are the causes of secondary Raynaud's phenomenon?

Ans: Causes of secondary Raynaud's phenomenon are tabulated in Table 3.

Q5. In which autoimmune conditions, Raynaud's phenomenon is most commonly associated?

Ans: The most common association is with systemic sclerosis (90%) and mixed connective-tissue disease (85%). It can also be seen in systemic lupus erythematosus.

Q6. What is the pathophysiology of Raynaud's phenomenon?

Ans: The complete understanding of the pathophysiology of Raynaud's phenomenon remains to be elucidated. However the recent reviews have described the mechanisms under three categories: (1) vascular, (2) neural and (3) intravascular abnormalities; based upon three major events, e.g. initial white (vasoconstriction), followed by blue (cyanosis), and then red (rapid blood reflow).

Vascular abnormality:

- A deficiency of vasodilatory mediators nitric oxide

- High level of endothelin-1, a potent vasoconstrictor which get triggered by vasoactive stimuli, including angiotensin, vasopressin and transforming growth factor-beta (TGF-β).

Neural abnormality:

- A low level of an important neuropeptide, a potent vasodilator secreted by nerves that supply blood vessels which is calcitonin gene-related peptide, in the skin of affected tissue
- Over activity of α_{2C}-adrenoreceptors; which enable cold-induced vasoconstriction of the blood vessels.

Intravascular abnormality:

- Increased platelet activation and aggregation
- An increased production of platelet thromboxane A_2, a potent vasoconstrictor
- High level of reactive oxygen species creating oxidative stress.

Q7. What is prevalence of Raynaud's phenomenon?

Ans: Internationally, the prevalence of primary Raynaud's phenomenon varies among different populations, from 4.9–20.1% in women to 3.8–13.5% in men.

Q8. What is the prognosis of patients of Raynaud's phenomenon?

Ans: The prognosis of patients with primary Raynaud's phenomenon is usually very good, with no mortality and little morbidity. In very rare cases, however, ischemia of the affected body part can result in necrosis.

Q9. Which are the primary investigations to be done in this patient?

Ans: She does not have features suggestive of any underlying disease condition. Usually Raynaud's phenomenon can be diagnosed clinically. However, laboratory investigations are required to know the baseline profile of patients and to rule out any secondary causes if at all present there. Special tests should be guided by clinical profile of the patient:

- Routine test: CBC, urine analysis, LFT, renal function test (RFT), blood sugar level, chest X-ray (CXR) posteroanterior (PA) view and electrocardiogram (ECG)
- ANA to rule out connective tissue disorder.

Q10. How are you going to treat the case?

Ans: The following measures should be taken:

Supportive therapy:

- Avoid contact with triggering factors
- Protective clothings

Table 3: Causes of secondary Raynaud's phenomenon

Parameters	*Causes*
Occupational or trauma	Vibration injury, vinyl chloride exposure, frostbite, lead exposure, arsenic exposure, organic solvent exposure (e.g. xylene, toluene, acetone, chlorinated solvents)
Hematologic/ malignancy	Paroxysmal nocturnal hemoglobinuria, polycythemia, cryofibrinogenemia, Waldenström macroglobulinemia, lymphoma, leukemia, myeloma, lung adenocarcinoma and other paraneoplastic disorders
Collagen-vascular (autoimmune)	Systemic sclerosis (scleroderma) including the diffuse and limited [formerly called CREST (calcinosis, Raynaud's phenomenon, esophageal dysmotility, sclerodactyly and telangiectasia) syndrome], systemic lupus erythematosus, mixed connective-tissue disease (and other overlap syndromes), dermatomyositis and polymyositis, Rheumatoid, Sjögren's syndrome
Medication-induced	Oral contraceptives, Ergot alkaloids, bromocriptine, β-adrenergic blocking drugs, Antineoplastics (e.g. vinca alkaloids, bleomycin cisplatin), cyclosporine, α-interferon, methylphenidate
Miscellaneous	Carpal tunnel syndrome, myxedema, Fabry disease, pheochromocytoma, acromegaly, diabetes mellitus

- Stop culprit drug
- Stop smoking.

Specific therapies: There is no single drug which is drugs of choice for Raynaud's phenomenon.

- Extended release tablet nifedipine is the first choice in varying dosage of 20–120 mg/day. Start with the lowest dose and titrate up as tolerated.
- Topical nitroglycerin cream (1% or 2%) to be applied locally twice.

Q11. Which other drugs have been tried in the Raynaud's phenomenon due to underlying systemic disease?

Ans: The following medications that have been studied in Raynaud's syndrome; however, none is currently approved for this indication by the US Food and Drug Administration (USFDA):

- Iloprost (prostaglandin analog)
- Selective-serotonin reuptake inhibitors (SSRIs): Fluoxetine, sertraline, etc.
- Phosphodiesterase-5 enzyme inhibitors (sildenafil, tadalafil and vardenafil)
- Losartan, bosentan (endothelin-receptor antagonist in systemic sclerosis)
- Botulinum toxin
- N-acetylcysteine (systemic sclerosis and digital ulcers).

CHAPTER 129

Corns and Callosities

Anagha S

Case study Corns and Callosities

Presenting Complaints

Doctor, I am having pain in my great toe during walking since 1 year. The skin beneath the great toe is also thickened.

Setting

Dermatology outpatient department

History of Present Illness

A 40-year-old lady, presented with complaints of pain and localized thickening of skin in the area below the great toe. The complaints are of 1-year duration. It is insidious in onset and gradual in progression. Patient complains of pain while walking. No complains of pus/bloody discharge from the lesion.

General Physical Examination and Systemic Examination

No abnormality detected.

Dermatological Examination

Solitary thickened and indurated localized lesion present on skin of soles under the left great toe. Pain present on vertical pressure. Skin markings maintained over the lesion.

Q1. What is the most likely diagnosis?

a. Corn
b. Wart
c. Morphea
d. Callosity

Ans: a. Corn.

Q2. What is corn most commonly confused with?

a. Plantar fibromatoses
b. Wart
c. Psoriasis
d. Secondary syphilis

Ans: b. Wart.

Q3. How will you confirm the diagnosis?

Ans: Diagnosis is made on clinical grounds. There is a localized area of hyperkeratosis with pain on walking. The skin over the lesion after being pared does not have bleeding points. The patient will not have pain after paring is done to a certain point. Dermatoglyphics (skin markings) are maintained. Patient complains of pain only on vertical pressure.

Q4. What are the definitions of a corn and a callus?

Ans: A callosity is a plaque of hyperkeratosis caused by repeated friction and/or pressure (Fig. 1). A callus is a broad-based diffuse area of hyperkeratosis

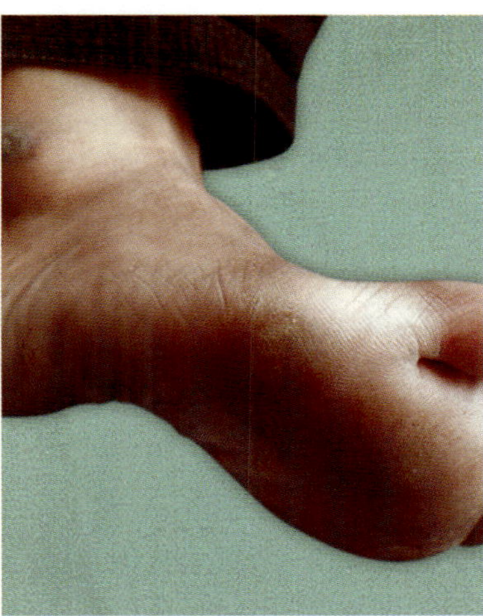

Fig. 1: Localized thickness on the soles

of *relatively* even thickness, usually under the metatarsal heads. A corn is a sharply demarcated callosity occurring over a bony prominence, usually on the hand or foot, and is painful.

Q5. What are the causes for corns and callosities?

Ans: Repeated mechanical trauma to the feet from poorly fitting footwear, anatomic defect, work or leisure activities, produces protective hyperkeratosis. This protective response to injury may result in the formation of uncomfortable thickened areas of skin known as corns or calluses.

A bony spur or exostosis may be present beneath both hard and soft corns of long duration. Corns are narrow based and sharply defined, whereas calluses are broad based.

Other causes include:

- Deformities due to rheumatoid arthritis, diabetic mellitus with neuropathy
- Habit of sitting with the foot tucked under the body with or without a prominent underlying talus
- Soft corn occurs when tight shoes press the condyle of a metatarsal or phalanx against the base of a phalanx on the adjacent toe
- An inherited disposition to callosities is an autosomal-dominant inheritance.

Q6. What is the pathogenesis?

Ans: Bony protuberances, such as the condyles of metatarsal and phalangeal bones, create outward pressure on the skin. Footwear and activities (walking, running) create counterpressure at these sites. The repeated friction and pressure leads to hyperkeratosis. The cycle of friction, pressure and thickening continues until a corn or callus develops.

Q7. What are the histopathological features of corns and callosities?

Ans: The histopathological features:

- *Callus:* Epidermal hyperplasia. The stratum corneum is thickened and compact, sometimes with parakeratosis over the dermal papillae. There is expansion of the granular layer. Dermis may show an increase in dermal collagen and fibrosis around neurovascular bundles.
- *Corn:* There is a thick parakeratotic plug set in a cup-shaped depression of the epidermis, usually with loss of the granular cell layer.

Q8. What are the usual sites of involvement?

Ans: Sites of involvement:

- Hard corns are found on the plantar aspects of the toes or on soles
- Soft corns are present in the interdigital web spaces
- In patients with bunions (hallux valgus), a callus usually forms at the medioplantar aspects of the hallux. Additional corn or callus forms on the second metatarsal head. Beneath the 1st and 5th metatarsal heads in cavus foot types
- Beneath the 5th metatarsal head alone in persons with tailor's bunions (bunionette)
- Erratic locations (e.g. beneath the 3rd and 5th metatarsal heads, isolated 3rd or 4th metatarsal head, 2nd and 4th metatarsal heads) in individuals with structural abnormalities, such as brachymetatarsia or dislocated metatarso-phalangeal joints
- Beneath the 2nd through 4th metatarsal heads when multiple hammer toes, hallux valgus, or an equinus deformity coexists.

Q9. What are the clinical features?

Ans: Hard corns (heloma durum) are firm, small, dome-shaped papules with translucent central cores, most commonly found on the dorsolateral fifth toes and dorsal aspects of other toes. The patient has dull/boring or sharp/lancinating pain by pressing on the underlying nerves.

- Soft corns (heloma molle) are painful keratoses in the interdigital web spaces; they often become macerated. Opposing toes may exhibit "kissing lesions".

- Broad-keratotic plaques, often under the metatarsal heads, are calluses.

Q10. What is tennis toe?

Ans: A callus is seen on the tip of the second (and sometimes third) toe, with associated transverse ridging, thickening and splinter hemorrhages in the nail. This is known as tennis toe or center's callus. Seen in tennis players due to repeated collision between toe tip and shoe with sudden stops. Also seen in gymnasts, soccer players, runners, football players and dancers.

Q11. What are the differential diagnoses?

Ans: Differential diagnoses:

- *Verruca vulgaris:* Warts interrupt dermatoglyphics, while corns do not interrupt. Calluses often demonstrate accentuated lines. Paring of a corn reveals a central translucent whitish-yellow core, whereas thrombosed capillaries and multiple bleeding points are seen in a wart on paring. Paring of a callus reveals layers of yellowish keratin, without the multiple punctate thrombosed capillaries of a mosaic plantar wart.
- *Porokeratosis plantaris discrete:* Sharply marginated, cone-shaped, rubbery lesion. Multiple lesions can occur. The lesions are usually painful.
- *Keratosis punctate:* They can be seen in creases of digits of feet which can be mistaken for a corn.

Q12. How do you treat corns and callosities?

Ans: Treatment of corns and callosities is explained in Table 1.

Table 1: Treatment of corns and callosities

Parameters	*Physical/injection*	*Topical*	*Surgical*
First line	Paring and padding	40% salicylic acid or 40% urea	
Second line	4% alcohol mixed with local anesthetic	Lipid extract with garlic	Osseous and/or soft-tissue procedures
Under investigation	Botulinum toxin to reduce digital contractures and thereby reduce local skin pressure		

Q13. What are the aims for treatment of corns?

Ans: Provide symptomatic relief, determine the source of abnormal mechanical stress relieve the cause by conservative means, consider surgery if these fail.

Q14. How does paring help in treatment?

Ans: Relief of symptoms caused by corns and calluses can be achieved by careful and regular paring. Regular paring reduces the pressure induced by corns. The initial procedure is best done with a scalpel and subsequent treatment with an abrasive device.

Q15. What is the role of keratolytics?

Ans: Salicylic acid (10–20%) keratolytic preparations can be of some help. Salicylic acid, lactic acid in collodion can be used. The collodion medication is carefully painted on the pared site of the corn and allowed to dry each day until cure. Soaking the foot for half an hour before reapplying the medication enhances the effect. This treatment is especially effective for interdigital soft corns. Salicylic acid and dichloroacetic acid can also be used in combination. 40% salicylic acid pads and plaster, 40% urea cream, and 12% lactic acid cream are usually used in combination.

Q16. What is the nature of footwear needed for corns?

Ans: Extra width with the toebox and a softer upper is needed. With marginal calluses, the shoe is likely to be too loose. The shoe needs to be adapted to receive an orthosis—a cushioning device designed to redistribute the mechanical forces causing the callosity. Examples are the metatarsal pad for localized plantar callus, and a medial wedge for the cavovarus foot. Another useful orthosis is the silicone sleeve that can be used on deformed toes that have corns on them.

Q17. Is cryotherapy useful for corns?

Ans: Yes.

Q18. What is the surgical treatment in corns?

Ans: Surgery to remove the bony prominences is indicated only if all conservative measures fail.

Surgical procedures include bunionectomy, syndactylization, osteotomy and arthroplasty.

Long-term improvement for lateral fifth-toe corns and interdigital corns has been achieved with partial and complete condylectomy.

Surgical enucleation of corns: A disposable biopsy punch, which encircles the central core, according to the size is taken. Very slow and gradual rotatory half circular motion is pushed into the tissue. Before applying the punch on patient's skin, the patient is explained that at the point when he or she feels pain sensation or an increase in the pain sensation, he or she should immediately inform to surgeon. If the punch is pushed deep into the tissue it may lead to severe pain, deep tissue injury and deep wound which may heal with a delay. The punched out tissue is held with Adson's toothed forceps and is gradually pulled without cutting. This leads to the complete extraction of the tissue with the central intact core excised. The pressure bandage is applied over the wound and the patient is instructed to use soft footwear.

Q19. What is the role of fillers?

Ans: Silicone injections to digital and plantar sites of corns are of significant value. Booster treatments are often needed. Injection of 0.1 mL of medical-grade liquid silicone below a clavus and above the bone has been performed. Hyaluronic acid gel injections are reported to be beneficial. The only complication reported is skin discoloration.

Index

Page numbers followed by *f* refer to figure and *t* refer to table

A

B

C

D

E

F

G

H

O

P

Q

R

S

T